First report on peds. June 30, 1956
Worked 3-11 c̄ M. Zepeda & Pearl, RN's
SN's V. Doyle & R. Anderson Working 11-7,

ESSENTIALS OF PEDIATRICS

PHILIP C. JEANS, A.B., M.D.
Late Professor of Pediatrics, State University of Iowa, Iowa City

F. HOWELL WRIGHT, B.S., M.D.
Professor of Pediatrics, University of Chicago

FLORENCE G. BLAKE, R.N., M.A.
Associate Professor of Nursing Education (Nursing Care of Children), University of Chicago

103 Illustrations,
Including 3 Color Plates

FIFTH EDITION

J. B. LIPPINCOTT COMPANY
Philadelphia and Montreal

Preface to Fifth Edition

The rapid pace at which medical knowledge advances creates a continual challenge to textbook authors. New discoveries in the field of antibiotics and hormone therapy have simplified the management of some pediatric disorders and rendered previous technics obsolete. Rapid strides in the surgical technics for dealing with congenital malformations of the heart have opened up completely new avenues. Changing points of view, such as the growing emphasis upon the emotional implications of disease for the child and his family, must be recognized also. For this reason much new material on the psychologic development of the child from birth through adolescence has been added. In revising a brief text the most difficult problem is what to omit. In the current revision decisions have been based mainly upon an estimate of the frequency with which a pediatric nurse is likely to encounter and be challenged by the situation in question.

Prior to Dr. Jeans' untimely death, he had already completed a revision of the section on nutrition and had indicated many of the areas in which modernization of the text was desirable. The succeeding authors have tried to preserve the wisdom of Dr. Jeans' long experience in the field of pediatrics while they were making the necessary renovations. The same principles which he set forth in his preface to the First Edition have guided the current revision.

A new chapter has been added to the unit on General Nursing Care, a chapter which describes the general principles of pediatric therapy. The chapter on disorders of the newborn has been rewritten with a view to helping the nurse to differentiate the important from the unimportant items of concern which surround the new baby. Material has been rearranged in several chapters, such as those on diseases of the nervous system and the infectious diseases, in the hope of providing a clearer concept of etiologic mechanisms. In the discussions of nursing care an effort has been made to view the illness through the eyes of the child and his family so that the nurse may better understand their reactions.

Our grateful appreciation is due to many members of the staff of the University of Chicago Clinics who have been kind enough to read and criticize several of the chapters and have assisted in the selection of illustrations. Our gratitude is also due to the members of the staff of the State University of Iowa who assisted Dr. Jeans in the preparation of previous editions.

F. HOWELL WRIGHT
FLORENCE G. BLAKE

v

Preface to First Edition

In preparing this textbook care has been taken to include all of the subject matter suggested in the curriculum for schools of nursing prepared by the National League of Nursing Education. Though the book contains the essentials of the technics which are peculiarly concerned with pediatric nursing and emphasizes the care of the child in health and in illness, more emphasis than perhaps is customary has been given to discussion of phases other than the technics of nursing. Many of the subjects are discussed in considerable detail, considering the space limitations of a small textbook. This is done with a realization that nurses usually are eager to extend their knowledge beyond that which is expected of them. A nurse should not be called upon to diagnose the nature of an illness and prescribe for a patient, yet a knowledge of these fields is an aid in understanding the reasons for those things which she is required to do. Better and more intelligent work results when the reasons for the task are understood.

The basic content of this book has been used as mimeographed text material in several training schools for some years and has thus been submitted to the searching criticism of classroom requirements. This plan provided a thorough checking up and has afforded a means of incorporating into the finished text all the valuable suggestions which have come through such a tryout. The text is illustrated by many cuts, each one of which has been carefully selected for its teaching value.

Chapters III and IV were contributed by Winifred Rand, R.N., Specialist in Parental Education, Merrill-Palmer School. The point of view presented by these chapters on child guidance and nursing care supplements in a useful manner that of the physician as represented by the remainder of the book. Knowledge of proper methods of managing children is fully as important to the nurse as knowledge of the physical aspects of the child in health and disease. When these fields of knowledge are combined, a more complete understanding of the child is attained.

P. C. J.

Contents

Unit Three

GENERAL NURSING CARE

Unit Five

NUTRITION AND THE NUTRITIONAL DISEASES

Unit One

ORIENTATION

CHAPTER ONE

Introduction to Pediatric Nursing

THE DEVELOPMENT OF PEDIATRICS AND PEDIATRIC NURSING

THE NEED OF UNDERSTANDING GROWTH

THE NEED OF APPRECIATING THE GOAL OF HEALTH

THE NEED OF ACQUIRING CERTAIN SKILLS IN PEDIATRIC NURSING

THE NEED OF CULTIVATING AN ALERTNESS IN NOTICING SYMPTOMS

THE IMPORTANCE OF ESTABLISHING AND MAINTAINING A CONSTRUCTIVE RELATIONSHIP WITH CHILDREN

THE CHALLENGE OF PEDIATRIC NURSING

THE DEVELOPMENT OF PEDIATRICS AND PEDIATRIC NURSING

A chapter introducing the subject of pediatric nursing might well begin with "once upon a time," that phrase beloved by all children at the beginning of a tale, for once upon a time there was no specialty of pediatrics and no pediatric nursing as we understand the term today.

Up until 1860, a very long time ago to any young woman studying nursing today, but in reality a short time ago when we consider the history of medicine, disease was taught as disease and little differentiation was made on the basis of whether the disease occurred in the youngest one or the oldest. Medical attention was centered on disease, and the patient as a person was of comparatively little significance to the physician, a fact reflected today in our tendency to speak of the patient as a "case." One should not read into that state-

ment the idea that physicians had no understanding of their patients as people, for that is far from true. Many of the physicians of the earlier days were intuitively psychologists and had deep insight into the personality of their patients and its relationship to the disease. But this type of learning came through living; it was not taught in medical schools or from textbooks. Diseases were taught as disease without reference to child or to man.

In 1860 pediatrics as a specialty came into being. Dr. Abraham Jacobi established the first children's clinic in New York and gave special lectures on the diseases of children. In 1888, the first department of pediatrics was established at the Harvard Medical School with Dr. Thomas Morgan Rotch as its first professor. It was Dr. Jacobi and Dr. Rotch who first taught that the diseases of children differed somewhat from the diseases of adults and were deserving of special consideration. Possibly this marks the beginning of our seeing the person as well as the disease.

Pediatrics, as a word derived from the Greek word *pais, paidos,* meaning child, according to dictionary definition means "the medical treatment of children."

Today pediatrics and pediatric nursing are concerned with the care of children through all periods of growth. Up until recent years the generally accepted medical meaning of the word *child* included only the ages from earliest infancy to early adolescence or the beginning of puberty. Pediatricians dismissed their patients at adolescence, and children's wards and hospitals made the upper age limit from 12 to 13 years. This left the adolescent at that important threshold, the period of transition when he is emerging from childhood and is not adult, without the special consideration he required. Today pediatricians are recognizing the adolescent's need for a continuing relationship with him until maturity is reached, and separation from home makes a change inevitable. As a result many pediatric wards are accommodating adolescents, and wards for adolescent patients are being opened in some children's hospitals. Today the adolescents' special health needs are being recognized to a greater degree than they ever have been before.

Special institutions for the care of children came into existence long before nursing ever was taught as a profession. The lovely Della Robbia plaques with which we are all familiar are found in the Hospital of the Holy Innocents built in Florence, Italy, in 1421, the first children's institution of its kind in Europe. This institution was in reality for the care of foundlings rather than for use as a hospital as we understand the word today, but within its walls were children who required nursing care. In this country the first hospital for sick children was built in Philadelphia in 1855, and the Children's Hospital in Boston followed in 1869.

Until Dr. Rotch was appointed as head of the pediatric department at Harvard Medical School, there were few schools of nursing and none in hospitals for children. In 1889, a year after Dr. Rotch's appointment, The Children's Hospital in Boston opened its school of nursing and became the first school in a hospital for children only. In 1880 The Children's Hospital in San Francisco opened its school of nursing, the first school west of the Rocky Mountains. This hospital is in reality a hospital for women and children, although the emphasis according to the name seems to be on children. There are many hospitals for women and children in this country, the first being The New England Hospital for Women and Children, which established the first school of nursing in the United States in 1872. Several hospitals for women and children still have schools of nursing, but at the present time only two hospitals for children only maintain schools of nursing. They are the Boston Children's Hospital and Denver Children's Hospital.

It is difficult to say when pediatric nursing came to be considered a specialty, for it developed gradually as nursing became a profession and as nurses recognized children's needs for nursing care which is adapted to their individual developmental requirements. One can glean some knowledge of society's concept of nursing through study of the definitions which have been given of the nurse. In the 1778 edition of Dr. Johnson's dictionary one finds this definition of a nurse: (1) a woman that has the care of another's child, (2) a woman that has the care of a sick person, (3) one who breeds, educates, and (4) an old woman—in contempt. In the Oxford dictionary the element of contempt has dropped from the interpretation of the word *nurse,* and the concept of education has appeared. The definition now given is a "person, generally a woman who attends or waits upon the sick, now especially one properly trained for the purpose." "To nurse" is defined as "to foster, tend, cherish, take care of, promote the growth or development of." In all its interpretations the word seems to imply caring for and promoting the growth of others.

The increased knowledge of children's developmental needs which has been acquired during this century has influenced nursing and made it a specialty. Pediatric nursing is recognized as an essential part of the course in all nursing schools, and postgraduate education is necessary for those who expect to specialize in the care of children. A century ago our knowledge of child development was limited. We did not know what children needed for sound personality development. Nor were we aware of the ways in which hospitalization affects children's feelings or of the psychological needs which arise in response to illness and its treatment and to separation from home and from all the security which the presence of protective,

loving parents represents. A century ago the care of the sick child consisted of food, fluid, treatments, medicine and physical protection. The hospitalized child was protected from cross-infection and from physical injury, but we had insufficient knowledge to recognize the child's need to be protected from emotional trauma which would jeopardize his potentialities for sound personality growth.

With increased knowledge, the pediatric nurse's responsibilities have increased. She needs preparation which makes it possible for her to prevent emotional trauma or injury and to promote the health of the children for whom she cares. In addition, her responsibility extends to parents. As the nurse works with parents in the home, the clinic and the hospital she again has the opportunity of promoting growth. If she is well prepared, understanding and skillful in her approach to parents, she can function in preventive health programs and make a valuable contribution to them.

THE NEED OF UNDERSTANDING GROWTH

The nurse promotes growth through the acquisition of knowledge, observation and meeting the needs of those in her care. The pediatric nurse cares for those who are in the process of growth. She needs to understand and meet the needs of the practically helpless and rapidly growing infant. She needs to understand the preschool child who is gradually acquiring the ability to control his asocial impulses, to socialize with children and adults outside his family, and to master his environment. She needs to understand and meet the needs of the school-age child with his widening intellectual and social interests and his drive to gain increased control of himself and his environment. The preadolescent and the adolescent are also in need of understanding for they, too, are in the process of growth and require supportive guidance which helps them surmount the developmental tasks essential for growth toward maturity. The pediatric nurse works with children in all stages of growth. To provide the physical and emotional support that growing children require, the nurse needs more knowledge of growth and child guidance than a textbook on *Essentials of Pediatrics* and any pediatric nursing experience can provide. For this reason supplementary reading and educational experiences are being suggested.

THE NEED OF APPRECIATING THE GOAL OF HEALTH

The profession of nursing grew out of a need for the care of the sick. Patients in hospitals needed care, and the nurse's education was concerned with knowledge and training essential to carry out those procedures which were necessary to restore people to physical health. Until recent years all the nurse's educational experience occurred in institutions established for the care of the sick. She did not have experience in homes, clinics and schools. In an institution usually filled with sick and oftentimes desperately ill people, it is little wonder that the nurse's education lacked the emphasis which would help her to become "health conscious" and to learn the meaning of optimal health.

Today the medical and the nursing professions devote a large fraction of their energies toward the prevention of illness and the restoration of sick people to a state of optimal health. If our goal for patients is health, we must not only know the characteristics of physical health but also that which in late years we have been accustomed to call mental health.

A knowledge of the so-called normal child is necessary for the nurse who is to care for the sick and convalescent child and for those who guide parents in the understanding of their children. Unless the nurse understands the characteristics of optimal physical and mental health she cannot possibly help an individual to achieve it. Through observation and participation in well-baby clinics, in nursery, primary and secondary schools and in organized recreational programs for boys and girls, the nurse will glean some concept of the goal toward which she is working.

Health involves the integration of the total personality; it is not limited to the physical body. For health the individual must experience satisfying, constructive relationships with other people, be free from exaggerated amounts of conflict and anxiety and confident of his ability to master himself and his environment. For the child who has not yet developed the inner resources necessary for independent mastery of himself or his environment, parents or satisfying substitutes are essential to maintain equilibrium and integration.

The nurse is an important part of her patient's environment. Her health—mental, physical and spiritual—influences her patient. This is especially true when the patient is a growing, impressionable, dependent child. Often we forget that we are a part of the child's environment and have the power to influence him for good or ill. The pediatric nurse needs to achieve integration of personality. What she is, as well as what she does, will have its effect on the child. If she is consumed with anxiety because she is unable to experience satisfying relationships with persons in her professional and social world, she will have little emotional energy left for her patients and will be inhibited in using the educational opportunities which could contribute to her personal growth.

THE NEED OF ACQUIRING CERTAIN SKILLS IN PEDIATRIC NURSING

There are certain nursing procedures which the pediatric nurse is called on to perform more often than the nurse dealing with adult patients; she needs to acquire special skill along these lines. Gentleness of touch and performance is necessary, as in most instances she is working with a smaller and more delicate individual and must employ smaller tools. Certain diseases are peculiar to infancy and childhood, e.g., many orthopedic conditions, certain nutritional disorders, prematurity and some of the communicable diseases. Furthermore, among those diseases which are common to both adults and children, there are some which have implications of greater severity and poorer prognosis for the child. All these circumstances make necessary special pediatric nursing knowledge which is the subject matter upon which the principles of physical care depends.

When the procedures of pediatric nursing are analyzed, certain fundamental guiding principles emerge which are accepted by the personnel in all hospitals. However, the actual performance of these procedures will vary somewhat in different hospitals. The maintenance of a sterile field may be the basic principle in one procedure; absolute accuracy, the essential factor in another; continuity of administration of a liquid at a given temperature may be the requirement in yet a third. The purpose of setting up procedures and working out routines and technics for the care of patients is to ensure safety and provide for the maximum comfort of the child. Ensuring safety requires adherence to the principles underlying the procedure. To succeed in bringing comfort to her patients, the nurse needs skill in observing the needs of her patient. She also needs freedom to utilize her creative imagination to find ways in which the procedure may be made acceptable to the child and a profitable experience for him. In this textbook, specific nursing technics will be discussed as they relate to the care of children with special diseases.

THE NEED OF CULTIVATING AN ALERTNESS IN NOTICING SYMPTOMS

The child, unlike the adult, cannot detect and report verbally every change in feeling to the minutest detail. The adult identifies pain, chilliness, nausea, or a feeling of uncertainty, rings his bell and reports his discomfort. This the small child cannot do. He *feels* changes in his physical and emotional status and reacts to them with changes in his behavior, but frequently he cannot locate his physical pain or identify the feeling which is bringing him anxiety. Through crying, restlessness, tempestuousness or the opposite type of reaction—withdrawal from emotional contacts—he signals discomfort from physical changes in his body. Through behavioral responses he also tells us of his need for someone who is alert to his wants and ready to attend to them to the degree which will restore his feelings of emotional security. Unlike the convalescent child who may express a dozen wants, loudly and lustily, the sick child will do little to announce his change in symptoms. The pediatric nurse must be ever alert to notice needs, for changes in children take place very quickly and often without warning.

The ability to observe and to feel with a patient, important in all nursing, is essential for a pediatric nurse. Experience in pediatric nursing should help the nurse to develop skill in noting signs which indicate changes in her patient's feelings, needs or physical status. Each day as the pediatric nurse goes about her work with her patients she needs to exercise her powers of observation not only through her sense of sight but also through her sense of hearing and touch and, perhaps most important of all, through that subtle sense of "feeling"—that sensitive quality which somehow tells her of changes in her patients which are not observed by the eye or the ear or the hand. She needs to be able to anticipate wants of the child of which he himself is hardly aware. She needs to be sensitive to the feelings which he cannot describe and be able to allay the fears which he cannot express. She needs to be

aware of his sources of comfort and pleasure, of his need for rest or for some form of constructive activity through which he can express himself, relieve tension and master his fears. She needs to perceive that the listlessness and the lack of appetite of the child with cardiac disease may be due partially to the fact that he is a homesick little boy who misses his parents, the noise and the laughter and even the scoldings of his home, which may be a poor one but is his very own.

The pediatric nurse who has developed skill in observation and a sincere interest in promoting optimal health learns to detect the signs which indicate physical or emotional distress. She notices the first evidence of a rising temperature, a drop in blood pressure, the beginning signs of increased intracranial pressure, the behavior that warns of an impending convulsion. She notices that in a group of children in the hospital playroom there is one who is evidencing fatigue or becoming overstimulated, which may indeed be a sign of fatigue. She also detects the child who is angry, fearful and grieving for a mother who is gone but he knows not where, and the child who has withdrawn, not because he is a quiet, "good" child but because he imagines that his new world is so scary or threatening that he dare not remain in contact with it. She makes these observations because her education and experience have made her sensitive to the needs of children and to the varied ways in which they may be expressed. Her education and experience have also made it possible for her to feel with them as they experience situations which are frightening or unfamiliar to them and to be alert to the slightest changes which take place in the child's appearance and behavior.

THE IMPORTANCE OF ESTABLISHING AND MAINTAINING A CONSTRUCTIVE RELATIONSHIP WITH CHILDREN

The ability to establish and maintain a constructive relationship with children is basic to the art of nursing. A child needs trust and confidence in those who are caring for him. This security comes only when his experience tells him that those who are caring for him *consistently* understand and meet his needs. A child who experiences emotional deprivation in the hospital loses trust not only in the nurses but in his parents as well. He reacts to painful experiences with resentment toward his parents who did not protect him from the predicament in which he finds himself. Without trust and confidence in his elders his opportunities for emotional growth are jeopardized.

In order to establish and maintain a good relationship with the child, the nurse must understand his developmental needs and possess the capacity to respond to his needs in a way which makes it possible for him to regain his physical health and master the emotional problems which hospitalization brings. The nurse must have interest in and sympathy for children as individuals who have certain rights and privileges. She must have an ability to see things from their point of view, to put herself in their places or, as psychologists say, identify herself with them. To succeed in this she must understand herself. By looking back into her own childhood and making a conscious effort to recall the events of her past experiences, she often furthers her understanding of the perplexities in the mind of the child who is in her care today.

THE CHALLENGE OF PEDIATRIC NURSING

Nursing is an art as well as a profession, that is, it must have in it the quality of creativeness. Creativeness is that subtle quality which gives the nurse the ability and the imagination to perceive in a given situation all the possibilities by which she may make a person more comfortable, more at ease in mind as well as body. Doubtless this quality is needed in all professions which deal with people but it is especially important in nursing children. Perhaps the reader questions the use of the word *creativeness* in relation to nursing when so much emphasis in the nurse's education must necessarily be placed on strict adherence to orders. Nevertheless, creativeness must exist in nursing if the profession is to meet the basic human needs of those in its care.

In pediatric nursing the nurse cares for a human being who is not only affected by a disease and all that is entailed in hospitalization but is also a growing, sensitive child. A human being is more than a physical body which is in good or bad condition; he is a person with a mind and feelings which are closely knit together and are reacting on each other constantly. The nurse is nursing a child, not a disease. True, she is nursing a person who is suffering from a disease and therefore she needs to know about that disease— its etiology, symptomatology and treatment—if she is to understand and meet his physical requirements when illness threatens his growth potentials. She also needs to understand, respect and care about children if she is to bring her patient's mind, feelings and body to their optimum pitch to combat disease and return to health.

A human approach which stems from understanding of the problems with which an individual child is confronted is an essential ingredient of pediatric nursing. To be a skilled technician in giving physical care is only a part of nursing. The most perfectly given bath, the most immaculate bed, medicines absolutely on time, the most punctilious restriction of effort are only partial treatment of a child. He has emotional needs which are equally important for his welfare. The nurse must have sensitiveness to those sometimes subtle but extremely important needs, as well as a knowledge of the physical requirements if she is to fulfill the functions of nursing and succeed as a pediatric nurse.

The nurse needs to understand the needs of all children, for she may have children in the ward who are not sick or are in the convalescent phase of a disease. The child who comes into the hospital for diagnostic purposes or for surgical repair may be a well child who needs experiences similar to those he has at home each day. It is so easy for a nurse in a busy ward to prefer to keep each child in bed, for there, she says, she "knows where they are." Keeping a well child in bed, however, does not meet his requirements. He needs guided experiences which help him to know what

activities are permissible and which ones must be restricted to protect him from cross-infection, from physical injury and from activities with which he is not ready to cope.

One only needs to view imaginatively the situation of 4-year-old Jimmy, who came into the hospital for operation on an arm misshapen because of an old and badly set fracture, to appreciate the dilemma he experienced when his capacities, interests and problems were not recognized. Jimmy's usual day at home was filled with a thousand and one interesting activities which gave him opportunity to practice his developing skills, solve his current problems in living and growing and obtain gratification. However, in the hospital Jimmy's situation was different. He was bathed and dressed, and most of the procedure was done by his nurse because it was quicker, although he might easily have done it himself. True, time is important, but other things become important too, when we understand a child's need for pleasure and independence. After his bath Jimmy was left more or less on his own resources—given nothing to play with and set down in a world that was utterly strange to him, to spend his day without direction and without the opportunities for satisfaction to which he had been accustomed at home.

Jimmy's new environment stimulated him to investigation, and he started on a voyage of discovery. In a short time he was found in the kitchen investigating the electric refrigerator and the gas stove. It was what he did at home, and he did not know that there were boundaries beyond which he was not allowed to go. Imagine the child's dilemma when he was punished by being put to bed for the day and being told he was a naughty boy for doing something which was natural, child-like and constructive in terms of his needs. He was in a strange environment, away from the security of his home, yet utilizing his well-developed inner resources to bring himself some satisfaction and keep himself comfortable.

Jimmy needed understanding and guidance which would help him to discover activities which were permissible; he also needed someone he could trust and depend upon for the satisfaction of his human needs. He received physical care without the personal interest and guidance that his emotional nature required. His nursing care was not creative; it was a series of technical procedures carried out with little imagination, feeling and understanding. No one discovered his motive in investigation; no one knew from whence he came or was aware that he needed an opportunity to become familiar with his new environment and discover that it was safe. His nurse did not know that he lived on a farm and never before had seen a gas stove or an electric refrigerator. She did not know that his mother always put wood in their stove and that his father cut ice in the winter and kept it in an ice house in their back yard. A few minutes of listening during the bath procedure might have given Jimmy's nurse some understanding of his curiosity about all the things that he viewed in his new environment. Through listening to his questions she might have discovered his need to investigate the strangeness of his world and realized the importance

of taking time to acquaint him with all that was different in the hospital.

Had Jimmy had the respect and the understanding that he required, he would have learned about his new environment, discovered the activities which were permissible and felt "good," trusting, accepted and safer than he had before. Instead, he undoubtedly felt "bad," misunderstood, angry and infinitely more threatened than he did earlier in the day.

Many adults care for children, shelter them, bathe them, feed them, put them to bed, guide and influence them, but to the pediatric nurse comes the special responsibility and privilege of seeing that they get the care that they need when they are ill. The mother, torn with anxiety and without the special knowledge of the nurse and knowing that she cannot meet some of her child's needs as the nurse can, steps aside and looks to her to do those things that she is unable to do herself.

The nurse's task is not easy, for she must not only know one child well but also she must have knowledge and imagination which give her an understanding of the many different types of children. She will not often have cared for and guided from birth the child whom she cares for in sickness. She must establish herself with the child and his parents and undertake the care of a child whose background of experience she has yet to learn. He may be a child who has had understanding guidance at home or he may be one who has been deceived constantly with false statements and consequently is suspicious of her every move. Quickly she must discover his needs, fulfill them and establish herself as an understanding, friendly person, for unless she can do that, his fears will prevent him from co-operating and utilizing his energy to fight his disease.

As the nurse reads this book with its discussion of the way various diseases attack children, doubtless she will be impressed with the fact of our great dependence on the body to heal itself and of its powers to do so. Diagnosis and treatment are only two of a necessary triad. The patient himself is the third tremendously important factor in the situation and may well tip the scales toward or away from recovery. Over and over again our greatest responsibility lies in helping the child to do his own fighting by keeping him at ease in mind and body. With understanding, the nurse can lessen the feelings of deprivation and anxiety which accompany illness and hospitalization; she can help to keep the child at ease in mind and body. She can understand the anxiety which comes to parents when their children be-come ill, and she can accept the different ways in which they express it in their relationships with nurses. She can alleviate parents' anxiety through understanding their need to keep in touch with their children and all that is happening to them in the hospital. She can also recognize the impact of the hospital experience on the child; she can discover his needs, fears and frustrations; she can prepare and support him as he meets new and frightening experiences; and she can provide the kind of care which gives the personal interest, the protection and the support that his ill body and emotional nature require. In doing so she can restore the child to physical health, prevent mental ill health by promoting the development of his personality, and make nursing an art. This is the challenge of pediatric nursing!

BIBLIOGRAPHY

Blake, Florence: The Child, His Parents and the Nurse, Philadelphia, Lippincott, 1954.

CHAPTER TWO

Preventive Pediatrics

INFANT MORTALITY
CHILD MORTALITY
MORBIDITY AND ITS EFFECTS

CHARACTERISTICS OF PHYSICAL
 DISEASE IN CHILDHOOD
PREVENTION OF DISEASE AND DEATH
SITUATIONS FOR FURTHER STUDY

Medicine once concerned itself only with curing human ills, but today it has changed its ideal to include the prevention as well as the cure of disease. In no field of medicine is this aspect of prevention so important as in the field of pediatrics. This is true because of the high incidence of death among infants and children, and because of the eventual effect of preventive measures on the adult population, since whatever can be done to protect the health of children should be reflected later in a healthier adult population.

In order to understand the problems of prevention, it is necessary to know the chief causes of sickness and death among infants and children, the proportion of children affected and the effects of the various illnesses on the subsequent health of the child. It is necessary to know also what measures may be taken in order to prevent these illnesses.

Promotion of health also entails an understanding of the growth process and the factors which foster healthy personality development.

This knowledge is essential in working with parents. It is equally important in our work with children in clinics, hospitals, schools and camps for the reasons which have been cited in Chapter 1.

INFANT MORTALITY

The infant mortality rate is the ratio between the deaths of infants under one year of age in any given year and the number of live births in that same year. The rate is usually expressed in terms of number of deaths occurring for each 1,000 live births. In other words, if the death rate is said to be 65, it means that 65 babies out of 1,000 live births die before the age of one year. The rate may also be expressed in percentages, e.g., 6.5 per cent in this case.

If the births within a given area are not fully recorded, the infant mortality rate for that area cannot be computed accurately. In 1915 only 10 states and the District of Columbia required birth registration, and not until 1933 was the goal of 48 states reached, primarily through the

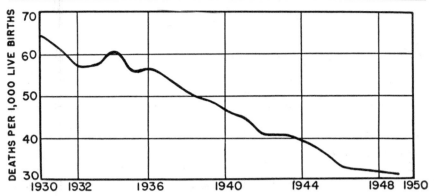

CHART 1. Infant mortality rates in the United States, 1930-49. (Children's Bureau, U. S. Department of Health, Education and Welfare, Statistical Series, No. 9)

efforts of national organizations concerned with child health. Since the birth rate remains fairly constant (except perhaps in war years), this method has been considered adequate for computing the infant mortality rate.

The death rate for the United States as a whole for infants under one year was 64.6 in 1930; 31.3 in 1949 (Chart 1). In the latter year the lowest death rate for a state was 23.1. The highest rate occurred in one of the territories—90.3. Among the 53 subdivisions of the United States Registration Area, only 5 states and 3 territories had infant mortality rates in excess of 40.

The infant deaths during the year 1949 were heavily concentrated among the very young. Almost exactly one third of the deaths occurred during the first day of life; a second third of the mortality was made up of infants who lived from 1 to 28 days; the remaining third of the deaths was among those surviving from 1 to 12 months. As Chart 2 demonstrates, the chief re-

duction in infant mortality over the years has been achieved among those who survive for a month. Almost no improvement in the rate during the first day of life has occurred.

Causes of Infant Deaths. The relative importance of the main conditions responsible for death during the first year of life are indicated in Chart 3. Since we have already seen that one third of the deaths occur on the first day and another third within the first month of life, it is not surprising to find that 70 per cent of the infant deaths are caused by abnormal conditions of pregnancy and delivery (prematurity, congenital malformation, birth injury, asphyxia and atelectasis). A more detailed view of the causes operative during the first month of life is given in Chart 4. The importance of premature birth is emphasized by the fact that more than half the deaths occurred in infants who were immature at the time of birth. Among the infants who died after the first month of life, the outstanding cause was infection, chiefly of the respiratory and the gastro-intestinal tracts. Congenital malformations were next in importance, and the remaining deaths were attributed to a wide variety of conditions.

Prevention of Infant Deaths. Analysis of the great strides which have been made in the reduction of infant mortality in the United States during the past 35 years

shows that the infectious causes of infant deaths can be controlled to a very large extent. In regions where the standards of public health and preventive medicine are high, it is possible to eliminate syphilis, tuberculosis, diphtheria and pertussis from the infant population and to reduce the incidence of diarrhea to a very low figure. Prompt and adequate treatment of the infections of

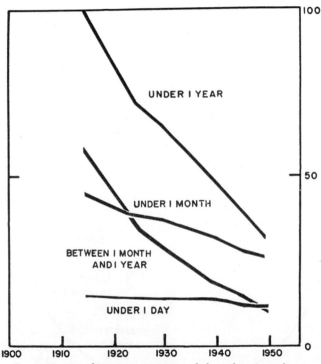

CHART 2. Trends in age segments of the infant mortality rate in the United States from 1915 to 1949. The top line shows the rapid decline of total mortality under 1 year of age. The bottom line shows the very slight decline of mortality for infants under 1 day of age. The intermediate lines show a moderate rate of decline in deaths under 1 month and a very steep fall in deaths among infants of 1 to 12 months of age. (Children's Bureau, U. S. Department of Health, Education and Welfare, Statistical Series No. 9)

the respiratory tract with chemotherapy and modern antibiotics has produced a considerable decrease in the number of deaths from this cause, although the complete elimination of respiratory disease is far from being realized.

Further reduction of the infant mortality rate will depend mainly upon our ability to prevent deaths during the early days of life (Chart 5). Although some progress has been made, it is less dramatic than the results obtained through the control of infections. Good obstetric judgment applied to all pregnancies can have an important effect upon the number of deaths due to birth injury, anoxia and asphyxia. A better understanding of the premature infant and improved facilities for his care have reduced the number of deaths from this cause. Little progress has been made in the prevention of prematurity and congenital anomalies and in the management of atelectasis of the newborn. Until these challenges are met and solved, substantial further reduction of infant mortality cannot be expected.

Sociologic Factors. In what has been said above on infant mortality, only the pathologist's or statistician's point of view is expressed. From

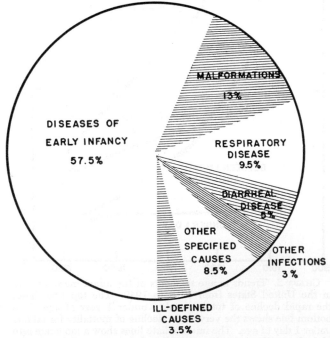

CHART 3. Causes of death among infants less than a year of age in the United States, 1949. (Drawn from data in Children's Bureau Statistical Series No. 9, U. S. Department of Health, Education and Welfare)

the sociologist's standpoint, an entirely different group of causes of death might be enumerated. For example, the economic and social conditions into which a baby is born may play a determining role in the state of his health, or in his death. Infant mortality is found to be related closely to housing congestion, employment of the mother away from home and low earnings of the father. Aside from all other factors, the infant death rate has been shown to vary inversely with the earnings of the father.

Such differences in the mortality rate as exist in this country among the various races may well be due to economic and social conditions rather than to race.

Public Health Factors. The quality of the milk supply is a most important factor in the infant mortality rate. As already stated, in former years diarrhea was one of the most serious menaces to the infant, due in part to an unsafe milk supply. Today, pasteurization of milk in all large communities and the increasing custom of boiling all fresh milk or using evaporated milk for infant feeding have been large factors in decreasing the incidence of dysentery. In general, in those states and

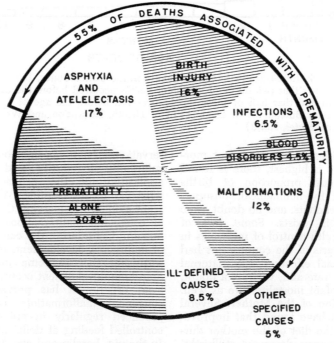

CHART 4. Causes of death among infants less than 28 days of age in the United States, 1949. (Drawn from data in Children's Bureau Statistical Series No. 9, U. S. Department of Health, Education and Welfare)

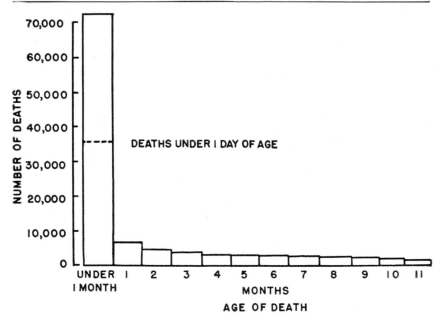

CHART 5. Infant deaths by age in months in the United States, 1950. The figure shows that two-thirds of all infant deaths occurred before the age of 1 month and that half of these deaths occurred before the age of 1 day. (Children's Bureau, U. S. Department of Health, Education and Welfare, Statistical Series, No. 9)

communities where the infant mortality rate is highest, there is found the greatest proportion of births managed by nonmedical, unsupervised attendants, and no doubt some relationship exists. Some sort of public-health control of midwives in certain parts of the country has had a beneficial effect on the maternal mortality rate and, without a doubt, on the infant mortality rate as well.

Nutrition of the Mother. Several observers have found that improvement of the diet of the mother during pregnancy decreases stillbirths, premature births and the incidence of disease and death after birth in babies born at term. Such ob-

servations have been confirmed sufficiently to justify widespread application of the principle by whatever means possible. We have scant evidence concerning the cause of congenital malformations in the human. Considering the complexity of embryonic development, it is not surprising that in some instances defects in development occur. However, experiment has proved that congenital malformations can be produced regularly in animals by controlled feeding of deficient diets. In the pig, harelip and eye deformities can be produced by feeding the mother a diet deficient in Vitamin A. In the rat, cleft palate and deformities of the extremities are produced by feeding the mother a diet deficient in riboflavin. Whether such observations can be applied to the human remains to be proved. However, the ingestion of an adequate diet by the pregnant woman can have no disadvantages, while the advantages may be manifold. It increases the vigor of the newborn baby, serves as a protection to the mother and, in addition, probably increases her ability to supply sufficient milk for the baby. The majority of deaths among infants after the first month are among those who are fed artificially.

CHILD MORTALITY

The mortality rate decreases very rapidly after the first year of life. During the year 1949 in the United States, 31 children out of every 1,000 under the age of 1 year died. But among those between the ages of 1 and 4 the rate was only 1.5 per thousand, and the older children between 5 and 14 suffered a rate of

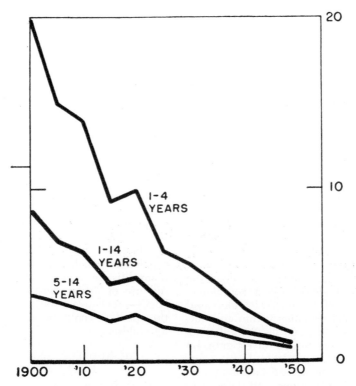

CHART 6. Trends in mortality rates of children of various age groups in the United States, 1900-49. (Reproduced from Children's Bureau Statistical Series No. 9, U. S. Department of Health, Education and Welfare)

CAUSE OF DEATH	PERCENTAGE OF DEATHS AMONG CHILDREN	
	1 to 4 years	*5 to 14 years*
All Accidents	26	35
(Motor Vehicle Accidents)	(8)	(14)
Respiratory Infections	15	5
Cancer and Leukemia	7	10
Congenital Malformations	8	3.5
Contagious Diseases	8	9
(Poliomyelitis)	(2)	(6)
Heart Disease and Rheumatic Fever	1.5	7
(Rheumatic Fever alone)	(.5)	(3.5)
Tuberculosis	4.5	3
Diarrheal Diseases	5	1
Appendicitis	1	2
Nephritis and Nephrosis	1	1
Other Causes	23	22.5

0.65 per thousand. During recent decades the rate of decline in mortality rate has been almost as dramatic among the preschool children as among the infants, but relatively little progress has been made among the older children (Chart 6).

Causes of Childhood Death. The important causes of death among children of the United States Registration Area for the year 1949 are listed in the above table. Approximate percentage figures are given in order to show the relative importance of the several causes.

A study of the table shows how, with his expanding environment, the preschool child faces a completely new set of hazards. His increased range of locomotion within and outside the home and his natural tendency to climb and investigate set the stage for accidents. His passage out of the home and into neighborhood social groups and later into school increases his exposure to infectious and contagious diseases. During the school years cancer,

heart disease and poliomyelitis each takes a significant toll of life.

While it is true that some cause of death always must head the list, we cannot feel complacent about the adequacy of our medical care until conditions over which we have no control predominate. The present pre-eminence of accidents as a cause of death beyond the first year of life requires repeated emphasis to parents, for many of these fatalities could be avoided by a little forethought. As a matter of fact, all of the fatal conditions mentioned except cancer, malformations and poliomyelitis are amenable to control if full use of modern medical knowledge—preventive, educational and therapeutic—could be extended to all children.

MORBIDITY AND ITS EFFECTS

Morbidity or sickness rates obviously are much greater than mortality rates. In the course of time, almost every person develops measles, for example, whereas the proportion of deaths from measles is small. The possible effects of illness other than death are manifold. In a general way, it may be said that children make remarkably rapid and complete recovery from most acute diseases, and that the deleterious effects of these illnesses are transitory and of no ultimate consequence to the child; but this is not true of all disease conditions.

Effect of Acute Illness. During acute illness, nutrition always is affected adversely: in part, by decrease in food intake; in part, by failure of utilization. The effect on growth is more noticeable in infancy than later, because growth normally is more rapid at this period. In those instances in which the illness is of brief duration and the recovery is complete, growth occurs at an increased rate until the normal again has been attained. During brief illnesses, the retarded growth rate may not be noted unless careful serial measurements are made. It seems likely that the seasonal growth of children, more rapid in summer and less so in winter, is dependent in part on the seasonal incidence of infection.

A few serious, acute illnesses leave evidence of their existence in developing teeth and bones. The scars in the bones, as shown by roentgenogram, tend to disappear in time. When the enamel formation of teeth is impaired by illness, the defect may not be repaired and may remain in the affected teeth for life as a transverse groove or larger area of thinned or absent enamel.

Effect of Chronic Illness. Chronic illness retards growth in the same manner as does acute illness, for the duration of the illness, and occasionally leads to permanent stunting of growth when the illness is greatly prolonged. Rather frequently it is observed that children who have had chronically infected tonsils and adenoids removed have greatly increased appetites and improved nutrition and growth.

Chronic or repeatedly recurring asthma is often associated with impaired nutrition and growth: in part, because of decreased food intake; in part, because of poor oxygen supply. Chronic, uncontrolled diarrhea, such as may occur in ulcerative colitis or in celiac disease, is likely to affect nutrition more seriously than most other conditions because of the greater difficulty of absorbing food.

Chronic, severe malnutrition, whether from anorexia and low food intake or from the secondary effects of disease, leads eventually to physical stunting and sometimes to mental lethargy simulating mental backwardness.

Permanent Damage of Certain Illnesses. Certain illnesses and abnormal conditions leave behind them permanent damage which may be a handicap throughout life. One of the important groups in this category comprises the conditions which cause damage to the central nervous system. This group includes intracranial hemorrhage at birth and some of the infections affecting the nervous system, either directly or indirectly. Recovery from encephalitis may be incomplete. Meningitis at times leaves residual defects. Syphilis of the nervous system may be devastating without producing death. Poliomyelitis may leave permanent paralysis. Cerebral accidents may occur as a result of whooping cough or of myocardial damage and weakness in various disease conditions. Mental deterioration may occur with uncontrolled convulsions. Deafness may be a result of some of these conditions, as well as of chronic suppuration of the middle ear.

In some of these conditions, nutrition—and therefore physical growth—is affected adversely. But even more important, and in a larger measure, mental capacity is decreased and in some instances abolished.

Another important group causing serious handicaps comprises those conditions affecting the heart, particularly congenital malformations of the heart, and rheumatic carditis. For some of these children, activity must be restricted more or less permanently. For others, nutrition is seriously impaired because of poor circulation.

Effect on Psychological Development. Chronic, crippling or frequently recurring illness can affect the child's psychologic development adversely. The normal growth from dependent, egocentric infancy to emotional maturity may receive severe setbacks through the experience of being physically handicapped or ill. The way in which such a physical handicap or illness affects the child's personality growth is determined by his parents' attitudes and feelings toward him and toward his physical condition, and by the quality of care that he receives when hospitalization becomes necessary. A sense of insecurity from the very presence of the illness or handicap itself cannot help leaving its imprint upon the mind of the child. In addition, he may be confronted with hospitalization which

brings separation from his parents, fear-provoking experiences, and a dearth of the kind of constructive relationships that he needs for personality growth.

The full effects of illness in childhood are by no means reflected by the mortality and morbidity tables. Illness and hospitalization can be a constructive experience or it can leave the child with emotional disturbances which hamper his opportunities for optimal personality growth. The effects of separation will depend upon his early relationship with his parents, the stage of development he is in at the time of separation, and the kind of experience with which he is faced. They will also depend upon the quality of care he receives in the hospital and at home after the period of hospitalization is over.

Separation from the mother during the earliest years of a child's life can injure the mother-child relationship upon which his personality growth depends. Young children who have been hospitalized frequently show symptoms of disturbed relationships with their mothers. The inevitable loss of the mother, of familiar surroundings, and of play activities, together with the painful experiences which accompany hospital care, often result in anxiety, exaggerated fears and regression to infantile modes of behavior.

The adverse effects of hospitalization are expressed in different ways. Some young children who have gone through the anxiety which follows separation from the mother during hospitalization become clinging, demanding and resentful. Others repress their feelings and withdraw from their mothers and associates because they have lost trust in people generally. Thumbsucking, night terrors, soiling, enuresis, negativism, eating and speech disturbances and increased aggressiveness are other forms in which the emotional effects of hospitalization may be manifested.

The nurse's task is to prevent emotional deprivation by providing care which meets the child's total needs and by helping his parents to understand the requirements for healthy personality development. The child's emotional needs in periods of illness have been cited already. Parental overprotection which commonly arises in response to chronic illness or deformity endangers the child's opportunities for personality growth. The nurse can help parents recognize their child's developing powers and assist them in discovering ways to provide him with growth-producing experiences. However, to accomplish this aim the nurse needs more than knowledge of the growth process and the needs of the individual child; she needs understanding of the problems and the anxieties which parents of chronically ill and handicapped children face, and she needs skill in timing her guidance to meet parental needs.

CHARACTERISTICS OF PHYSICAL DISEASE IN CHILDHOOD

The outstanding characteristics of disease and abnormalities in infant and child, in contrast with those in the adult, may be included briefly in a few large groups.

Congenital malformations of any part of the body may be noted at birth. Some—for example, malformations of the brain and the heart —may constitute grave handicaps throughout life. Others—such as intestinal malformations with an obstruction—demand prompt surgical relief. Still others do not permit continuance of life.

Diseases of the newborn and abnormal conditions incident to birth form a large and important group. Some of these represent difficulty in adaptation by the infant to changed conditions of living, as in the case of premature birth or congenital weakness; some are caused by various types of birth injury; some result from infections of a type peculiar to the newborn period. It is obvious that both this and the preceding group are peculiar to or have their greatest importance in infancy.

Abnormalities of nutrition assume their greatest seriousness in infancy, but they occur also in the older child, and to a greater extent in the child than in the adult. Growth makes greater nutritional demands than does the more static state of the adult. The more rapid growth of infancy creates the more serious problem.

Infections in general are not peculiar to childhood, although many of their serious effects are. The communicable diseases occur more commonly in childhood than later, and the serious complications and the mortality from them are preponderantly in this age period.

Miscellaneous Diseases. A large miscellaneous group of diseases peculiar to infancy and childhood do not lend themselves to easy classification. Some of them are dependent on normal physiologic, anatomic and psychologic differences between the child and the adult. The conditions which produce a chill in the adult are likely to cause a convulsion in the young child. Intussusception occurs almost exclusively in infancy. On the other hand, certain degenerative diseases of the adult, such as arteriosclerosis and coronary disease, have no counterpart in childhood. The neoplasms and the tumors of infancy and childhood in general differ conspicuously from those found in the adult. Carcinoma and sarcoma, common in the adult, are rare in childhood. Most of the childhood tumors are congenital in their origin. They may be present at birth, or more often they become manifest later, but they arise from misplaced or abnormal fetal tissue or developing tissue. The common tumor of the kidney is an embryonal adrenosarcoma (Wilms's tumor). The most common tumor of the brain is an astrocytoma (glioma). Second in frequency of the brain tumors is neuroblastoma (medulloblastoma). The common tumor of the adrenal is neuroblastoma. A neuroblastoma is a malignant tumor of developing neuroblasts of the sympathetic nervous system. It may arise in various places, but most commonly it starts in the adrenal. A large tumor of the liver in a young child is most likely to be metastatic neuroblastoma, with its origin in the adrenal. A hemangioma (birthmark) is a blood-vessel tumor, most commonly of the skin. A lymphangioma is a similar tumor of the lymphatic vessels. Both hemangioma and lymphangioma are congenital in origin and usually are benign. Sexual precocity encountered occasionally in childhood is caused most often by adrenal tumors in boys and by ovarian tumors in girls.

PREVENTION OF DISEASE AND DEATH

PREVENTION OF DISEASE IS A PUBLIC RESPONSIBILITY

In approaching the problem of the measures to be taken to prevent disease and death, we are justified in considering the lowering of the death rate first, as that was in fact the historic approach to the problem. There was a national organization "To Study and Prevent Infant Mortality" long before there was a national association whose aim was to keep babies and children well, although the latter organization in part grew out of the former, and the former broadened its scope long before it changed its name.

We know that infant death rates may be lowered, that they have been lowered. In other words, a large proportion of the deaths of infants, when the infant death rate was 150 or even 250 in some cities of this country not so many years ago, were preventable. Slowly but surely the infant death rate has decreased until, in 1949, it stood at 31.3. How has this been brought about? Can we do better than 31.3? Without doubt! The fact that a death rate of 20 or less has been achieved in some cities of this country is evidence of the possibility. Public-health effort directed to this end is becoming constantly more extensive and more active on the part of the nation, the state and the community, and on the part of private local and national associations not a part of these political units. As the public conscience has become aroused to a sense of responsibility in regard to the welfare of children, there has been a definite trend toward an assumption of health effort by the public (tax-supported) agencies. Private agencies (supported by private funds) have been in many instances the pioneers in this field of endeavor. But when the need is demonstrated and the public becomes aware of it, public funds tend to become available for the work. The private agency has served one of its purposes in demonstrating, and the public agency carries on. Infant and child mortality and morbidity are being combated today by legislation, by welfare stations for prenatal and postnatal care, by corps of school nurses and physicians, by community-health nurses, by nutritionists, by press, television and radio, and by many other means.

METHODS OF PREVENTING
ILLNESS AND DEATH

The means available for the prevention of disease might be classified in various ways, but, however classified, all should be employed. As one group of prophylactic measures, we have such proceedings as would normally be carried out by a local board of health aided by community laws. This group would include supervision of milk and the water supplies and disposal of the sewage and the garbage, isolation of those with communicable diseases, and similar activities designed for the general protection of the community. Then we have those measures which are carried out with the individual child, either by the physician in the course of his practice, or in the public-health clinics by the physician, the public-health nurse and possibly the nutritionist and the child-guidance worker. The efforts for the individual child always imply

an educational program with the mother, aiming to teach her those things which maintain and improve the physical and mental health of the child.

The points to be stressed in our method of attack are: (1) periodic examinations, (2) nutrition, (3) application of prophylactic measures against specific diseases, (4) accident prevention and (5) child guidance or, we might say, parent guidance. Each important factor in the mental and physical health of the child should be studied, and to each should be applied our medical, social and economic resources.

Periodic Examination. Perhaps the importance of periodic examinations is more generally recognized for the infant than for the older child and adult. By such examinations, abnormal states may be detected in their incipient stages; or, better still, trends toward abnormal states may be observed before definite abnormalities exist. Periodic examinations must not be permitted to prevent the seeking of medical advice earlier if it is indicated.

More important than the physical examination is the guidance which is given pertaining to the subsequent time period. This, if followed, should help toward assuring normal growth and development and a good state of health. The examination is a check-up on past performance; the guidance given looks to the future. The periodic consultations could well be held at least monthly during the first year, the interval then being increased gradually to 6 months. In the latter half of childhood, an annual physical examination usually is sufficient, although in any program attempting to guide the parents in the training of children there should be more frequent consultations, through either home visits or visits to a child-guidance clinic.

Nutrition. The nutrition during each period of infancy and childhood is important for general health, not only during the period under consideration, but for all later periods as well. Good prenatal nutrition produces more vigorous infants. Good infant nutrition gives the baby a better start into childhood. Some of the defects which are discovered later at school, which may persist through life, may be contracted in infancy and the preschool period, often to a degree which affects the stamina and the learning capacity. Dental caries is as yet an uncontrolled human scourge and is caused in large measure by improper diet.

Specific Protective Measures. An important part of the periodic consultation is the protection of the child against the serious infectious diseases which he may encounter in later life. Practices differ somewhat, depending upon the health circumstances of the community. It is almost universal practice to give all infants protection against smallpox, diphtheria, whooping cough and tetanus as a minimum. Smallpox vaccination is usually given during the latter half of the first year of life. It is ineffective if the procedure fails to result in a "take," i.e., the production of a blister and a scab. For the other 3 diseases a triple toxoid is now in general use which permits simultaneous administration. A basic course of 3 injections spaced about a month apart is required. Although the immunity produced is somewhat better if this procedure is delayed until after 6 months of age, many physicians feel that it is preferable to establish some degree of protection earlier in life. Frequently, initial immunizations are begun at 2 to 3 months of age and sometimes even earlier. Booster injections are added at the age of a year or 18 months when early immunizations are given. Periodic stimulation of the immunity should be continued through the childhood years about every 3 or 4 years.

Protection against other diseases is also available. In regions where typhoid fever is prevalent, active protection by the administration of vaccine during the first year of life is desirable. Under special circumstances, active protection against typhus fever, Rocky Mountain spotted fever, mumps and rabies may be desired. Effective treatment with penicillin has made vaccination against scarlet fever obsolete.

In certain instances it is desirable to give a child or an infant temporary protection against a disease to which he has been exposed recently. Immediate but transient protection is available for many infectious diseases through the administration of preparations of convalescent serum or adult blood products. This type of protection is called passive immunization and should not be confused with the previously mentioned immunizations which are designed to give long-lasting protection. Passive protection against measles is desirable for infants and children between the ages of 6 months and 3 years when known exposure has taken place. Gamma globulin is the most widely used preparation for this purpose. Convalescent serum is desirable for protection of unimmunized infants who are exposed to whooping cough within the family. Tetanus antitoxin must be given following certain injuries if the child has not been previously immunized.

Of the preparations used for passive protection against disease, those which are manufactured in animals such as the horse or the rabbit, carry the disadvantage of serum sickness and the induction of sensitization to animal proteins. Human convalescent serum and gamma globulin do not have this disadvantage.

Accident Prevention. The increasing prominence of accidents as a cause of death and disability among infants and children has emphasized the need for better safety education of parents and of the children themselves. Such a program requires a concerted attack from several directions with an emphasis which shifts according to the age of the child. According to figures of the Children's Bureau for 1949, accidental deaths among infants are due most commonly to the inhalation or the ingestion of foreign materials. The potential danger of small objects, medicines, and poisons which may be reached by the exploring infant can be discussed profitably during the sessions of a periodic examination or a well-baby conference. Fire constitutes the second most frequent hazard for the infant. The preschool child who is beginning to explore beyond the confines of his home runs his greatest risk from motor vehicle accidents, with fire and drowning next in order of importance. Within these age groups accident prevention is primarily a problem of parent education and of es-

tablishing safe habits in the child through parental discipline.

Among children of school age the hazard from motor vehicle accidents increases with age until within the teen-age group 1 out of every 4 deaths is due to this cause. In addition to parental influence, the school can exert some constructive effort through driver training and safety programs for older children. The major campaign for reduction of deaths through traffic accidents must be a broad one, striking at all age groups striving for better self-discipline and safer operation of motor vehicles.

Drowning is the second most common cause of accidental death among children of school age. The schools, the camps and the youth organizations can assist in accident prevention by offering instruction in swimming and water safety.

Parent Education. One of the most important aspects of preventive pediatrics is the education of parents. Until those who have immediate responsibility for children are informed and convinced of the need for protective measures, results will be disappointing.

In the early part of this century efforts were directed toward the reduction of the infant mortality rate, and success was achieved. Education was focused upon the provision of a safe milk supply, for much of the infant diarrhea was due to ignorance about the preservation of infant formulas. Prophylaxis against smallpox and diphtheria was soon added as another objective of parent education. Later, the emphasis shifted toward improving the nutrition of infants and children with specific campaigns against rickets, scurvy and anemia. The results of these efforts are gratifying, for the diseases enumerated have been virtually abolished in communities which have good programs of parent education.

But the task is never finished, for new generations of parents are continually arising to be instructed in the established technics of prevention, and the scope of activity continually broadens. As the task of saving lives and preventing physical disease becomes simpler with modern facilities and a better informed group of parents, more time and energy can be devoted to considerations of physical and emotional growth and development and the manner in which they affect the individual child's adjustment to his environment.

The nurse's role in parent education is changing with the newer concept of health which considers not only physical disease but the child's social and emotional adjustment as well. Previously, the nurse's role in parent education was largely concerned with the physical care and health of the child. Now she is becoming involved in preventive health programs which assist parents in gaining increased understanding of their children's developmental needs as well as functioning in the realm of preventing physical disease.

In each period of personality development there are developmental tasks which the child must surmount if he is to continue to grow emotionally. A child can master the tasks of development if he is emotionally and physically prepared for the experience and is guided through them with the understanding support of his parents or their substitutes.

The nurse's role in preventive mental health programs is one which requires keen observation, understanding and an ability to interpret children's developmental requirements without being judgmental or authoritarian. The nurse needs knowledge of the factors which promote optimal physical growth and the signs which indicate deviations from normality. Early detection and treatment of physical defects provide the physical preparedness necessary for mastering the tasks of development. She also needs understanding of the developmental process and the factors which support healthy personality development. To function in preventive health programs, she needs preparation to do what Levy calls "anticipatory guidance."

Anticipatory guidance is that guidance which prepares parents to understand their children's needs for growth. It gives parents understanding of the changes in behavior which come with growth and assists them in recognizing their children's readiness for the new growth-producing experiences. It also helps them to prepare themselves to support their children so they can master the tasks that are necessary for growth with comfort and a feeling of accomplishment.

Providing anticipatory guidance requires understanding of oneself and parents as well as children. The nurse's success in guiding parents is dependent upon her attitudes and feelings toward them as persons. It is also dependent upon her ability to appraise their readiness for guidance and upon her skill in interpreting knowledge to them. Self-understanding, objectivity and clear recognition of her own limitations are equally essential, for a nurse's efforts may do more harm than good if she permits herself to become involved too deeply in the complexities of emotional disturbances of parents or children. She can interpret the findings of those who have studied the needs of children; she can utilize her knowledge in her relationships with children; she can be alert to symptoms which manifest emotional distress, but the treatment of serious emotional disturbances must be left to someone with special training in this area. Emotionally disturbed parents and children need the help of someone who has special training in the dynamics of human behavior and in the use of the therapeutic measures which are required to restore individuals to mental health—a physician, a child-guidance worker or a pediatric psychiatrist.

SITUATIONS FOR FURTHER STUDY

1. What does the promotion of health entail?

2. What are some of the reasons why the infant death rates are so high in some states of our country? What preventive health measures would be necessary to reduce the high mortality rates existent in some states?

3. Why is the mortality rate during the first month of life so high?

4. How could the mortality rate during childhood be reduced? How can the nurse assist in programs which are planned to reduce the mortality rate in children of the school-age period?

5. How may illness affect a child's physical development? His psychologic development? How may care during illness affect a child's psychologic development?

6. Observe children in the ward. Observe a child that you believe has been affected adversely by illness and hospitalization. Describe his behavior and indicate why you feel his personality growth has been affected by his illness and hospitalization. How might it have been prevented?

7. What is the nurse's role in preventive health programs? What preparation does the nurse require to function in preventive health programs? Is theoretical preparation sufficient to ensure successful parent education? What else is required?

BIBLIOGRAPHY

Charts on Infant, Childhood and Maternal Mortality, 1949: Children's Bureau Statistical Series, No. 9.

Childhood Mortality from Accidents 1949: Children's Bureau Statistical Series, No. 17.

Lemkau, Paul: What can the nurse do in mental hygiene?, Public Health Nursing 40:583, 1948.

Unit Two

GROWTH, DEVELOPMENT, CARE AND GUIDANCE OF THE INFANT AND THE CHILD

CHAPTER THREE

Growth, Development, Care and Guidance

GENERAL CONSIDERATIONS

The Child a Growing and Developing Organism. There is an important difference between nursing children and nursing adults of which the pediatric nurse needs to be aware. When nursing children, she is caring for a child in which growth changes are taking place at a rate so much more rapid than is possible in an adult that the adult seems like static material in comparison.

Growth is the most pre-eminent characteristic and the most vital of all the tasks of childhood. The most important thing one does is to "grow up," and "growing up" implies a much more complex process than adding inches to one's stature or pounds to one's weight. Many other phases of development are closely related.

The Interrelatedness of Growth. Inherent in the word *growth* is all that is implied in the phrase *growth and development* so frequently used today, for growth is, according to a

dictionary definition, "the progressive development of an organism." In the minds of many, growth always has had very much of a physical connotation. The definition of growth means infinitely more than physical growth. The newborn baby is a complexity of interrelated growth forces — physical, mental, emotional, social and spiritual — which through an ongoing and inevitable progression result in the adult.

Every individual has within him the impulse for growth. If the infant lives, he will grow, but the nurturing he receives, that is the care and the guidance that he is given, may foster optimum growth or it may stunt or warp his physical and psychological growth in some or all of its aspects.

A General Pattern of Growth. Physical growth proceeds in an orderly fashion; each stage of growth is preparation for the next. The baby does not talk, for example, until he has gone through the so-called "babble stage," when he experiments with many sounds, and not until some of the sounds he has heard come to have some meaning to him. He does not walk until growth of his nervous system and exercise make it possible for him to balance his head, to sit, usually to creep and then to stand.

Growth is individual; no two children grow exactly alike. Children will show individual differences in their patterns and tempos of growth. Therefore, it is impossible to say, "This child should be doing exactly thus and so at this time and should weigh so much and be so tall."

Norms of growth represent a range rather than an exact point; they should be used as guides rather than standards. To obtain a fair evaluation of a child's development, he must be measured against himself, as well as against the norm.

Understanding of the Child Reached Through a Study of the Whole Child. To understand a given child, the total picture of that child must be viewed, for many factors entered into making him what he is. His background of experience within his family and community must be known. Physical characteristics also influence his personality and development. Growth is a complex matter, and no one aspect of it can justifiably be isolated and considered by itself. His height and weight, for example, may possibly be an underlying cause for promoting the social pattern of aggressive behavior or its reverse. The very short child may attempt to compensate for being smaller than his playmates of the same age by being overaggressive or "cocky." On the other hand, his shortness of stature may be a reason for his retreating from the group or seeking companions younger than himself. His physical make-up and the environmental factors to which he has been exposed doubtless will affect the behavior patterns that he has developed.

In attempting to discover the dynamics of an individual child's behavior all factors must be studied and evaluated. The whole answer is not always found in reviewing his physical condition; emotional and social factors also must be considered. Poor eyesight may have caused a child's withdrawal from active play. Possibly poor motor co-ordination and a lack of vigorous outdoor play may have an effect on the child's appetite, and that in turn may be a contributing cause of malnutrition and underweight. Is the child who seems to be a troublemaker in the ward one who has been a troublemaker in school because he felt himself inadequate to the requirements of his teacher and the group? Or was he really mentally inadequate as the teacher may have thought? Or had he come from an unhappy home where he felt insecure? Or had he done poor work in school because his eyesight was poor? Always the fact of the interrelatedness of growth must be borne in mind in attempting to reach an understanding of the child. Unless this is done, those factors which are blocking his full potentialities for growth may never be corrected. Yet for the sake of simplicity and clarity it is probably wise to present the subject of growth and development under the headings of physical and psychological growth.

PHYSICAL GROWTH

GENERAL CONSIDERATIONS

Variability in Normal Growth. Childhood is the bone-growth period of life; both heredity and environment are influencing factors. By 20 to 25 years of age, one expects that the adult pattern so far as height is concerned will have been acquired. The 6 ft. 4 in. man does not grow over a greater number of years and thereby gain his commanding stature; he grows at a more rapid rate than the man who is a foot shorter. The growing time has been the invariable factor; the rate, influenced doubtless by heredity and environment, has been the variable factor.

There are two periods of more rapid physical growth in childhood: one during infancy, especially the first 6 months; and the other during the pubescent period, which usually begins somewhat earlier for girls than for boys. Therefore, the child will meet the first demands of formal school life (6 years) at a time when less energy is being given to the business of growing physically, but he must meet the increased demands of high-school life at the same time that he undergoes his prepubertal spurt in growth.

Not only do individuals vary from other individuals in rate of growth, but each individual varies within himself in his own rate and emphasis on growth. At one time he tends to grow tall; at another time he increases more rapidly in weight.

Seasonal variation, uncommon in infancy but frequently apparent in children past this period, gives the picture of growth increase above the average in the late spring, summer and early fall, and below the average during the remainder of the year. However, these seasonal variations do not occur when an adequate diet and exposure to sunlight are constant and when infections are absent or of a mild type. Therefore, they are related to environmental factors and are not necessarily a part of the expected growth pattern.

Differential Growth. The infant is not a miniature man, but by different rates of growth within his body he changes from the contour of an infant to that of a man. From birth to adulthood he changes from an individual whose head represents one fourth of total body length, whose trunk is about the same length as his legs, to an adult whose head is about one eighth of the total body length, whose legs are long in comparison with the trunk. At birth, the middle of his body is 1 inch above the umbilicus, but as his legs increase in length faster than the trunk, the midpoint of his body gradually lowers. At 2 years of age it is about an inch below the umbilicus; at 6 years, halfway between the umbilicus and the pubes; and at maturity it is at the pubes. At birth his arms are longer than his legs. The reverse is true in adult life.

Not only is the infant's head larger in proportion to his body in contrast with adult proportion, but the relation of cranium to face is different. The ratio of the size of the cranium to that of the face is 8:1 in the case of the baby, 5:1 at 5 years, and 2:1 in the case of the adult. In infancy, the upper portion of the face is more completely developed than the lower. But during the growth years, the rate of growth in the lower part of the face is accelerated. The room is provided for the first, and then the second, set of teeth, and eventually the strong line of chin and jaw is attained for the adult.

The upper jaw may grow faster or slower than the lower jaw, affecting the contour of the face and the development of the teeth. Such dental difficulties as malocclusion or crowding of teeth may occur, and the orthodontist of today can do much to correct them.

At birth the head and the chest are little different in circumference; in adulthood the proportions have changed markedly. At birth, the circumference of the head is (33.1 to 35.4 cm. or 13 to 13.9 in.); the circumference of the chest is (32 to 34 cm. or 12½ to 13½ in.). In adult life, the chest has more than doubled its circumference, the increase in size having continued through adolescence, whereas there is relatively little increase in the circumference of the head after 5 years, when its approximate circumference is 55 cm. or 22 in.

Therefore, the differential aspect of growth is an important element in the developmental picture and is reflected in the changing proportion of weight given to organs and blood, as well as bones, muscle and fat, in infancy and adult life. In the newborn, the organs and the blood represent about 35 per cent of the weight; bone, muscle and fat, about 65 per cent (bone 10 per cent, muscle 20 to 25 per cent, fat 30 to 35 per cent). From the second to the fourth years, the muscles undergo very rapid growth, about 75 per cent of the weight gain at this period being due to such increase. The rounded contour of babyhood with its dimples and curves disappears, and the more slender child emerges. After 6 years, the relative increase in the musculature is gradual, and at about 12 years the adult value of 40 to 45 per cent of the total body weight is reached. During adolescence, the amount of muscle increases, but in proportion to the increase in total body weight. The upper extremities contain about 15 per cent, and the lower extremities 60 per cent of the entire musculature.

In the actively growing years of childhood, the organs and the blood concerned with the nourishment and the functioning of the organism have a greater proportion of the total weight than in the adult years, when growth has been accomplished, for then only 20 per cent of the weight is needed for organs and blood, instead of 35 per cent.

The body framework or skeleton, serving as the storehouse for calcium and supporting the entire musculature, will constitute about 20 per cent of the adult's weight in contrast with the 10 per cent of infancy.

The muscles, which give man his power of movement and vigorous effort, and likewise store proteins and carbohydrates for him, will constitute about 40 per cent of adult weight, about twice the percentage of weight attributed to the infant's muscles.

The fat, which is a nonconductor of heat and serves as a storehouse for the energy demanded by growth, must be had in abundance by the baby, because his heat regulatory mechanism is not well established, and he must expend much energy in growing during his first year. The fat covering needed for the adult is between two thirds and one half as much as that needed by the baby, and even that sometimes seems too much for the dictates of fashion in our culture!

Influences of Sex on Growth. Girls average somewhat less in height and weight than boys at birth, but on the whole the differences are slight and of little importance until the onset of the pubescent period (9 to 14 for girls, 11 to 16 for boys), girls averaging about 2 years' acceleration over boys. The second rapid growth period which begins at this time of life is definitely related to maturing sexuality. Girls usually begin to grow rapidly taller within the year before the onset of menstruation, and a boy's spurt in growth occurs shortly before puberty. Children who have reached sexual maturity tend to be taller and heavier than children of the same age who may still be in the prepubescent period. Although for a time during prepubescence and early adolescence girls may be heavier and taller than boys, usually the relationship of infancy is re-established after 17 years, and the average young man is both taller and heavier than the average young woman.

Measuring Growth

Height and weight are the usual measurements of growth. For many years attempts have been made to compile tables of growth which would serve as guides to the expected measurements at various ages. Such tables have a definite field of usefulness, but it is important to realize that they represent only averages reflecting our present standards of nutrition and may be changed materially as our nutritional standards continue to improve.

If the height-weight tables published in the past 20 years are reviewed, it will be noted that the average rate of growth now is greater than that reported in earlier studies. This is particularly true of infants and young children. The 1921 tables of Baldwin show definitely slower growth than those of Stuart in 1933. This difference—an interesting one to note—is attributable almost exclusively to improved nutrition. The data of Baldwin were collected during a period when neither cod-liver oil nor orange juice had come into use in the routine management of infants. If the Baldwin tables are no longer representative, as indicated by the data of Kornfeld and of Stuart, what reason have we to believe that the more recent tables should be set up as standards? Babies and children fed nutritionally adequate diets grow at a rate more rapid than is indicated by any of the currently available growth tables.

However, skeletal height and body bulk, the two aspects of physical growth measured, are only the most obvious manifestations of growth. Anthropometrists have at least 16 measurements, not of equal reliability, which they take in attempting to study the growth pattern. Measurements of hip and chest, for example, give us a picture of body build. Some of the measurements give the picture of differential growth, such as the measurements taken of the jaw. Some measurements are taken over a longer period of time than others. Height will be measured for perhaps 25 years, weight doubtless for life; but the circumference of the head, which holds that important organ, the brain, is not measured routinely after 6 years. Obviously, the brain, although the seat of continuous mental processes, reaches its mature size many years before intellectual maturity is reached.

The physician in examining the child's growth considers such factors as musculature, bone structure and blood hemoglobin. The nutritional status is determined by numerous criteria other than height and weight. To ensure accuracy in judgment of the physical status, a physical examination should be made, and the weight and the height measurements should be included as a part of the examination. Also, the regimen of diet should be compared with that recommended. When examined in this way, some children will be found to be malnourished, although they are little, if anything, below standard average weight. Even though normal in weight, they may be flabby and obviously in poor nutrition. However, it is usually found that if a child is more than 10 per cent underweight or 20 per cent overweight, the chances are that he is not normal.

The Use of Growth Tables. All current growth tables are divided on a sex basis and compare height with age and weight with height, thereby giving a more nearly accurate picture of the child's status than if weight were compared with age. However, the size of the skeleton is not entirely a matter of length but is also a matter of bone circumference; that is, we do find the child

of so-called "slight frame" and the child of sturdy frame or large bones. In other words, children differ as to body build, and that difference is reflected in their weights; but for practical purposes the weight-to-height comparison is relied on to give the proportion of weight to size of skeleton.

Babies vary greatly in length at birth, and considerable variation in height may be found at any given age of the child. This variation we should expect to see reflected in the weight; that is, the taller child would be expected to weigh more than the shorter child of the same age. If their weights were the same, it might well be that the tall child would be rated as undernourished and the short child as well nourished. Length is less quickly or markedly affected by short periods of illness or dietary deficiency, and therefore it can be expected to continue at about the established norm, whereas the weight is quickly and often markedly affected by illness. During infancy, however, the height measurement is frequently omitted, and only the weight gains are noted. Perhaps this is chiefly because the picture of growth that it gives seems to be more impressive to the parent than the somewhat less dramatic growth in height, as we may expect a baby to double his weight at 5 months, but not until he is nearly of kindergarten age will he be twice as tall as when he was born.

Although, as has been said, growth tables are useful, and many have been developed from studies made of children's growth in various parts of the country, they must not be taken too seriously in relation to any one child. A table which is as nearly as possible the result of a study of children comparable with the child to be considered is preferable to one made from a study of children living under different conditions or coming of different stock. Then, too, as previously stated, the child always should be measured against himself, as well as against a growth table.

The Children's Bureau Growth Table, the outcome of the weighing and the measuring of preschool children all over the country in 1918, was the earliest table for preschool children to come into general use. It took no account of socioeconomic factors, of stock, of previous illnesses or of other factors which are now recognized as important. However, it served as a tremendous impetus to the public's interest in the health of children.

Some of the growth tables in use today are those of Stuart, the Merrill-Palmer School and of Meredith, tables which are the result of careful studies. The growth curves reproduced in this text (Charts 7 to 12) are those of Jackson, based on the data of Meredith. The curves show a mean value at the different age levels represented by the middle line of the three lines shown. The other two lines represent one standard deviation* on each side of

---

* A standard deviation is the amount of variation above or below the mean which will include ⅓ of all the observations made. Thus, between the lines which represent plus 1 S.D. and minus 1 S.D. will be found exactly ⅔ of the observations from which the graphs were drawn. At a given age, the heights or the weights of ⅙ of normal children will be above the top line; ⅓ will fall between the top and the middle lines; ⅓ will fall between the middle and the lower lines; and ⅙ will fall below the bottom line.

the mean. Heights and weights falling within the ranges shown are considered to be normal, provided that certain criteria are met. Growth may be considered normal if it parallels the general course of the curves, even though the height or the weight may be above or below the median curve. Change in position in relation to the curve may represent abnormality of growth, especially if relative decrease is found from one observation to another. From these curves it is apparent that the norm consists of a range of values. A tendency exists to discontinue the use of "average" in relation to growth and to consider growth only in terms of the normal range. A general picture of the expected growth in height and weight is useful as a guide, although it must be remembered that the word *approximate* may represent a wide range.

GROWTH IN HEIGHT. Growth in height may be expected to follow somewhat this picture for the first 5 years:

	APPROX. IN. EACH YEAR
At birth	20
Increase first 3 mos.	4
Increase second 3 mos. ...	2¾
Increase third 3 mos.....	1½
Increase fourth 3 mos....	1¼
Total gain for year	9
Increase 1 to 2 yrs........	4
Increase 2 to 3 yrs........	3¼
Increase 3 to 5 yrs........	2½

From the growth charts included in this chapter it may be calculated that a boy who is 43 in. (110 cm.) tall at 5 years will be about 60½ in. (154 cm.) at 13 years, and about 65 in. (166 cm.) at 15 years.

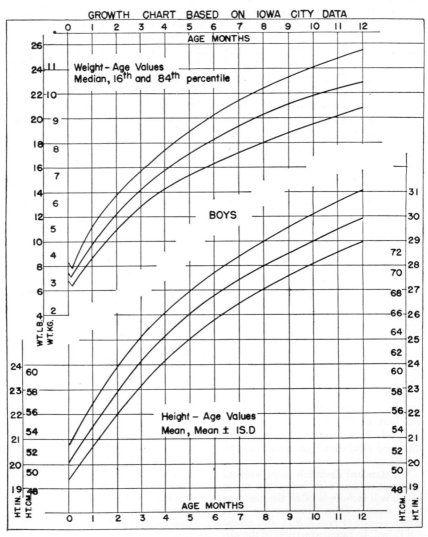

CHART 7. Average measurements of boys from 0 to 12 months of age.

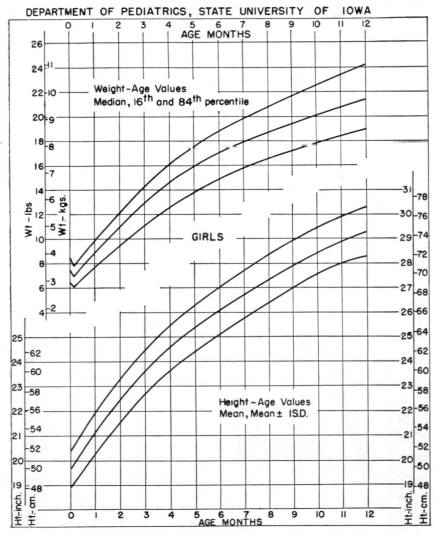

CHART 8. Average measurements of girls from 0 to 12 months of age.

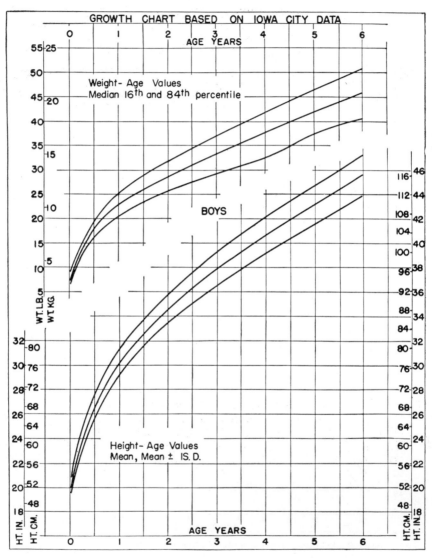

CHART 9. Average measurements of boys from 0 to 6 years of age.

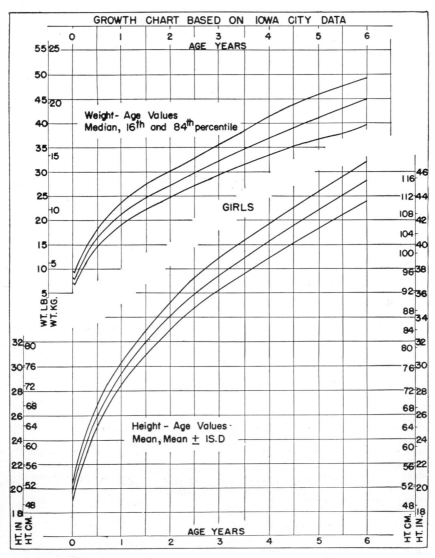

CHART 10. Average measurements of girls from 0 to 6 years of age.

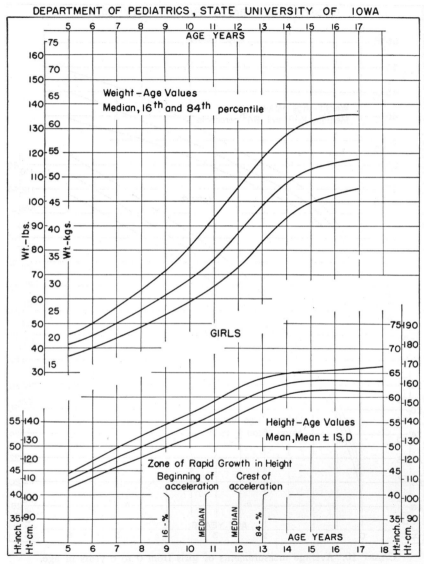

CHART 11. Average measurements of girls from 5 to 18 years of age.

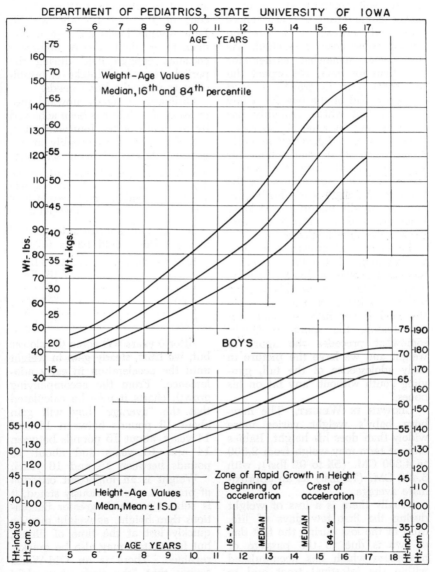

CHART 12. Average measurements of boys from 5 to 18 years of age.

There is an appreciable slowing up in growth after one year, and growth will continue at an even slower tempo during the early school years and until shortly before the age of pubescence is reached. As this comes somewhat earlier for girls than for boys, we expect the pubescent spurt in growth to send the girl ahead of the boy for a few years, a fact which probably has some bearing on some of the social differences and difficulties in early adolescence. At dancing school, for example, the still little boy avoids the girls of his age and seeks the younger girls more nearly his height, and the rapidly maturing girl looks longingly, and not always in vain, toward the older adolescent.

The increased growth preceding and accompanying puberty requires increased intake of food. Usually, appetite takes care of this needed increase. When it does not, or when the food is not fully adequate for any reason, the spurt in height somewhat precedes the spurt in weight and we have the picture in early adolescence of the tall, gangling youth without "any fat on his bones."

GROWTH IN WEIGHT. The newborn baby's weight varies more widely than does his height. Babies born at term may weigh from 2,500 to 4,300 GM. (5½ to 9½ lbs.), with 3,400 GM. (7½ lbs.) as an approximate average.

Usually there is a loss of weight during the first few days of life. Most of the loss during the first day or two is due to the passage of meconium which has accumulated within the intestinal tract and to the delivery of edema from the subcutaneous tissues. The magnitude of this early loss is quite variable from one infant to another. It may amount to as much as 10 to 15 per cent of the initial body weight. Later weight losses are due in the main to metabolic loss or failure to consume enough fluid during the period when food intake is insufficient to meet the body needs.

Ordinarily a steady upward progression of weight has been achieved by the tenth or the fourteenth day, and the child gains steadily at approximately the following schedule:

```
4 mos.........double the birth weight
1 yr...........triple the birth weight
2¼ yrs......multiply birth weight by 4
4 yrs..........add birth weight again
```

In terms of approximate general average, this would be as follows:

```
Birth weight ............ 7½ lbs.
4 mos. .................15   lbs.
1 yr. ...................22½ lbs.
2 yrs. .................28½ lbs.
4 yrs. .................37½ lbs.
5 yrs. .................42   lbs.
```

After 5 years will come the slower but, we trust, steady gain in weight until the acceleration in early adolescence. From the accompanying growth charts it may be calculated that the "average" boy will gain about 13 pounds between 13 and 14 years, about 15 pounds between 14 and 15 years and about 13 pounds between 15 and 16 years.

Weight is an important criterion of progress. As previously stated, it is subject to much greater fluctuations than height, as weight may be quickly lost at the time of illness, but fortunately may also be quickly regained. There is an Old-World saying that "the flesh of a child does not fly far," a reassuring statement for the mother who sees with alarm the rapid loss of flesh that accompanies a sudden severe illness. Even during the slower period of growing there should be a constant gain, and any loss of weight or stationary weight over a long period should be investigated.

Bone Growth. Growth in length is dependent entirely on bone growth, and bone growth is largely dependent on the mineral supply which the body is given and can use. During growth, bones change in composition, number and size, and the skeleton as a whole increases in size about 20 times from birth to maturity. Bones consist of an organic matrix, cartilage, fibrous tissue, mineral salts, fat and water. The fat is largely in the marrow cavities.

At birth, the amount of mineral matter in the bones (chiefly a complex calcium phosphate carbonate) is relatively small and the amount of water large (75 per cent) in comparison with that existent in the adult. As growth progresses, the amount of mineral increases, and the water decreases. At one year, the skeleton is about 60 per cent water, at which level it remains for the next 2 years. After this time, the mineral gradually increases, and the water decreases until the adult level of 40 per cent mineral and 10 to 25 per cent water is reached at about 12 years if the nutrition has been good. As the amount of mineral increases and ossification takes place, the pliant bones of infancy, easily subject to changes due to muscle pull and pressure, become the rigid bones needed to protect the organs of the child and to give the adult his sturdy framework.

In the cartilaginous and membranous structures destined to become bone, mineralization starts at one or more points and gradually spreads throughout the bone from these points. Approximately 800 of these points or ossification centers exist, more than half of them appearing after birth. During growth, the epiphyses of the long bones grow independently of the bone shaft and have their own classification centers. It is chiefly by the growth in the length of the bone shaft that growth in body length occurs. This growth takes place at the end of the shaft, between the shaft and the ununited epiphysis. Growth ceases when shaft and epiphysis unite. Union of the epiphyses with the neighboring bones begins in the innominate bone at about 12½ years in girls and 14 years in boys. It ends in the upper end of the humerus at from 19 to 20 years with good nutrition, but often later with poor nutrition.

THE USE OF ROENTGENOGRAMS IN STUDYING SKELETAL DEVELOPMENT. Roentgenograms have become an important implement in studying skeletal development. By their use we can study bone growth and so are able to talk of bone age as well as chronologic or mental age. For example, a 5-year-old child whose height and weight indicate him to be within the average range expected for that age might be shown by x-ray examination to have a bone age of a much younger child in that ossification has not taken place in some of the cartilaginous and fibrous tissue to the extent that would be expected. Roentgenograms of the hand and the wrist which have been found to give a reliable picture of the skeletal development of

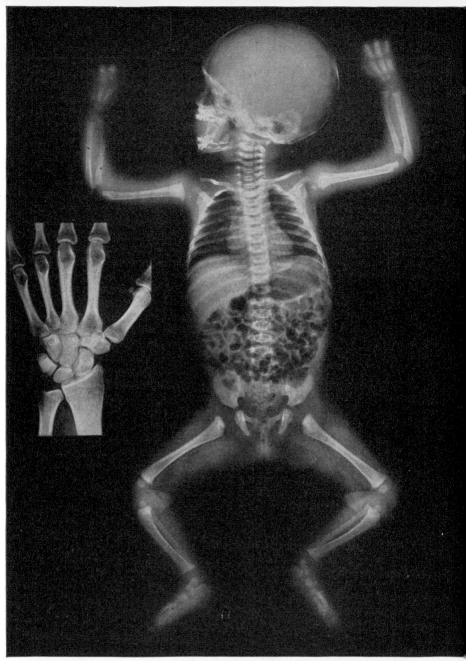

Fig. 1. Roentgenogram of a normal infant 6 months of age. The thinness of the skull and the presence of partially mineralized but unerupted teeth are to be noted. Relative lack of ossification of the skeleton is shown by the wide spacing between the calcified portions of many of the bones, especially in the pelvis and at the larger joints of the extremities. The wrist of an adult is shown for comparison; it is approximately twice as large as it should be to compare with the infant's wrist in relative size. (Medical Division of the Eastman Kodak Company)

the young child show no carpal bones at birth and no epiphyses. Succeeding roentgenograms will trace the appearance and the development of these bones and epiphyses. Here again, as in other aspects of the child's growth, a knowledge of the child's life and environment may be the key to our understanding of a retarded skeletal development that might be observed. For example, the child whose diet is habitually low in minerals and vitamin D may be lagging behind in his skeletal development. Infectious diseases also may hinder skeletal development, as scars can be noted in roentgenograms of children who have experienced some acute infectious process.

Since growth in length is so largely dependent on the mineral supply, and since that in turn is so dependent on the food we eat, it is to be expected that those with an inadequate or poor food supply, through either poverty or ignorance, will not reach their optimum growth in stature, and certain studies have borne out this supposition. It has been noted that when the mineral intake is only moderately decreased, growth continues at the normal rate, but the bones have a low mineral and high water content. With a still lower intake of mineral, bone growth is slowed, and with greater deprivation it is stopped.

Roentgenograms not only give us the picture of the appearance and the growth of bone, but they also indicate the differences in density of bone. It is not uncommon to find greatly decreased density of bone during adolescence. Since this is a time of rapid growth, it may be that the food supplied the child is deficient in minerals and that the store of calcium already in the bones is called on for formation of new bone —an indication of the extreme importance of a diet adequate in calcium during adolescence and a fact that school lunchrooms might well take into consideration!

THE BONES OF THE SKULL. The upper part of the skull is made up of 7 "membranous" bones still separate and ununited at birth. The boundary lines between them are known as sutures, and the point of juncture of 3 or more bones is a fontanel. Six fontanels exist at birth, but only 2 of them are normally palpable in a full-term baby—the anterior fontanel and the posterior fontanel. The posterior fontanel closes at approximately 2 months. The average time for closure of the anterior fontanel is usually stated at 18 months. However, in many robust, well-developed babies, it may be closed at one year or even earlier. The most common cause of delayed closure is rickets. Closure is delayed also in mongolism and cretinism. The sutures become ossified at from 6 to 9 months of age, though still capable of expansive growth. Premature closure of some of the sutures leads to growth of the skull in other directions, with consequent deformity. Separation of the sutures occurs with hydrocephalus.

Teeth. Although a newborn baby rarely shows any erupted teeth, the 20 deciduous teeth (first set) and the 6-year molars of the permanent teeth (second set) have begun to develop before birth. The enamel (outer portion) and dentin (inner portion) formation of the crowns of the first teeth begins as early as the fourth month of fetal life, and that of the first permanent molars begins shortly before birth.

Since tooth formation is a part of the picture of fetal development, the mother's health, diet and nutrition play a considerable role in the character of the early teeth. The health, the diet and the nutrition of the infant in the years before the eruption of his second teeth likewise play a considerable role in the character of those second teeth.

TOOTH DEVELOPMENT. The age variability, found in other aspects of development is also found in relation to the eruption of teeth. It must be remembered always that there is not a set pattern for growth and development, but rather an approximate pattern, from which the individual child may vary. Many a mother has become unduly anxious because she has had in mind a set pattern to which she has felt her child should conform.

However, in tooth eruption, as in other aspects of growth, we do have an approximate developmental picture. There are 20 deciduous teeth, all of which we generally expect to have put in their appearance by the time the child is 2½ years old. The usual order of appearance and approximate age of appearance are as follows:

2 lower central incisors	6 to 12 mos.
2 upper central incisors	
2 upper lateral incisors	
2 lower lateral incisors	12 to 15 mos.
4 anterior molars	
4 canines ("eye and stomach teeth")	15 to 30 mos.
4 posterior molars	

Subtracting 6 from the age in months will roughly approximate the number of teeth which should be present during the first 18 months.

The eruption of teeth is a physiologic process, and in most normal well babies is not associated with illness. There is often a certain amount of discomfort from swollen, tender gums which may cause restlessness and loss of appetite, but even this disorder is very temporary. Occasionally, however, illness occurs due directly or indirectly to teething. Along with irritability, the infant may have a slight fever and a lessened digestive capacity; possibly this is a good illustration of the effect of the emotional life on the physical. If his usual diet is continued, diarrhea results. However, many mothers are too much inclined to atttribute illness to teething, thus leaving the real condition undiagnosed and untreated. Much harm has been done by the promiscuous lancing of gums.

The seemingly excessive "drooling" which is evident at about the time the teeth erupt is not due to teething, but to the fact that the salivary glands are becoming active, preparatory to the time when saliva will assist in the digestion of solid food, and the baby has not learned to swallow the saliva.

The teeth of the first set are shed as the teeth of the second set which replace them push against them, causing absorption of their roots and consequent loosening. Therefore, the age at which the first teeth are lost corresponds closely to that stated subsequently for the eruption of the second set.

The permanent teeth are 32 in number. They begin to erupt at about 6 years and are completely erupted at from 17 to 23 years. The following is an approximate schedule

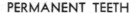

PERMANENT TEETH

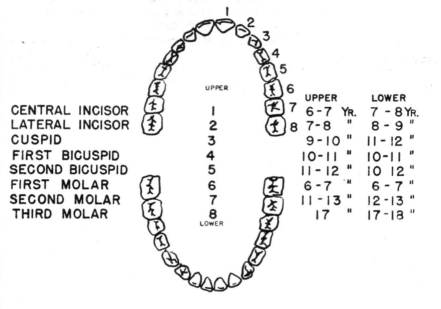

		UPPER	LOWER
CENTRAL INCISOR	1	6-7 YR.	7 - 8 YR.
LATERAL INCISOR	2	7-8 "	8 - 9 "
CUSPID	3	9-10 "	11 - 12 "
FIRST BICUSPID	4	10-11 "	10-11 "
SECOND BICUSPID	5	11-12 "	10 12 "
FIRST MOLAR	6	6-7 "	6-7 "
SECOND MOLAR	7	11-13 "	12-13 "
THIRD MOLAR	8	17 "	17-18 "

DECIDUOUS TEETH

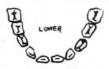

		(LOWER)	
CENTRAL INCISOR	1	8 - 12 Mos.	5 - 9 Mos
LATERAL INCISOR	2	8 - 12 Mos.	12-18 Mos
CUSPID	3	18-24 Mos.	
FIRST MOLAR	4	12-18 Mos.	
SECOND MOLAR	5	24-30 Mos.	

FIG. 2. Showing time of eruption of the teeth.

for the eruption of the permanent teeth (Fig. 2):

4 first molars
("6-year molars") ... 5 to 7 yrs.
4 central incisors .... 6½ to 8 yrs.
4 lateral incisors .... 7 to 9 yrs.
4 first bicuspids .... 9 to 11 yrs.
4 second bicuspids ......10 to 12 yrs.
4 cuspids ("canines") ....11 to 14 yrs.
4 second molars ....11½ to 13 yrs.
4 third molars ....14 to 23 yrs.
or more

The four first teeth of the permanent teeth to appear, the so-called "6-year molars," do not replace any of the first set but come in back of the deciduous posterior molars and are exceedingly important teeth. Too often they are neglected because they are thought to be some of the first set of teeth, and caries in them remains untreated. Seventy-five per cent or more of school children are said to have caries of the first molars. It is around these teeth that the whole denture develops, and their loss affects the relation of all the teeth to the skull and the shape of the face. The jaw from which these teeth have been lost prematurely remains much shorter than it would be normally, and the teeth do not meet effectively for mastication. Premature loss of the first teeth, often due to neglected caries, is a common cause of poor alignment of the second set. The child with carious or lost first teeth will not and cannot chew food well, thereby suffering a disadvantage in regard to nutrition as well as in regard to jaw development.

Thorax. The chest of the young infant is soft and flexible, chiefly because of the large amount of cartilage at the sternal end of the ribs. Deformities occur more easily then than later when the chest is more firm. In infancy, the chest is almost circular. It is narrow at the top and widens below where it meets the abdomen. In its growth, the chest becomes relatively larger at the top and widens throughout to approach the adult proportions at from 5 to 7 years. At birth, the ribs are almost at a right angle to the long axis of the body. The change in position to the adult angulation of approximately 25° is very gradual, being only about one third of the adult angle at from 4 to 5 years.

PHYSIOLOGIC CHANGES

Lymphatic System. The lymphatic tissue of the body is relatively well developed at birth, and its growth is rapid during the early years. After puberty, the lymphatic organs decrease in size. Much of the growth of the lymphatic organs, particularly the nodes, seems to be in response to infection rather than the result of maturation of the body. Lymphatic response to infection is characteristic of childhood and occurs much more in early childhood than later. Because of the relative lack of immunologic defense, infections are much more likely to reach the lymph nodes in early childhood than later, when a greater degree of immunity has been attained. Because of their accessibility, it is easily noted that the tonsils and adenoids tend to undergo retrogressive changes in late childhood.

The thymus is a lymphatic organ which follows much the same rate of growth and retrogression as the nodes. It has been set apart from other lymphatic structures because of supposed endocrine functions, but the evidence that the thymus has any function other than as a lymphatic organ is unconvincing, as is also the evidence that it has any relationship to sudden death attributed to lymphatism or status lymphaticus. It is now well known that the thymus atrophies rapidly in any illness, even though brief. Therefore, at necropsy, it is only in cases of sudden death of children previously well that the full-sized normal thymus is found. In the past, the relatively large normal thymus has been considered as abnormally enlarged because of the contrast in size with the thymus usually found at necropsy.

Skin and Hair. As part of the picture of physical growth we should note the changing picture in regard to skin and hair. At birth, the skin of the Caucasian is dark or bluish red, changing to a light pink in 2 weeks. "Rosy cheeks," a part of the traditional picture of healthy childhood, are not always present in the older child, since they seem to have a relationship to other factors as well as health, such as general coloring and racial inheritance. The newborn baby's color may be modified by jaundice, a not uncommon occurrence in the newborn. A certain amount of desquamation is normally present during the first month, the amount and the depth varying widely with different babies. The sweat glands, as well as the salivary glands, are inactive at birth. Their function gradually increases, and many babies are able to perspire freely after one month. "Goose flesh" is not an accomplishment of the very young baby.

Newborn babies present various pictures so far as hair is concerned, from the bald-headed baby to the one with hair that is relatively abundant and long. The hair at birth is very soft and usually dark. Loss of the first hair may occur soon, either because it falls out or because it is rubbed off by friction against the bed. The new hair, which will come in slowly, is of a firmer texture than the first, and usually lighter. The very fair hair of early childhood tends to darken as the child grows older, although it may stay very fair without aid throughout the growing years and for some years after maturity is reached.

At birth, fine downy hairs (lanugo) are often thickly distributed over the body, especially on the back and the legs. These disappear largely by the end of the first week. Occasionally excessive hair is found, particularly on arms and legs in early childhood, but usually there is no noticeable hair on a child's body until puberty is reached.

The condition of the hair in childhood often gives us a clue to the child's nutrition. The child who is in good nutritional condition reflects it in glossy, strong hair. Dull, lifeless-looking hair is often part of the picture of poor nutrition.

Body Temperature. The ability of the very young infant to maintain the body temperature constantly at the normal level is not well developed. The smaller and more delicate the infant, the more this is true. Even the older baby, whose temperature-regulating mechanism is reasonably adequate, is helpless to overcome without assistance the handicap of prolonged exposure to extremes of temperature. Consequently, it is necessary for the responsible adult to see that the clothing and the environment of the infant are such that the body temperature is maintained at the proper level.

The body temperature of no child is constant, regardless of age. The temperatures, when charted, never produce a straight line. Variations of ½ to 1° F. from the assumed normal of 98.6° usually are not to be considered as abnormal. Mothers frequently need reassurance on this point.

The temperature taken by rectum represents more nearly the true body temperature than does that taken by mouth. The general belief that rectal temperature readings are 1° F. greater than those taken by mouth is not strictly correct. As shown in the following illustration, rectal temperature readings may differ from oral readings by amounts varying from –1.0 to +3.2° F.

Pulse and Respiration Rates. The rates of pulse and respiration vary in the same child under different conditions. Even when such factors as excitement and exercise have been eliminated, these rates vary considerably in different children of the same age and size.

Despite all the variations, however, it is evident that a relatively high rate is present at birth, and that the rate gradually diminishes with age until the adult values are reached.

It has been observed that the ratio of respiratory rate to pulse rate usually approximates 1:4. The approximate respiration and pulse rates to be expected at the various ages are shown in the table on page 55:

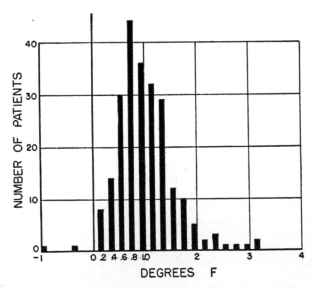

CHART 13. Variations of rectal from oral temperature readings, using the oral readings as a base line. (J. Iowa M. Soc., January, 1942)

PULSE AND RESPIRATION RATES

| AGE | RATE PER MINUTE | |
	PULSE	RESPIRATION
First mo.	120 to 150	34 to 45
First yr.	100 to 140	25 to 35
1 to 2 yrs.	90 to 120	20 to 30
2 to 6 yrs.	90 to 110	20 to 30
6 to 10 yrs. . . .	85 to 100	18 to 25
Over 10 yrs. . .	75 to 90	18 to 23

Blood Pressure. The determination of blood pressure in infants is a difficult and often inexact procedure. In small children care must be taken to use a cuff of suitable width. One which is too narrow may give falsely high readings; one which is too wide may give an artificially low reading. The cuff should be approximately 2/3 the width of the child's upper arm. Blood pressures taken from a struggling, excited or fearful child are unreliable. Fear increases the blood pressure. To get accurate readings and to help the child accept the procedure, explanations and demonstrations are necessary. The following table gives the range of values which can be expected at various ages when suitable conditions prevail:

BLOOD PRESSURE IN MILLIMETERS
OF MERCURY

AGE	SYSTOLIC	DIASTOLIC
4 to 6 years	60 to 110	40 to 80
7 to 10 years	70 to 120	45 to 75
11 to 14 years	85 to 125	45 to 85

(Modified from data of Downing, E. M., Am. J. Dis. Child. 73:293, 1947)

Growth of the Reproductive System. During the conversion from functionally sexually immature child to fully developed adult, pronounced changes occur in body size and in social and emotional development. The latter will be considered subsequently in this chapter. The infant at birth possesses a full complement of the reproductive organs which mark him definitely as male or female. These organs, the primary sex characteristics, are small in size and remain functionally dormant until the second decade of life. Then, under the stimulus of hormones secreted by the pituitary gland, profound changes take place which convert the child from an individual who is relatively sexless in appearance to one who displays the distinctive appearance (the secondary sex characteristics) of his sex and is able functionally to play his part in reproduction.

The pubertal changes which occur in girls affect all tissues of the body. In girls, such changes may begin as early as the tenth year. Under the influence of estrogens produced by the developing ovaries, the bony pelvis enlarges and broadens, and the hips become rounded. First the nipples and then the breasts begin to bud. Later the nipples become pigmented. Hair appears in the pubic region and later in the axilla. The vagina enlarges, and its secretions become more profuse and acid in reaction. While these external changes are taking place, the ovaries and the uterus are enlarging and are beginning to acquire the periodicity of function which eventually produces menstruation. The first menstrual period is termed the menarche and is the official onset of puberty. In the United States it occurs most commonly between 11 and 15 years but occasionally is seen earlier or later. Irregularities in the appearance and the duration of the periods is not uncommon during the first 2 years. At some point during this time interval the girl acquires the ability to reproduce. The estrogenic substances not only influence the skeleton by stimulating growth in height, but they also limit this growth by fostering closure of the epiphyseal lines. Consequently, while the girl initiates her spurt in growth earlier than the boy, she is likely to approach her ultimate height early in her teens, whereas the boy may continue to grow into his twenties.

The pubertal changes which occur in boys are equally marked. In boys, pubertal changes begin about 2 years later than in girls. Under the influence of androgenic substances produced in the testes, the penis and the testes begin to enlarge. Hair appears in the pubic region, then on the face and in the axilla. Changes take place in the larynx which make the voice more resonant and lower in pitch. For a time the control over pitch may be uncertain so that sudden breaks occur during speech. The skeleton is not only influenced to grow in length, but it tends to become broader and more sturdy and there is a dramatic increase in the mass of the skeletal muscles. There is no externally apparent point at which reproductive ability is signalized. Production of spermatozoa probably begins at 13 to 15 years of age but cannot be determined readily.

PSYCHOLOGICAL DEVELOPMENT, CARE AND GUIDANCE DURING THE GROWING-UP PROCESS
THE IMPORTANCE OF THE PRENATAL PERIOD

The prenatal period is of vital importance to the unborn child and his parents. It is a period in which the fetus is growing from a minute cell into an individual who is capable of life physically apart from his mother. *To cope with the adaptations required by extra-uterine life and to realize its full growth potentials, the fetus needs essential nutrients. It also needs a peaceful, parasitic existence and a mother who is prepared to receive him with unconditional acceptance and motherliness.*

The capacity for parenthood does not come automatically with pregnancy; it evolves out of the complex of each parent's experience with his own parents during his childhood. The prenatal period is the time during which expectant parents are making their final preparation for parenthood. In our culture better preparation of individuals for parenthood could be achieved if all children were protected from physical disease and provided with the kind of relationships which foster wholesome personality development. Successful marriage and parenthood requires emotional maturity. Preparation for marriage is a problem for the home, the school and the church.

In addition to preparation from their parents and teachers during childhood and adolescence, expectant parents need the help of professional workers throughout the maternity cycle and in the years while they are guiding their children toward maturity. Although attitudes and feelings toward the unborn child will have been formed already from past experiences within their own families, evidence exists which shows that expectant parents can profit from the guidance of professional workers. With interest in people, knowledge, skill and understanding, the nurse can help them to become prepared for the new experiences which are a part of the maternity cycle. She can also help them to anticipate and prepare for the changes that come with growth.

Alleviating anxiety and building up expectant parents' confidence in their own abilities bring satisfaction which help to prepare them for their future roles in the care and the guidance of their child. *The expectant mother needs help in learning about her health requirements during pregnancy. She needs help in understanding the emotional and physical changes which occur. She also needs preparation for labor and the care of her newborn infant; she needs comfort and freedom from anxiety so that she has energy available to prepare herself to receive her infant with readiness to minister to his individual requirements.*

The expectant father also requires consideration. *He needs to feel that he is a part of the experience. He also needs to understand the emotional changes which come with pregnancy and to become prepared to support his wife during labor and in her role as a mother.* This is essential for his security; it is also important for his unborn child and for his wife. Her motherliness will be influenced by the support, the security and the understanding that she receives from her husband not only in the period in which she is establishing her relationship with their child but also in the years to come.

Guidance during the maternity cycle motivates parents to seek the help of professional workers in the guidance of their children. When a family's needs have been met during the maternity cycle, they become aware of the values of health supervision. They continue to use the health supervision resources of their community not only for physical examinations but also to obtain guidance which increases their insight into the needs of their children.

DEVELOPMENT, CARE AND GUIDANCE DURING THE FIRST YEAR OF LIFE

A full-term, normal infant is born after 9 months of intra-uterine existence which ideally fulfilled his requirements and prepared him to adapt to extra-uterine life. In utero, the fetus experiences a parasitic existence. Essential nutrients for growth are supplied without any effort being required to obtain them. It experiences a close symbiotic relationship with its mother and presumably is free of frustration, pain and fear. It is secure because it is protected from exposure to cold, from inappropriate stimuli and from psychologically traumatic experiences which would come if it were born before term. By the end of 9 months of gestation, the fetus is ready to meet the frustrations which come with physical separation from his mother. He is also ready to adapt to life outside the uterus.

The Meaning of Birth to the Infant. Sometimes birth is called a traumatic experience because it abruptly separates the infant from his source of security (mother's body) and forces him to participate immediately in his own adaptation to extra-uterine existence. He is expelled from a warm, dark place where he has lived and grown completely surrounded by water. He comes into a world where air, not water, is the element which surrounds him; a world of light and darkness; a world full of other people upon whom he is completely dependent and in whom he needs to find trustworthiness and security.

The infant reacts to the birth experience as though it had affected him both emotionally and physically; his behavior expresses frustration and fear. His cry serves a physiologic function; it forces air into his lungs and initiates the breathing process. It manifests his feelings. It also communicates his need for supportive measures which help him to adapt with ease and a maximum amount of pleasure.

Equipment for Adaptation and Learning. Thrust into his new environment, the infant must begin to adapt himself to it immediately. He must oxygenate his own tissues, signal his need for food, suck, swallow, digest and excrete. He must also signal his distress which arises when needs other than hunger remain unmet. He must communicate his discomfort from inappropriate temperatures, painful internal or external stimuli, an uncomfortable position, physiologic insufficiency or from the loneliness which comes with separation from his mother.

Fortunately, the normal infant has been prepared adequately for this, as his brain at birth is one of the farthest advanced in size of any of the organs of his body. The body increases approximately 20 times in size from birth to maturity, the brain slightly less than 4 times. This growth of the brain occurs in the first 7 or 8 years of life. Even by the fifth month of fetal life the individual has the 12 million or more nerve cells with their nerve fibers which make up the vast nervous system which will control every function of his total complex physiologic

make-up. He is equipped with the network which controls every move which his body makes, be it under voluntary or involuntary control. He is equipped normally with the neurons which will make it possible for him to communicate with others by means of language, to remember, to think, to learn, to imagine, to reason —in fact to function as an intelligent human being. He is equipped to respond to the world about him, to people and things, to develop attitudes toward them; in other words, to develop a personality from the rudiments of personality with which he is born. Life in the extra-uterine world does not start at zero in personality as it does not start at the zero mark physically.

This intricate and vast nervous system upon which functioning and learning depend has begun to operate before birth. In the fifth month of fetal life, his mother will report that she "feels life" because the fetus has begun to move his arms and legs. Before birth he has acquired many motor abilities. The newborn baby is able to suck, swallow, cry, sneeze, yawn, hiccup, and respond to painful stimuli with motor activity.

Pleasure Is an Essential for Adaptation and Personality Growth. At birth the newborn infant's brain is not developed functionally, and his personality is unformed; he is a demanding, uncontrolled, dependent individual. He wants what he wants when he wants it. He seeks the pleasure which comes when his biologic and emotional needs are completely satisfied. He cannot wait for satisfaction because he has no power within himself to control his wants or to understand why their fulfillment and the resultant pleasure is not forthcoming. He has not developed the inner resources, or ego strength as it is often called, to get gratification through his own activity as a way of withstanding frustration. Ego strength comes from mutually enjoyed experiences with his mother and from the acquisition of new powers which come as a result of nervous system development and guided constructive experiences with others who are important to him personally.

The newborn infant is unorganized and unstable; his responses to environmental changes are immediate, automatic and intense; he *needs* what he wants when he wants it. *He requires consistently satisfying experiences with his mother to become organized and secure in his new world.* During the earliest months of his life he requires the pleasure which comes from fulfillment of his biologic and emotional needs. He needs pleasure not only to achieve optimal physical growth but also for sound personality development.

Growth in later stages of personality development is dependent upon the kind of foundation he acquires during the earliest months of his life. Acquiring feelings of trust in those who provide him with care and feelings of confidence in his power to summon someone to his aid in times of stress provides the security that he needs for personality growth. These emotional feelings provide the foundation upon which his personality must become structured or built.

The newborn infant is born with the power to signal his needs, and he feels and responds to the emo-

tional attitudes that are reflected in the care which is provided for him. His personality grows as life begins to speak to him through his sense organs and he comes to understand the meaning of these sensory experiences. When his signals of need are heeded and his physical requirements are provided for lovingly, he feels safe and cherished; his vital energy is available for growth and adaptation to his new world. When the infant's signals of need for food and closeness to his mother are interpreted erroneously as tempestuousness or a sign that he is "spoiled," he experiences frustration, anxiety (pain) and is without the security that he needs for biophysiologic and psychological growth.

Frustration traumatizes the young infant and threatens his potentialities for growth. Frustration in the earliest months of life is injurious because he cannot understand it and because it brings anger and anxiety when he has no inner resources to handle it constructively. It also utilizes the energy that he needs for adaptation and growth.

Individual Differences. No two babies are alike; their drives differ in intensity, rhythm, mode of expression and the way in which they can be satisfied. The first responses which the newborn infant makes to the countless impressions that immediately come rushing in upon him; his first ways of adapting to his first frustration and to the world about him show individual differences in relation to perceptivity. Each infant responds in his own way to internal and external stimuli —to hunger and pain and to his need for sleep, love and stimulation. He is not a personality if one thinks of the word as associated with an awareness of self. But he is an individual with his own characteristic ways of behaving.

The infant will grow and develop physically; he will also develop a personality which will be the outgrowth of his constitutional make-up (his inherited characteristics) and the environmental factors which impinge upon him in infancy, childhood and adolescence. His personality growth will depend upon his relationships with his parents, brothers and sisters, or siblings as they are often called, and with his playmates or peers, teachers and others who become important to him. If hospitalization becomes necessary during the formative periods of his life, his potentialities for personality growth will be influenced by the kind of experiences he encounters with nurses and doctors within the institution.

The child's personality growth will be a progression, following a general pattern of development but it will have its own individual characteristics. Both heredity and environment will have a share in making the infant what he is and what he is to be. His environment will be a complexity of the cultures into which he is born and will live, his family, the care and the guidance that he receives, people and the other phases of life that keep impinging on him from the moment of his birth.

Each child in a family has a different constitutional make-up; each one also has a different environment. Each individual's place in the family in itself influences his environmental milieu, and there are countless other factors which make each child's environment different from that which is experienced by his siblings.

Rest and Age-adequate Stimulation Are Essential for Growth. The infant's schedule of care needs to be planned in accordance with his individual needs. The newly born infant sleeps most of the time because he is fatigued from the process of birth. *He requires periods of undisturbed rest to gain the energy that he needs for adaptation and growth.* His behavior will provide the clues which are necessary to formulate his schedule of care. During the first month or two of life, his need for food and rest will be variable from day to day. Gradually, however, his patterns of need will become more regular. He will establish a schedule of his own— sleeping when he is tired, and eating and playing when he requires food and stimulation. With growth his needs will change. When his needs change, he will establish new patterns of behavior which require change in his schedule of care.

As the child grows and is carried away by his new-found powers and all the joys of activity and exploration, the mother needs to provide conditions that are aids to sleep and conditions that are favorable for activity. His need for age-adequate stimulation will be considered subsequently. In this section his need for protection from overfatigue which comes from inappropriate stimulation will be considered.

During the first 3 months of extra-uterine life, *stimulation should be given at the time his biologic needs require satisfaction.* He is ready to be held and loved during his feedings; he is ready to be fondled and caressed at bath time. Stimulation given at other times is fatiguing. If it is excessive, observation will show his feelings about it. He will either scream or respond by withdrawing, showing his rejection of the experience. He is saying "Leave me alone. I have had all I can take. I must rest now to become ready for the experiences that I really need."

There is little agreement as to how much a child should sleep at different ages. Gesell has recorded observations of a 2-month-old child's sleeping 14 hours and 14 minutes and being in a state of quiescence 2 hours and 5 minutes and of a 6-month-old child's sleeping 14 hours and 50 minutes but being quiescent 39 minutes. Statements are found in medical and nursing books which recommend a longer period of sleep than those recorded by Gesell at 2 and 6 months. They suggest from about 20 to 22 hours for the first 4 months, 18 to 16 hours at 6 months, and 15 hours at 1 year. Requirements for sleep are more variable than any of these figures suggest.

Until 5 years of age, most children cannot get enough sleep without the daily nap. Few children after infancy actually sleep from 7 P.M. to 7 A.M. To provide 12, 13 or 14 hours of sleep most infants need naps as well as a long night's sleep. A child gives up the nap gradually, sometimes by shortening the nap period, sometimes by skipping the nap more and more frequently.

There are individual differences in sleep needs, and for this reason it is essential to follow the child's cues in providing care. The child should have enough rest for health and happiness. He should show no signs of undue fatigue, he should be gaining, he should be refreshed after sleep, his color should be good, his eyes bright and he should be happy, composed and productive. If he has no undesirable symptoms like irritability, loss of appetite, hyperactivity or apathy he probably is getting sufficient sleep to meet his daily requirements.

As the child grows older, he becomes increasingly more needful of help in recognizing his need for rest. With the development of sensory perception and motor skill, the child becomes increasingly more stimulated by the things within his environment. He has difficulty in relaxing because his mind is stimulated with all the new discoveries that he is making.

Guarding against overfatigue is an important responsibility of the adult. When beginning signs of fatigue are noted, the adult must kindly but firmly help the child to accept his need for rest. This is done by preparing him for rest with quiet activities and with behavior that helps the child to know that the time for rest has come and that nothing will distract his mother or nurse from providing what she knows he needs at the moment. Many times little children become overpowered with their drive for exploration. They do not recognize their need for rest. In such instances it is the adult's responsibility to help them learn through experience that rest periods bring more enjoyment than frustration. When a child discovers through experience that playtime is more fun when he is rested, he will accept resting time amicably.

Fresh Air and Sunshine. TEMPER-ATURE, VENTILATION AND HUMIDITY. The need for fresh air and warmth is accepted so universally that it is hardly necessary to discuss it as something which the adult must provide for the child. However, the temperature and the ventilation of the infant's room is often the subject of parents' questions. Only one factor is important. The child should not become chilled or overheated. Either extreme has its bad effect, since the infant's heat-regulating mechanism is not perfectly developed, and he cannot adjust to sudden changes in temperature as can an adult. In the daytime the infant's environment should be warm enough (about 70° F. to 75° F.) and he should have on enough clothing so that he does not need to be wrapped in a blanket when he is awake. His arms and legs should be free to move about so that he may have the pleasure of using them.

At night or during the nap the temperature may be from 10° to 15° lower for the little baby and from 15° to 20° lower for the older child. The child should be in a well-ventilated room and should be warm enough for relaxed sleep. It is important to remember that one is ventilating a room that is inhabited by a little person who cannot get up and close the window when he feels cold. One needs to ventilate the room without allowing the baby to get chilled by having a direct draft blowing on him. Screens and window boards which can be bought or home-devised are helpful in protecting a baby from drafts.

The amount of covering needed over a baby or a child at night is difficult to gauge. A baby's extremi-ties should be warm, but he should not have so much covering that he perspires or is restless. A child who is too hot tends to be restless in his sleep, although that is not the only cause of restlessness. Sometimes it is difficult to keep the active baby covered at night, and there may be devised sleeping bags of flannel which give the child freedom of movement yet protect him from becoming chilled. The sleeping bags which permit him to use his hands are better than blankets which are wrapped tightly around him.

Adequate humidity is as important as fresh air. The tendency in the heating of many homes has been to provide an atmosphere with too little moisture. In such an atmosphere the child's body must give up moisture which he should be retaining. The mucous membranes lining the nose and the throat suffer, as do other skin surfaces. Many nose-and-throat specialists are especially insistent on the importance of a sufficient amount of humidity in the room. Various devices for supplying moisture are on the market. The principle of most of them is to supply a fairly wide surface of water which will evaporate rapidly. Humidity is tested by a hygrometer, and the amount present should be about 55 per cent of saturation.

FRESH AIR AND SUNSHINE. A baby is almost always provided with a baby carriage as a means of being taken out of doors. The baby born in the winter cannot get out of doors at as early an age as the baby born in summer. He must get all his fresh air within the shelter of the home for his first few months of life. Weather below freezing is not suitable for taking a baby under 3 months outdoors for any length of time. In warm weather, a baby a few weeks old can spend much time out of doors. Two things must be provided—steady warmth and fresh air. If weather permits and the baby is put out in the carriage for his nap, the hood of the carriage should not be pulled down in such a way that he is almost hermetically sealed in space made hot by the sun which is pouring down on the leather hood.

A baby should be comfortable in the carriage. After he has learned to sit in a chair, he is uncomfortable sitting with feet outstretched in a carriage. At that time a go-cart is more suitable. Children find pleasure in riding, and new scenes are opened up to them by their ride in a buggy or go-cart.

Sunshine, the greatest source of vitamin D, was recognized as important to the health of human beings long before science taught us just what it gave individuals besides heat and light. Vitamin D is important for the utilization of calcium and phosphorus, two minerals essential to bone development. It is needed especially throughout the growth period. Appropriate exposure of the body to the sun will supply ample vitamin D. However, adequate exposure can be made only in the summertime. At other times, and when outdoor exposure is not feasible, vitamin D must be obtained from some other source.

The ultraviolet rays which produce vitamin D do not penetrate ordinary window glass or several layers of clothing. Smoke and dust also filter out the ultraviolet rays. Several varieties of glass and transparent materials which allow passage of ultraviolet rays are on the market. None is completely efficient, and all deteriorate with age. For most of them replacement each year is desirable. They have their greatest usefulness in the winter. In many parts of the country, the amount of winter sunshine available is relatively meager, and consequently an insufficient amount probably is given even with a glass which transmits ultraviolet. It is not practical to rely on winter sunshine in the house as a source of vitamin D.

Protective measures need to be carried out when the infant is exposed to the direct rays of the sun. The child's eyes need protection from strong light. Every precaution needs to be taken to protect him from becoming sunburned. The skin of infants is tender and burns easily. Only a small area of skin should be exposed initially. Exposure can begin at the feet and be increased gradually. At first the time of exposure must be short—only 5 minutes. Gradually, the time of exposure can be lengthened until the infant's skin is pigmented or tanned.

Children as well as infants can become overheated and badly burned by undue exposure to the sun in the summer months. Hats which shade the eyes should be worn. Children should drink freely of cool water and be protected from long periods of play in intense heat. Sunstroke and heat prostration can occur, although the incidence is lower in children than in adults. Gradual exposure to the intense heat of summer is equally important for children. Sunsuits should be used for only short periods of time during the first hot days of summer, as shoulders, arms and backs can be burned so badly as to make the child ill and miserably uncomfortable.

Sensory Equipment. The special organs of sense through which the outer world is to reach the child are present at birth but as yet are not completed functionally. As his sense organs present him with impressions of the world around him, the infant gradually learns to associate certain emotional feelings with some of these experiences. Thus he begins to react very early to his mother's touch. If this touch usually brings comfort to him, his response is eventually one of pleasure just to the touch itself. At a later age he will react with similar pleasure even to the sight of his mother who is about to touch him. By such a process the infant gradually accumulates a group of emotional reactions toward many of the sensory experiences of his everyday life.

SENSE OF TOUCH. Although the extent to which there is sensory perception before birth is not known, the sense of touch seems to be the most highly developed at birth. It is certainly the most extensive of all senses, for the total body is the organ of the sense of touch. The child sees with his eyes, hears with his ears, smells and tastes through his nose and mouth, but his sense of touch, to which pain and the feeling of temperature are related, comes to him from every part of his body. Some areas of his body are more sensitive than others, and at birth he is less sensitive to some stimuli than he will be later. A touch on the lips causes the reflex of sucking in the newborn, and a light touch on the nose will cause the eyes to close.

Sensitivity to pain and temperature is present in early infancy. Sensitivity to physical pain is existent at birth but it is less acute than it is in the older child. The newly born infant tolerates physical pain fairly well if he can suck on a nipple or a sugar tip and be fondled during the procedure. The temperature sense is developed early. An unfavorable reaction to bath water which is too hot or too cold is often observed. If the temperature of the bath water brings discomfort, a fear of the bath may arise which will be difficult to overcome. Bath water of 95° to 100° F. usually brings comfort to the baby. If he is put into the water gradually, he will adapt much more readily to the experience of being bathed.

The child's first impressions of life in this world will come to him through the sense of touch. He feels the touch of hands at the moment of his birth. He feels the crib in which he lies and the touch of his mother's hands and body before he is aware of anything of the world beyond his touch. Later, sight and sound will bring to him those experiences of the world beyond.

After 3 months the sense of touch is well developed over the body, and for many years the child will seek to understand the world close at hand through this sense. The mouth and the lips are sensitive tactile areas. The infant will do much investigating by putting things in his mouth. From these experiences he will get pleasure and learn the properties of the objects in his environment. He will discover which things are edible and which are not; he will learn the difference between softness and hardness, warmth and cold, sharpness and smoothness.

Mouthing is the natural avenue of investigation. Through the use of his mouth he takes in food and love from the person who feeds him. He also makes discoveries concerning the physical properties of objects.

The sense of touch, as is true of all the senses, comes to have meaning to the child through the variety of experiences that he will have. He will learn about the people in his world through his sense of touch long before he is aware of them as persons. The infant who is lifted and held lovingly and gently develops warm feelings toward people. His mother's hands will come to mean comfort to him. In fact, his mother's touch will contribute much to his eventual concept of his mother as a person who gives him care and loves him, one whom he will love in return.

The infant who does not receive understanding care cannot develop warm feelings toward those whom he needs to trust and love. The infant who is left to cry it out and is deprived of comforting and gentle handling develops feelings of hostility and insecurity instead of trust and confidence in himself and others. Long before he recognizes his mother as a person, he may develop hostile feelings toward the person whom he needs most to trust.

Warm feelings toward his mother are essential for both physical and personality growth. The child learns to master his infantile impulses in the process of becoming a socialized individual through his relationship with his mother and eventually through interpersonal experiences with his father. If he has warm feelings toward those who are guiding him and if he feels that they are

expecting only that which he can accomplish, he will want to please them. He will also be willing to forfeit infantile pleasures like sucking, biting, hitting and indiscriminate soiling. He will try to win his parents' approval, remain secure in their affections and develop the ability to imitate the things that they do.

The child identifies with or imitates the behavior of those he admires and trusts. He wants to be more grown-up, to acquire self-mastery and to gain gratification through his own accomplishments. The impulse toward growth is within each child at birth. *Trust in his parents and understanding from those who guide him support the growth impulse and give it the opportunities that it needs to guide the child toward its goal—maturity.*

SENSE OF SIGHT. The extremely delicate organs of sight, the eyes, equipped with their 12 delicate muscles, seem from a functional point of view to be the slowest in development. A fine muscle control must be learned after birth before the baby is said to "see." The eyes must learn to move together. For some months, and occasionally for much longer, sometimes the eyes may move independently, especially when trying to focus on a near object. This natural characteristic often makes mothers fearful. They think that their babies are cross-eyed because they do not know that it takes time for fine muscle co-ordination to develop.

Development of the organs of sight shows patterned progression. At birth, the baby's eyes move about without fixing themselves on a given object. There is a vague reaction to a moving light, and by the time the baby is about a month old he will fix his eyes on a bright object dangled above him and will follow it for a brief moment. As he grows and has the practice and the stimulation that he needs, he increases the arc of following. His horizons widen, and when he masters the ability to sit up, they will broaden further, thereby increasing his opportunity to see more of the things within his environment. By 3 to 4 months of age he is able to fix and follow well. At this time he enjoys and profits from new sight experiences.

Between 4 and 6 months of age the baby begins to recognize the person who constantly cares for him and objects such as his bottle which have become important to him. He has learned through many experiences with persons and objects to fix and follow with his eyes. His mother begins to emerge from the as-yet-unknown world about him into something seen and recognized. If she has come to mean comfort and pleasure, he focuses on her, follows and responds to her smiles, words and gestures. He knows her only in part, but he is building those associations which eventually will mean a person called Mother. As his vision improves and he recognizes that she is the giver of comfort, he becomes more discriminating and prefers her to others who are less important to him personally.

Because the eye does not reach its full development until the child is 7 or 8 years of age, protection from eye strain is essential. The preschool child's play equipment should be large because his visual powers are incomplete and also because he

has not developed the fine muscle co-ordination essential for delicate manipulation. For example, beads that the small child will enjoy stringing should be large and have large holes. Pictures should be large and simple in design to prevent strain and discomfort.

SENSE OF HEARING. Soon after birth, babies respond to sharp, loud noises. At birth, babies apparently are deaf to ordinary sounds. The deafness is caused in part by absence of air in the eustachian tubes but perhaps in a larger measure by the persistence of embryonic epithelial tissue within the middle ear. Fairly soon, however, responses to sound can be observed. A pleasurable response is often elicited with kindly spoken words or song; a fear response is elicited from sharp, harsh or sudden sounds. Association between some sound and its meaning may come as early as the second or the third month if it is a sound which has occurred frequently and been associated repeatedly with the same experience which has come to have meaning for the infant.

The recognized sound of his mother's voice will come to be associated with the meaning that she has come to have for him. If she has provided attention and comfort, the sound of her voice will bring a pleasurable response; he will smile and respond with his entire body. But if she has punished natural behavior (crying when he has urgent needs which are clamoring for satisfaction), the infant's response will be totally different. He may scream or withdraw because he has associated pain with what he hears. Thus sounds do their share in building up the concept of Mother.

SENSE OF SMELL. The sense of smell seems to be present in young babies and grows more acute during preschool years. Young babies show some reaction to extremely strong odors. By 3 years of age, the preschool child shows definite preferences and dislikes for odors. If one listens to preschool children's comments and observes their behavior, one will discover that there are marked variations in sensitivity to different odors.

SENSE OF TASTE. Taste and smell are closely associated in infancy. The year-old baby, for example, who has learned to sniff in response to the stimulus of something fragrant held before him will open his mouth sometimes even later than that, as if he expected to taste the fragrant flower. He does this because he has not yet learned complete discrimination between smell and taste. Doubtless, too, his interest in investigating by mouth plays a part in this reaction.

The sense of both taste and smell develop somewhat slowly in the first months of life. Although rejection of bitter and acceptance of sweet have been noted in very small infants, on the whole there seems to be an attitude of indifference toward taste in infancy. This fact has a bearing on the development of positive attitudes toward different kinds of food.

First rejections of solids, such as cereals and vegetables, in the diet seem to be more closely related to their consistency—a function of touch rather than of taste. Other factors, too, may impede his acceptance of solid food. The muscle activity which is required to get solid food from a spoon is more laborious

for him than the sucking movements which are instinctively present at birth. In addition, the solid food is obtained more slowly than milk from the breast or the nipple, a fact which doubtlessly tends to frustrate him in his early attempts to eat this new variety of food. He spits because he has not yet learned to accept slowly coming food and to manipulate his tongue muscles to get it into the back of his throat from whence it can be swallowed. It is not the taste to which he is reacting; it is the new experience with which he has had insufficient time to become familiar.

Toward the end of the first year of life, the infant becomes increasingly more discriminating in his taste. He also becomes more positive in his likes and dislikes and expresses his feelings more vehemently. In addition, he is beginning to respond to and imitate his parents' reactions toward specific foods. The combination of these factors often leads to a decline in apparent appetite during the last quarter of the first year. It also tends to increase the amount of contention which accompanies his meal periods.

Because of the above characteristics, it is wise to accustom children to a variety of foods and consistencies before the eighth or ninth month of life. Adult reactions to different foods probably are a more important influence on the child's reactions than taste, as children in a nursery school unexposed to the adult reaction of dislike will take cod-liver oil as if they like it!

Throughout the first year of life the infant's feeding experiences are of prime importance in personality development. Earlier the importance of prompt satisfaction of hunger and a need for closeness to the mother during the earliest months of life was cited. At the time the introduction of solid food is indicated, understanding of the infant's need for time in becoming accustomed to new foods and new methods of feeding is essential to sustain the mother-child relationship. An understanding mother accepts her infant's reactions to new foods, consistencies and methods of feeding and finds ways to help him gain pleasure in the experience; she remains poised throughout the learning period. She neither forces food nor gives up her responsibility in teaching. She also rewards her infant's efforts to withstand frustration with expressions of pride in his accomplishments. When feeding time continues to be a mutually enjoyed experience the relationship between mother and child becomes strengthened. In the feeding experience all his senses are utilized. He feels, hears his mother's voice, sees her facial expression and gestures and gets a taste of the outer world in the form of food. As was discussed above, the quality of these sensory experiences may condition his attitudes toward the food which is being presented to him.

Motor Development in the First Year of Life. MOTOR RESPONSES OF THE NEWBORN. The earliest responses which the infant makes to the sensory stimuli that impinge upon him in such countless numbers after birth are motor responses. The seemingly helpless infant can do a number of things. Many of his actions, such as sucking, winking, knee jerk and corneal and pupillary movements, are reflex. All of these reflexes continue throughout life.

Other reflexes appear after birth and some of them disappear.

The newborn infant's movements are random and un-co-ordinated. He wriggles, stretches, spreads his fingers and brings them together. His arms and legs move together, for he does not have the control necessary to inhibit the action of any extremity. When lying on his stomach, he can hold his head up for a brief moment, but for 3 or 4 months he must be held in such a way that support is given to his head and back. He has neither the skill nor the strength to hold his head or spine erect.

Development of muscle control comes rapidly during the first month of life if he is healthy and is permitted to exercise his developing powers. Much of the learning during the first year of life is in the field of motor control, i.e., acquiring the ability to make the body respond to the individual's will. This implies motivation, which is the impulse or the desire to do something.

MOTOR DEVELOPMENT AN INTERRELATED PHENOMENON. Motor development does not progress independently of development in other areas; it is an interrelated process. The child is growing physically, mentally, socially and emotionally; maturation is taking place; he is getting ready in various ways to sit, crawl, walk, climb, run and master objects in his environment. The infant must grow bigger and stronger before he is ready to learn to control his body. His mind must learn to co-ordinate his movements into the complicated pattern of sitting, crawling, walking and using his body. He must also have an eagerness and a desire to learn to use his body functionally.

People and his relationship to them are important factors in learning to master his body and environment. They must keep him physically fit and provide the encouragement and the support that he needs to learn to use his body. *The infant needs permission to grow more capable of independent activity; he needs play equipment and protection while he is discovering the use of his body and the properties of the things within his environment.* Unless his need for new experiences is understood and encouraged, he will not only have insufficient exercise but he will feel thwarted and resentful toward those who inhibit his drive for self-mastery.

To appraise a child's progress in motor development, the interrelatedness of growth and the differences between individuals need to be considered. Standards of development must be flexible and must be used cautiously because there are wide variations in rate of growth and in the ages when children develop given skills. The sequence in which developmental milestones are reached is more definitely fixed than are the chronologic ages at which they are reached. Individual differences exist; heredity and environment are both influencing factors.

Aldrich and Norval[1] studied the neuromuscular development of 215 normal infants from birth to the early part of the second year and recorded the time of onset of various accomplishments. The infants were

from all strata of society in Rochester, Minn. However, it is recognized that the population of Rochester is made up of more professional people than is usual in many other cities of its size. Each mother was informed about the usual sequence of neuromuscular development. Each was also advised to encourage her baby to use each new skill as it appeared. The investigators tested the infants at monthly intervals and instructed the mothers to observe the onset of achievements which would be elicited less easily in the clinic. The following steps in neuromuscular growth were chosen for study:

1. Smile—the baby begins to smile in response to an adult or to his voice.

2. Vocal—the infant utters such sounds as "ah," "eh," and "uh" spontaneously or on stimulation.

3. Head control—when the infant is lifted by his hands from the supine to the sitting position, the head does not lag but is supported by the anterior muscles of the neck.

4. Hand control—when a toy is dangled in the midline above his chest, the infant is able to close in on the toy with one or both hands and to grasp it.

5. Roll—the baby makes a complete roll from back to abdomen.

6. Sit—the baby sits alone for several moments.

7. Crawl—the baby is able to move across the room or pen toward some distant object; this may be accomplished by rolling over and over, pushing himself along on his stomach or back, or by any individual modification of progression.

8. Prehension—this is the bringing together of the thumb and index finger to pick up a small object. This can be tested with a bright-colored button.

9. Pull up—the infant pulls himself to a sitting position.

---

[1] Aldrich, C. Anderson and Norval, Mildred A.; A developmental graph for the first year of life, J. Pediat. 29:304-308, 1946.

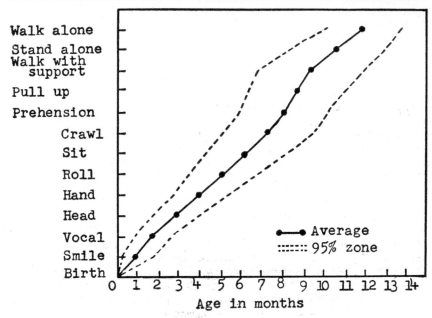

CHART 14. A developmental graph for the first year, showing the average age for the beginning of the achievements selected and the zone in which 95 per cent of the infants' developmental graphs fell. (Aldrich and Norval: J. Pediat. 29:304)

10. Walk with support—the infant walks by holding to his playpen, a piece of furniture, or an adult.

11. Stand alone—without any support, the infant stands for several moments.

12. Walk alone—the infant takes several steps alone.[2]

Chart 14 is the developmental graph that Aldrich and Norval prepared. It is useful in following the neuromuscular growth of infants and in appraising their maturity.

THE EXPECTED SEQUENCE IN MOTOR DEVELOPMENT. The ran-

[2]Aldrich, C. Anderson and Norval, Mildred A.; A developmental graph for the first year of life, J. Pediat. 29: p. 304, 1946.

dom, un-co-ordinated movements of the newborn gradually organize themselves and form patterns which result in the motor skills essential in our daily living. The newborn's movements *seem* to be without purpose, although within the first month one sees his hand make contact with his mouth, especially when he is hungry. It seems as if he had some dim perception of the fact that hunger is assuaged by the putting of something into his mouth. His first random movements are probably in response to internal tensions. Through the activity he obtains relief from tension (comfort) and a pattern of behavior which serves his need.

Finger sucking has purpose; it is a natural way for a baby to obtain pleasure. Sufficient sucking at the breast or on the bottle combined with closeness to the mother helps to prevent prolonged thumb-sucking. However, some babies seem to have an intense need for sucking which cannot be satisfied during the feeding experience. They use their fingers or objects to obtain the satisfaction that they require. Curtailing this natural activity with restraint, nagging or punishment does not eliminate the need for this kind of pleasure; it merely serves to intensify the drive and thwart the sucking activity which he needs during early infancy.

The infant needs freedom to satisfy his sucking needs; it exercises the muscles of his jaw and gives him the oral satisfaction that he needs for personality growth. It also prepares him to relinquish this pleasure for more grown-up modes of behavior. Finger sucking continues until the infant discovers new ways of obtaining pleasure and relief from tension. When his sucking and other emotional needs are satisfied and he is given opportunities to use his hands in play and in learning new skills, he discovers substitute activities which are more satisfying. Under these conditions, relinquishing finger sucking comes about through a natural sequence of events. Permissiveness in the early months of his life gratifies his urgent need. It also prepares him for enjoyment of more grown-up modes of behavior when growth brings new powers which make it possible.

Many people become concerned about thumb-sucking because they fear permanent deformity of the child's jaw. Studies have shown that thumb-sucking may be a cause of malocclusion in the deciduous teeth, but that this malformation tends to correct itself if the habit is broken before 5 years of age. However, persistence in the habit beyond that age tends to make the malformation permanent.

Prolonged thumb-sucking is a symptom of insecurity; it is a symptom which says that the child's life and living is not as emotionally satisfying as he needs it to be. Finding the cause of his discomfort and eliminating it is the only effective method of cure. This is true in all realms of therapy—psychological as well as physical.

By 3 to 6 months of age nervous system development increases the infant's powers of control. During the first months of extra-uterine life the infant learns to hold his head up for a longer time, and by 3 months of age usually he can hold it fairly steadily, although he still needs support for it. When lying on his stomach, he begins to lift his chest as well as his head. During this same time, he has been learning to control the tiny eye muscles and look at things. When lying on his stomach, his hands are brought into view without active volition, and he plays with them. As yet he does not know that they are his, but he is beginning to exercise some control of them. He also finds them interesting playthings. In this period he attempts more control of his body, usually achieving first the ability to roll from back to side or side to back. Then will come the ability, at approximately 6 months, to roll completely over, a fact of significance to those caring for babies.

When a baby is approaching the stage when he will be able to roll over it is no longer safe to leave him lying on a bed, a bathinette, or a davenport. In fact, a baby never should be left without the protection of crib sides or a railing because new skills are developed rapidly when physical readiness is attained.

Nervous system development and exercise prepares the infant for more complex achievements. The infant is in a constant state of experimentation, waving arms and legs and moving his body during his waking hours if freed to do so. Little by little the motor skills which will be necessary for the complex skill of walking become developed. The 4-month-old baby cannot sit up but he is getting ready for that accomplishment. He is being held in the sitting position and moving his legs and arms with good co-ordination and strength. By 5 or 6 months of age he is pushing vigorously and springing up and down when held in his mother's arms. Within the next month or two he will develop the power to sit alone. At first he will lean forward to hold himself up, and even then it will be evident that his sitting position is not a very steady one. In approximately another 4 weeks, he will have mastered thoroughly the ability to sit up straight.

During the early months of growing, the infant makes those movements which predict the power of locomotion when lying down. In other words, he has been getting ready for the creeping, crawling or hitching stage of locomotion. Most children creep, crawl or hitch before they walk, but occasionally one observes a child who walks at a very early age and does not creep or crawl at all. During the first 6 or 8 months of life, he stretches his legs with increasing vigor and pushes himself up toward the head of the bed when lying on his back. When he is in his bathtub, he makes swimming motions with arms and legs and finds the greatest pleasure in the experience. Through these experiences he acquires the motor skills which make it possible for him to move about, although still in the prone or half-sitting position, if he is going to be a "hitcher" instead of creeping or crawling.

In the last quarter of the first year the infant will pull himself up on his feet. He has enjoyed stretching his legs out straight; he has felt their increased power. He has been held upright and has been allowed to press his feet against the bed, the table, or someone's lap. He has begun to make stepping motions when doing so. The inevitable next step in the orderly progression is that some day he will pull himself to his feet by taking hold of the side of his play-pen, crib or something which gives him an anchor toward which to pull.

Learning to stand upright and walk is a triumphant feat of accomplishment. At this moment the child begins a new way of life; he is a different person with increased feelings of confidence and self-respect. He can stand upright; he has mastered a feat in bodily control. He feels accomplished! One can detect his new feelings about himself in his behavior. He beams, chuckles and looks self-satisfied. From now on he will look at the world from a new angle.

Experimentation soon brings into his category of motor skills the ability to sit down from a standing position and to walk. When a baby first gets onto his feet, he often does not know how to sit down and may stand until he tumbles in a heap. However, with experimentation and his mother's help he will become agile and self-sufficient. Soon he begins to take a few steps when holding someone's hand. Then comes the day when he takes a few steps alone, and then more and more until he is off on his own adventuring about his home and yard. In learning to walk he has acquired the skill which will take him out into the world. At first he is awkward. He stands with a wide stance and wobbles as he walks, but with experience he gains the skill to walk smoothly and the assurance that comes with practice.

No definite date can be set for walking, for there may be a variation of months between the walking time for normal babies. Some babies walk before they are a year old; some cannot accomplish the feat until they are 18 months of age. But the months 12, 13, 14 or 15 probably will find most babies walking, and by the time a baby is 2 years old he will have mastered the skill to the point where he can run, and even run away!

When the infant begins to walk he will need shoes that have a flexible sole and give support to an undeveloped foot. At birth, the bones of a baby's feet are cartilaginous and incompletely formed. Because the child's foot is in the process of development, it is important that only well-fitting stockings and shoes be put onto his feet.

After the toddler learns to walk and run, he begins to experiment with climbing. In a short time he learns to climb up and go down stairs. If he is allowed to practice, he will also climb up onto almost anything that will offer some chance of success. He needs supervised opportunities to experiment to discover his capacities. Overprotection by anxious adults brings fears and inhibitions which slow the learning process.

Supervision should protect the child from trying feats that he is not ready for and provide the encouragement he needs to overcome difficult obstacles. Bumps and tumbles are inevitable during the experimentation period. They are a part of growth. The child takes them in his stride and learns to tolerate them if the adult refrains from offering sympathy and coddling except when he is hurt.

Learning to walk and climb is a complicated process. First the child develops gross motor power. Then nervous system growth and exercise bring the control which makes it possible for him to use his legs for walking.

Development of the muscles of the arms shows similar progression. At birth the infant has no control over the smaller, more delicate muscles of his hands. The newborn infant cannot reach out to grasp and draw things toward him. Only random movements give him the experience of making contacts.

After the fourth month of life progress in the use of his hands is rapid. At about 4 months of age, the infant holds a rattle and enjoys waving it about, but he cannot get it unless it is placed within his hands. With growth and experience he learns which movements bring him in contact with objects and give him pleasure. He repeats these pleasurable activities over and over again. Exercise increases the size and the strength of his muscles. Soon he is able to reach out and get the thing that he wants if it is within his reach. But when he gets the object he lets it drop from his hand with no realization of his part in the release process. The automatic grasp reflex present at birth has disappeared, but now he can grasp and reach more or less voluntarily.

Between the fourth and the eighth months of life the infant develops many new powers in the use of his hands. By 7 or 8 months of age, or possibly earlier, the baby can reach for his bottle and hold it. He can also take it out of his mouth and put it in again, showing how skillful he is in hand-mouth co-ordination. He can bang noise-producing toys, and he revels in the sounds that he creates. He learns to bring thumb in opposition to finger—the "pincer technic" Gesell calls it—a definite advance over grasping with the whole hand. Seeing, desiring, and with the ability to pick things up with thumb and forefinger, he can pick up tiny objects undesirable as well as desirable, and these, too, will go into his mouth for investigation.

The infant needs a mother or a nurse to be on hand to provide security and protection. She must keep undesirable objects out of reach. She also needs to encourage his accomplishments with her interest in his absorbing, important activities.

In the last quarter of the first year, the baby uses his hands constantly during his waking hours. He picks things up and puts things down, pushing them away from him, drawing them toward him, putting one thing on top of another or putting one thing into another. Over and over again he does these things, and day by day his skills increase. He practices until he masters the skills of manipulation which are so important to work and play.

Play has purpose; it is the child's business. Through the use of toys and social play with his parents and siblings, he learns many skills and valuable lessons in living. He gains motor skills and develops sensory perception and experiences the joy of having others interested in his activities. With his siblings he probably will experience some measure of frustration as well. He will discover that they are fun to have around and contribute to his happiness. He will also discover that they are an annoyance because they thwart many of his desires.

The adult who understands the purposes of play selects the play equipment that furthers learning and provides opportunities for self-expression. Low shelves or cupboard space in which the child's toys and books are within his reach facilitate self-directed activity. The child is free to get his things when he wants them, and very soon he will also enjoy helping in the process of putting them away. Respect for this space for his things helps the child to learn property rights. To learn property rights, the child needs the experience of having his own things and having his rights to ownership respected. Infants are not discriminating; their only requirements are equipment and freedom to experiment. Experimentation helps the infant to master himself and the things within his environment. If he is provided with sufficient play materials and is encouraged to use them he will discover the ways which are best for his personal learning. Not all children learn in the same way. Self-directed activity serves his purposes most effectively.

Suggested play materials for the young child are as follows: tin pan, a small saucepan, a set of measuring spoons, small wooden bowls, a string of spools and napkin rings, clothspins, boxes—these will give the baby as much delight as the expensive silver rattle, or one of the commercially made educational toys. Bathtub toys are also a delight to the baby and incite him to reach out and splash when in the tub. As the baby learns to walk, things he can push or pull about will interest him. Large blocks, a small wagon or a doll carriage, animals on wheels or other pull toys will stimulate pushing and pulling activity. Nests of blocks, or cans which have been made safe with can-openers designed to remove cutting edges, sand toys which can fill and empty over and over again, are other toys that the child will enjoy and profit from before he is 2 and for many months afterward as well.

MAKING USE OF THE SKILLS ACQUIRED. There are many ways that adults can help children to utilize their new skills to advance their powers of independence. If an infant's mother follows a general pattern of giving care, he soon begins to co-operate, expecting to have his hands washed at a certain time, to be turned over at another time or to put his arms up, when his mother is about to get his arms through his shirt sleeves. Between the eighth and the eleventh months of life the infant uses his hands to get food to his mouth and reaches for the spoon in an attempt to feed himself. The 11- to 12-month-old infant pulls at the toe of his sock and attempts to get his clothing off. Simultaneously, he enjoys using the washcloth and the soap and tries to imitate his mother's technic of bathing him. In the second year he enjoys putting away his toys, getting into his clothes, doing simple errands and hanging up his clothing.

Self-help clothing and well-placed equipment facilitate the child's learning. Clothing of a simple design, simple to put on and take off, should be used to encourage his interest in learning to dress and undress himself and to acquire independence in waiting upon himself. Elastic bands, which are not too tight, zippers, large buttons and buttonholes make garments easier for the child to manipulate himself. Low hooks encourage the child's learning to hang up his tooth brush, towels and clothing. Steps that can be used at the wash bowl and the toilet and to get into the tub are enjoyed by the young child.

The child's attempts at self-help should be utilized to prevent him from clinging or regressing to babyish modes of behavior. Often his interest in learning to do things for himself goes unnoticed. His readiness to learn is not recognized because his mother or nurse enjoys doing for him or because it is easier to carry out the procedure than to teach him to do the things that he is capable of doing. Self-feeding does bring messiness, and self-undressing and dressing does take time, but practice is necessary to perfect skills. Teaching a child to do for himself is a rewarding experience for both the child and his teacher! The child demonstrates his interest in learning. If his teacher is interested in promoting growth in independence, she will observe his cues and utilize his interest in learning in each experience with him. The adult needs wisdom in teaching a child to do things for himself. Failure which incites the child to further effort is a wholesome experience; constant failure which discourages is not.

When a child's interest in learning to do for himself is not utilized, he is thwarted and reacts in a way which is characteristic for him. He may fight to use his powers, or he may acquiesce to his mother's desires to do for him and regress to the stage of dependence. Later when his mother or nurse wants him to take over the responsibility of self-care, he resists. He does so because he has lost interest and become overly dependent upon his mother's solicitation.

With each new accomplishment the infant's inner resources (ego) are strengthened; his personality grows. Acquiring increased mastery of self and environment brings pleasure, and increased awareness of himself as a person. He also acquires resources which prepare him to withstand small doses of frustration. During the earliest months of his life he was an independent being yet totally dependent upon others for gratification of all his needs. In the last half of the first year he acquires motor skills, has sensory experiences which teach him the property of things and grows increasingly more able to obtain pleasure through his own activity and play. His pleasure in self-directed play makes it possible for him to wait a little while for gratification. If his mother is within sight and he is pleasantly occupied, he can wait while she prepares his food; he does not have to have it the minute stomach contractions signal his need

for food. Learning to get pleasure through self-directed activity prepares him for the first crucial step in adaptation to the socialization process.

Weaning as the First Crucial Step in the Socialization Process. BOTH PLEASURE AND FRUSTRATION ARE NECESSARY FOR PERSONALITY GROWTH. *The child needs age-adequate frustration to help him become increasingly more independent and self-directing.* Each new experience in socialization will bring some measure of frustration; also, it will bring pleasure and inner strength— the satisfaction and the power that come when one surmounts a difficult task in growing-up. Continuation of unconditional acceptance beyond the stage when the child is ready to adapt himself to a step in the socialization process is as depriving as withholding pleasure when he has no resources to cope with the frustration that it brings.

The timing of socialization experiences and the methods that are utilized in helping the child surmount the tasks are important factors in personality development. *The child needs readiness to master the experience and guidance which provides understanding and support in surmounting his problem.* The methods that the adult uses to guide the child will depend upon his knowledge of the developmental process, his understanding of the complexity of each problem from the child's point of view and his attitudes toward the child and the learning process. An ability to appraise an individual child's readiness to cope with a new learning experience is an essential quality of guidance. If he is coerced into meeting demands before he has had optimal gratification and has developed interest in learning, he will become filled with rage. He will also resent those who deprive him of that which he continues to need urgently. Well-timed and thoughtfully guided socializing experiences promote personality growth; ill-timed frustrations, introduced without heed to the child's ability to meet them, stunt growth. They either bring regression or fixation at the stage in which deprivation was experienced.

GROWTH AND SATISFYING EXPERIENCES WITH HIS MOTHER PREPARE THE INFANT FOR THE WEANING PROCESS. A period of fulfillment and rapid physical growth prepares the infant to adapt himself to the weaning process. Satisfying experience gives the infant feelings of trust in his mother and a desire to emulate her way of drinking. If he has been held for feedings, has been given ample opportunity to meet his need for sucking and has been talked to while eating, he will have acquired pleasant associations with words, smiles and gestures. Because words, smiles and gestures have come to mean love, interest and expression of his mother's pride in him, the infant will need less physical demonstrations of affection. He will be ready to utilize substitute satisfactions in mastering a new experience. If he has had opportunities to use his developing skills, he will have acquired increased ability to obtain gratification from his own accomplishments. He will seek self-directed activity and prefer it to the confinement which bottle or breast feeding necessitates.

After the sixth month of life, the infant begins to show interest in learning to drink from a glass. Accustoming the infant to drinking water and sips of milk from a small glass from the fifth month onward teaches him the use of eating utensils. It also stimulates his interest in accomplishing a new feat. Soon after he learns to sit independently, he begins to reach for eating utensils. He picks up a cup, brings it to his mouth and looks to the adult for help in learning. It is his cue of readiness to learn. His mother's delight in his developing ability and his own thrill of accomplishment heighten his interest in perfecting the skill. When he takes a goodly quantity from the cup, the bottle or the breast can be eliminated at that feeding. When he shows less ability to accept the cup, the breast or bottle feeding can be resumed. With this method, weaning is a gradual process which is adapted to his individual requirements. He regulates the amount of frustration that he can tolerate; he is not abruptly or heartlessly deprived of something which has been one of his greatest sources of pleasure.

Readiness for weaning coincides with a period of seeking new play and social experiences. The infant is awake for longer periods of time and delights in social experiences with his mother. If this need is met, he will not feel deprived, even though he has his beloved bottle less frequently than he did before. He will have obtained substitutes which are more valued than the bottle or the breast—a feeling of being more grown-up and a new kind of social relationship with the person to whom he is becoming more attached each day.

When weaning is done gradually after a period of sucking satisfaction, many babies wean themselves by the end of the first year. Successful mastery of the weaning process marks the end of the period when the primary satisfactions come from the mouth and from closeness to the mother.

DEVELOPMENT,
CARE AND GUIDANCE DURING
THE TRAINING PERIOD
(1 TO 3 YEARS)

When the infant relinquishes his need for sucking and develops skill in the use of his body, his concept of himself changes, and his interests broaden. *He becomes more aware of himself as a person; he becomes increasingly more interested in independent activity; he develops increased capacity to communicate with words; and he begins to gain control over his impulses to explore and to soil and wet indiscriminately.*

Language Development in the First Years of Life. FACTORS INFLUENCING LANGUAGE DEVELOPMENT. Growth must occur before the infant is able to communicate both feelings of pleasure and discomfort with his organs of speech. At birth the infant can communicate discomfort only with his organs of speech. The welcome cry of the newborn will develop fairly soon into sounds which express hunger, pain and anger. The babbling sounds of comfort, the coos, the laughs out loud do not come until the infant is 3 or 4 months of age. The so-called "talking" increases with varying intonation. He squeals with delight in his bath, he crows, he responds with various noises when one talks to him. He becomes

increasingly more aware that sounds come from his mother's mouth. He watches her as she talks, imitates the movement of her lips and attempts to "talk back" to her.

The child's speech development depends on various factors—on his ability to hear and retain what he hears and on his desire to understand and to talk. Social experiences with his mother give the infant a model and motivate him to learn to understand her and to speak with her. Understanding of his mother's words precedes his ability to communicate with her verbally. Between the ninth and twelfth months of life the infant begins to understand his mother's verbal communications with him. At about 9 months of age the infant begins to utter sounds which seem to mean certain people or things. He has come though the cry-and-babbling stages of speech development and has entered into the third stage of imitative expression. Certain words are understood, especially those that name concrete things and have been associated with them repeatedly. By the time that he is a year old, he responds to his name and to simple directions. He also understands the words associated with certain activities. "By-by" connected with the pleasure of going outdoors, and "No, No" connected with inhibition are understood by many infants before they are a year old.

In the second and the third years of life vocabulary increases rapidly. Because many factors influence learning, there are wide variations in the vocabularies of different children. Some children at 2 may have a vocabulary of 300 or more words; others may use less than a dozen.

The child who is credited with a vocabulary of 300 words is doubtlessly using a much smaller number than that, but he has been recorded as having said that number. Some words may be said once, possibly in direct imitation, and then may not be used again for months. Without doubt many of the words used are not spoken with the clearness of enunciation necessary to be understood generally, but to the adult caring for the child they are intelligible.

The child needs help in acquiring vocabulary; he also needs an interested listener who strives to understand his verbal communications with her. If there is no hearing or mental impairment, learning to communicate verbally develops naturally when child and mother or nurse have consistent, mutually enjoyed experiences together. The interested mother or nurse talks to the child, helps him to associate words with things and activities and listens to the way in which he expresses himself. She soon discovers that he is "parroting" her words and attempting to use them in appropriate ways. She rewards his efforts with her responsiveness, and soon his quest for vocabulary begins.

LANGUAGE FOSTERS UNDERSTANDING. The baby will have been exposed to countless words as people enter his life, not only the name words (nouns) but the words describing action, space, time, relationships, feelings, etc. He will acquire an understanding of all those aspects of life. He will learn to reason and to solve problems. At first, his comprehension will be what might be called gross understanding. Through experience he will become more and more sensitive to meanings and be more discriminating in his choice of words. For example, he will understand "big" as a 2-year-old, and "bigger than" and "biggest of all" as a 4-year-old. "Gone" can only be "gone" out of sight. It will be months before the words "not here" become associated with the idea of "downstairs" or "downtown." As children are learning to talk, they necessarily must hear much more than they can understand. Such circumstances challenge them to greater understanding if their need for attention is not slighted.

Young children need their language limitations considered in their guidance. Unless directions are given simply and are accompanied with the act itself, understanding is often impossible. In times of stress the child's limitations in self-expression also need understanding. When the child is experiencing strong emotional feelings, he cannot communicate them verbally. He jumps with joy; he also screams in anger or in moments of fright. To say "Don't cry" or "Stop moving your arms about" communicates lack of understanding of his nature. The young child cannot say "I am scared of that needle and syringe. You make me angry when you approach me like this. Why didn't you tell me what you were going to do? If you had I could manage myself a little better." Nor can the young child control himself unaided when he is scared or angry. He has not yet gained that degree of control.

In situations like the above the mother or the nurse needs to be able to accept the way the young child expresses his feelings. "Don't cry" makes him feel misunderstood. "Of course you're scared, Timmy. All children are when it is time for their hypo. Some children are angry, too" recognizes the child's natural feelings and supports him in times of stress. The child not only needs understanding; he needs help in holding himself still. If he is held by a nurse who understands his inability to control himself, he will welcome her helpfulness.

Acquiring Mastery of Bowel and Bladder Functioning. In this period from 1 to 3 years of age the toddler develops readiness to learn the toileting customs of his society. His mother is his guide and teacher. She needs to be ready to watch for signs which indicate a readiness to learn. She also needs to interpret the customs and to make learning a satisfying, growth-producing experience.

When the weaning process is completed the child's interest shifts to himself, his body, its products and functioning. As he toddles about the house he views the toileting facilities and becomes fascinated with the way they work. He becomes keenly interested in all his mother's activities, including those which take place in the bathroom. He seems to be more aware of his body; he views and explores every part of it and delights in his excretory products. He sees nothing shameful about urine and feces. They are interesting substances because they are the products of his body and activity. He examines them just as he explores every other substance or object that is within his reach. He is not born with the idea that urine and feces are wastes and inappropriate play materials. He must learn this through carefully guided experiences with his mother.

The child needs help in finding socially acceptable outlets for his natural urge to explore and mess. If the mother or the nurse understands his feelings about the products of his body, she will accept his interest. In addition, however, she will help him simultaneously to obtain satisfaction for his urge to explore from play with appropriate materials. Sand, water and eventually clay and finger paint are appropriate play materials. He can explore and discover outlets for his urge to mess with these materials. When he is given substitute materials, he feels understood and lovable. The understanding mother or nurse knows that scolding, shaming or rejecting punishment result in fear and anger and make him feel "bad" and unlovable. He cannot understand such management, and it is obvious that it is detrimental to personality development.

PHYSICAL AND PSYCHOLOGICAL READINESS ESSENTIAL FOR MASTERY. The child must learn the customs of his society through experiences with his mother. Our customs place inhibitions on the individual and make definite requirements of him. The young infant is completely unaware of these expectations. He passes his urine and moves his bowels whenever the urge comes. He has no inhibitions and can exercise no conscious control over his sphincter muscles. He relieves himself, irrespective of time or place— in the drawing room, in the lap of the haughtiest visitor, no matter how it may embarrass his mother— if the inclination comes. It is more comfortable to relieve himself as soon as the inclination comes. But it is considered more civilized in our culture to control one's inclination in this respect and to relieve oneself only under certain conditions.

The child can meet the requirements of his culture if both physiologic and psychological readiness for learning have been attained. After a period of pleasure from unrestricted soiling, wetting and exploration which gives him awareness of his family's toileting customs, he develops interest in excretory activity. He shows his readiness to master bowel control when he shows his awareness of his need to defecate. This usually occurs when nervous system growth makes standing possible. His signs of awareness of a full rectum are individual. Some children make grunting sounds or strain; others communicate their interest in learning control by pulling at their diapers or saying self-formulated words which express the feelings they are experiencing.

The ability to co-operate is essential for self-mastery. The child's behavior is his cue—his way of telling us that he is interested in learning. It is our responsibility to help him find pleasure in learning. If we do, he will not feel angry or resent society's restrictions; he will use the experiences for growth, feel adequate, accepting and giving. He will do this if we respect his autonomy and expect functioning on the toilet only when he is ready to co-operate.

Learning excretory control is a social experience which should foster personality growth. The mother observes his cues, kindly interprets her expectations and provides substitute satisfactions when he withstands frustration to meet her requirements. He gives in return for all he has received. He also derives pleasure from his mother's pride and approval and from his own self-mastery. Toileting becomes a give-and-take experience which fosters personality growth. He gives because he is ready to give, and he gets satisfaction in return for his efforts. With this method there is no coercion and no deprivation that he is unable to tolerate. As a result he *feels* satisfied with his experience, and his relationship with his mother is sustained at an optimal level.

Readiness to develop bladder control is equally essential for personality growth. When physiologic functioning has progressed to the stage where a child's bladder can retain urine for a 2-hour period, he is usually ready to learn that the toilet is also a place to deposit his urine. Preceding this stage of development (15 to 18 months) the child will show awareness that he has already urinated. He will point to his wet panties or show us the puddle he has made. This is growth in awareness; it needs understanding. Just because he can tell us he has wet, it does not mean that he has matured sufficiently to tell us *before* he urinates. This requires more growth and will come at a later date.

Helping the child to learn to use the toilet for urinating should be a gradual process. Again his autonomy needs to be respected. When his bladder has held urine for a 2-hour period, the chances are that he will be able to co-operate. Then it is wise to take him to the toilet, interpret the custom with simple words that are within his understanding and maintain faith in his capacity to function independently. The child will respond to his mother's or nurse's confidence in him and will welcome approval for his efforts.

Successful functioning on the toilet will be influenced by the child's current emotional and physical state. Illness brings regression because it utilizes energy that he needs for adaptation. Anxiety does the same thing. When a young child is separated from his mother, the source of all his security, he regresses to infantile modes of behavior. If he is anxious about his mother's love, regression may also occur. This can happen when a new baby arrives in the family. It can also happen when his mother's interest becomes diverted away from him to a new apartment or to herself during pregnancy, for instance.

Gradually, the child will take his mother's standards into himself and desire cleanliness as she does. This is accomplished slowly, a step at a time. At first he will be able to function successfully only when his mother is with him. However, gradually control will come from within and when it does, he will have attained real self-mastery. In the interim accidents are bound to occur for they are the natural outcome of stress or absorption in play. They are nothing about which the adult needs to feel discouraged. If there is a good relationship between adult and child, if successes are commended and failures ignored and treated in a matter-of-fact manner, the goal of mastery will be attained eventually. Expecting complete independence before 3 years of age

is expecting behavior which is incompatible with a child's nature.

After the child has attained mastery of excretory functioning during the daytime, he becomes ready to learn night-time control. Usually diapers are worn at night for some time after they are discarded for daytime use. When daytime control is achieved, it is wise to discard the diapers at night. Discarding the diapers with teaching like the following interprets the standard and motivates his interest in his growth: "You don't need diapers at night any more. Soon you won't need to urinate while you sleep. You will wake up when you need to urinate. You can use the potty chair which is next to your bed."

Taking the child to the toilet during the night may keep the child's bed dry but it teaches little of lasting value. The child who has become accustomed to urinating into the toilet and does not go through the night without urinating may be taken up sometime between 10 o'clock and midnight and placed on the toilet with some degree of success. If he is not awakened, however, it is not valuable as an aid in learning. It may save wet beds— and that has its values, to be sure— but the important lesson of subconscious control of the sphincter muscles of the bladder is not achieved. The child is still continuing to urinate in his sleep. It is difficult to waken a soundly sleeping child, and if the attempt to do so creates antagonism or long periods of sleeplessness, it is wiser to discontinue the attempt.

If there are neither physiologic abnormalities nor disturbances in the parent-child relationship, night-time control will evolve eventually with growth and with a better understanding of the social requirements of his culture. Sometime between 3½ and 4½ years of age, physical and psychological growth makes night-time control a reality. It will come about naturally if the standard is taught with understanding and if the family interpersonal relationships continue to foster personality growth.

CLOTHING AND TOILET FACILITIES AID THE CHILD IN LEARNING. When a child develops readiness for learning control of bowel and bladder functioning, he needs to be kept dry. This is essential to accustom him to a feeling of dryness. Diapers are usually given up in the daytime, sometime before they are discarded at night. Daytime use of diapers should be given up as soon as the child seems to have some understanding of the use of the toilet. Diapers are infantile clothing and presuppose the infantile habit of emptying the bladder and moving the bowels without heed to time or place. The very fact of discarding the diapers helps in the learning process. The child feels more grown-up and is motivated to want to master himself. The use of training pants is equally necessary in the care of hospitalized children. It is depreciating to keep a preschool child in diapers unless he is acutely ill. If they must be used because of an inadequate nursing staff, care must be taken to protect the child's feelings of self-respect.

Clothing which a child can manage easily is a help in a child's learning. For girls, there should be panties that slip down easily. Boys need trousers with few and large buttons and buttonholes, and with wide legs that can be pulled up for urinating. The trousers with zippered flies are intriguing to boys because they can manage them independently. One-piece rompers that have to be removed every time a toddler is taken to the toilet are enough to make any child rebel at the procedure, and rebellion retards learning.

A toilet chair is most advantageous from the child's point of view because eventually he can use it independently, and there is nothing of which to be afraid. Small seats placed on the adult toilet are also useful if movable steps with a good base are available. Any possible experience of fear by being placed for the first time on a large toilet should be avoided. Unless the noise of flushing is anticipated for children, fear reactions are the outcome in many instances. In institutions, small, low toilets should be available because they prevent fear reactions and foster learning. When the toilet is accessible to the child, a boy of 2½ or 3 years of age can learn to stand for urination.

Self-Discovery and Assertion— an Important Phase of Development. SELF-ACCEPTANCE, A NECESSARY PERSONAL QUALITY FOR GROWTH. The young child is an egocentric person who is concerned primarily with himself. He loves those who care for him and make him comfortable and happy. However, that love has little evidence of a concern for the feelings of others. He takes at this stage of development; others give. He says "Mine" and clutches his toys, holding them away from the child who approaches. He is selfish, possessive and feels himself to be the most important person in his universe. It is the natural way for him to feel. He is in an important phase of growth. *He needs to identify himself and his powers.* Before he can share and be concerned with others, he must feel the joy of possession, self-expression, personal power and the self-respect that comes when one is accepted as he is. He will become concerned with others and will develop into an adequately socialized person through guidance and life experiences which help him turn outward the love that he feels for himself and for those who minister to his personal needs.

In the years from 1 to 3 the child discovers himself and expresses his feelings, wishes and thoughts more potently than he ever has done before. Between 12 to 18 months and 3 to 4 years he goes through a negativistic stage of development. It is so natural and easy to assert one's independent self by saying "No" and "I won't" that one cannot be surprised that this occurs. After all, "No" probably was one of the first words that he ever came to understand.

NEGATIVISM, DAWDLING AND RITUALISTIC BEHAVIOR CHARACTERIZE THE YOUNG CHILD. A period of negativism is natural, desirable and important for growth toward maturity. It comes when he begins to work out his dependent needs. It is a short period if he is understood and if he is guided with wisdom. The child in this stage of development has new-found powers, and he is aware of his capacity to assert himself. He does it in a negativistic way. He does it impulsively; it springs from a drive to be powerful,

controlling and independent. Often it may be only by saying "No" and doing the thing which is asked. Simultaneously with his drive toward independence, he feels a great need to be dependent upon his mother. One minute he asserts his independence; the next he begs to be held and manifests the most infantile dependency.

The child needs guidance which assists him in finding ways to use his new-found powers in constructive and socially acceptable ways. Overcoming negativism never is accomplished by opposing him. He needs to be guided by suggestion and teaching rather than by command: "It is time to go to bed now. You can bring Teddy with you and help to open your bed." A 2-year-old needs a certain amount of physical direction as well as verbal, taking him by the hand as we say the above. When children are in good rapport with adults, they are eager to please. When we express our pleasure in their helpful co-operation they gain status and self-importance. When we recognize their ability and desire to learn to do things for themselves, their egos become strengthened. They acquire a wholesome concept of themselves which is basic to their acceptance of others.

Dawdling and ritualism are also characteristic ways in which children express themselves during this stage of development. These characteristics come because the child is in a transition period; he does not know right from wrong; he cannot make one choice, so he makes two. We call him and say, "It is time to go to the clinic now." He dawdles; he does not know whether to come or go so he does both. He needs help to know what is expected. When he learns this through repeated experiences, he can make a decision more quickly, and the dawdling will cease to be a predominant characteristic of his behavior.

Ritualism comes in response to his deep need for self-mastery. He formulates ritualistic ways of doing things because then he knows what to expect and can master himself and his environment more effectively. Ritualistic behavior is at its peak at 2½ years of age; it is less pronounced at 4 because he is surer of himself and can adapt to changes in routine with a greater degree of ease. It is wise to utilize his self-devised rituals within a framework of the limits which he is able to tolerate, which he needs for growth. It saves time and energy and gives him the security that he requires during this phase of his development.

Discipline Which Provides Freedom and Appropriate Limits Is Necessary for Growth. Discipline Is a Continuing Process of Guidance Which Fosters Personality Growth. Discipline is education; it is guidance which helps the child grow increasingly more self-controlled, self-respecting, self-reliant and independent. Discipline is concerned with the preparation of the child to take his self-reliant place in the world, ready to live in harmony with his fellow beings. *The child needs to acquire controls gradually from within.* Acquiring self-control, self-reliance and independence is a slow process. It is a matter of growth, development and guidance. It begins in infancy and

ends when emotional maturity is reached.

Limits Which Change with Growth Are Essential for Security. The young child has no controls from within; he must get them from the adults within his environment. The mother is the young child's ego. It is she who must determine the inner strength that he possesses to meet restrictions. She is also the one who must guide him patiently and kindly in learning acceptable ways of expressing himself and attaining his goals. She must teach him what activities are safe and appropriate and which ones are dangerous and unsuitable for his growth or for the protection of others and of things within his environment.

The child wants and needs limits which are geared to his capacities to meet them. It is the only way that he can feel safe in his parent's affection; it is the only way that he can learn to be a more self-directing, confident person. Overindulgence frightens a child and gives him no help in getting controls from within. When he is unsure of what is expected he wants to know what is permissible and that which cannot be done. He feels loved when there is someone who cares enough to teach him the ways of his world and helps him to find socially acceptable outlets for his feelings and powerful drives. He wants this help because he is torn between two potent forces which are pulling against each other—the drive to explore, to give vent to his impulses, and the drive to learn to control himself more effectively. Limits give security. The child learns parental requirements; he also discovers that if he meets them he will remain safe in the affections of his parents. Limits also provide freedom. He has learned that certain things are not permissible, but with the exception of these limits he is free to express himself. He *knows* the limits; he is not fearful lest he exceed his parent's patience and bring their wrath down upon him.

Because the ego of the child from 1 to 3 years old is weak and his powers of control are limited, he needs protection from frequent thwarting. His drives to explore and to learn to do things for himself are powerful; he has little control over the expression of his feelings and impulses. For these reasons his environment needs to be made safe, and valuable objects need to be placed out of his reach. His ego is too weak to tolerate excessive frustration. He has toilet training and locomotion tasks to surmount. In addition, he is utilizing energy in learning to communicate verbally with others and in becoming more independent in self-feeding, dressing and play.

As the child acquires ego strength through successful accomplishment, he becomes more capable of withstanding frustration. When he is ready to tolerate frustration it should be introduced, for growth comes through mastery of difficult situations. *The child needs limits which change as he grows.* This requires flexibility of character and imagination in those who guide him. Successful guidance depends upon the adult's intuitive capacity to sense the child's capacities for new learning experiences and responsibilities. It also depends upon the

adult's ability to help the child find ways to express his emotions and drives in ways which protect his mental health and the safety and the comfort of others.

DEVELOPMENT AND GUIDANCE DURING THE EARLY PERIOD OF SOCIALIZATION (3 TO 6 YEARS)

Development from 3 to 6 years is a period of marked psychological growth. Gradually the child acquires the ability to communicate with language his feelings, wishes and thoughts. His curiosity expands, and with questions and exploration he strives to understand the world of events which touch him personally. In this phase of development the child's relationships with his parents change. He also becomes more social and seeks friendships with children and adults outside his family. He develops increased security; he learns to do more for himself; he gains more inner controls; and he discovers many new ways of obtaining gratification through hours of important play each day. He tolerates separation from his mother, if there are no difficult problems with which to cope. *Through interpersonal experiences within his home and the outside world, he gains increased understanding and acceptance of others and of himself as a boy or a girl. He finds his place with his parents. He also acquires knowledge and attitudes toward every aspect of life within his society.*

Language Development and Growth in Understanding. During preschool years the comfortably adjusted child increases his vocabulary by leaps and bounds, and probably averages about a yearly 600-word increase between the ages of 2 and 6. Children acquire their vocabulary through "parroting" what they hear, through association and through the answers that come from their questions. The 2-year-old begins with the "what" question: "What's dat?" "What are you doing?" It is his way of learning about his world. At 2 years of age his talking is largely made up of nouns and verbs, with possibly a sprinkling of pronouns, adjectives and prepositions. But as perception, understanding and experience expand, they become reflected in his speech. Adjectives, descriptive and qualifying, appear; these are followed by more prepositions, adverbs, words indicating some understanding of time and space relationships, of human relationships, of cause and effect.

The 3-year-old uses longer sentences, and his questions become when, where, why and how questions as he seeks increased understanding of the complex life about him. The 3-year-old uses sentences like "I want to go to the playroom after I've had my hypo and bath." His questions are often incessant and run something like the following ones: "Where's Mommy gone?" "How does that syringe work?" "Why can't I go to the playroom now?" "When is my Mommy coming?" *His questions reveal his needs and require answers which give him increased understanding of what is happening to him and what is going on about him.* The child needs the events of life interpreted to him. From observation and the adult's interpretation, the child gleans feelings, attitudes and ideas which will influence his feelings about himself and others, religion, sex, school, hos-

pitals and all the other aspects of life to which he becomes exposed.

Before questions are answered, the adult should try to discover the need which has motivated the question. There are many reasons why children ask questions. The most obvious reason is to obtain information or to discover how things work or how they may be used. However, many more questions are asked to obtain relief from anxiety. Some queries are bids for attention and companionship. The child feels lonely and is seeking a social relationship with someone who will be interested in him as a person. When questions are asked the mother or the nurse needs to interrogate herself before she responds: 'What is this child trying to understand? How can I respond in such a manner as to meet his needs?"

The questions at 4 or 5 years are more complicated and require more detailed explanations. They want to know how things work: "What makes them do that?" "Where have the icicles gone that were hanging on the roof?" Often the adult is puzzled as to how to answer their searching questions. The one guiding principle should be to give the child the truth to the best of his ability and as simply as possible. Often the question is so far from simple that this is difficult. If the adult does not know the answer he should acknowledge that fact to the child. It will not bring loss of respect. The adult who answers a child's question with "I don't know, Skipper, but let's find out together" is nurturing the eager spirit of learning. Telling the child untruths and deceiving him undermines his sense of trust. It brings suspicion of adults and a sense of insecurity which have far-reaching consequences for personality development.

The 4-year-old child chatters as he plays. A vocabulary of 1,500 or more words is fairly adequate equipment for communication. As he plays house, creating all aspects of family experience—store, policeman, fire, hospitals, school, flying, even all the tragedies which are a part of life—he has at his command the language for each situation.

The 4-year-old child is also acquiring number concepts. When 3 he knew 2, but now that he is 4 he can count 3. Within the next year he probably will learn to count to 10. A child often learns to say the numbers by rote before this, but that is a feat of memory and does not indicate an ability to make use of the numbers to count.

The 3-year-old, or even the younger child, apparently has been interested in color, and he differentiates colors, putting objects of the same color together. The 4-year-old begins to name colors, and by 5 he can be counted on to be accurate in regard to the primary colors and even to some of the other colors. Some children may name colors at a much earlier age.

The concepts of time, size, space and shape slowly become more clearly defined. A 3-year-old child has some conception of present, past and future. "Today" has some meaning for him, "yesterday" comes to mean a time that has gone, "tomorrow" a time that is to come. When a 3-year-old child is with his mother, waiting until "tomorrow" is usually comparatively easy. But when he is separated from all that

means security, "tomorrow" must seem like an eternity. Often we glibly say, "Tomorrow, your mother will come." "Tomorrow" is a word which to us means a relatively short time, but to a young child experiencing the pain of separation anxiety "tomorrow" brings little comfort.

The understanding of gradations in time is slow in developing and far from perfected even for the 5-year-old. The 4- or 5-year-old becomes interested in "week" as a unit of time and is also desirous of learning the days of the week. A child of 4 years and 8 months at the nursery school was heard to say on a Friday in haughty reproof to a child who had said, "I'll see you tomorrow," "No, I won't see you tomorrow, Janet, I'll see you Monday." The 4-year-old child can also tell how old he is, and if 4½ the ½ is equally as important as the 4.

The preschool child grows in understanding of space relationships. The 2-year-old, with no comprehension of size or shape, may try to put the big square into the small hole. An understanding of difference in size will come first, and later shape will be understood; the square and the circle first and then the more difficult shapes. A 4- or 5-year-old may enjoy the simply formed puzzle, fitting the 6 or 8 pieces into which the figure has been cut into the inset shape of the figure. But he still relies largely on the trial-and-error method because his perception of shape is not yet accurate enough to be a completely reliable guide. Johnny, 2 years and 8 months old, identifying the white moon of the evening said, "Moon up too high. Johnny needs a chair to get it down." The 4-year-old will know that it cannot be done, for he has grown in his understanding of space relationships. He will not only know that it cannot be done, but also he will be able to express his knowledge with words.

The 4- or 5-year-old child becomes increasingly interested in the matter of relatives. He has known his mother for a long time as "Mother," but now he comes to know that she may be a daughter, a sister or an aunt as well, and that he too stands in various relationships to other people.

Sex Education. SEX EDUCATION IS PREPARATION FOR SATISFYING MARRIAGE AND PARENTHOOD. The child's sex education begins at birth and continues until emotional maturity is reached. Sex education is more than the transmission of the biologic facts of growth, reproduction and the sexual relationship. It is guidance which prepares the individual for satisfying marriage and parenthood. To be sure, specific knowledge must be imparted, but of even greater importance is the creation of wholesome attitudes and feelings toward the self and toward others as male and female personages.

Preparation for marriage and parenthood requires the kind of parental guidance which makes emotional maturity a possibility. It begins with acceptance of the child as a boy or as a girl and is influenced by all the care and the experiences of the growing-up process. Well-guided experiences within his home and community foster self-respect, the capacity for love and acceptance of responsibility for himself and others. Wholesome sex education is achieved more readily when the child has two parents who respect each other, who are satisfied with their life together and are ready and desirous of sharing their life and love with him in ways which are appropriate for his emotional growth.

If the reader reviews the relationship experiences which are cited on the foregoing pages and thinks through the ways that they can influence the child's feelings about himself and others, it will become evident that sex education is a continuous process which begins even before the child is born. The feelings that the child acquires about himself and others will become reflected in his marital relationship and in his relationship with his children. For example, the woman who respects herself and those of the opposite sex will have better chances for marital and parental satisfaction than will the woman who depreciates masculinity or feels inferior because she is feminine.

GROWTH HEIGHTENS CURIOSITY. In preschool years the child's curiosity becomes heightened, and he seeks answers to the many problems which perplex him. The 3-year-old knows that he or she is a boy or a girl, and soon inevitably there will be an interest in the differences between boys and girls, and between men and women. He also ponders about his origin, and eventually he will raise questions pertaining to reproduction and birth. It is right and natural that he should be interested in his body and find pleasure in it. Every child explores his body and experiments with masturbation. It need not cause any concern unless he consistently chooses it instead of play with others, or instead of interesting activities which are available to him.

It is also natural that the child should be curious about his origin and the origin of others and seek to understand what he is feeling, hearing and seeing. *The child needs to grow up with the feeling that sex is an important quality inherent in his personality and in the personalities of all other people.* He needs to grow up feeling that sex is something which is right to think and talk about. Only then will he get his fantasies or thoughts clarified and the understanding that he needs for growth. In each stage of growth new questions will arise. Sex education cannot be given in one lesson; it must be given a step at a time as growth creates a need for deeper understanding of life in a bisexual world.

When a child shows curiosity or verbally communicates his questions, it manifests his concern and a need for help. Before factual information is given to the child over 3 years of age, it is wise to encourage him to talk about the thoughts he has been having. This can be done with sympathetic listening and with attitudes that communicate one's acceptance of any thoughts he might have. Often children have fantasied answers to their queries and more often than not they are unrealistic. These erroneous concepts need to be ventilated to an understanding listener and corrected *before* factual information is given. When erroneous fantasies are repressed, emotional understanding of truths is nigh to impossible.

GROWTH BRINGS CHANGES IN FAMILY INTERPERSONAL RELATION-SHIPS. In the third year of life the child becomes more strikingly masculine or feminine. Growth also brings changes in his relations with his parents. The little boy acts more masculine; he imitates his father and strives to do the things he does. The little girl delights in "playing mother"; she dresses up in her clothing and dramatizes her activities in her play. The boy's attachment to his mother becomes intensified, and he manifests rivalrous feelings with his father for his mother's love. The girl shifts her center of interest from her mother to her father. She may say to her mother, "I love Daddy more than I love you," or "I'm going to marry Daddy when I grow up." This phase of personality development brings conflict, fear, disappointment and confusion. The girl may wish her mother away so that she might have her daddy all to herself. However, simultaneously she feels a deep need for her mother. The boy is irritated with his father. He, too, may wish his rival parent away, but simultaneously he loves his father and wants to be like him. It is obvious what losing a parent might mean to a child in this stage of development. Repeated experiences are necessary to learn that wishes cannot destroy. They are also necessary to learn that wishes are different from deeds.

The above changes in family interpersonal relationships further the child's personality growth and influence his sex education. Frustration and disappointment come because he is denied that which he desires. Loving one's parent of the opposite sex and conflicting feelings of love and hate for one's rival parent also bring fear. *The child needs his im-*

pulses of love accepted. He also needs help in renouncing his desire for his parent of the opposite sex. He needs help to find and accept his place within his family. It is a step in development which is important for his growth. When he has parents who love each other and respect his need for growth, he gets the help that he needs to solve his complicated problem. He represses his sexual feelings. Instead of wanting *to be* mother or father, he changes his goal to a desire to be *like* his parent of the same sex.

In this stage of development social experiences with children help the child to solve his problems. Through satisfying experiences with children he finds outlets for his feelings of love. He also discovers ways of alleviating his feelings of frustrations and ways of mastering the many fears which come in this developmental phase of growth. In play he *can* be father or mother and do some of the things that he or she can do. In fantasy he *is* mother or father. This type of play helps the child to withstand the frustration that he feels and prepares him for his masculine or feminine role in his society. In the years to come he will emulate his parent of the same sex and gradually acquire the characteristics of his own sex. His play prepares him for marriage and parenthood. It does so because it helps him to accept his place within his family and provides experiences which promote social and emotional growth.

By 3 years of age the child should have acquired inner resources which make it possible for him to broaden his horizons and feel safe in the company of those outside his family.

If he has had a continuous warm relationship with his mother, he has gained trust in others and some measure of security within himself. The 2-year-old is not ready to separate himself from his mother. He continues to need her as a constant companion. He may venture away from her into the next room for a few moments of play but soon he returns to her. He does this because he gets anxious when she is out of his sight. He is dependent upon her, loves her and wants her constant attention. He is lost without her. She gives comfort and protection; she helps him to learn; and she makes it possible for him to master himself in ways which bring him satisfaction. The 3-year-old child feels safer in his world. He is ready too for a nursery school or play-group experience.

A 3-year-old child can profit from a nursery school or play-group experience if he has gained security in his relationship with his parents; if he is familiar with the teacher and the school environment; if he knows why he is being placed there and what is going to happen while he is there; if he knows that his mother will return to take him home; and if he is sure that his needs will be fulfilled in her absence.

The above are the emotional requirements which are necessary to master any experience which brings separation from the security which the presence of Mother represents. These requirements are equally important for a hospital experience. Unless the child's emotional requirements are met in each new situation he meets, his psychological growth can be seriously jeopardized. It will be jeopardized because he will be confronted with problems that he is unable to master constructively.

During this period children have great concern about their bodies and fear bodily injury. For this reason many physicians postpone operations if there are no contraindications which would make delay injurious to physical health. When a child must undergo an operation, he needs careful guidance to prepare him for everything that he will consciously experience. Knowing what to expect helps the child prepare himself for the experience and prevents emotional trauma.

Growth Through Supervised Play with Others. MOTOR DEVELOPMENT. In the years from 2 to 5, motor skills that show themselves in play and daily living are acquired and perfected. Learning to skip, hop and jump becomes engrossing activity. The 3-year-old will jump from a low height, e.g., a stair or a low stool. Between 4 and 5 years, he is ready to jump from a greater height, say, 3 or 4 steps. He learns during this year to skip and hop as well, and to run lightly on tip toes.

Balance is acquired with growth and practice. At 2 he did not have sufficient control of body balance to stand on one foot. Before he is 3, he tries to do it, then accomplishing it for a brief second or two; and by the time he is 5, Gesell reports that he can do it for 8 seconds.

Learning to use a Kiddy Car and a "bike" absorbs the interest of the preschool child. The 2½ year old goes about on a Kiddy Car with the greatest of ease. Soon he wants to try the 3-wheeled "bike" with pedals, and between 4 and 5 years

of age he can ride around the playground with speed and dexterity.

Opportunity and encouragement to practice using his body during these early years brings self-confidence and prepares him to compete favorably with others. The 5-year-old usually has excellent motor control if he has been given opportunities to practice. The child who has been inoculated with adult fears which are manifested with "Look out," or "Don't fall," etc., probably will be slower in learning and possibly may never acquire skill in some of the more complicated and daring activities. All this practice in learning to use his body during these early years will help him when later he starts to learn to skate, ski, etc. In the school-age period physical skills are necessary to compete favorably with one's group of age-mates. Especially is this true for boys.

Not only has the 5-year-old child learned to use his large muscles more skillfully, but also he has become more skillful in the use of his hands. Even before he was 2 he may have enjoyed making marks with crayons. He can hold the crayons because he learned before 1 year to bring thumb in opposition to finger. The 3-year-old paints with great pleasure and begins to show evidences of design with lines or masses of color. The 2-year-old cannot cut with scissors, although he begins to become interested in learning. The 3-year-old begins to use scissors with some success. The 5-year-old has had a year or more of enjoying cutting, pasting, stringing beads, building with blocks and doing puzzles. The baby's banging with his rattle has slowly organized itself into the skill of "hitting the nail on the head." The 3-year-old is fairly accurate in hitting big pegs, and the 5-year-old learns to use a real hammer and nails and even a saw.

The child needs supervision to learn to use materials. Supervision should guide him in the use of paints, brushes, scissors, hammers and other equipment; and it should provide him with opportunities for free expression within the limits which are necessary to protect himself and others and the physical environment he is in. Supervision is not adult domination; it is leadership and guidance. Children need help in learning the use and the care of the tools of the craft. When the adult has completed the task of teaching the use of the tools and the places where they may be used, she needs to leave the children free to express themselves in their own way. Setting standards of adult performance stifles creativeness. Children cannot compete with it or measure up to standards that adults inadvertently set when they do this. Children need opportunities to learn. Learning comes from within and should be a creative experience which brings feelings of accomplishment. Children feel no accomplishment if their activities are directed or interfered with by adults who "want to help" by doing the task for them.

PSYCHOLOGICAL GROWTH. Social and emotional development comes with growth and supervised activities with others. The 2-year-old child wants to make friends but he usually does not know how. Often his aggressive methods of approach need redirection, for we may find him punching or pushing the new acquaintance. Two-year-old children do not play together—they are not advanced enough in development for that. They enjoy being together; they may have successful physical association, take each other by the hand or hug each other (possibly too violently for one of them) and sit side by side at the table in the playroom and do the same thing; but there is no co-operative play. The toys may be snatched from the newly admitted child sitting across the table and called "mine."

The adult who understands that guidance is necessary for growth does not condemn the child who snatches as selfish or force him to give up all his toys. Instead she gives him an opportunity to share and find that playtime is happier when this is done. She knows children are not born unselfish and ready to share. They learn to share, to control their aggressive impulses and to consider the rights of others gradually through their desire to please their mothers, teachers or nurses.

It is obvious that a good relationship between the adult and the child is necessary for psychological growth. Unless the child values the adult's approval, little real social and emotional growth can take place. He may inhibit impulses out of fear, but this kind of learning is not mastery or growth.

Between 3 and 6 years of age the comfortably adjusted child learns to play with other children. At 3 years of age, there is evidence of playing together which may develop into the delightful and imaginative play of the 4- and 5-year-olds and of school children. Playing together means that the child is old enough to co-operate with another child, each one doing his part toward making the play successful. In the early stages of playing together, it will be a simple and probably short time of co-operation between two children, perhaps of piling blocks together. Between 4 and 5 years of age, observation shows social and emotional growth. The play of these children is more elaborate and continues for a longer period of time. They dramatize the activities of the home and the community. Several children play together, and often new ones are permitted to join them.

Learning to play together is probably never an entirely unruffled experience. There are clashes of will and storms of anger, especially as two dominant personalities come into opposition with each other. This kind of situation may be especially evident as the 4-year level is reached. Anger in the young child is accompanied by physical reactions of violence, screaming, kicking, hitting, etc.

Gradually, with understanding guidance the child can be helped to express his aggressive feelings in socially acceptable ways. Anger is a natural response to frustration. *Guidance is necessary to help the child direct his aggressive feelings into constructive channels.* Little by little he can find ways to work through his feelings in play, and eventually he will be able to express his anger verbally. Being able to express anger verbally manifests growth. It is a constructive way for the child to vent his feelings.

Growth in the ability to handle anger constructively is observable in preschool children. The baby screams with anger if he is thwarted by having his hands held down, for example. The 4- or 5-year-old says, "I hate you when you put that needle in my arm. I'd like to grind you into mincemeat." The 5-year-old may be enraged by seeing another child knocked down. True, he may come to the rescue by first knocking down the culprit, but the reason for his anger is concern for another, not himself, and we know that psychologically he has grown.

Opportunities for learning to share, to take turns, to help each other, to make plans about their play, to control the expression of their emotions all come as part of learning to play together. All the qualities that make for harmonious living may be guided and fostered in the play of preschool children. With understanding guidance the 6-year-old has become a co-operative, gregarious person who is beginning to recognize and respect the rights of others.

Through guided experiences in the home, the school and the community the child's personality becomes formed. His ego becomes strengthened, and he incorporates the standards of his parents and teachers. By the end of this period these inner standards have become a part of his personality—the super-ego or conscience. These standards function automatically; they keep him from doing that which he has learned to be unacceptable; and they motivate him to do those things which he knows are acceptable to his parents and teachers.

PLAY EQUIPMENT FOR PRESCHOOL CHILDREN. With an understanding of a child's growing skill, knowledge, interests and needs, it becomes a comparatively easy task to make a selection of toys for hospitalized pre-school children. Play equipment that promotes motor skills, sense percep-tion, physical development and en-courages imaginative, creative and social play are needed by the pre-school age child. Much discarded household equipment makes excel-lent play materials for children. The list of equipment which appears below includes those things which would be desirable to have in a hospital playroom.

Blocks, big and little
Simple puzzles
Sand box on wheels, pail, shovel, etc.
Galvanized tub on wheels for water play, or rubber wading pool
Inflatable water toys
Wagon, kiddie car, tricycle
Teeter totter, seesaw
Record player and records
Hanging blackboard
Books
Piano
Large wooden beads for stringing
Packing box, planks, sawhorse, ladder
Balls, large
Toys for dramatic house play—wood people dolls, baby dolls, doll buggy, doll bed, toy cooking set, tea set, tele-phone, toy cleaning equipment, toy laundry equipment, bottles and nip-ples, overnite cases, adult clothing to dress up in.
Equipment for dramatic hospital play—baby crib, rubber dolls, bedside table and equipment, doctor's kit, bandage, bandage scissors, adhesive tape, equip-ment which could be used to play doctor and nurse.
Toys for dramatic transportation play—trains, trucks, automobiles, airplanes, fleet of boats, fire engines, toys for store play, farm and barnyard animals
Pounding toys
Painting easel for brush, paints and crayons

Raw materials for creative self-expres-sion—crayons, paint, chalk, clay, finger paint, scissors, construction paper, bells, rhythm sticks, tambou-rines, cymbals, xylophones and drums
Pets—birds, rabbits or hamsters

DEVELOPMENT AND GUIDANCE DURING THE SCHOOL-AGE PERIOD (6 TO 10 YEARS)

Physical and Emotional Prepared-ness Is Essential for Success in School. The basis for the child's adjustment and success in school lies in the first years of his life. His rela-tions with teachers and peers will be determined by the character structure that he has acquired through interpersonal experiences with his parents and siblings. His adjustment in school will be deter-mined by his feelings about him-self, siblings and parents, by the degree of independence and security that he has acquired, by the degree to which he has gained control of his sexual and aggressive drives, by the extent to which his sexual curi-osity has been satisfied and by the way he has learned to relate himself to his playmates.

Intelligence and the emotional climate of his school environment are factors which influence success in school, but more important is the way in which he approaches the learning process. His approach to his teacher and scholastic activities is not only determined by what he meets in the school situation; it is influenced by all that has gone before. Many normal and superior children fail in their first years at school because they are physically unfit or are unprepared emotionally to use school activities effectively.

Life in the school-age period brings conflict and new difficult developmental tasks to surmount. Physical growth slows down and frees energy for personality growth. *To succeed in this stage of growth the child needs emotional freedom to acquire intellectual and physical skills (ego), to break away from parental dependence and become a part of a group. He also needs energy available to gain increased control over his sexual and aggressive drives through strengthened inner controls (conscience). In addition, he needs to learn the laws of his society through play and school activities.* All of these tasks are difficult ones requiring effort, perseverance, and the capacity to give up many personal desires that involve frustration. To surmount the tasks he also needs confidence in himself and trust in those who are guiding him. Acquiring mental skills is an important developmental task, but the other ones are equally essential for personality growth.

Growth and Experience Prepare the Child for Acquiring Mental Skills. MENTAL GROWTH. So much of what might be called basic learning has been accomplished before the child enters formal school life that this latter seems to be a time of expansion in the fields of knowledge that he has already acquired. He can learn arithmetic because he has the number concept. He can learn to read because he can recognize the shapes of things. He can learn geography because he has a sense of shape and direction. He can learn history because he has a sense of time. He can acquire his own vocabulary and learn another language because he has one already.

He has learned to use his mind, to reason, to solve problems in his preschool years; and he can go on to more complex problems in this stage of his development because of previous experiences and because growth of his nervous system makes him biologically ready to begin to learn to read and write.

Mental growth or the learning to function as an intelligent human being will take place according to a general pattern. The sequence of this general pattern and the approximate ages when mental skills are acquired can be outlined. However, widely varying individual differences must be expected, for they are as characteristic of mental growth as they are of physical.

THE USE OF INTELLIGENCE TESTS. Standardized intelligence and personality tests provide understanding of a child's mental and personality development. These tests have come to play an important part in helping adults toward an understanding of the child in home, in school and at work. There has been a mistaken tendency on the part of some individuals to regard them as infallible, an oft-repeated reaction to new developments in many fields of endeavor. They are not infallible, but they are extremely useful tools when employed by those who are skilled in interpreting their results and in recognizing their limitations.

Intelligence tests are divided into group and individual tests. The group tests are less reliable than are the individual ones. However, they are practical in school situations. They aid teachers in understanding the child's capacities for achievement and guide them in formulating plans for their education.

Intelligence tests are usually reported in terms of I. Q. (intelligence quotient), which is arrived at by dividing the mental age by the chronologic age and multiplying by 100. A child who has an I. Q. between 90 and 110 would be said to have shown the intelligence to be expected of a child of his age. The child's mental age is arrived at by listing his ability to perform those items in the test which have been found possible for most children of his age. If he can perform those at a higher age level, his mental age is correspondingly higher. It may be that he can perform some items at a higher age level and others at a lower. The system of scoring is such that the mental age can be computed in spite of the marked individual difference in performance.

One isolated test is of far less value in studying a child than is a series of tests given at different age levels. By doing this, it is possible to check the child against his own development as well as against the standardized picture of development. Tests for infants and those at the preschool level covering motor development rather than language, as well as tests for school-age children and adults, have been worked out.

Personality Growth, the Result of Experience in the Home, the School and the Community. There are problems for the child to face in school, but there are also many opportunities for gratification. As the mental skills of the period are accomplished, the child feels strength in his personality. His feelings of confidence and self-esteem expand, and he revels in his new knowledge, and the things that he learns to do. In this period the child's curiosity expands from the subject of himself and his parents to other aspects of life about him. He is avidly interested in the activities of school and in learning about the world in which he lives. His interests take him away from home—to museums, airports, parks, clubs, playgrounds—to the country to fish, swim, hunt and to learn about birds, animals and vegetation.

His interests and impulses toward growth compel the child to seek friendships with his peers. No longer is he satisfied with the attention of his parents. After he has surmounted the task of adjustment to his teacher and the learning process, his interests expand. He feels a need to find security, satisfaction and a way of life from experiences with his peers. The groupings change in this period. The preschool child played with both boys and girls; the school-age child wants a "gang" of his own sex. They draw off into little groups and follow their particular interests. Through identification with those of their own sex, they acquire characteristics of masculinity or femininity. They also have opportunities to find their places in a group, to learn the laws of fair play, to respect the rights of others, to work through the feelings of rivalry, to find outlet for their aggressive feelings and to master their fears.

Growth during this period of development entails conflict and frustration. Parental standards are different from those of the child's group. He wants both parental acceptance and security and satisfaction in his life within the group. As a result he experiences conflict and anxiety. If he succumbs to parental standards, he will remain dependent and be deprived of the experiences he needs for growth. If he identifies with his group and follows their codes; he experiences anxiety because his newly formed conscience or inner voice says, "This is wrong." He feels guilty and he has a problem to solve. The way he solves it will depend upon past experiences with his parents and upon their attitudes toward him in this stage of development.

The child needs freedom to venture forth and become a part of the group outside his family. When his parents understand his needs for growth, they will provide this freedom. They will know that he needs their love expressed in new ways. They will continue to give him their undivided attention when life in school or within the group brings more frustration than he can bear; they will continue to give him security for his emotional needs. But they will also recognize that his teacher and peers need to become increasingly more important to him. They will accept the changes in behavior which come through association with his gang. They will let him wear the togs the group approve of and permit him to do most of the things the other kids do. They will accept his moments of rebellion and devaluation of them as important people because they know it is a necessary phase of his growth. If he continues to do as Mother says, his conscience cannot become modified by peer interaction. And he will miss experiences which help to turn his interest away from his parents and to learn to get along with his contemporaries.

Play with others provides opportunities for mental, social, physical and emotional growth. Through play the child learns new skills, gains knowledge and self-confidence. He learns to sacrifice his wishes for the benefit of the group; he learns to conform to their self-imposed rules and regulations; he learns to depend upon the emotional satisfactions that come from relations with contemporaries; he learns to adapt himself to the outside world—to discover the meaning of life in his own way.

Observation of school-age children at play shows what takes place as a result of interaction with peers. The play of school-age children is different from the play of preschoolers. They are concerned with skill and perfection, with rules and regulations and in learning to become self-directing individuals. They feel a need to learn to control themselves, to abide by the rules of the game and the group. Instinctively, they are trying to master their fears and gain control of their sexual and aggressive drives.

Personality growth is the outgrowth of parental and teacher guidance and group interaction. Parental and teacher guidance is necessary to help the child sublimate or redirect his impulses into constructive activities. With wise discipline the child's capacity to control impulses becomes strengthened in this period, and he develops increased independence and new powers of self-direction. *As a result he needs less direction and needs permission to be as self-directing as he is capable of being.* He enjoys and is proud of the independence that comes from being able to take care of himself. He feels depreciated when adults fail to recognize the many things he is able to do for himself. No longer does he need the directives essential for the preschool child who has not yet learned what is expected of him. The school-age child *knows* when it is time to go to school, time to go to bed or to get ready for his daily trip to the physiotherapy departments. And he feels respected when his mother or nurse recognizes the inner strength of character that he possesses.

Broadened social experiences also bring personality growth. Through group experience the child acquires new strength within himself. He gains new physical and social skills which give him security and a place in the affections of his peers. He also acquires stronger inner resources which prepare him to accomplish the developmental tasks of adolescence which are the most difficult of all tasks to surmount.

In addition to the play materials listed above, the following equipment is needed to meet the play needs of the older child:

Puzzles of graded complexity
Construction blocks for making buildings
Construction equipment for making airplanes, space ships, vehicles and mobiles
Tinker toys, erector sets, etc.
Materials for pottery, leather, papier-mâché, jewelry, block printing, crepe-paper crafts
Materials for making doll clothes
Materials for scrapbooks of collector's items
Paper dolls
Costumes—policeman, Indian, baseball players, etc.
Marionettes

Card and table games, including Anagrams, Animal Lotto, author and travel games

DEVELOPMENT AND GUIDANCE DURING PREADOLESCENCE (10 TO 12 YEARS)

Psychological Growth Brings Purposeful Changes in Behavior. Preadolescence, the 2-year period prior to the onset of puberty brings changes in behavior. By 10 years of age the comfortably adjusted child has acquired superb mastery of himself and of his environment. He is sympathetic, well-mannered, courteous, diligent, co-operative and self-directing. These accomplishments make both the child and his parents secure and satisfied with themselves. However, this period is one of short duration. Parents no sooner relax and revel in their accomplishments than they begin to be aware that changes in behavior are occurring. His composure, control and thoughtfulness gradually diminish. His activity increases as he redoubles his efforts to master reality in preparation for the physiologic changes which he intuitively knows are going to come.

The change in behavior which comes in preadolescence has purpose; it loosens up the child's character, provides further opportunities to resolve old conflicts and problems that were incompletely solved before; and it makes reorganization of personality during adolescence a possibility. *Preadolescence is a period during which the individual needs to gain the ego strength that he will need to make healthy solutions to the conflicts of adolescence.*

The preadolescent is filled with abounding energy. He is full of ideas and experiments with every conceivable project known to children. He is active incessantly and seems to recognize the behavior which annoys his elders the most. Part of his activity is the result of his driving need to assert himself and impress others with his independence. Part of it stems from the supply of energy that he has at his disposal. He uses most of his energy in constructive activities that help him to master reality. However, some of it spills over into finger drumming, feet tapping and impulsive behavior of one kind or another which relieves his tension.

There are other characteristics of preadolescent behavior which are often criticized because the purpose of the newly developing behavior is misunderstood. The preadolescent is preoccupied because he is absorbed in himself, his development and in the activities of his important "gang." He shuns his parents' interest in his growth and excludes them from his innermost thoughts. The controls that he had formerly seem to vanish; he becomes exhibitionistic, unsympathetic, greedy, annoying, sloppy and negativistic temporarily. Chores that he formerly enjoyed become bugbears — "the things his parents hate to do," "unimportant," "rot," "the result of the old-fashioned parents he happened to acquire." His interest in school work often diminishes, and he conveniently "forgets" to do those things that his parents want him to do first and foremost. Old problem behavior reappears which his parents thought had been outgrown forever. He devalues his parents,

seeks an adult friend of the same sex to identify himself with, emulate, idealize and obtain satisfaction for his continuing dependent needs. He looks longingly on the family situation of his friends. He is unappreciative. Nothing his parents do seems to please him. His parent of the same sex is the object of most of his criticism.

Sustaining Good Adult-Preadolescent Relationships With Democratic Guidance Is Essential for Growth. The changes in behavior bring anxiety to both the preadolescent and the adults unless the adults who live and work with him understand his needs for growth. It is infinitely easier to accept and work with the preadolescent if one realizes that he *needs* to assert himself, rebel and depreciate others in the process of working through his conflict between dependence and independence. He does not hate the adult he depreciates; he is merely trying to prove to himself and his world of associates that he is grown-up—that he really does not need them as much as he did before. He continues to have powerful dependent needs but he cannot tolerate having them satisfied in the same way that he could when he accepted himself as a child. Now accepting dependent gratification from his parent makes him feel infantile. His behavior manifests the way that he obtains his goal without accompanying anxiety.

Sustaining adult-preadolescent relationships with democratic guidance is imperative to support the youngster in surmounting the developmental tasks of the period. His changing behavior needs acceptance. He continues to need limits and the strength of his parents' support. He cannot completely direct himself by any means. His impulsiveness is heightened in this stage of development. He needs help in accepting himself as he is and in finding ways to channelize his feelings and energy. Recreational therapy provides outlets for his feelings, builds self-respect and provides a way to use the influx of energy that he has at his disposal. He accepts guidance which considers his new preadolescent status and helps him to handle himself more independently. He loathes the kind that he has experienced as a child and rebels at autocratic discipline which fails to recognize his personal powers. He is approaching adolescence. The more the adults in his environment can do to build up his self-esteem, the more adequately he will be prepared to solve the many personal problems that are a normal part of adolescence.

Development and Guidance During Adolescence

Adolescence is the crucial stage of personality development which begins with the onset of physical maturity and merges gradually into young adulthood. Among all the age periods adolescence creates the most difficult problems to solve. During the space of a few years the adolescent must make his preparations to take his place as an interdependent member of society. *To attain emotional maturity, the adolescent needs to find and accept himself and his sexual role, resolve his conflict between dependence and independence and emancipate himself from his attachment to his parents. He also needs to choose and become prepared for his future career.*

The adolescent's past experiences influence the way he will approach and resolve his problems. All that he has experienced prior to adolescence will become reflected in his behavior. The adolescent who has trust in himself and others will approach his problems with courage, hope and confidence. He also needs a character structure that is strong enough to master the increased potency of his sexual and aggressive drives. If he has these personality traits, he will waste less energy on anxiety over the problems he faces and will be able to solve them in a manner more satisfying to himself and society.

The child who has been deprived of supportive relationships prior to adolescence will be less well prepared to tackle new tasks. He will be encumbered with a multitude of old problems and conflicts and have excessive anxiety to master. He will have fewer inner resources to use in solving his problems. As a result he will need more understanding and support than the individual who enters adolescence prepared by growth-promoting relationships within his family.

Self-Discovery, Self-Understanding and Personality Reorganization Are Essential for Maturity. The hormonal changes which mark the onset of physical maturity stimulate physical and psychological growth. The adolescent has a rapidly changing body and new bodily functions to which he must become adjusted. He also has new feelings, attitudes and interests. His impulses are stronger, and old patterns of behavior cease to keep him in emotional equilibrium. These changes bring anxiety and uncertainty which are manifested in vacillating, unpredictable and oftentimes impetuous behavior.

The adolescent's anxiety, uncertainty and searching for mature patterns of behavior also become manifested in behavior which is paradoxic. One minute he is bursting with pride in his newly formed body; the next minute he is embarrassed with it. He desperately needs advice on all manner of things but when it comes he flies into a rage. One moment he loves his parents deeply and values their way of life and their qualities of parenthood. In the next breath he loathes the ground they walk on and can see no good in anything they think or do. He is daring, brash and courageous; simultaneously he is cautious, fearful lest his body is weak or abnormal. He is often hypochrondriacal. He forges ahead toward those of the opposite sex and then runs away from them, denying any interest whatsoever in their persons. He criticizes with abandon but simultaneously conforms like an automaton and wants to be exactly like those he berates. His ideals express utopia. He wants to change the world, yet he wants it to remain exactly as it is. One minute he is abounding in energy, the next he is completely depleted and finds the easiest of tasks an insufferable burden. Is it any wonder that his parents say, "I just can't understand him?" And does not the teen-ager's behavior spell a mental state of confusion and turmoil?

The adolescent's behavior is not only trying to himself but it is also frustrating to his parents. It is not easy to live with an unpredictable, vacillating teen-ager. His parents never can anticipate his reactions, and 99 times out of 100 they get a response different from what they expected. Parents of a teen-ager never can be right for long, no matter how hard they try. It takes secure, stable parents to maintain their equilibrium while they are living with an adolescent.

Many parents of adolescents need understanding as much as their children do. Many parents have repressed their adolescent trials, heartaches and bouts of rebellion and view their teen-ager's behavior with acute apprehension. Some are not emotionally ready to handle the problem of guiding their teen-agers. They get confused, anxious and uncertain. They need help in understanding themselves and their youngsters. Unless they get it they may inflict an unreasonably strict regimen of discipline on their teen-agers or give up in despair, leaving them alone and unsupported.

Learning to understand a new self requires self-examination, exploratory experiences, knowledge, parental acceptance and guidance. To solve his problems, the adolescent becomes absorbed in himself, daydreams and tests himself out in competition with others. He also seeks security from associations with his age-mates and struggles to find solutions which relieve his anxiety and help him to feel more competent.

The adolescent needs acceptance as a growing individual and guidance which helps him to discover his powers and his limitations. He needs the help of strong parents and professional workers who understand his anxiety and support him with their strength. He needs interest in himself as a person and faith in his capacity to find solutions to his personal problems. The adolescent must find his own solutions to his problems. He will, if he is counseled in a way which increases his self-esteem, confidence and understanding of himself and others of both sexes. Those who guide the adolescent also need patience, tolerance and the intuitive insight which is necessary to appraise his capacity to utilize freedom constructively.

The adolescent continues to need limits which are set by his parents, teachers and by his nurses if he is a patient in the hospital. The young adolescent's personality is disorganized from the changes of preadolescence. In addition, he has powerfully strengthened drives to master and an intense desire to become independent of his parents immediately. But he is not psychologically ready to be independent. He does not have inner controls which provide consistent mastery of himself. Until he acquires a new set of inner controls which permit socially acceptable and personally satisfying emotional outlets, he needs wisely chosen and diplomatically imposed limits. These limits on the one hand must be sufficiently flexible so that he has opportunities for growth. Yet on the other hand they must constrain him from actions which will merely serve to enhance his anxiety. For example, it is reasonable to encourage a 15-year-old to go to adequately supervised social parties, but it is unwise to subject him to the temptations of an unchaperoned house party. The adolescent who is not con-

fined within reasonable limits is left unsupported and unprotected. The unsupported adolescent may respond with impulsiveness which leads to delinquency or other signs of mental ill-health. Or he may defend himself from anxiety by becoming so overcontrolled that he blocks his opportunities for legitimate satisfactions and further personality growth. There are adolescents who respond to unrestricted freedom as if it had given them license to express themselves fully. Such behavior neither meets their needs for growth nor considers the needs of others. There are other adolescents who become frightened when they are given more freedom than they know how to utilize. In an attempt to find their previous comfort they return to preadolescent relationships and modes of behavior.

The adolescent needs limits which change as experience promotes growth in self-understanding and mastery. Guided experiences which foster feelings of success, self-esteem and security in his relationships with others prepare him to handle increasingly larger amounts of freedom. Unless he is given freedom to explore increasingly more difficult tasks, his opportunities for personality growth will be thwarted. He is likely to wind up in unwholesome rebellion or equally unhealthy submission.

Emancipation from Parents Is Essential for Maturity. Growth of the child's love life normally progresses through stages which begin with simple love of himself, in which full personality development ends with a love of humanity. The newborn infant is incapable of loving anyone else but himself. As he grows, the recurrent satisfying relationships with his mother permits his capacity for love to extend so as to include her. Later, his father becomes an object of his affection. Girls become deeply attached to their fathers, who represent their first male sweethearts and the objects of their tenderest feelings. Boys during early childhood tend to direct their warmest feelings toward their mothers. For a time the boy's father and the girl's mother become rivals and objects of their hostility — feelings which make them feel anxious. To alleviate this anxiety they repress their hostility and permit only warm feelings to remain in their conscious minds. This makes it possible for them to imitate their rival parents and begin the long process of becoming a man like father or a woman like mother.

Rivalry with brothers and sisters within a family is a natural part of the growing-up process. Children within a family enjoy each other as playmates. However, they also find that the presence of siblings results in friction and rivalry for their parents' love. Gradually, through constructive experiences in the home, children outgrow their rivalrous and ambivalent feelings toward their brothers and sisters.

When the child acquires increased security in his relationships with his parents, his love interests expand to include those outside his immediate family. Playmates of either sex become the object of the preschool child's affections. His relationships with them help to wean him from the consuming love he feels for his parent of the opposite sex. In the school-age period, the child turns his love interest to those of his own sex. These attachments provide security at a time when he has an urgent need for companionship but is as yet unready for friends of the opposite sex.

When puberty comes, the adolescent's love for his parent of the opposite sex is revived, and he has to struggle to emancipate himself from it. He must free himself of this tie in order to develop relationships with members of the opposite sex outside his family. In the process of weaning himself from his parent he becomes attracted to persons of the opposite sex who are often years older than he. The next step in development is general interests in age-mates of the opposite sex. He dates many persons. This experience gives him understanding of the opposite sex, brings security in his capacity for acceptance and should sharpen his powers of discrimination. After he has gained security in his capacity for popularity, he begins to focus on one person. He "goes steady," "gets pinned" or engaged and makes plans for marriage. After the individual has become adjusted to marriage, his love expands, and he wants children to nurture. When parenthood is accomplished successfully, his interests expand to the needs of humanity.

The above sequence in normal development takes place through wholesome relationships within the adolescent's family. His parents are the objects of his greatest attachment. He must free himself from his attachment to them before he has energy available for a mature, heterosexual adjustment in marriage. Therefore, it is logical to assume that emancipation must take place within the adolescent's home. Moderate degrees of rebellion are natural. He has to find fault, defend himself against his unconscious love for his parent and search for standards and a philosophy of life which are his very own.

Emancipating himself and becoming emotionally free to develop mature adult relationships is an arduous task which precipitates a repeated series of advancement and regression to childish modes of behavior. The sequence of development outlined above may give the impression that progress is simple and that the individual merely moves from one level into the next. Progress in personality development is not this rapid or as smooth. Often there is forward movement toward the opposite sex, then withdrawal to the more comfortable relationships that he has experienced before. There are bursts of independence, braggadocio and exaggerated competitiveness—then periods of dependence which are more pronounced than during the school-age period.

The adolescent is in conflict; he wants both independence and the comfort that he has known before. One part of him wants adventure, adult pleasures and responsibilities; another part wants to cling to childish pleasures and escape from the trials of adulthood. Conflict generates anxiety and uncertainty of his capacities. He moves forward to explore and test himself and then becomes fearful of the responsibility that growing-up entails. Anxiety makes him regress. Babyish modes of behavior make him feel inadequate. This feeling is less tolerable.

To alleviate his anxiety he asserts his independence and tries again. Over and over again this cycle of behavior repeats itself! Gradually his powers expand. As they do he gets pleasure, security and trust in himself. He discovers that adulthood is more pleasurable than childhood. When he makes this discovery he is on his way to becoming an emotionally mature member of his society.

The adolescent is fortified when the adults in his world understand the reasons why he is erratic, rebellious, competitive, self-concerned and contradictory. The adolescent is in the process of becoming reorganized, integrated and goal directed. When his parents and professional workers believe in him and understand the many problems that he is facing in the process of growing up, he will have the strength that he needs for healthy personality reorganization.

Preparation for a Career Is Essential for Success. It is obvious why an adolescent needs to know himself to find a career that will bring satisfaction and productivity. When a person is fitted for his work, selects it independently and enjoys it, the possibilities of creativity and success are infinitely greater. *The adolescent needs help in appraising his abilities, and the opportunities presented by the different fields of endeavor. He also needs freedom to make his own decisions concerning his career.* He will need guidance in learning how to prepare himself for his chosen career. With understanding help, he will be able to think through his needs and plan his preparation wisely.

The adolescent is emotionally ready for help in becoming prepared for marriage and parenthood. Logically, preparation for marriage and parenthood should be provided in the home. However, the school and the church must be ready to supplement his preparation, for many adolescents are in need of it. A well-prepared school nurse can contribute to a program of education for family living.

SITUATIONS FOR FURTHER STUDY

1. Why should pediatric nurses be concerned with the prenatal period?

2. When does preparation for parenthood begin? What are the factors which influence an individual's capacities for parenthood? Of what value is preparation for parenthood to the child and his parents?

3. What is the nurse's role in helping expectant parents become prepared for the experiences of the maternity cycle?

4. Of what value to the nurse is a knowledge of personality development?

5. Select a child under 3 years of age for whom you are caring in the ward. Read the section on development which pertains to the stage of growth he is in. Read similar discussions in other books which are listed in the references at the end of this chapter. Observe the child each day and record what you see, hear and feel. Use the following questions to guide your observations and study.

A. Describe your patient and his behavior.

B. What is the child's background of experience within his family?

C. What did you learn from reading that helped you to understand this child?

D. What are the needs of a child in this stage of development?

E. How does his behavior differ from that described in the texts you read? What factors do you think have influenced these differences?

F. What are his problems? How have they been intensified by his illness and hospitalization?

G. What kind of adjustment is this child making to his illness, treatment and separation from his family? Is he making a healthy adjustment to hospitalization? What are the factors which have helped him to make a healthy adjustment in the hospital? If this adjustment is unhealthy, what are the factors which are preventing him from mastering the experience?

H. Describe his behavior toward you and the care that you give him.

I. What have you observed about his relationship with his mother? His father? From observation of his behavior with other children and of his verbal communications with you, what kind of relationship do you think he has with his siblings?

J. How has observation of his behavior influenced the way you care for him? What care and guidance does he need? Have you been able to meet his needs? Describe ways in which you have met his needs. If you have not been able to meet them, think through the factors which prevented you from doing so.

K. Visit the child's home after he has been discharged from the hospital for 1 week. In the home, observe the following:

(1) How did the child and the mother respond to you as a visi-

tor in the home? Describe their behavior toward you.

(2) How did the child respond to returning home? What changes in behavior did his mother observe? What changes in behavior did you observe? What do you think evoked these changes? What do you think these changes in behavior mean? How do you think they will influence his relationship with his mother? How do you think his mother feels about the changes in behavior that she has observed? What did she say and do which indicated her feelings toward the child and his change in behavior?

6. Why is need satisfaction necessary during the earliest months of life?

7. What changes would be necessary in hospital policies to meet the basic emotional requirements of infants and preschool children? What prevents these changes from being made?

8. Describe a newborn infant who is assigned to you in the ward. What are his physical and behavior characteristics?

9. What are the needs of the infant during the adjustment period (birth to 3 months)?

10. If a year-old child received little or no social stimulation during the first year of his life, what effect do you think it might have upon him?

11. How can an adult tell when a baby is ready for stimulation? What value is stimulation to him?

12. How do an infant's needs change during the first year of life? What brings these changes?

13. What are the 6-year molars? Are they part of the deciduous set of teeth?

14. When would you take a child to the dentist for the first time, and what would be your reasons for taking him? How would you prepare him for the experience?

15. Observe infants of 1 month, 6 months and 1 year of age. Indicate some of the differences in their social, motor and emotional responses. Observe 2 or 3 infants of approximately the same age and indicate the differences in their responses, describing them as to personalities. Have you any clues as to the factors affecting their differences in behavior?

16. What types of toys do infants need during their first year of life? Why do they need the types that you suggest?

17. What might some of the reasons be why a 4-year-old child sucks his thumb in the hospital? What would you do if this 4-year-old were your patient?

18. What purpose does play serve in the life of the child? Illustrate with use of observational material from your experience with children in the ward.

19. How does growth in independence affect personality development? Describe a situation in which you observed the effect of teaching in a child.

20. How does weaning affect personality development? What might be the effects of early weaning (before 6 months of life)? How can a nurse use knowledge of the effects of abrupt weaning on personality development?

21. What are the developmental tasks of the 1- to 3-year-old child? How can you use knowledge of the problems of the 1- to 3-year-old and of the way in which he can be helped to surmount them in your care of young children?

22. What results might coercive toilet training have on a child's personality development?

23. How is personality growth in the training period influenced by the guidance that he received during the first year of life?

24. How can the adult help the child pass through the negativistic stage of personality development?

25. Of what importance is it for the child to acquire a good concept of himself? How can the adult help the child to acquire a feeling of power and yet learn his limitations?

26. How do the needs of the 3- to 6-year-old child differ from those of the infant and the toddler?

27. Why would death of a parent during preschool years be more potentially traumatizing than in a later stage of development?

28. What are some of the questions that children have asked you in the ward and what did they reveal to you as to the child's development and personality? How did you handle his questions, and what guided you in behaving as you did?

29. What is the significance of the preschool child's questions pertaining to sex? How do you think they should be handled? What influences your thinking? Of what value is wholesome sex education?

30. What do preschool children learn from playing together? Observe a group of nursery school children playing together. List the things that you consider the children have learned during the play period. What did you learn that would assist you in planning for the play of hospitalized preschool children?

31. Why does the child of preschool years need help in learning to relinquish his parent of the opposite sex? What help does he require?

32. What are the reasons why preschool children have fears pertaining to bodily injury? Of what significance to you is this knowledge in giving nursing care to preschool children?

33. What factors play a part in determining the kind of adjustment that a preschool child will make to hospitalization?

34. Observe a teacher in a nursery school. What attitudes do you think that she has toward the children? What do you think her philosophy of guidance is? How did she encourage independence, self-expression and personality growth? How can you use the knowledge that you gained from observation in your care of hospitalized children?

35. What does emotional preparedness for school entail?

36. How does guidance during the first 5 years of life influence the child's opportunities to surmount the tasks of the school-age period?

37. How does the care of a school-age child differ from the care required by a preschool child?

38. How do the play interests and activities of the school-age child indicate his development from the preschool-age level? What play materials would you provide for well school-age children? How would you modify your list for ill and convalescent school-age children?

39. Observe school-age children on a playground. Describe their behavior. How does their play differ from the play of preschool children?

40. What are some of the possible reasons why bright children have difficulty in learning to read?

41. What behavior changes occur

in preadolescence? What is their purpose? Describe a preadolescent whom you have cared for in the ward. What problems did you have in caring for him? How did you handle them? How did his behavior differ from the behavior of 8- or 9-year-old children?

42. What behavior during preadolescence would indicate the child's need for expert guidance?

43. What are the developmental tasks of adolescence?

44. What are the common fears of the adolescent? How can the adults in his environment help him to master them?

45. What is entailed in the nursing care of the adolescent?

46. Why is adolescence such a conflictful period of development?, How does the adolescent manifest his confusion and anxiety?

47. How does guidance before adolescence affect the way an individual solves the conflicts of the final stage of personality development?

48. What behavior would manifest an adolescent's need for more skillful guidance than he was receiving?

BIBLIOGRAPHY

Aldrich, C. A., and Aldrich, Mary M.: Babies Are Human Beings, New York, Macmillan, 1946.

Bakwin, Harry: Loneliness in infants, Am. J. Dis. Child. **63**:30, 1942

Blake, Florence G.: The Child, His Parents and the Nurse, Philadelphia, Lippincott, 1954.

Breckenridge, M. E., and Vincent, E. L.: Child Development, ed. 2, Philadelphia, Saunders, 1947.

Burlingame, Dorothy, and Freud,

Anna: Infants Without Families, New York, Willard, 1934.

Caplan, Gerald: The mental hygiene role of the nurse in maternal and child care, Nursing Outlook **2**:14, 1954.

Dagliesch, Alice: First Experiences with Literature, New York, Scribner, 1937.

Duval, Evelyn Millis: Facts of Life and Love for Teen-agers, New York, Popular Library, 1953.

Erickson, Erik: Childhood and Society, New York, Norton, 1950.

Frank, Anne: The Diary of a Young Girl, New York, Pocket Books, Inc., 1953.

Gesell, Arnold, et al.: The Infant and Child in the Culture of Today, New York, Harper, 1943.

Glantz, Evelyn: Scrap Fun for Everyone, New York, Larch Book Co., 1944.

Goodrich, Frederick W.: Natural Childbirth, New York, Prentice-Hall, 1950.

Gruenberg, Sidonie: The Wonderful Story of How You Were Born, Garden City, N. Y., Hanover House, 1952.

Hartley, Ruth E., Frank, Lawrence K., and Goldenson, Robert M.: Understanding Children's Play, New York, Columbia, 1952.

Hymes, James: Understanding Your Child, New York, Prentice-Hall, 1952.

Isaacs, Susan: The Nursery Years, New York, Vanguard, 1929.

Josselyn, Irene: Psychosocial Development of Children, New York, Family Service Association of America, 1948.

————: The Adolescent and His World, New York, Family Service Association of America, 1952.

Kawin, Ethel: The Wise Choice of Toys, ed. 2, Chicago, Univ. Chicago Press, 1938.

Newkirk, Louis V., and Zutter, LaVada: Your Craft Book, Scranton, Pa., Internat. Textbook Co., 1946.

Redl, Fritz: Pre-adolescents: what makes them tick, Child Study 21: 44, 1943-1944.

Ribble, Margaret: The Rights of Infants, New York, Columbia, 1943.

Smith, Anne: Play for Convalescent Children, New York, Barnes, 1941.

Spock, Benjamin: Common Sense Book of Baby and Child Care, New York, Pocket Books, Inc., 1946.

————: The middle-aged child, Pennsylvania M. J. 50:1045, 1947.

Staff of The Child Study Association of America: When children ask about sex, (pamphlet), ed. 3, New York, Child Study Association of America, Inc., 1953.

Swift, E. H.: Step by Step in Sex Education, New York, Macmillan, 1946.

Weng, Lorraine: Group feeding for hospitalized children, J. Am. Dietet. A. 25:620, 1949.

Problems of Infancy and Childhood, Tr. of the first, second, third, fourth, and sixth conferences, New York, Macy, 1947, 1948, 1949, 1951, 1952.

Your child from 6-12 (pamphlet), Washington, Federal Security Agency, Children's Bureau, 1949.

Proceeding of the Midcentury White House Conference on Children and Youth, Raleigh, N. C., Health Publications Institute, 1951.

Infant care (pamphlet), Washington, Federal Security Agency, Social Service Administration, 1951.

The Child Health Conference as a Means of Guidance

GOALS, FUNCTIONS AND METHODS
ORGANIZATION AND PERSONNEL
CONDUCTING THE CONFERENCE

FUTURE GOALS IN HEALTH
   SUPERVISION
SITUATIONS FOR FURTHER STUDY

GOALS, FUNCTIONS AND METHODS

The need for adequate health supervision and child guidance has been shown to be essential. It is valuable both for the purpose of lowering mortality and morbidity rates and for the less tangible but possibly more far-reaching effects of increasing the health and the happiness of the children of the nation. The general methods have been outlined and discussed in the orientation chapters. In this chapter the nurse's functions will be considered.

The study of infants and children has progressed rapidly in recent years. The main problem which confronts nurses is to make available the results of child study to those who have the immediate responsibility for the care of infants and children. Obviously, the most important of these are the parents. The nurse has a tremendous responsibility for interpreting to them the wealth of material now available about the normal infant and child.

One of the most satisfactory means of communicating this knowledge is the Child Health Conference. The technics of the Child Health Conference can be applied also to other health-interpreting situations in which the pediatric nurse finds herself.

The forerunners of the Child Health Conference were the milk stations which were started in New York City just prior to the opening of the twentieth century in order to provide safe, properly prepared formulas for babies in an attempt to reduce the very high morbidity and mortality from gastroenteritis or summer diarrhea. Maintaining a safe milk supply for babies reduced the morbidity and mortality rates. The milk stations also became centers to which mothers could bring babies for examination and for advice.

As the mother's needs were felt, gradually they were met more and more adequately. Today there are Baby Health Stations, Well-Baby

Clinics, or Child Health Conferences throughout the country. The Child Health Conference is the name which probably best expresses their function and goal—optimum mental and physical health for every child through planned health supervision.

Planned health supervision of the child starts with good prenatal care and continues until he reaches school age. Good prenatal care is becoming more and more widely available. A mother who has had good prenatal care is better prepared to recognize the importance of continued health supervision for her child. When a child reaches school age, his health supervision ideally is taken over by the school system.

The nurse is often the person who interprets the child's need for health supervision. In the clinic the baby is immunized against diphtheria, whooping cough, tetanus and smallpox during his first year. He also receives other prophylaxis as may seem to be necessary or valuable. Often evidence of disease or abnormality will be discovered very early and referred to a doctor or a hospital, where early treatment may affect the prognosis favorably. In addition, guidance concerning feeding and readiness for learning experiences is available. The opportunities available to mothers require interpretation. Once a mother has attended a well-planned Child Health Conference, she usually discovers how much help she can find for the many problems which confront her when she begins to assume the responsibility of child-rearing. When she has made this discovery, her use of the conference undoubtedly will broaden.

The Child Health Conference is set up for the children who are not directly under the supervision of a physician elsewhere. Many mothers bring their children to the Child Health Conference for health supervision even though they may have a private physician when the child is ill. The Child Health Conference is introduced to mothers in many ways —during prenatal care, in the hospital when the baby is born or by a public health nurse who delivers the birth certificate of the baby and invites the mother to the conference at the same time.

It is the responsibility of every nurse to know the facilities of the community for well-baby health supervision so that she can interpret such services to mothers. The nurse caring for newborn babies needs this information. A nurse caring for sick babies needs equal preparation. The mother whose baby is discharged from the hospital is receptive to suggestion because she is doubly aware of the need for keeping her baby well. Hospital personnel need a definite well-worked-out plan whereby any baby discharged from the hospital inpatient or outpatient service is referred automatically to the most accessible Child Health Conference in order that his health supervision may be uninterrupted.

Places for the Child Health Conferences are chosen so that they are convenient, either by proximity or by easy transportation, for those who will come. The conferences may be held in a school, a church, or any other available place where the facilities can be made adequate. There is a growing tendency toward making the hospital a community-health center. Many times the Child Health Conference becomes one of its functions. Often such a Child Health

Conference is called a Well-Baby Clinic, distinctive from the usual connotation of the word *clinic,* having to do with illness.

ORGANIZATION AND PERSONNEL

The Child Health Conference may be voluntary in its organization and financial support, or, as it becomes recognized as a necessary public-health function, it may be taken over by the tax-supported or official agencies. In either case, the personnel requirements are the same.

The two essential members of the personnel group are the physician and the nurse. The physician, when possible, should be a pediatrician, or at least one who has had experience with children. The nurse in charge should have had work with children and a broad public-health experience. If other nurses are assigned to her, especially students, she will have the responsibility of interpreting to them the public-health aspects of the Child Health Conference. It is also her responsibility to plan for the public-health-nursing visits which follow the work of the conference. In some places it has been found possible for the nurse who makes visits in a certain district to be in charge of the Child Health Conference when the mothers and the children from her district are given their appointments. This has proved to be very valuable.

In addition to the nurse in charge, and possibly other nurses, other very desirable members of the personnel group are a nutritionist, social workers, a child-guidance advisor, a dental hygienist, a secretary and volunteers. Usually the volunteers are trained by the nurse in charge to carry out certain procedures during the conference. They relieve the nurses and others for the functions requiring their professional skill. The well-planned use of volunteer help serves also to interest and educate the community in the functions and the work of the Child Health Conference.

CONDUCTING THE CONFERENCE

THE PHYSICAL SET-UP

The physical set-up has certain prerequisites. The nurse is usually responsible for the best use of the physical resources. It is necessary to have at least 3 rooms, or partitioned spaces if several rooms are not available: (1) a reception and waiting room; (2) a dressing and weighing room; and (3) a room in which the doctor examines the child and holds his conference with the mother. Other rooms are desirable and can be well utilized, if available, for other conferences, for teaching exhibits and for play and office space. All these rooms must be light, as well as adequately heated and ventilated. Some source of water is necessary.

THE WAITING ROOM

The waiting room must be large and equipped in a way that is comfortable for all who attend at one time. It should be remembered that the waiting room is not only for adults but also for well children for whom play space needs to be provided. Small furniture is very desirable. Even young children would rather be independent enough not to be held on their mothers' laps during the waiting period. Also, the waiting room should be thought of as a room where learning can take place. Posters, charts, exhibits and demonstrations are utilized if they are well presented. People waiting are more likely to observe and absorb new material than people who are in a hurry.

A friendly, pleasant atmosphere is more important than elaborate equipment. Mothers must want to come. The hostess, a volunteer or a nurse, needs to be ready to help them feel welcome. The value of the visit, or even future visits, may depend on the first contact. It is very desirable to have a "play nurse" or "play teacher" for the preschool children. A "play nurse" not only makes the waiting period pleasant for the children but she also gives their mothers an opportunity to take advantage of the educational exhibits. She also makes it possible for the mothers to have an opportunity to talk with each other. In addition, mothers may have an opportunity to learn ways of handling a tempestuous, negativistic or withdrawn child by observing how a "play nurse" finds ways to help him feel more secure in a strange environment.

WEIGHING AND MEASURING ROOM

The room where children are weighed, measured and have their temperatures taken should be separate. A place should be available for undressing and dressing. A basket or bag for each child's clothing to prevent loss is also required.

Mothers will have many questions at the time their children are being weighed and measured. They will be interested in height and weight tables and will want to know how their children stand in relation to others. They will need to know that height and weight tables are interpreted with caution; that a steady rate of growth is more important than the total height or weight; that growth and development show wide variation in different babies but that the patterns are similar. The mother may learn a new skill from watching a skillful nurse—how to lift the infant onto the scales, take his temperature or how to utilize safety measures in handling, etc. Mothers will ask many questions. Some the nurse can answer by interpreting the knowledge that she has gleaned from specialists. Others she will refer to the doctor to whom the mother will talk next.

THE DOCTOR'S CONFERENCE

The doctor's examination and conference are the focus of the visit. Whenever possible the nurse should be present at this conference. When this is impossible, she will have to rely on the notes which the doctor added to the record. The doctor makes a general physical examination in which he notes growth and development and points out significant aspects to the mother. He observes the child's state of nutrition and his general condition and looks for any abnormality, defect or evidence of illness. If there is any need of correction or therapeutic management, the child is referred to the proper source, i.e., a private physician or hospital clinic. Frequently, early evidence of defect or illness may be found on routine health-supervision examination. As a result the child is cared for more promptly.

After the examination the doctor confers with the mother. He interprets the findings of his physical examination. He gives her an opportunity to talk about any problems that she may have. Together they discuss the way in which previous suggestions for care have been carried out. Also, the mother is given suggestions for any changes in the baby's care, such as addition of new foods into the diet, increased exposure to sun, readiness for help in learning bowel control, weaning, etc.

Any immunization, test or blood work which is needed is usually done at this time. The nurse prepares the equipment. She also prepares the child and gives him attention while the needle is being inserted. The mother should be the provider of comfort as soon as the procedure is completed. Blood for a serologic test for syphilis may be taken. After a tuberculin test, some arrangement must be made for the return of the child for reading of the result.

The Nurse's Conference

After the conference with the doctor, the mother needs an opportunity to talk with a nurse. The conference with the nurse serves to amplify and interpret the doctor's suggestions for care. It also serves to give the mother an opportunity to talk further about the problems which are concerning her. Many times a mother will be more at ease with a nurse and feel free to ask questions which she has hesitated to ask the doctor. However, her ease in asking questions or revealing her problems will depend largely upon the nurse's approach to her. The effectiveness of the conference will be dependent upon the confidence that the mother has in the nurse and upon the degree to which she feels accepted by her. If the nurse is truly interested in the mother and is motivated to want to understand her, she will reflect her attitudes in her approach. The nurse's attitudes and feelings determine her capacity to establish the kind of relationship which helps the mother to feel comfortable and gives her the support and the constructive help that she needs.

The purpose of the nurse's conference is to meet the mother's need. To accomplish this objective, the nurse needs to be ready to listen with a genuine desire to gain understanding of her as an individual. Ideally, the mother should see the same nurse each time she comes to the Child Health Conference. When such a plan is in effect, the benefits of the experience for both individuals are multiplied. If the mother finds interest, a nonjudicial and nonautocratic attitude, it will be easier for her to disclose the problems that are troubling her. They may be in relation to the doctor's suggestions or to some aspect of development or behavior which she does not understand. When a mother discovers that the nurse is interested in her problems, eventually she will look to her for help in gaining understanding of her child. In the meantime the nurse will have obtained increased understanding of the mother and of her situation. As a result she will be in a better position to help her.

Mothers come to the Child Health Conference seeking satisfaction of varying kinds of needs. Many times a mother is only seeking reassurance and security in knowing that her judgment is sound. Some come seeking information, some only to have their children examined medically, and others because they feel that it is the thing to do. There are mothers who use the Child Health Conference for a social experience. They enjoy meeting other mothers, sharing their problems and dressing their youngster up for inspection. Many mothers come feeling discouraged, perplexed and fatigued. An opportunity to talk often helps them through a period of confusion. If they find genuine interest and understanding, they will leave the conference more relaxed and with increased strength to solve their problems more effectively. Some mothers come with realization of their mistakes. They feel guilty, inadequate and insecure. The nurse's task is to lessen their guilt and provide the understanding that they need to feel more competent in the maternal role. The nurse should remember that the mother who fails to discharge her duties well is probably an individual who in turn has received insufficient mothering during her childhood. She needs understanding and respect, help and approval. The nurse does not need to feel that a conference is a failure because she does not do any direct teaching. Often the nurse's greatest contribution lies in her ability to alleviate anxiety and guilt and provide supportive help. This will be the inevitable outcome if she is accepting, generous with her interest and objective in her feelings toward the individual.

A mother may come to the Child Health Conference feeling hostile toward her child and yet be exceedingly guilty because she feels that way. All mothers get angry at their children sometimes. Many mothers

long for the days when they were free of the responsibility of child-rearing. The feeling is natural. Child-rearing 24 hours a day, 365 days a year is a responsibility of great magnitude. It is also a tiring and oftentimes perplexing job. Negative feelings which arise upon occasion are inevitable, normal and understandable. Mothers need help to accept such feelings when they arise. If they can accept them as universal, they will have less guilt and anxiety. Also, they will be able to accept their children's angry feelings and the "I hate you, mother" that comes from their offspring in moments of frustration. When mothers can express their hostile feelings and air the burdens that they are experiencing, pleasanter relationships with their children are usually the outcome. Feelings which are kept suppressed bring guilt and tension. Energy, which should be available for loving, is used to keep unacceptable feelings under control.

Mothers also come to the Child Health Conference with questions concerning thumb sucking, negativism, rivalry, masturbation, etc. There are no formulae that nurses can give mothers which will solve their problems. The cause of prolonged thumb sucking, for instance, varies in different children. The nurse can help the mother think through possible causes of the "problem" behavior. Often in talking about the problem with a sympathetic listener, the mother's anxiety becomes dissipated. As a result she is more capable of recognizing and meeting her child's needs. In many instances the mother is worrying about behavior that is common to all children during the age period which her child is traversing. Often the mere knowledge that study of children has disclosed the fact that certain behavior is universally found in children of her youngster's age helps the mother to gain perspective. Understanding the above fact often decreases the emotional tension which has contributed to the child's insecurity and hence has increased his problem.

Anticipatory guidance is a preventive measure. It alleviates anxiety and prepares parents to understand the developmental problems which come with growth. When the nurse-mother relationship is constructive, the mother will welcome guidance which prepares her to recognize and handle developmental phases of growth. The nurse can interpret the growth changes which are to come. She can give the mother insight into the problems that the child will be experiencing. Then when changes in behavior come, the mother will be more able to recognize their normality and understand their role in personality growth. The mother will be freer of anxiety because she is prepared to understand and guide the child in a way that helps him to surmount his problems. Her understanding will prevent problem behavior from developing.

Many serious problems arise because parents are unaware of the behavior changes which must occur if the child is to become an increasingly more independent person. Often a parent interprets a child's behavior as abnormal. The father or the mother communicates this anxiety to the child. This increases the child's burdens. It also robs him of the energy that he needs to solve

his current problem. Behavior that might have been transient and phasic becomes exaggerated and fixed. Instead of support which helps him through a particular stage of his development, the child gets criticism, rejection or punishment. These nonconstructive modes of guidance have their effect upon the production of personality distortions.

The ability to interpret growth changes and developmental needs in a nonauthoritative way is a skill of great import. It is important because it fosters more constructive nurse-parent relationships. The nurse needs knowledge. She also needs the capacity to interpret it in a way which makes it possible for the mother to accept and utilize it. Guidance which makes the mother feel that the nurse is a transmitter of knowledge rather than a supporting helper blocks the nurse's opportunities to be of service to families. The nurse can interpret the knowledge that she has acquired from those who have done research in the field of child care; but it is the mother's right and task to apply the knowledge in her own way to the individual needs of her child. This privilege needs to be granted to her in a wholehearted, supportive way. The nurse's task is to help the mother become more competent and find increased satisfaction in her relationships with her child. This result cannot be accomplished if the nurse assumes a superior role and gives the mother little freedom to develop her own inherent capacities for self-direction and motherliness. It is in the realm of anticipatory guidance that the nurse can and should function, for she has a real contribution to make to preventive health programs. Her effectiveness can do much to alleviate children's anxiety and provide them with what they need for sound physical and mental health.

When serious problem behavior occurs, the nurse must recognize her limitations and be prepared to help the parent feel a need for seeking the services of a therapist who is specially trained in the treatment of troubled children. She can interpret the functions of the child-guidance worker. She can also alleviate the fears that come when a mother recognizes that her child has a problem which requires psychiatric therapy. Mothers who have disturbed or troubled children usually experience feelings of frustration and incompetence. They are often fearful of psychiatric therapy because they expect condemnation from the therapist, or from those in the community where they live. In referring a child to a child-guidance clinic, the nurse needs understanding of these natural feelings. When a mother learns that therapists have special skills which enable them to help children and parents solve their problems, often her fears are dispelled. As a result, she becomes motivated to seek help.

From this conference, plus the entire report of previous conferences and home visits, the nurse plans for the future needs of the family. Often a home visit for a demonstration of a new skill may be provided for, or suggestions of observations to be made before the next visit will be outlined. If the mother needs help from other members of the conference group, the nurse will take her and introduce her to the social worker, the child-guidance advisor, the nutritionist, the dental hygienist,

or any other specialist who may be available for the needs of the patient. Then the mother is given a return appointment. This is made according to the needs of the child.

FUTURE GOALS IN HEALTH SUPERVISION

The Child Health Conference movement has spread rapidly, in cities and in rural areas. In some rural areas there are clinics which go from place to place, stopping long enough to hold a Child Health Conference and then moving on. Child Health Conferences have proved their value in reducing mortality and morbidity. Good attendance illustrates the value that mothers have found in them. However, more than half the counties in the United States still do not have Child Health Conferences available. To remedy this, more work is required: better education of the public, favorable legislation, financial support, and constant effort on the part of those who realize the value of health supervision of infants and children to the nation's well-being.

Not only is there need for more facilities and for health supervision but also for more effective use of those already in existence. An unattended conference ceases to have value. Those in the nursing profession need to recognize an outstanding trait in human nature: people tend to do things the easy way, the way they are accustomed to doing them and the way that brings the results that they are seeking. If attendance at Child Health Conferences can be made easy, pleasant and helpful, the habit is formed. The mother who gets constructive guidance and support when she needs it will continue to come, even though she never may comprehend the far-reaching effects of the whole movement. One unpleasant visit, a few uncertain, uncomfortable moments may be enough to discourage a mother and prevent her from returning. It cannot be stressed too much that everyone who comes into contact with these mothers should realize the necessity for their wanting to return because they have found it to be a valuable experience.

SITUATIONS FOR FURTHER STUDY

1. How is infant health supervision provided for in your community? How are appointments made?

2. What play equipment would be practical and useful in the waiting room? How much play supervision is desirable?

3. Arrange an exhibit for a Child Health Conference waiting room on any pertinent subject you choose. Explain your choice and methods of presentation. If possible, present it and observe results.

4. If attendance is falling off in the Child Health Conference, what might be some of the reasons for it?

5. Describe a conference between a mother and a nurse which you observed. How did the nurse approach the mother? Did she encourage her to talk about her problems? How did she do it? Was she successful? Why? If she failed, what do you think were the reasons? What questions did the mother ask?

6. Describe a conference that you conducted. What were your feelings concerning it? What did you learn about the mother, the child? How do you think the mother felt about

you? Did you feel adequate in giving the mother the help that she required? If not, what further preparation do you feel that you need?

7. Describe a conference that you observed between a doctor and a mother. Did he show interest in the mother's problem? How did he show it? How did he approach the child? What technics did he use to gain the child's co-operation? What specific help did he give the mother? What was her attitude toward him and his teaching?

8. Describe a situation in which you observed a nurse offering anticipatory guidance. What was the mother's reaction to it? Had she anticipated the change in the child's behavior that the nurse described? What were her questions concerning it? Do you think that the mother received enough insight into the behavior and her feelings concerning it to be able to handle it wisely when it arises?

BIBLIOGRAPHY

Foster, Mary L.: Reasons for attending child health station, Pub. Health Nursing 44:123, 1952.

Gilbert, Ruth: The Public Health Nurse and Her Patient, ed. 2, Cambridge, Harvard, 1951.

Ginsburg, Ethel L.: Public Health Is People, New York, The Commonwealth Fund, 1950.

Hawley, Eleanor: Our stake in the future, Pub. Health Nursing 44: 447, 1952.

Lemkau, Paul: Mental Hygiene in Public Health, New York, Mc-Graw-Hill, 1949.

Levy, D. M.: Observations of attitudes and behavior in the child

health center, Am. J. Pub. Health
41:182, 1951.

Levy, Julius: An experiment in training nurses to help mothers in preventive mental hygiene, Ment.
Hyg. 23:99, 1939.

Richmond, Julius: Health super-

vision of infants and young children, Am. J. Nursing 52:1460,
1952.

Wishik, S. W.: Parents' group discussions in a child health conference, Am. J. Pub. Health 43:888,
1953.

Unit Three

GENERAL NURSING CARE

CHAPTER FIVE

The Nurse-Child and Nurse-Parent Relationship

THE PEDIATRIC DEPARTMENT OR HOSPITAL

THE ADMITTING ROOM

The admitting room should be attractive and friendly, for here the child usually gets his first impressions of the hospital. Pictures on the wall, colorful print curtains at the windows, low shelves with toys and small tables and chairs help the child feel that hospitals are comfortable and safe places for children to be. For the children who can be permitted candy, lollipops communicate friendliness and affection. When the waiting period is prolonged and extends into mealtimes, the child will need more substantial nourishment to keep him comfortable. The use of volunteers to help children enjoy play activities while they are waiting and while their mothers are being interviewed is an invaluable asset to both the children and the parents.

For years the use of colored uniforms for pediatric nurses has been suggested. They add color and eliminate the starched whiteness which has become the traditional aspect of the hospital. Furthermore, they are more practical, for the nurse does not have to guard herself as rigorously from becoming wrinkled or soiled. Thus some of the regimental cold dignity can be eliminated from an atmosphere which should be warm and friendly. Most important of all, the children enjoy seeing their nurses in colorful uniforms which are not so unlike the dresses that their mothers wear at home.

ISOLATION

Protection of the children from cross-infection always poses a complex and difficult problem. It must be remembered that the dissemination of additional disease to the relatively well or convalescent child may serve to prolong his period of hospitalization, and that the seriously ill or debilitated child may be completely unable to tolerate such an insult. Each hospital unit formulates general rules for the protection of its children, rules which must be adapted to the physical facilities and to the nature of the patient clientele. On the other hand, it must be recognized that for many children isolation and segregation are psychologically very undesirable for they exaggerate the adverse effects of separation from the home and the family and make it difficult or impossible to provide adequate substitutes for them. Isolation should be regarded as a generally undesirable procedure which ought to be imposed only by medical necessity and should be kept as brief as possible. The nurse is obligated to abide by the decisions of the medical staff for they have the ultimate responsibility for the patient's welfare. However, she can do a great deal to ameliorate the lot of the unhappy isolated child if she comprehends his needs.

The need for the company of other children varies with the character of the illness and with age. During severe illness, isolation may be needed to protect the child from the disturbance of the general ward activities and to ensure sufficient sleep and rest. Some children must be segregated because their appearance or behavior is too disturbing for other children to observe. At the onset of acute illnesses the exact nature of the disease may not be immediately apparent, and isolation has to be imposed as a protection to others until the illness is better understood. Small infants have little need for the company of other children and are best placed in separate rooms to protect them from the casual infections which may circulate.

The older infant or toddler-age child primarily needs the company of his mother. Of all ages these are the ones in which hospitalization is most damaging from the psychological point of view. If adequate companionship and stimulation from other children cannot be provided, the child is likely to regress in his development, to withdraw or become tempestuous. Sympathy, understanding and patience are required to tide the child over this period of unhappy loneliness. False promises, threats and disciplinary actions are out of place for they merely serve to accentuate the child's unhappiness and sense of distrust in his environment.

The school-age child is better able to cope with isolation for there are many ways in which he can amuse himself and exploit his inner resources between visitors. For him, too, prolonged isolation becomes dreary, boring and even depressing. Special measures must be employed to sustain his interest. Radio and television sets form an important link with the outside world.

Fortunately, the necessity for isolation is declining as antibiotic treatment shortens the infectious period of many of the transmissible diseases. The practice of isolating children for 2 or 3 weeks after admission in order to be sure that they are not incubating contagion is losing favor. Gamma globulin and convalescent serum afford means of control for many of the contagious diseases when they appear accidentally in a hospital ward.

ATTRACTIVENESS OF THE WARD

Children need to be in a happy place if emotional suffering is to be prevented. In pediatric wards one sees too often the tragedy of suffering which might have been avoided, or of mental illness emerging while physical illness is being cured.

A children's ward should be decorated in soft, warm colors and furnished in a way that appeals to children. Children enjoy pictures if they are at the level of their eyes and simple in design and coloring. It is questionable whether the permanent decoration on the wall is as satisfactory as the plain wall. A change in pictures from time to time is more desirable from the child's point of view. Bulletin boards of beaver-board are highly desirable in each child's unit. Pictures, the child's greeting cards and art productions can be placed on his bulletin board. And he can have a part in their selection! Plants and living creatures always interest children. Birds, bulbs, blossoming plants or an aquarium of fish offer children opportunities for enjoyment. Their delight will recompense the ward attendants for any time that they may have to expend in caring for such additions. Music, too, has its place in the children's ward. If it is regulated to meet the needs of all children, including those who are convalescent and those who are acutely ill, it will bring pleasure. Also, it will provide opportunities for self-expression.

Each child needs to have some of his toys from home close to him. They are an emotional tie to all that has given him comfort before coming into the hospital. As the child's stay in the hospital lengthens, his number of cherished possessions increases. He needs to have some place to keep them. A cupboard in his bedside table or a bag hung on his bed serves the purpose for most types of toys. Toys and objects from home are precious possessions. None of them should be thrown away without the owner's permission. The toys of children who are on isolation technic must be kept separate. Otherwise the sharing of toys is an important social experience for those who are mature enough to do so.

SELECTION OF TOYS

Selecting the toys, play materials and books, which are a necessary part of the ward's equipment, requires insight into the interests and the needs of individual children. Toys should afford children something to do. There may be a few treasures of childhood at which a child merely looks. However, in some way these treasures must be stimulating to the imagination of the child. The successful toys are those which provide opportunities for independent and group dramatic and imaginative play. The toy may be as simple as a square of cloth. Individuals, who have observed children at play, know that a square of cloth may become a blanket, a tablecloth, a dress, a tent, or merely something that is pleasant to touch. Even then its possibilities are not exhausted. Many of the toys must necessarily be of the sort that can be handled by children in beds. These toys should be selected to suit the needs of the individual child. For example, the child lying on his bed strapped to a Bradford frame cannot use all toys that a child lying on his stomach can. Small, simple toys, light in weight, which give opportunities for dramatic play, are better than complicated or mechanical toys. They are better because more than one thing can be done with them. A suggested list of toys and play materials which

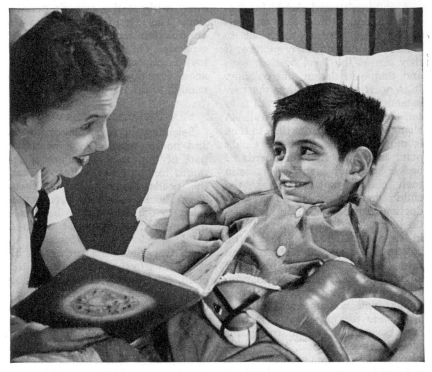

Fig. 3. Nurse reading to a child as part of a program to keep children contented and growing.

are appropriate for children of different age levels appears in Chapter 3.

The Playroom and Activity Program

Ambulatory and convalescent children require a playroom for play, recreational activities and meal service. In the playroom they will not be subjected to necessary restrictions of a ward where doctors are making rounds and treating patients. Nor will they be interfering with the rest needs of acutely ill children.

The need for play is present in all except the acutely ill children. Providing play activities tells children that their needs are being understood. It helps to assure them that friendliness and thoughtfulness govern life in the hospital even though the situation that they experience is bewildering and oftentimes painful. Play diverts their minds from the emotional and physical stresses which they are experiencing. It relieves tension. It also gives them a chance to master their fears and induces relaxation. Furthermore, play fills the time between visiting hours — time that would seem endless and almost unbearable to the homesick, frightened child if he were left unoccupied and alone. The playroom should be amply supplied with toys and raw materials which are suitable for children in different stages of development. Low shelves where toys are accessible to young children are desirable. When toys are accessible, children can choose the play materials which they have a need to use at the moment. Raw materials like sand, clay, construction paper, boxes, crayons, paint and blocks are the most appropriate of all play materials. There are many pieces of scrap materials in hospitals which children can use; empty boxes, old magazines, adhesive containers, cartons, etc., are useful objects with which to play. Some children who feel aggressive may tear up the magazines and smash the boxes. There is value in having materials that children can use for this very purpose. It is far better that they smash boxes and tear old magazines to shreds than hit at others or turn their aggressions in upon themselves.

Activity programs are essential in the care of children; they are a part of every program of nursing care. Play programs do more than divert and amuse the children and keep the ward peaceful and quiet. *A play program is therapeutic; it is essential for mental, social and emotional growth; it is important in restoring the child to physical health.* Without satisfying play, regression increases. Regression occurs because the child has no way to release tension and master his fears. Nor has he the opportunities that he

needs for psychological growth when he recuperates and has energy available for it. As soon as the child's physical condition permits, he needs the stimulation which play activities and association with other children foster.

Prolonging dependency, or infantilization as it is often called, encourages regression. When a child is acutely ill, he needs the gratification that comes from comforting, dependent care. He needs it not only because he is physically ill but also because he is anxious and uncertain. However, when he recuperates and his anxiety has been relieved through discovery that his needs will be fulfilled, he requires guided experiences which help him to meet the realities of life. The child who has been acutely ill needs help in discovering that independent and shared activities are more satisfying than complete dependency. Vander Veer* says

Everyone, at every age, has some secret longings to escape from the responsibilities of the present into the less demanding existence of earlier years. Bed rest tempts the individual to yield to his backward-looking trend because it legitimizes his dependency on other people. The longer the rest, the stronger the temptation.

Nurses need to be aware of this tendency in children, and they should be able to relinquish the satisfaction that they derive from having children dependent upon them. They need to learn ways of

---

* Vander Veer, A. H.: The psychopathology of physical illness and hospital residence, *in* Personality Development and Its Implications for Nursing and Nursing Education, Springfield, Ill., Dept. of Public Health, 1948, p. 62.

obtaining gratification through the help that they give children in growing in their capacity for increased independence. With experience nurses can learn to help children find satisfaction in play with other children. When they develop skill in teaching they will obtain satisfactions which exceed those they obtained from routinized care.

The child who has been acutely ill needs opportunities to regain his independence gradually. First, he needs to discover that being with other children for play and meals is enjoyable. When he finds group experiences are fun, he will grow from the regressive state that his illness produced. At first he may only want to play with his nurse; but gradually, if the nurse gives him freedom to develop his independence from her, he will find more pleasure in activities with children in the ward. The preschool child will continue to need his nurse close by. However, his need of her will be different from that which he experienced before he found pleasure in play with peers.

Older children need opportunities to continue their school work and to learn to take responsibility while they are in the hospital. Doing things is an important part of the child's life. Children learn by doing. They also obtain pleasure from taking responsibility. No child in a hospital should be cheated of any opportunity to do what he is able to do. Learning from self-directed and teacher-directed activities in school is the school-age child's responsibility. If he is physically able, he should go to school in the hospital, not only to occupy his time but also because he should be helped to take the responsibility that he is able to assume. From school activities he will get the satisfaction that comes from keeping up with his classmates.

The child loves to help in the ward. The thoughtful nurse will find opportunities to give this pleasure. She will know that happiness is an essential part of his treatment. The ambulatory child enjoys sharing in the process of "picking up" in the playroom. It gives him activity and the feeling that he is a responsible, helpful person. Children enjoy putting away supplies, stamping ward stationery, helping to pass fluids and making cotton swabs and balls. Many school-age children will delight in reading stories to or playing with the younger children in the ward. It gives them a feeling of worth and thereby helps to restore their self-confidence.

Meal hours offer opportunities to give the child a homelike and happy social experience each day. Eating is an important social activity. Mealtimes in the hospital should provide a social experience for all those children who are physically able to participate in it. If the playroom is large enough, bed-ridden convalescent patients can be moved in to enjoy a group meal experience. Children enjoy setting the table and playing host or hostess. A nurse or two can share the meal period with them. This experience can be of educational significance to the nurse. It can also provide a happy, satisfying experience for the children. More and more hospitals are instituting this form of meal service. Hospital personnel have found that both the children and the nurses profit from the experience. Appe-

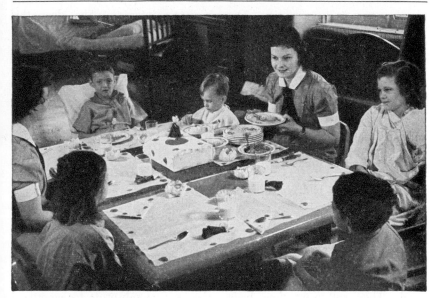

Fig. 4. Nurses eating with children as a means of providing a homelike and happy environment.

tites are improved, and the spirit of good will and comradeship is furthered when children share an enjoyable experience together.

Children need play therapists and nurses who work together in providing an environment that is suitable for those who require a period of hospitalization. In some hospitals play or occupational therapists direct the activity program. Nurses need opportunities to assist in the program because it is a valuable training experience. They also need it to learn ways to co-operate in making the program successful for all the children in the ward.

PLAY AN ESSENTIAL PART OF NURSING CARE

Planning for the child's play needs is as much the responsibility of the nurse as of the play therapist. It is as important for the nurse to see that her patients are occupied constructively as it is for her to provide them with nourishment, medication and treatment. The nurse needs to observe her patients at play, to see that they are progressing in their relationships with other children. Observation will give her clues concerning their adjustment to hospitalization and also will provide the data that she needs to plan ways to make their present situation a more satisfying one. From observation of her patients' play, the nurse has many opportunities to learn about her patients. It will help her understand them as persons and to be more successful in meeting their needs.

Adult standards of order and tidiness cannot be maintained when a play program is in operation. Orderliness which facilitates work, and cleanliness which safeguards health are essential. However, they can be maintained without inhibiting children's interest in and need for play activities. Requiring beautifully smoothed bedclothes, absolute alignment of beds and chairs and military precision in the placement of furnishings and equipment are unreasonable standards to expect of a pediatric nurse. They are also a hindrance to the children's happiness. Such order may be restful and beautiful in the eyes of visitors and hospital administrators, but it contributes nothing to the child's peace of mind.

A children's ward is for children, and their interests need to be fostered. They will want their beds moved closer to other children or moved into the doorways where they can view the activity of their nurses —or watch hopefully for their mothers to arrive. They will drop things on the floor and not bother about it. The ambulatory children will use play materials and then suddenly be diverted to a new interest which catches their attention. What seems like disorder to the adult is orderly and satisfying to children. They cannot keep their beds and bedside tables tidy and play in a way that brings satisfaction and release of tension. A nurse who is perpetually tidying up a child's surroundings brings him little comfort. Inadvertently she is telling him that play is not acceptable to her. Children should learn to take care of their play materials. This learning can become a part of preparation for meal and rest periods.

The nurse needs to encourage her patient's interests. She does this when she provides him with play materials and gives him permission to meet his needs through self-chosen activities. When she is motivated to help him find comfort in his new surroundings, her interest will be centered in the way he uses play materials rather than in the untidiness his play creates.

THE ATMOSPHERE OF THE WARD

A pediatric ward needs an emotional atmosphere which gives children the feeling that they are enjoyed and protected and that their needs will be fulfilled consistently. Equipment and an attractively decorated pediatric unit are helpful aids in the care of children. However, they are no substitute for emotional satisfactions. When a child is ill and away from all that has given him comfort and security before, he needs an interpersonal relationship which proves that he has not been abandoned, that he will be taken care of and will have the support, the understanding and the protection that he needs in a strange, fear-provoking situation.

The *feelings* of hospital personnel toward the child, his parents and co-workers set the emotional tone of a pediatric ward. When the personnel's interest is child-centered they are more able to see their patients' needs. They also learn to respond in ways which bring relief from both physical and emotional discomfort. It is the nurse's feelings and attitudes which motivate her to do what she does and determine *how* she will do it. It is her *feelings* toward each child and his parents which determine the quality of nursing care that she is able to give. The child's adjustment in the hospital will be influenced by a multitude of factors. One of the most important factors is concerned with the quality of care and interest that he and his parents receive within the hospital. The child is a dependent individual who is in need of a continuous relationship with a warm, giving mother throughout the growing-up process. *When hospital policy does not permit the presence of the mother in the ward, substitute care must be provided.* The child needs some one upon whom he can depend. He needs a nurse who will do those things that a mother ordinarily would do for him. Case method of assignment is the only method of assignment that can begin to fulfill the hospitalized child's emotional needs. It provides personal interest and emotional and physical support.

Case method of assignment is necessary to safeguard the child's mental health; it is also an essential educational experience for the nurse. Assignments which center the nurse's interest in illness, treatments and duties to be performed foster ward efficiency. However, they deprive the child of what he needs most—a relationship with some one person who is able to respond consistently to his basic human needs. Assignments which are changed before the nurse and the child have developed understanding of and importance to one another are equally frustrating. The child has no one person to whom he can relate himself and from whom he can gain the supportive care that he requires. The nurse loses the satisfactions that can come from experiences which help her to gain understanding of children.

Placing Children in the Ward

Placement of children in a ward requires sensitivity to the needs of each child. Placement should be on the basis of the child's psychological needs as well as on the basis of the type of disease from which he is suffering. The acutely sick children, who need quiet and rest, may be grouped near each other. The sociable convalescent children should be in another section where they can visit with each other without harm to others.

Children need each other. Unless a child is so ill that he is unaware of his surroundings, he will adjust with greater ease if he is placed near children who have become familiar with their new environment. Introductions help children become acquainted with each other; they also help them feel recognized and important in their strange environment. The children in the ward can be of assistance to the nurse. They can help her make the newly admitted child feel more at home in his new environment. The atmosphere in a ward should be that of a friendly neighborhood where each child has status and is a member of a group.

Clothing

Hospital clothing should be attractive and foster self-dependence. When the child's illness is acute and he is in a recumbent position, the usual night clothing is practical. However, when he becomes able to sit up, he will need extra clothing to take the place of the bedclothing which no longer covers him. Children like to wear bright-colored bedjackets over their nightgowns. They can be slipped off easily when they lie down for rest hours and for the night. Jackets, dresses and suits of different colors and styles provide opportunity for choice. Choosing their clothing is an experience which brings children a great deal of pleasure. If the child is not incontinent from acute illness, he should be provided with training panties or trousers which he can manage independently.

Bathrobes, shoes and slippers from home are a source of great comfort to children. They should be permitted to have them, even though it entails more responsibility for the nursing personnel. When ambulatory children require hospitalization over long periods of time, clothing from home is highly desirable from the child's point of view. Whenever possible the wish for their own clothing should be granted.

Bedclothes covering children should be light in weight and tucked in loosely on each side of the bed. Children's extremities need to be kept warm. However, they should not be covered so tightly that they feel inhibited in the use of their bodies. Children do not lie as still as adults do. It should not be expected that they should. In some hospitals today, the nurses dress the children warmly enough so that they do not need to be covered with bedclothes. This procedure gives the child more freedom of movement. It also saves time and linen, for there are no upper bedclothes that require adjustment.

PROTECTION FROM FEARFUL SIGHTS AND SOUNDS

Every ward needs a room to which children can be taken for treatments which are painful or for experiences which could easily be misinterpreted by other children in the ward. Children need to be shielded from sights that are disturbing. Things which hospital personnel take for granted are often fear-provoking to the imaginative, anxious child. If he sees another child having a paracentesis, for instance, he may well wonder if that will also be done to him. Likewise, children should be protected from seeing children who are critically ill or dying.

When a child cannot be protected from the experiences cited above, he will need a great deal of help in understanding what he has seen, heard or felt. The nurse needs to be alert to signs of anxiety. She also needs to be ready to try to discover the child's interpretation of the event that he has witnessed. Often he has interpreted it erroneously. Sometimes he suspects that it will happen to him also. Reassurance given before the nurse has discovered the child's fears is rarely effective. It must come *after* she has helped the child feel comfortable and safe enough to verbalize his fear. This is the reason the young, nonverbal child needs to be protected from sights and sounds which he is unable to understand.

VISITORS IN THE HOSPITAL

Children and parents need each other. More and more hospital personnel are beginning to recognize the effect of separation on children. They are growing more observant of its effects on young children who have not as yet developed sufficient independence to understand why hospitalization is necessary or to tolerate the frustration that it brings. As a result of their understanding, hospital personnel are increasing and lengthening visiting hours. In some hospitals they are also permitting mothers to give care to their children while they are with them. In a few instances mothers are also permitted to bring food from home.

Visiting hours are disrupting to ward personnel but they are important for the child and his parents. The daily arrival of his parents relieves the child's anxiety lest he has been abandoned. It also helps to assure him that he has not been placed there as punishment. The child feels hostile when he is left in the hospital. He feels this way because he is deprived of the security to which he is accustomed. Visiting hours give him an opportunity to ventilate his feelings. They also give him the comfort for which he longs, which he deserves to have.

Crying at the time of his mother's arrival and leave-taking is not damaging; *it is therapeutic*. It does disturb the peace of the ward. It also makes the nurse's task more difficult. However, it provides an emotional outlet which the child apparently needs. If he did not need it, the presence of his parents would not evoke a tempestuous response. Repressed hostility and grief disturbs the child's relationship with his mother. Many little children are so grieved and angry that they have to deny their need for their mothers. Many also are forced to deny their need for mothering to alleviate unbearable anxiety. Some must forget the image of their mothers because remembering them makes their longings too intense to bear. Failure to

recognize the mother after a period of separation is frequently observed. It is an ominous sign. The child who "forgets" his mother needs more frequent visiting hours, not fewer. The example which follows serves to illustrate the reasons why some children reject mothering.

Bill was 4 years old when he came into the hospital with leukemia. He sat in a big chair hour after hour in deep thought. A nurse attempted to establish a relationship with him. She told him she wanted to play with him. Then she sat down to give him an opportunity to relate to her. Almost immediately he yelled, "Get out of here. I don't want you here. I want to be alone." The nurse said, "Billy, I want to stay with you and take care of you." Billy's screaming "Get out," etc., continued. It was evident that Billy did not want a nurse to stay with him.

During the remainder of the morning the nurse acceded to Billy's request. However, simultaneously she made herself available to him. She placed him in the doorway where he could see her sitting at the desk. She said, "Billy, I'm going to be at the desk. I want to help you; when you need something you call me." But Billy never called her! He sat watching—yet he did not seem to see what was going on about him. After lunch, he permitted the nurse to put him to bed. However, he rejected the nurse when she expressed her wish to read him a story. Again he screamed, "Get out of here. I don't want you here." Why did Billy want the nurse to leave? Why did he reject her offer to care for him?

The next morning Billy's resistance to the nurse was equally pronounced. To discover the meaning of Billy's behavior, the nurse said, "I wonder why you don't want me to stay with you." His response was revealing. It was as follows: "Do you know why? It's because you make me lonesome, that's why. Get out." The nurse said, "You want your mommy here. You need her so much and she can't be here. All children want their mommies in the hospital. When a nurse is here, it makes you want mommy more. That's the way lots of children feel." Billy's response was filled with longing. He said, "My mommy is the *goodest* mommy in the whole wide world." Then his feelings broke through. He cried piteously and was able to accept comforting in the arms of the nurse. It began a constructive relationship which helped Billy accept the care that he needed desperately. At first he resisted the nurse's offers of help. However, gradually he became more receptive to her nearness and care.

When an adult is frustrated because his most valued friend does not visit him, he also reacts to his disappointment. He either expresses his feelings to the person who brought his discomfort or to some sympathetic friend. Or he may brood and take his anger out on himself; or he may be hostile to someone who has not provoked his anger. He may say or think, "I don't ever want to see that person again. The quicker I can forget him the better." It will not be difficult for the nurse to remember how relieved she felt when she vented her feelings after she had been disappointed or hurt. Or if she suppressed her feelings of disappointment, undoubtedly she can remember the misery she experienced.

The child responds in the same way as an adult, but his need for a continued relationship with a loved object is urgent because his growth is dependent upon it. If a child rejects the person who has disappointed or angered him, his personality cannot grow. The adult's personality is formed. He can continue to grow without the inter-

est of a valued friend. It will be a difficult and painful feat but it is within the realm of possibility. The child cannot grow if he represses his hostility and anxiety and denies his need for his mother or for mothering. He continues to need his mother because his ego is too undeveloped to make it possible for him to be an independent person.

When a mother visits her child, it is natural for her to want to bring him food and toys. Many times this disturbs hospital personnel. They know that he is provided with food and play materials by the hospital. The nuisance of taking care of his possessions often blinds hospital personnel to the significance that his mother's presents would have for him.

Parents have needs as well as children. Most mothers long to take care of their children when they are ill. It is not easy for a mother to leave her child in the hospital. Nor is it a simple matter to turn the care of her child over to someone else. Bringing food and toys to her child has emotional significance for her. It also has significance for the child. A bit of mother's food is infinitely more delectable than the food that comes from the hospital kitchen. And taste is not the only reason why the child feels this way! His mother's food has deep significance to him. Associations pertaining to comforting experiences with his mother come into play; the taste is of minor significance. Perhaps the nurse can recall her feelings when she received a box of food from home during the first weeks of her experience in the school dormitory. Was it the taste that stimulated her feelings or was

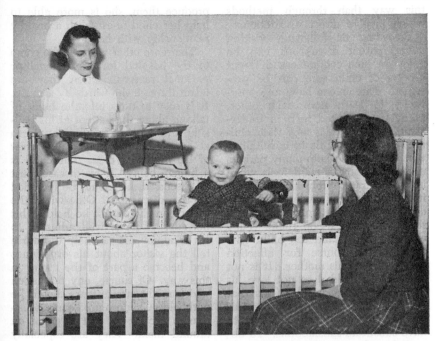

Fig. 5. A nurse who recognizes a child's needs for his mother minimizes the discomforts that are associated with hospitalization.

it the idea that someone important had remembered her?

Nurses can help parents select gifts for their children. This can be done indirectly with the use of posters or toy displays. Or it can be done directly in conference with them.

Nurses can use visiting hours to great advantage. During visiting periods nurses have an opportunity to develop relationships with parents. Nurses can learn a great deal from parents which will help them to become better nurses. They can also observe parent-child relationships and use what they see in planning the care of their patients.

They can also do something for parents in this period. If a mother discovers that the nurse is interested in her child and herself, she will be more apt to seek guidance which will help her increase her capacity to meet her child's needs more completely. A mother never will be receptive to help if she feels unwelcome in the ward. Nor will she be receptive if her need to care for her child is thwarted by the nurse. Sometimes the most effective teaching is done indirectly. When nurses are skillful and understanding in their care of the child, the parent sees the effect that it has on the child. Often more is accomplished this way than through methods which involve direct instruction. Preceding or following visiting hours, parent discussions can be held. In such conferences different aspects of child care can be presented. Parents can have an opportunity to learn from each other. Many parents need help in understanding the reasons why their children react as they do to hospitalization. Insight can help many parents understand how a child feels when he is separated from them. With insight they will understand why children withdraw from them—and sometimes even forget them. They will also understand the child who turns to the nurse for affection rather than to his mother. It is not because the child does not love his mother; it is because he feels that she has punished him. As a result he is angry and hurt. He has to have substitute satisfactions. To obtain them he turns to the nurse as a possible source of satisfaction. Many a mother feels rivalrous with the nurses. She demonstrates her anxiety in her behavior toward them. Her anxiety will be relieved if she can be helped to see the situation from her child's point of view.

Conferences can also help the mother anticipate her child's reactions when she comes to visit and when she takes him home. Insight will help her handle the child's withdrawal or tempestuousness. It will also prepare her to understand the reasons why he may cling, regress and display feelings of hostility overtly or by withdrawal when she gets him home. Anticipating changes in behavior prepares the mother to meet them. When she understands the dynamics which

produce them, she is more able to help her child re-establish a healthy relationship with her.

There are other visitors who come to the hospital for professional or personal reasons. Often they are taken through the wards by a nurse. It is easy to drop into the habit of talking about the patient at his bedside and perhaps of holding forth at length as to the special interest of his particular case. The child is a human being. If his disease must be discussed, he should be included in the discussion. Otherwise, the discussion should not be held at his bedside. If he is well adjusted to his condition, he can help the nurse tell the visitor about his experience and become a part of the group in this way. Of course, any discussion which might arouse fears should be withheld. Children are keenly sensitive to everything that is going on around them. They are especially aware of conversations that concern them. When they cannot understand all of what is being said, they become anxious just as adults do.

ADMISSION OF THE CHILD TO THE HOSPITAL

The nurse who is going to help a child and his parents through the admission routine of a hospital is confronted with a responsibility of great magnitude. When she goes into the waiting room she will find a child with one or both parents. All of them need her understanding and help. Both the child and his parents may have been prepared for the experience at the time hospitalization was recommended. But in many instances, unfortunately, this probably will not be true.

Perhaps in the future some ingenious person will produce a film which graphically illustrates all that admission to a clinic or a hospital entails for a child and his parents. It would be an invaluable method of helping a mother become prepared to help her child. When she brings her child in for a clinic visit or for admission, the film could be shown to the child in his mother's presence. It would reinforce his trust in his mother. In addition, it would prepare him further for all that he will experience. In museums there are films that go into action the minute a button is pushed. No attendant is required to operate the machine. Only apparatus, a room and motivation to inform the public are required. These automatically run films are principally for advertising purposes. They could be used equally well as an educational tool.

The way in which the admitting routine is carried out is of great significance to the child and his parents. It is important because their attitudes and feelings toward hospitals, their personnel and procedures are influenced through the experience. The child and the parent who are greeted immediately upon arrival feel differently from those who spend long periods in waiting. No parent or child feels confident when he is unnoticed by hospital personnel. When the child and his parents get to the ward feeling that they are in the hands of understanding people, the child's adjustment to his illness and hospitalization is better ensured. The attendant trauma for both mother and child is also lessened.

Even though the child and his parents have been verbally prepared, adapting to the new experience will be a difficult process. *Preparation is essential.* It assists the child in preparing himself to meet the situation. *However, of equal importance to his adjustment is the understanding guidance that is available to help him understand and accept all that is happening to him.* The nurse must be emotionally ready to supply the guidance that both the parents and the child require. Coming into the hospital is a routine experience to the nurse. However, it is anything but routine to the child and his parents. They do not know what is going to happen to them. The admission procedure is only one of the many things to which they must adapt themselves. There is illness and the anxiety that it generates. In addition, there is the thought of separation which looms large in the mind of every parent and every child if he is old enough to comprehend that it is what hospitalization requires.

Children utilize preparation for hospitalization in many different ways. Some children cannot utilize it at all. It may be that they were too young to see into the future and anticipate what it will hold. Or it may be that the thought was so painful that they had to repress the idea and the feelings that it evoked. Some must produce fantasies that make the experience different from what they will experience in reality.

Children's individual ways of handling the anxiety which arises from anticipation of a fearful situation are determined by the personality structures that they have acquired in the growth process. Some children will come ready for the experience. However, there will be others who may have been totally unable to assimilate the preparation. Jessner and Kaplan studied the emotional responses of children to tonsillectomy and adenoidectomy. They concluded that preparation for hospitalization and operation was necessary. They also made the following statement pertaining to children's use of information.

The factual information is sometimes not accepted by the child, but is replaced or remodelled by fantasies. Fantasies are often indicative of the fact that earlier anxieties or anticipations are mobilized by the operation or expectation of the operation. On the other hand, fantasies may also represent another method utilized by children to assimilate the new experience, to translate it into their own picture language and to integrate it into their former experience and body conceptions.*

If the parent and the child have been prepared for admission and seem ready to meet the experience, the nurse can proceed soon after she has introduced herself, established rapport with them and explained the first things that they will need to do together. Situations in the admitting room, however, will not always be so ideal. There will be many types of patients, parents and illnesses. Each situation will be different. Each person will need individual consideration.

Need of Parents for Understanding and a Sense of Security

An understanding of people and their problems is essential for successful pediatric nursing. What are the influences in life that have made a parent what he is? In Chapter 3 the developmental process has been

traced briefly. In many individuals development has been retarded or has become distorted in one way or another. Their background histories contain the reasons for their problems. Their early childhood experiences often explain their current behavior. If nurses knew the antecedent life experiences of parents they would be in a better position to understand their behavior and accept them as persons. Behavior has purpose. It is not only a response to the current situation which the individual is meeting but it is also the outgrowth of all that he has experienced previously. This knowledge should help nurses to be more sympathetic and less quick to form judgments. Also, it should help them to understand all behavior, including that which seems to be infantile, demanding or unreasonable.

A mother in the hospital needs to have interest directed toward her as well as toward her child for a number of reasons. First, the child coming into a hospital needs his mother's help to adapt himself to the new experience. The mother is the child's source of security and his protection. If she is anxious, he will be frightened and less able to adapt himself to the demands of the situation. He will be frightened because the source of his support is gone. Secondly, the mother is under stress, either because her child is acutely ill or because his illness or

---

* Jessner, Lucie, and Kaplan, Samuel: Observations on the emotional reactions of children to tonsillectomy and adenoidectomy, in Problems of Infancy and Childhood, Transactions of the Third Conference, New York, Josiah Macy, Jr., Foundation, 1949, p. 115.

condition in some way threatens her security.

Emotional reactions to a child's illness or deformity show wide variation. Many mothers feel guilty because their children have become ill. Often their oversolicitude and exaggerated fears reflect these conscious or unconscious feelings. Some mothers are in terror lest hospitalization arouse their child's hostility toward them. Others are concerned about leaving the child in the hospital. Some resent the fact that they are not permitted to stay and take care of the child. Some feel rivalrous with nurses and fearful lest the child transfer his affections to a nurse. Often their behavior in the admitting room and at visiting hours is a response to these feelings. Self pity is a predominant feeling in some parents. They see their child's illness or deformity as something which is a catastrophe to them. They dwell on the effect of the illness or deformity on them rather than on the effect that it has on the child. Some of these mothers are intensely resentful because illness or deformity has befallen them. Others feel ashamed of the child's deformity; others have been stigmatized by the attitudes of society and are angered by them. Other parents are grief-stricken, panicky and unable to control their feelings.

The mother needs a nurse who is responsive to her feelings and ready to understand the meaning that illness of her child and hospitalization has to her. If the nurse gives the mother an opportunity to talk, she will get clues that will help her to understand both her and her child. The nurse cannot assume that everyone feels as she does about a child's illness or deformity. The nurse may take illness and hospitalization in a matter-of-fact way. She may take it casually because she knows that the condition is not serious or because she knows from experience that an operation can correct the deformity. She can know that the mother has no realistic cause to feel guilty. However, this does not mean that the mother feels the same way about it. Mothers often express feelings of guilt to nurses. Instead of reassurance, mothers often sense attitudes which make them feel misunderstood. Some mothers clearly demonstrate their anxiety in the admitting room. The nurse may not see any cause for concern. However, if she listens to the mother she will discover that there are reasons why the experience is frightening to her. Her reasons may be irrational in the nurse's eye but to the mother they are real. If they were not real to her, they would not be precipitating anxiety in her.

The nurse needs understanding that will prepare her to work successfully with many kinds of people. She needs to understand how abysmal ignorance can be and to be ready without any note of scorn in her voice to explain in the simplest of terms. Fear of the unknown is a terrific fear! And many mothers as well as children are in the throes of this fear when they enter the clinic or hospital. Many mothers are guided more by superstition than by reason. Some have had unhappy experiences in hospitals. They assume that all hospitals are alike. Some of these mothers have been forced against their will to bring their children to the hospital. They have irrational fears that block their capacity to learn. The mother who is frightened needs to know that her child is in kind, gentle and wise hands. Her anxiety will decrease when she gains faith in hospital personnel.

There are, on occasions, women in the admitting room who are terrified of the unknown, and sometimes they are hysterical or belligerent as well. These women are trying. They tax the nurse's ingenuity to the utmost. They will leave her feeling frustrated, antagonistic and critical unless she understands the reasons for their emotional instability and can provide the support that they require.

In instances like the above, time and the help of an additional person are essential. The nurse must protect the child by establishing rapport with him. She needs to be ready to give him the emotional support that his mother is unable to give him. The terrified, hysterical mother needs calming, support and kind, firm, positive and consistent treatment. She is like a child—in need of a sense of security. Had she had it in her childhood, she would be ready to give it to her child. Before she can give it to him, she must receive it in abundance from hospital personnel. It will take time and the help of an additional person, but it is the only human thing to do. She, too, is a sick person who is in need of understanding.

Then there is the mother who recognizes the true seriousness of the situation. She knows that her child is seriously ill. She has observed his change in behavior and recognized the onset of more ominous symptoms. She is acutely anxious. And there are rational reasons why she feels this way.

The mother who recognizes the seriousness of her child's condition needs the support that comes from understanding of her concern and from skillful, sympathetic care of her child. Denials of the seriousness of the child's illness will not alleviate her anxiety; it will increase it. Denials will make her feel that the nurse is an incompetent observer. They will also make her skeptical of her capacity to care for her child. In addition, she will feel misunderstood because her feelings have not been accepted. A mother gets relief from anxiety when hospital personnel recognize the seriousness of the situation and share their concern with her. In addition, she needs to know that everything possible is being done by sympathetic, skillful persons. Words alone will not convince her of this. She must *see* and *feel* that everything is being done. She will gain this feeling not only from seeing her child scientifically cared for but also from the attitudes and the feelings that are being communicated to her and to her child. It cannot come from efficiency or scientific treatment alone. It comes when the hospital personnel's skillful work is motivated by a genuine concern for other people's feelings and needs.

Words, attitudes and feelings that convey understanding and explanations that assist people in meeting the unknown are a necessary part of hospital care. They are not a waste of time; they are timesavers. They ease the mother's mind, win her confidence and prepare her to be supporting to her child. A friendly greeting and an opportunity to talk to someone who can share her burden will do much to allay the mother's anxiety. In doing so the child is also benefited, for he will be protected from the contagiousness of his mother's anxiety.

TALKING WITH PARENTS OUT OF THE CHILD'S HEARING

The child needs protection from hearing what he cannot understand. Certainly he should not be within hearing distance when his personal history, disease, treatment and condition are being discussed. Nor should he hear his mother talk about her feelings pertaining to his illness or deformity. In fact, it is better if he does not hear any conversation about himself which he cannot understand. The unknown so often means fear to the child. Matters of everyday occurrence to nurses and terms that fall easily from their lips are strange to the imaginative child and full of portent to him. "A shot in the arm" means a hypodermic injection of medicine to a nurse but to a child it might have a totally different meaning.

When a mother attempts to discuss her child's personality and habits of behavior within his hearing, the nurse can suggest that she wait until she can get someone to attend the child during the conference. Curiously enough, in some instances, the mother's comments about her child are derogatory. When a child hears his mother criticizing him, he may become frightened lest he start a new experience handicapped by a reputation that he feels he does not deserve. Information about the child can be obtained while the child is being examined by the doctor. When it is

possible, both parents should be encouraged to bring their child to the hospital. Then he will not need to be separated from a parent so soon after he enters the hospital. In this conference the nurse can obtain information that will help those caring for the child to understand him. Knowledge of the child's history and background as a human being are essential in giving him ease of mind and sympathetic understanding. Wilkins° constructed the following form to collect data about preschool children:

NAME OF HOSPITAL

Name ....Age...........
Date of Admission...............................
Birthday...
By what name does the child like to be called?....................
Are there other children in the family?
    Brothers: Ages ....
    Sisters: Ages..............................

Eating Habits
How is the child usually fed?
    Bottle?..........Cup?..........Spoon?..........
Feed self independently?.....................
Feed self with help?.....................
Food disliked?.....................
Favorite foods?.....................
What is his appetite like?.....................

Elimination
Is the child independent in toiletting?....
    ....To what degree?.....................
What is the term used to refer to urination?.....................
Bowel movement?.....................

° Wilkins, Gladys: The Role of the Nurse in the Admission of Preschool Children to Hospitals, Unpublished Master's paper, University of Chicago, Dept. of Nursing Education, 1950, p. 61.

Is the child accustomed to a toilet chair?
.................Bathroom?...........................
What is the approximate time of daily
bowel movement?...........................
Is the child taken to the toilet at night?
....
Is so, at what time?...........................

Sleeping Habits
Does the child take a daily nap?.............
What is his usual bedtime hour?...........
....
Does the child sleep alone?.....................
If not, with whom?...............................
Does the child sleep in a bed with sides?
...........Adult bed?...............................
Does the child have a prayer that he
says at bedtime?...............................
Does the child have a special bedtime
routine?...
Is so, what is it?...................................
....

Play Interests
What type of play does the child like
best?..
Is the child accustomed to playing
alone?...............With other children?....
...........With adults?...............Does he
have a favorite pet at home?...............
If so, state name and kind...................
....
Favorite type of toys?...........................

Personal Habits
Does the child brush his teeth?...............
Comb his hair?.....................................
Bathe himself?.....................................
Dress himself?.....................................

Miscellaneous
Does the child know why he is being
admitted to the hospital?.....................

What information did you give him?
....
....
....
How did he respond to it?.....................
....
....
When was he told?.................................
Has the child fears, such as fear of
unfamiliar adults?...............................
People in white uniforms?...................
Needles?...............Surgery?.................
Other?...
Do the parents live together?.................
If not, divorced?...................................
Deceased?...............At what age was
the child when the parent died?........
....
Have any new experiences occurred in
the home recently such as birth of
a sibling?...........When?.......................
Other?...
Has the child attended nursery school?
...............Kindergarten...............Grade
school?...............Sunday school?...........
Mother's remarks:

[Record on the reverse side observations
which describe the mother-child relationship, the child's response to admission, and the kind of adjustment that he
made in the ward.]

After the nurse has learned about
the child from his mother, she can
help her to become prepared to
participate in the hospital experience. The admission routine can be
described to the mother so she
knows what it entails. Then she
can help interpret the steps of the
procedure to her child. Mothers
need to know that the nurse understands how difficult the experience
is for both of them. When a mother

recognizes that the nurse does not expect complete compliance from her child, her anxiety is relieved. The nurse can also explain visiting hours and interpret the child's need for them. She can anticipate and help her to understand the possible responses that may come at visiting hours and at the time of her leave-taking. Some mothers may express dread of parting from their children. It helps a mother to know that she will be able to go to the ward and remain with her child until he begins to become more comfortable in his new surroundings.

Many mothers need help in knowing how to carry through leave-taking. Many mothers cannot face telling their children the truth about their leaving. They may fear the anger that comes when a child is irritated with his mother's behavior. Or they may not know that children need a truthful explanation of why they are being left in the hospital. Explanations that give mothers understanding of the impact of the experience on the child usually help them to be supporting. Many mothers will need help in learning that their children will be helped most if they truthfully prepare them for their leave-taking and for the time of their return and then quickly leave their bedsides. Mothers should know that at this point nurses will be there to support their children.

Information collected on a form like the one above and from a conference with the mother can be used to provide individualized care. It should be readily available for the nurses who are assigned to the child's care. It is not enough to report the admission of Johnny Smith,

aged 3, diagnosis—hydronephrosis —and follow it with a reading of the doctor's orders. *Each nurse caring for Johnny Jones needs to know the history of his disease, its symptomatology and treatment. She also needs information that helps her to understand him.* The nurse receiving Johnny as a patient can report the observations that she has made pertaining to his reaction to her, to his mother, ward mates, treatments and the adjustment that he is making in the ward. In this conference the nurse assigned to Johnny could report the plan of nursing care which she has formulated from the knowledge that she already has acquired about him.

NEED OF CHILD FOR HIS MOTHER AT THE TIME OF ADMISSION

The child needs the help of his mother throughout the admission procedure to assist him in adjusting to the strangeness of the situation. In the conference with the mother, the nurse can evaluate the mother's capacity and interest in assisting. She can use these clues in planning ways to meet both the mother's and the child's needs at this time. The mother can help undress, bathe, weigh and reclothe her child. With supervision she can also take his temperature and obtain a specimen of urine. At such times most mothers long to do for their children. They need to be permitted to do everything for their children that they are capable of and interested in doing.

A co-operative project increases the child's security. He has his mother near-by for support and he can adapt himself to the nurse more slowly. The child's comfort is increased when he observes that a friendly feeling exists between his mother and the nurse. If he recognizes that his mother accepts the nurse, he will be more ready to do so. In addition, he will be less apt to feel guilty if he likes the nurse. A co-operative project can give the child a "we" feeling. It will foster his trust in those who are going to give him care.

A co-operative project also gives the nurse time to observe the mother-child relationship and their response to the total situation. Observational material gathered throughout the admission procedure is vital in understanding the child. The newly admitted child needs help in adjusting at once. Observational material is helpful in understanding his needs.

Hospital routines need to be flexible enough to allow for changes in procedure when they are indicated. There will be times when a child is unready to co-operate in some of the admission procedures. To force a child into having a bath, or in being weighed, for instance, may condition him negatively to nurses and to the hospital. When a child indicates a need for variation in procedure, his feelings should have thoughtful consideration. Nurses need to ask themselves the following questions: Is this procedure absolutely essential for his safety? Would the child be benefited if the procedure were postponed until he has become more familiar with his surroundings and with the personnel? Are there ways in which the procedure could be modified to gain the child's co-operation?

The child needs to have his mother accompany him to his room or ward and remain with him until he begins to feel comfortable with the nurse to whom he has been assigned. The time will vary with different children. Only when rules are flexible can they be of service to children. Parting at the bedside does much to foster a sense of security in both the mother and the child. If the mother and the child have not been able to find security in their new situation, for their sakes and the sake of other patients in the ward, they may have to be separated temporarily before the child is taken to the ward. Then the mother and the child should be helped independently. They should be reunited after better equilibrium has been attained. To send the mother away before she sees where her child is located is an inhuman thing to do. The child needs to see that his mother knows where he is. Otherwise he may live in dread lest she not find him. Feelings of being lost are minimized after he sees that his mother knows where he is.

NEED OF THE CHILD TO BE
ADMITTED TO A NURSE RATHER
THAN TO A HOSPITAL UNIT
OR WARD

The child needs to have the security of knowing that he is not alone and unprotected in a strange new world. When a mother and a child enter the ward, they should be introduced to the head nurse, who has the responsibility of introducing the patient and his mother to the nurse whom she has assigned to the child's care. Children know the people in their homes and neighborhood by name. It is also important that they have that added sense of intimacy which comes from knowing their nurse's name. When the nurse meets the child, an interpretation of her role will help to relieve his anxiety concerning his welfare. When a child knows that he is going to be separated from his mother he wonders who will take care of him. It is one of the first questions that a child usually asks. He may say "Are you my nurse?" Or he may express his uneasiness more directly by asking, "Who is going to take care of me?"

After the nurse has interpreted her role to the child, she needs to proceed by proving through all she does that she *is* the person who will take care of him in his mother's absence. Telling him that she is going to take care of him will be of little value to him unless he finds through experience that it is true. When his nurse goes off duty it is her responsibility to inform the child whom he can turn to for help and care. Until the young child is assured that there is someone who is his own protector, he will be uncomfortable and afraid. He knows that he needs help in controlling his inner drives. He also senses that he needs support in meeting what is to come in a new situation. The child is not an independent being. When the young child's mother is not with him, mastery of himself and his environment is often an insurmountable task.

The newly admitted child, sick, or arriving in the hospital for some operation, is forlorn and scared. This is especially true if it is his first experience in the hospital. He has had to part from his parents, perhaps for the first time in his life. He has come into a room, the like of which he never has seen before.

The student nurse's first days in the hospital ward may not hold one tenth the terror that hospitalization does for a child. Perhaps recollection of the way the student nurse sought the support of her classmates in a new situation will serve to help her identify herself with the newly admitted child's feelings. Vander Veer* says,

The situation might be disastrous, were it not for the fact that children can displace their dependent needs fairly readily from parents to other adults. Time and contact are essential for this process to occur. Only through attention to and interest in, the individual child, can nurses, doctor or attendant be accepted as reliable parental substitutes.

The child's first emotional need is relief from anxiety. He needs energy to combat his disease and also to adapt himself to all that hospitalization entails. The nurse's task is to minimize his anxiety. To do this she must *first know what is making him fearful.* If she has insight into the emotional life of the child, she will be sensitive to many of the things of which children are afraid. Fears differ in children. The nurse needs to discover the particular things that are frightening to her patient. Many of his fears may be irrational. The nurse can help him discover that they are unreal. She does this by standing by to prove to him that the world that he is in now is less frightening than he had imagined it to be. Trying to explain irrational fears away with words is useless. It is the nurse's protectiveness, interest and understanding of his need for personal

---

* A. H. Vander Veer, *op. cit.*, p. 60.

reassurance that bring him relief from irrational fears.

Some of the child's fears will be realistic ones which can be alleviated by preparation, by support and by freedom to express the feelings which are stimulated by new or painful experiences. Preparation *before* he must meet the experience helps him to mobilize his energy to master it. It also provides the basis for a trusting relationship. If he is approached for a treatment before he is prepared, he cannot help distrusting his nurse. Imagine how a child must feel when without warning, a nurse and a doctor carrying a foreboding-looking tray of equipment arrive at his bedside to do a gastric lavage! Without a word of preparation, they overpower him with their strength as they restrain his arms and legs. They thrust a tube into his esophagus, manipulate a syringe and talk about the possibility of finding microbes in his stomach contents. Then without warning they pull the tube out from his throat, unfasten his restraint and leave him alone feeling attacked, angry, overwhelmed with anxiety and perplexed as to what will happen next. Is it any wonder that children become unmanageable in a hospital? Would not the adult respond to the situation similarly? He probably would not act out his anger but he would have hostile feelings with which to cope.

Support during the procedure and permission to express his feelings are equally important in preventing trauma. Explaining every step of the procedure and helping him find ways to co-operate make him a helpful participant and motivate him to master the experience in the best way that he can. There are always parts of the procedure that the child can do. There are also choices that we can help him to make. We can increase his interest in the procedure by telling him why it is to be done. He needs to know when it will hurt. He also should receive permission to give vent to his feelings. New or painful treatments evoke hostile feelings; these the child needs to express. He also needs to discover that expression of feeling is acceptable. Repressed hostility increases anxiety; the nurse's task is to alleviate it.

Support comes from the nurse's approach and from the strength that she possesses. If the nurse is secure in her ability to do the procedure and to obtain the child's confidence, he will sense it. He will feel reassured that he is in skillful hands. If the nurse approaches him with a comment like the following, he will be doubtful as to her ability and to his own: "Now you are going to be a brave boy, aren't you?" In addition to putting doubts in his mind, the foregoing question fails to recognize the natural fear that inevitably arises when a child is confronted with a new hospital procedure. One cannot be brave unless one is prepared and thoroughly convinced that he is not in danger. Often the first seed of doubt is sown when the nurse says, "Go to the doctor. Don't be afraid. He won't hurt." The child may not have thought of being afraid. When the adult says, "Don't be afraid" and follows it up with "He won't hurt," fear will inevitably arise. If he is going to be hurt, telling him it will not hurt is untruthful. If it is not going to hurt, it is better that the word not be used, even though it is used in a negative fashion.

A child will not ask the questions that can give the nurse some insight into his fears until a bond of friendliness is established between them. Learning to establish a friendly relationship with a child is a skill of great import. It is important because it is the quality of the nurse's relationship which determines her effectiveness in meeting the needs of her patients.

Establishing a Relationship with the Child

There is no sounder way to establish a relationship with a child than by meeting his emotional needs and by relieving his physical discomfort. When a nurse discovers a child's needs and meets them, she lessens his frustration and gives him gratification. Because the nurse has given him relief from his discomfort, he recognizes her as a person to whom he can turn with confidence that she can meet his needs. Repeated experiences of gratification heighten his warm feelings toward her. Gradually, he displaces his dependent needs from his mother to his nurse. When the child feels confident of her interest and support, the nurse is well on her way toward helping him meet his situation constructively. At first the child may be excessively demanding because he has quantities of anxiety and an illness that has produced regressive symptoms. To establish a relationship the nurse must meet him at his current emotional level. If he is demanding, it needs to be accepted. When the needs which he is seeking to satisfy are met, his anxiety and tension will decrease. Then the nurse on whom he has come to depend can help him gradually to become more independent of her.

The child needs an opportunity to become familiar with his surroundings. A tour about the ward and the playroom affords the child this opportunity. A child is less fearful if he knows what is down the corridor and behind closed doors. He also needs to know that there is a place in that ward which belongs to him. The following introduction to the ward gives the child increased feelings of belonging: "This is your unit, Johnny. This is your bed and table. This is where you can keep your toys and the things you brought from home. Inside the table are the things I will use to take care of you when your mother cannot be here with you." When a child enters nursery school, the teacher shows him his locker and explains its use to him. His locker is important to him! It is not unusual to hear a child saying, "This is mine. It's my special place."

In this period when the child is becoming oriented to the ward, the nurse can watch for clues that will tell her how to establish a relationship with him. The more the nurse can follow his lead, the more successful she will be. If the child does not need to be put to bed at once, freedom to investigate his surroundings as he so desires will facilitate adaptation. If the nurse is interested in him, he will sense it. Gradually, as he becomes adjusted to her presence, he will reach out toward her emotionally. He will show her in words or actions what he needs from her. If he is a child who has little trust in people, he probably will test the nurse out in many ways.

In this way he attempts to discover her responses to his behavior.

Knowledge of the child's preparation or lack of preparation for hospitalization is helpful in orienting the child to his surroundings. Often the newly admitted child does not know why he has been brought to a strange place or why he has been put to bed before night-time. Often a question like the following brings information that helps the nurse to know how to help a child understand his current situation: "Johnny, why are you here?" or "Children stay in their beds here. Do you know why?" If the nurse discovers that he does not know why he is in the hospital, she should explain the reason for his admission just as she explains everything else that is new to him. Such explanations should be given gradually so that he can assimilate them.

One must rely more on deed than on word to give the young and the very sick child peace of mind. They can get comfort only from knowing through experience that they are among friends who understand their need for comfort.

The child will also require help in learning the routines of the hospital. This is as important for the child who comes in for a tonsillectomy as it is in the case of a prolonged stay. The way children go to the toilet, summon their nurse, have meals, rest hour and playtime in the hospital are all things about which the newly admitted child needs information. Hospital routines are different from those that he has known before. These he will question either verbally or nonverbally. He will feel safer if he knows what the nurse is going to do, what is ex-

pected of him and what he must anticipate in the immediate future.

A child's need "to be in the know" is no different from the nurse's need. Nurses probe new situations to discover what is expected of them. Perhaps the nurse can remember how she felt the day she went to a new ward. She probably can also remember how she felt when a doctor arrived in the ward ready to do a treatment for which she was unprepared. She may remember thinking, "I don't understand what he wants. Why didn't he call the head nurse and tell her he was coming? I wonder if I will know what instruments he will want. I wonder how he will expect me to assist him?" The hospitalized child is in a similar predicament. He, too, wants to be ready to participate. He, also, dislikes being caught unawares. He wants to feel competent and accepted. But he does not have the past experiences to draw upon as does the nurse!

The principles involved in approaching the child who must be put to bed immediately upon arrival are the same; methods of carrying them out will require modification. The child's adjustment will be facilitated if his nurse postpones painful procedures until he begins to become more secure with her. In the meantime the nurse can give him toys, sit beside him quietly and attentively and wait until he approaches her. Presenting play materials tells the child that the nurse is a friendly person who understands his need for play. Merely placing toys on the newly admitted child's bed is not sufficient because he needs more than toys. A newly admitted child requires emotional gratification before he has energy available for play. Through play with his nurse a relationship can be established, after which the child will be more prepared to co-operate to the best of his ability. The situation which follows subsequently serves to illustrate one way in which a relationship can be established.

Billy was 18 months old when he came into the hospital with cystic fibrosis of the pancreas. When his mother left, he stood in his crib and screamed. He tossed every toy onto the floor. When the nurse showed her willingness to hold him, he ran into the corner of the crib like a frightened baby animal. He seemed to be both panic-stricken and furious. The nurse sat quietly by his bedside. His screaming continued for many minutes. Then tempestuously he tore a rubber washer from the movable cribside and threw it onto the floor. The nurse picked it up and put it back in place. Billy repeated the performance not once but a dozen times. Each time the nurse replaced the washer on the cribside.

Gradually, Billy's behavior began to change. His tears vanished; he relaxed and began to smile. Then the nurse placed a ball on his bed. For several minutes the above kind of play was repeated. Then a pyramid of rings was placed on his bed. Again the nurse watched for clues which would indicate ways in which he needed her. Billy began to play. He removed the rings from the stick, handed one to the nurse and then held out his hand to have it returned to him. Before long Billy moved himself closer to the nurse. Soon he scrambled over onto her lap. In a few minutes Billy's need for closeness lessened. He reached for the toys and began to play. Soon he indicated a desire to be put back onto his bed.

Later when the nurse said, "Billy, I must go now. I'll be back," she left a child who was more at peace than he was when she arrived. And his nurse did go back very soon. When she did she said, "Billy, I came back. I'll always come back when I tell you I will." A relationship had begun and Billy had made a start in his struggle to master his new situation.

BEHAVIOR OF A CHILD IS DEPENDENT UPON TYPE OF ILLNESS AND PAST EXPERIENCES

The nurse in the admitting room, the clinic, the wards and the private rooms of a hospital will have experiences with many different types of children who are well, ill or convalescing from various types of disease. There will be those who have not had intelligent care, some who have not been well fed, others who have had little wholesome discipline, some who have been deceived and some who are filled with fears which were instilled in them by an unfortunate type of guidance. However, there will be many who come from homes where they are loved and have had wise care. They respect authority because it has been reasonable. They trust others because they have not been deceived. They expect friendliness and care because they always have had it. This latter group of children are fortunate in times of illness. They will experience intense grief when they are separated from their mothers but they will approach their new situation with less anxiety, with trust and with belief in the friendliness of others. They will have more inner resources available to adapt to the treatment and the care which they require to become restored to health.

There will be children in all degrees of sickness: the chronically sick and weak children; those who are acutely ill, medically or surgically; and children with physical handicaps which require correction. The latter group come into the hospital crippled in some way but usually are comparatively well until after they have had their operation. They recuperate rapidly from the immediate effects of the operation. However, they are often faced with long periods of convalescence in plaster and splints.

THE FRIGHTENED CHILD

All children are anxious when they come to the hospital. Preparation lessens anxiety and helps children to meet the experience. *However, until they meet the experience and discover that their needs will be fulfilled with friendliness, they will be anxious and uncomfortable.*

Children handle their anxiety in many different ways. Many frightened children scream in terror and fight rebelliously. Some are provocative to gain security or freedom from guilt. Regression and self-comforting behavior are commonly observed in infants and young children. Some children withdraw into themselves like frightened little animals and become depressed. Denial of fear is not unusual. Some manifest their denial with aggressive, overly brave behavior.

Crying is the young child's way of communicating his feelings; it needs interpretation, for its meaning may vary in different children. The nurse should learn to view children's crying with serenity. Crying is inevitable in hospitals. The young child is grieved when he becomes separated from his mother. He needs to express his grief in the presence of a friendly, understanding person. The child also cries when he is scared or frustrated and angry. Naturally, he cries when he is hurt physically. It is the only way in which many children can express their feelings. The nurse's task is to discover the cause of a child's crying and meet the need that he is seeking to satisfy.

There are children who come into the hospital ready to fight because they expect the worst, having been deceived on many previous occasions by their parents. They assume that they are being deceived again. Some have been threatened with hospitalization as a punishment. Such children are fearful and suspicious of the unknown. They look upon the nurse as an enemy. They are ready to use their fists and fight at the slightest provocation or without any provocation. *But there has been provocation,* even though the nurse has not been a party to it. Already, these children have been threatened or deceived; their reaction is understandable, even though it is difficult for the nurse to handle.

The child who comes into the hospital mobilized to fight needs an immediate experience which shows him that the situation he is in is not as fearful as he imagined it to be. If the mother is threatening the child, the nurse should help her to see that such a course is unnecessary. Usually her threats become ineffective in the face of the nurse's statement that they never would be carried out in the hospital. Following this, the nurse might add: "Sometimes mothers do not know that nurses and doctors want to help children. I will tell you and your mother exactly what I am going to do. Then you both will know all about it. And you can help me."

Many times a child kicks and screams because it is the only way he knows how to meet a new situation. Through experience he has learned that it is a successful method of avoiding the unfamiliar and the unpleasant. If so, the mother is usually trying to kiss and soothe the child. Or she is offering candy or some other bribe or is promising to take him home from "this horrid hospital very soon." The child who responds to new situations in this way needs help to learn that his temper tantrum is an ineffective way to handle his frustration.

In a situation of emotional tension the calm, firm, positive voice carries weight. There are voices, low rather than high in pitch, full rather than thin in tone which can express kindness and understanding at the same time that they communicate expectancy of reasonable behavior.

The mother who, with promises of candy, begs her child to stop crying or kicking, needs her own anxiety alleviated. She requires help to see that blandishments are an ineffective way of helping a child to meet a difficult situation. But first her co-operation must be won. Undoubtedly, she is anxious and frustrated. She bribes and threatens because she does not know better ways of helping her child. In most instances temporary separation of the mother and the child is indicated.

The first approach to the child should be one that helps him to know that the nurse is friendly, honest, understanding and unperturbed even in the face of a temper tantrum. If a few friendly gestures are not effective, it is wise to sit down beside him and wait until he has become calmed. If nothing happens for a few minutes, a frightened child has time to realize that there is little to be afraid of. When he re-establishes his equilibrium, friendly words will assure him further that his interests are being considered. Familiarizing him with his new surroundings will also provide reassurance. The nurse's behavior should demonstrate that she respects him as a person; that she will be honest in her dealings with him; that she can be depended upon; and that she will not make him the victim of her moods or become the victim of his. This type of guidance increases his sense of security.

Some children defend themselves against anxiety with provocative behavior. It may be a way of testing out the limits of the adult's tolerance or of relieving their fear of their own consciences. The child who has not had consistent discipline at home is insecure. He does not know the limits of his environment. He is constantly afraid lest his behavior precipitate physical punishment or loss of love. To get the security of knowing the limits of his environment, he persists in irritating his mother until he learns her tolerance. He gets relief from anxiety because he discovers how far he can go without being punished.

A child may use provocative behavior to get relief from fear of his conscience—in other words, from guilt feelings. The child who is provocative is often unable to sublimate his aggressions into constructive channels. He cannot channelize his aggressions because he has not had the help of consistent, unwavering

discipline. Instead of getting help
in channelizing his aggressions, he
received condemnation which made
him feel that he was a bad child.
Experience taught him that punishment relieved him of discomfort.

If a pattern of behavior like either
of the above has been established at
home, the child undoubtedly will
use it in the hospital, both because
it has become a habitual way of relieving his tension and because his
illness often serves to intensify his
feelings of guilt. In the ward there
are often children who literally ask
for punishment—not in words because their need for punishment
is unconscious — but in behavior.
Johnny used provocative behavior
to rid himself of guilt feelings.

Johnny was 7 years old and in the
hospital with rheumatic fever. Every
time the nurse came to give him care,
he would knock the equipment off the
table. When she pulled up his cribside
he would leap over the side of the
bed. He did not wait until she had left
the room; he did the jumping in her
presence.

Punishment merely serves to encourage the child with provocative
behavior to repeat his misdemean-
ors. Punishment relieves his guilt
and brings relief from anxiety. Under these circumstances he naturally
does the things that he is forbidden
to do. When he is not punished for
his provocative behavior, he will be
less apt to repeat it because it brings
no satisfaction. Instead of punishing
him, the nurse should use her energy in trying to help him discover
that he is not the bad child that he
believes himself to be.

The child who defends himself
against anxiety with provocative behavior requires *consistent,* kind and
firm guidance. He should know
what is expected of him and what
he can and cannot do. Only then
will he have the security which
comes from knowledge concerning
the limits of his environment. The
child who is under compulsion to
provoke adults to anger is a difficult
child with whom to deal. He is the
way he is because he has been made
that way. When he discovers that
his behavior brings a response different from the retaliatory kind he
previously has been accustomed to,
his behavior will begin to show signs
of change. If it does not change, it
probably indicates his need for psychological therapy.

Situations like those cited above
call heavily on the nurse's store of
patience and poise. Handling
frightened, angry or grief-stricken
children is not easy. It usually
evokes anxiety in the nurse. As a
result she has to cope with her own
feelings as well as help the child
to handle his. It is natural for a
nurse to feel aggressive in the presence of an angry child. It is
equally natural for her to feel her
anxiety mounting in the presence of
a panic-stricken child. Grief-stricken
children evoke painful feelings in
the sensitive nurse. These, too, are
difficult feelings to handle. They
may reactivate feelings that the
nurse had herself in a similar situation. Or they may make her feel
inadequate or uneasy because she
does not know how or does not have
the time to ease the child's distress.
Sometimes the nurse defends herself
from anxiety by not seeing the
child's anguish. This solution meets
her immediate needs but it leaves
the child with a problem that he

cannot master without the aid of an understanding person.

The nurse needs serenity which can be maintained in the face of many trying situations which are bound to arise in pediatric nursing. Her patience should be the *patience of understanding* and not merely self-control which holds the expression of impatience in check. It takes time for the nurse to gain understanding of her feelings and to learn to handle them constructively. It will also take time to acquire patience and tolerance. Before knowledge can be used in relationships with others, it has to be integrated or digested. Often this is a slow process. The nurse should be patient with and tolerant of herself. If she is, she will learn more rapidly. She will also communicate less anxiety to her patients. Poise and understanding of others will come when she discovers through experience that all persons including herself behave in the light of their past experiences and require new relationship experiences to change attitudes, feelings and behavior.

Many children have not learned to trust and co-operate with others; and many have regressed and therefore are unable to accept the frustrations that they might tolerate otherwise. Their bodies are often pain-racked. They are also using tremendous amounts of energy to fight their diseases and adapt themselves to separation from their mothers. Changes in behavior will come if their feelings are understood. In addition, they will require time to orient and adapt themselves to the changes which they are experiencing physically and psychologically.

Many children regress and utilize self-comforting methods to alleviate their anxiety and tension. Some suck their thumbs, masturbate, bump their heads or rock their bodies to and fro. In addition, they may pick their noses, scratch their fingers or faces or sit fingering a lock of hair. These children are anxious. They are getting what comfort they can by themselves. This kind of behavior pattern is symptomatic of distress. Unless the child's anxiety is alleviated, he will continue to get relief from anxiety by these methods.

A child who manifests his anxiety by excessive use of the foregoing symptoms needs his mother. If his mother cannot be with him, he should have a continuing relationship with a nurse so that his security can be restored. When he becomes reassured and comforted by the care and the interest of another, the nurse can help him find pleasure in play and in association with other children. Scolding or rejection of him or his behavior will serve only to increase his anxiety. It will also increase his need for self-comforting behavior.

In hospitals there are children who manifest their anxiety by withdrawal symptoms. Many of these children have experienced excessive frustration and rigid discipline in the early years of their lives. Past experiences have made them feel that anger was "bad." They also feel that anger is punishable, either by physical means or by loss of love. As a result they have acquired a punishing conscience. Their conscience makes them fearful of people and of their own aggressive feelings.

The strictly disciplined child who is unprepared for separation from his mother is often unable to express his hostility overtly. Lack of preparation may be due to inability to understand because of his age or to failure to anticipate for him what going into the hospital entails. Feeling hostile toward someone he is supposed to love is often unbearable. If he thinks that it is his fault that he is ill, his anger at his mother is not justified. Therefore, he feels it is "bad." If it is "bad," he cannot direct it at her. Instead, he keeps it bottled up inside of himself. In doing so he punishes himself instead of his mother. Or he may be afraid to express his aggressive feelings because previous outbursts of feeling brought loss of love. He defends himself against fear of his own aggressiveness by becoming withdrawn.

The depressed child often behaves as though he thought that his treatment was punishment. Often he also acts as though he thought he was deserving of discomfort. Each time the nurse came to give Timmy his intramuscular injection of penicillin, he whimpered quietly and said, "I be sorry. I be good." Timmy seemed to think he had done, felt or thought something "bad" or wicked. The needle and the syringe seemed to represent punishment to him. When asked why he is in the hospital, some children say, "I naughty" or "I bad." The depressed child often goes unnoticed for he is quiet, withdrawn and unusually accepting of everything that is done to him. Unconsciously, some of them want punishment. If they feel guilty, punishment relieves it.

The withdrawn child is not as comfortably adjusted to his new environment as he appears to be.

Closer observation discloses abject misery and unhappiness. He does not smile, eat or play. Nor does he relate to children or adults. Instead, he sits or lies still. His facial expression betrays the depth of his inner turmoil. Much of his energy is being used to keep his hostile feelings and anxiety under control. As a result, he has a smaller quantity of energy available to combat his illness, to play or to relate to others.

The depressed child is in great need of sympathetic understanding and interest. He requires permission to express his anger overtly. This can be accompanied by guidance such as the following: "Some children get very angry at their mothers for leaving them in the hospital. Some children get angry at the things I do to them. They tell me when they feel angry. And I am glad that they do. I don't like them less. I know they need to holler and cry when they are hurt. I know being in the hospital makes them feel angry." When a child responds to treatments as if they were punishment, their interpretation needs correction. "I wonder what Timmy did that makes him feel sorry" often brings a response which furthers the nurse's understanding of his withdrawal. If the child cannot verbalize his fantasied misdeeds, something like the following communicates understanding and encourages expression of feeling: "Sometimes children think injections are given to punish them. They aren't given to punish you, Timmy. They are given to make you well. And when you are better, you will be able to go home again."

The nurse not only needs to give

the withdrawn child permission to be angry but she also should be ready to accept a tempestuous response. Words and deeds which prove that his expression of aggression will not bring punishment are imperative. A response like the one which follows is reassuring: "I know how you feel. You are angry and unhappy. You need your mother and she isn't here. That makes all children mad."

When the child is able to express his anger and discovers that his illness is no fault of his own, depression symptoms begin to subside. Gradually, a change in behavior becomes observable. He has energy to play because his hostility has become released and accepted. His anxiety is relieved. He begins to eat and resist things he formerly accepted in a compliant way. *This is progress; it is not undesirable behavior.* The following example serves to illustrate the above principles.

Sally was 3 years old when she was brought from the South for surgical repair of extrophy of the bladder. She never had been away from home before. She found herself surrounded by a multitude of strange people and subjected to experiences that she never had had before. Her malformed body was viewed repeatedly. She had many treatments which were painful and restricting. She complied submissively. She showed no overt response to pain, restraint or to the unknown.

The day after her operation, Sally was more silent and withdrawn. She never whimpered when the doctor changed her dressing or inserted the needles for intravenous therapy. She did not relate to her nurse who was in constant attendance each morning. The third day her dressing was changed again. The doctor

probed her wound and inserted a drain. Pain and anger were stronger than her controls. She shrieked at the top of her voice, "No more, I hate you. Go away." Simultaneously, she reached for the doctor's hands. Sally's face was contorted with terror. She looked as if she expected to be demolished.

Instead of being punished, Sally got immediate understanding and praise. The nurse did not say "Don't do that. Keep your hands down." Instead, she looked at Sally, smiled acceptingly and said, "It does hurt Sally. It hurts terribly when the doctor uses the instrument. I'm glad you can tell us how you feel." Simultaneously, the nurse stroked the hand that reacted to her aggressive feelings. Sally looked up at her nurse and nestled her hand into hers. It was Sally's first personal contact since admission. Previously, the nurse had held her hand and stroked her head, but Sally's hand was limp. There was no response that indicated that she even had felt the nurse's interest in her.

Sally's nurse encouraged expression of feeling. She provided reassurance which proved that her interest would not be withdrawn because of tempestuousness. A bond was established between them. Later, Sally continued to express her anger. She became more resistant to treatments. Temper tantrums also began to appear. Expression of feeling was welcomed. Her nurse knew that pent-up feelings would retard her physical progress and disturb her relationships with others. Gradually, Sally's anxiety and depression lifted. She began to play and became interested in all the activities that were going on around her.

Denial of fear is another way in which children handle their anxiety. Sometimes they cover it with aggressive, overly brave behavior. Vander Veer* cites the case of a boy who used a pocket knife to try to out-bluff a person he fantasied to be an

---

* A. H. Vander Veer, *op. cit.*, p. 65.

attacker. As the child entered the doctor's office, he drew a pocket knife from his pocket and opened it up. When the doctor asked him what he was doing, he said, "I'm going to cut the doctors before they can cut me." Vander Veer interpreted this behavior as a defense against his fear of being injured.

The situation described subsequently serves to illustrate denial as a method of handling anxiety. It also describes the nursing care which is essential to help a child face a situation of which he is fearful. Davy was prepared for hospitalization and for operation by his parents. However, his behavior showed that the details of preparation were too scary to think about. Davy needed further verbal preparation by his nurse. He also needed support both before and after the operation to face what he wanted to deny would ever happen.

Davy was a 5-year-old, red-haired, well-built and unusually bright and vivacious youngster. He entered the hospital for surgical repair of squint. Outwardly, Davy seemed to be quite self-contained. He was sociable and friendly with his nurse and the children in his 4-bed unit. He co-operated well when he was permitted to express his ideas and suggest how things should be done. He resisted breakfast in bed. He could not wait until his temperature was taken and he could be out of bed. His nurse anticipated that he would be reluctant to have a bath in bed. She suggested using the bathtub. He was delighted with the suggestion. He bathed himself and talked constantly while he was doing so. He mentioned his red hair and showed pride in having hair "just like Daddy." He talked more about his father than about his mother. It was his daddy who was going to do things for him. He would bring him things, etc.

The nurse and the doctor met resistance when they attempted to discover how Dave had used the preparation that his parents had given him. When the nurse asked him why he was in the hospital he said, "To get a patch on my eyes to fix them up." He ran away from the nurse when she began to prepare him for some of the forthcoming events of the day. The doctor arrived and said, "Dave, do you know that today is the day you are going to sleep and have a patch put over your eye like you had put on in the clinic?" Dave answered, "Yes" and went immediately out of the door. Davy acted as though the subject of surgery was anathema to him.

To prevent Davy from being overwhelmed with the event, the nurse continued to help him understand the treatments which were forthcoming. She told him about the medicine she would give him with a needle. She explained its purpose. She also told him that it would hurt and that it was scary to many children. He said, "I don't want it." Then he ran away again to his play. To prepare him further, she showed him how hypodermics of medicine were given. She used a doll to demonstrate the procedure. His interest became stimulated. Independently, he took the syringe and the needle and returned the demonstration on the doll. He handled the equipment skillfully and seemed to have observed every detail of the technic. However, one experience of hypo-giving was not enough! Davy gave hypos to every toy in the room that had arms, legs or tails. He even went down the corridor to the playroom in search of the huge elephant that he said had "great big ears." He stuck the elephant in the hip and in the ear. His face was serious while he manipulated the syringe. When he finished, his face became transformed with a glow of self-satisfaction.

The nurse used an alcohol sponge and a clown doll to show Davy how a mask and medicine would be used to put him to sleep. Davy paid no attention. He looked as if he was not hearing a word that she was saying. She told him that he would be unable to drink or eat until after he had been put to sleep and his eyes had been fixed. Again his facial expression was blank. He appeared as if he was thinking of other things than the current subject of conversation. His only verbal response was "I am thirsty." Then he ran away again.

Davy was active constantly. His attention span was short and he did not concentrate on any activity for long. Once he wanted a playmate's toys. He proceeded to take them away from her against her wishes. When she clung to her possessions he said, "You ought to be ashamed of yourself for not giving them to me." Later in the morning the nurse again tried to help him face the forthcoming events. He would not listen. He changed the subject or ignored her completely.

At noon Davy's parents arrived bringing him a record player, a new gun and holster and bedroom slippers. The nurse told him she would play the records for him the next day. He responded with, "No you won't. I'll play them myself." (Davy continued to deny that an operation was a reality which he must face.) When the nurse brought the hypodermic of medicine his anxiety was evident. His daddy said, "It won't hurt." His father's words seemed to redouble Dave's efforts to control himself. He submitted complacently. He did not seem to hear the nurse when she said, "All children are scared when they have hypodermics. Lots of them get angry, too. They tell us that it hurts." Immediately, he wanted to show his parents how well he could give a hypodermic. This time he gave a toy kitten a hypo in its tail.

Until it was time to go to surgery Davy sat with his parents in the playroom watching television. When it was time to leave the ward, he waved goodbye to his parents. But first he said, "Give me my gun." En route to the operating room Davy shot every person in sight. During the waiting period, Davy continued to shoot. As he shot he talked incessantly about gangsters, cops and robbers. His nurse stood by supporting him with her presence and interest. To try to help him face his fear, she said, "Davy, soon the lady doctor will come. All children get scared when they know that they are going to be put to sleep. They don't know that the doctor and the nurse are going to tell them everything that they are going to do. I am going to stay here and help you go to sleep."

When the anesthetist arrived, she explained every step of the procedure to him. She also suggested that they play a game together while he went to sleep. He asked about the smell in the room and said, "I 'spose it's alcohol." He was also curious about the purpose of the tanks which were beside the anesthetist. Just before the mask was put over his face he said to his nurse, "Tomorrow you play my records for me, will ya?" The nurse assured him that she would. She also told him that she would be beside him when he awakened. He was more receptive at this point. He listened when she said, "Your eyes will hurt when you wake up. And you won't be able to see because there will be patches over your eyes. I'll be there to help you. In a day or two the doctor will take the patches off. Then you will be able to see again."

Davy's tension was evident, but his powers of control remained intact until the anesthetic and its discomfort made it vanish. Restraint was not necessary until the excitement stage.

THE ACUTELY ILL CHILD

The way in which the nurse establishes a relationship with an acutely ill child will depend upon his physical condition. Factors, which do not exist in children who come to the hospital for corrective work, will need to be taken into consideration. The acutely ill child is often apathetic to his surroundings. He is too sick to reach out to the nurse to indicate the ways in which he needs her. He has pain, anxiety and a feeling of helplessness which brings marked regression. Immediate transportation to the operating room or ward is often indicated. Frequently, danger is imminent. Both the acutely ill child and his parents feel intensely the danger in the situation.

The sick child must get immediate emotional security because his survival depends upon the energy that he has available to fight his disease. Every word and act needs to communicate strength to him and his parents. Many times the nurse must work quickly and deftly. Combined with efficiency, there should be sensitivity to the fact that the child *feels* even though he is unable to make any overt behavioral response to the care that he is receiving. The sick child's relief from anxiety will come from medical treatment that supports his body in its fight against disease. It will also come from gentleness, sympathy and the strength that he feels in the touch of the nurse's hands, in the tone of her voice and in the manner in which she regards his parents. Both he and his parents need to feel confident that he will be cared for; that he will be made more comfortable; and that his pain will be eased. Both medical treatment and understanding care are imperative in promoting emotional security; one without the other leaves the child unsupported in his struggle for survival.

Conservation of energy is the foremost principle in the care of the acutely ill child. He should receive quiet, consistent supportive care which anticipates his every want. The nurse needs to be alert constantly to symptoms which indicate physical or emotional distress. She should plan her care to avoid interruptions in rest. This will require careful timing of feedings, medication and treatment, as well as consideration of his parents' need for help in handling their anxiety.

Most of the serious illnesses of childhood are acute. The child is usually desperately ill during the acute phase of an illness. He reacts to disease intensely. He is a sensitive little person who has not yet developed the physical or psychological stamina to withstand disease without being grossly threatened. The balance may tip quickly in one direction or another. For this reason every detail of care which conserves energy and helps him towards recovery needs to be provided.

Fever. One aspect of many acute illnesses is a high temperature. A child's temperature rises much more readily than does an adult's. Therefore, a high temperature in a child does not have the significance that it has in the adult. A temperature of 104° or 105° F (40° to 40.5° C) from an illness that is ordinarily of short duration, such as tonsillitis, usually requires no interference. However, the same temperature in a child with a more serious and protracted illness may require that something be done to lower the fever. The high fever should be reduced if it causes irritability, restlessness and loss of sleep. These symptoms are incompatible with rapid recovery. The presence or the absence of these signs is more of a guide than the degree of temperature in deciding whether or not to interfere. Hydrotherapy and anti-pyretic drugs are the most satisfactory method of combating fever.

Alleviation of Pain. All legitimate measures should be used to reduce the amount of pain that children are called on to endure. In caring for adults there are doubtless many situations in which the patient has something to say about the amount of pain that he can endure. However, in caring for children, this is seldom the case. An adult says that he cannot tolerate a treatment without something to alleviate the pain. His feelings are considered. A sedative is administered unless it is contraindicated. A child has nothing to say about what he can or cannot withstand. He probably has not had experiences which make him competent to judge.

Those who have the matter to decide need to consider his needs from his point of view. If a sedative or anesthetic can spare the child unnecessary pain without causing complications, it should be given.

Nourishment an Important Part of Treatment. One of the most important factors in maintaining the body in condition to combat disease is to keep it well-nourished. Although the nurse has nothing to do with planning the meals in the hospital, she should know what food materials the body requires. She also should know the foods in which the various components are found. Providing food that the child needs is an essential part of nursing care. However, it is equally important to provide an atmosphere that helps the child to feel like eating.

Nurses and dietitians should work together in helping the child to maintain adequate nourishment.

Food has deep significance to a child. Often its significance is connected with religion and race. Nearly every race has developed its characteristic dishes and diet. It is not a matter of wonder, therefore, that the proper nourishment of patients is a very real problem to hospital personnel. It is entirely possible to plan well-balanced meals and yet not nourish the children adequately. Nurses should know their patients' likes and dislikes. These should be communicated to the dietitian just as symptoms are reported to the doctor.

The acutely ill child's lack of appetite or refusal to eat needs to be accepted and handled in a way that encourages co-operation. Lack of appetite is the usual response to an acute illness. It may be a protection against his lessened digestive capacity or a response to the emotional distress that he is experiencing from separation. The acutely ill child cannot digest the amount of food that a convalescent or well child can. The amount of his feeding should be lessened; he should be fed at shorter intervals; but he should receive those food components which the tissues of his body require. He should be given amounts of food that he can take easily. The food should be made tempting and should be served as attractively as is possible. Dishes of attractive design and color, or special dishes set aside for a special child are often intriguing to him. The element of surprise also makes an appeal to children. It is an excellent device for making the meal hour pleasant. The acutely ill child should not be expected to feed himself. He needs every ounce of energy, and self-feeding is a difficult process for a small child. On the other hand, if the child resists the nurse as she tries to feed him and expresses a desire to feed himself, he should be allowed to do so unless all physical effort is forbidden. Enough time should be devoted to meal periods to give the child sufficient help and encouragement and the company that he requires.

The child who has learned to eat a well-balanced and varied diet is far better equipped to fight his illness than the child who has endless food prejudices. Discovering the child's reactions to food at home is helpful knowledge for the nurse to acquire. Does the child refuse his food because of loss of appetite due to illness and hospitalization, or is it his usual reaction to food? The cause of poor appetite needs to be found and rectified. If his disinterest in food is the result of his illness, patient waiting until he feels better is necessary. If he is lonely and grieving or filled to overflowing with rage because he has been left in the hospital, the nurse's efforts should be directed toward supplying him with the comforts that he requires. Until his security is re-established, he probably will express his feelings of resentment by refusing to eat.

When a child enters the hospital with many food prejudices, he will require help to learn to accept an increasingly larger variety of food. The nurse will be more successful if she serves initially only those foods that she knows the child likes. Gradually, she can introduce *minute morsels* of disliked food with an approach that communicates her expectancy of co-operation. He probably will say, "I don't like it." This

the nurse needs to face with him by saying something like the following: "I know it isn't one of your favorite foods. Lots of children do not like it when they first taste it. I know you'll try it. I'd like to help you try it." Each bit of co-operative effort should be encouraged. Learning to eat new foods is a difficult process for the child who has missed experiences in learning during the first year of his life. Therefore, it is wise to indicate understanding of his problem by commending his willingness to participate in a new learning experience.

A small amount of food eaten without friction and with a certain degree of pleasure is better than large amounts forced on an unwilling and tearful child. Forced feedings never are justifiable with a sick child or a well one. Some children who come into the hospital have already been in combat with an adult over food. Such children may even have resorted to vomiting a disliked food and so have convinced an unsuspecting adult that he cannot digest food. There are many children who come into hospitals whose inner conflicts are expressed by behavior problems in relation to food. Forcing food will not solve these problems; it will only increase the child's resistance toward food and his need to refuse.

The nurse can help the child if she does everything possible to make mealtime a happy period of the day. Conflict and the expression of resentment when the child refuses food slow the learning process. The child needs to feel that the nurse wants to help him learn to eat even what he thinks he does not like. If the relationship between the child and the nurse is constructive and if she understands the reasons why he has refused food in the past, the food situation will cease to become a major problem. Serious cases of refusal to eat with no physical basis indicate some deep emotional difficulty. These children usually require intensive treatment by a psychiatrist or child guidance worker. When the child is acutely ill and he is not taking enough to sustain him, fluid and nourishment must be given either by gavage or by intravenous route. The emotional trauma resulting when an acutely ill child is forced to eat probably has more long-lasting psychologically damaging effects than the technic of gavage or intravenous fluid administration. The acutely ill child's need for fluids is urgent. Consideration to the administration of fluids is given in Chapter 6.

THE CHILD REQUIRING OPERATION

The child who enters the hospital for an operation needs care which is adapted to his special requirements. For the time being he is not a sick child whose illness requires special attention. It is easy to forget the child who has been admitted for diagnosis or future operative procedure. He is not sick and needful of symptomatic treatment. Nor is he convalescent and so much at home that he has no inhibitions about making his wants known. However, undoubtedly he has a sense of insecurity, for he is in a new situation. He cannot help but sense that something unusual is going to happen to him. *Before operation, the child should become familiar with the nurse who is going to help him through the critical experience which he is to meet. After a relationship has been established the child needs gradual preparation for everything that he will experience before and after operation.* A 2-year-old will not understand everything that he hears but he will catch the nurse's feelings as she talks. He will recognize that she is trying to help him. When he meets new experiences bits of her preparation will have its effects. He will know that she had forewarned him. Therefore, his trust in her will be heightened. If the time of waiting is longer than the actual time needed for preparation, he should be up and occupied with constructive pursuits.

If the nurse knows that the child has been prepared for operation by his mother, she should attempt to discover his concept of what is to happen to him in the hospital. Children interpret explanations in the light of their own needs, as has been stated already. Often a child's ideas are unrealistic. If he has interpreted his mother's explanations erroneously or dressed them up with fantasies of his own making, the nurse should help him understand what is really going to happen to him. Often what he imagines is more gruesome than reality. When he knows the truth, his anxiety is relieved. A way to help the child who handles his fear with denial has been presented already. There are physicans who would not operate on a child unless he showed evidence that he was ready to accept the realities of what he is to meet. There are others who do not feel acceptance is necessary. Therefore, many times the nurse will be confronted with children who obviously have repressed or denied knowledge of what is to occur. When she does she should explain what she is doing and tell him what is to come, even though her words go unheard. The child who has repressed or denied the event to handle his fears needs more help and more support because he is unprepared to meet the situation in which he finds himself.

After operation the child needs an opportunity to master the anxiety which was evoked at the time of the experience. His nurse needs to spend time with him helping him to know that she is interested in all that he has experienced. If he feels her interest, he will be encouraged to talk. Many times his concept of what occurred is unrealistic. Again she can help him understand reality. Everyone, including children, needs to talk about disturbing events to understand and to assimilate or digest them. The young child who cannot communicate his thoughts and feelings verbally will disclose them in his behavior. He needs play activities as soon as he is physically able. Through play he will be able to obtain mastery of his anxiety. The following situation describes one child's response to operation. It also shows the way he was helped to master his fear and to co-operate in the process that was necessary to make him well.

Jimmy, aged 7 years, had just experienced a pneumoencephalogram and was lying in a tiny room waiting to be anesthetized for a craniotomy. He was strapped down and alone; he was in anguish! He knew that he was going to be operated on but there was no one present to help him meet the painful, frightening reality. He knew that "op-eration" meant anesthesia because he had experienced that before. He also knew that they were going to do something to his head because it had been aching constantly for days and days. His conversation ran as follows: "I don't want to go to sleep. I don't want a mask. I want to go back to my room. Why isn't my mother here? Don't people around here know that I need her? My mother and doctor said I could go to sleep from a needle or by taking deep breaths from sweet smelling stuff on a cloth and blowing it out again. How will they put my head back together again? They are going to cut through the bone, aren't they?"

Jimmy was in no condition to be anesthetized. He was unready to meet the experience before him. He needed honest answers to his questions, as well as reassurance that his head would be put back together again after the doctor had fixed the inside so his headaches would cease. In addition, he needed to know that his head would be bandaged and painful when he awakened; that he would have fluid running into his veins; and that he would be just as he is now after new hair has grown on his head. The following questions showed the problems which were concerning Jimmy: "Where will I be when I wake up? Why do I have to go to sleep to have the operation?"

Relieving a child's fears, reassuring him that he will not be alone in moments of stress takes time, but it is time that the child has a right to and needs. In a half hour Jimmy had relaxed. He accepted the idea that the operation had to be. He knew exactly how the anesthetic would smell. He also knew that the nurse and his mother would be with him when he awakened. Jimmy had been helped to meet a fear-ridden experience. At the same time his confidence in nurses was strengthened, and he was better prepared to adjust to the pain of the postoperative period which was to come.

THE CHILD WITH CHRONIC ILLNESS AND THE ONE PHYSICALLY HANDICAPPED

There will be children in the hospital who probably will go through life with some physical handicap. There are those whose lives will be circumscribed by a disease that sets them apart from the normal life of childhood. Many of these children perhaps will spend much of their time in hospitals or convalescent homes. These children lose their childish look and become wise about so many things that do not seem to be a rightful part of childhood. They grow pathetically old before their time. They become the little old men and women who are seen in many children's hospitals.

The children described above cannot do all that well children can do, but effort should be directed toward making it as constructive as possible. Everything possible needs to be done to help them look out rather than in upon themselves and their symptoms. This is no easy task. The chronically ill child's needs for normal personality development are difficult to satisfy— especially the deepest need of all— a continuous relationship with a warm, giving mother who recognizes his physical and psychological readiness to adapt to increasingly more socialized modes of behavior and to become independent gradually through his own accomplishments. *A plan of nursing care which includes growth-producing experiences is essential if he is going to be helped to make a constructive adjustment to life.*

Another group of children who need help in growing more capable and secure are the physically handi-capped whom the public call "crippled." These children have physical limitations. Many times they have severe personality handicaps as well. Many tests have been devised and used to discover whether or not children with a designated handicap have a special kind of personality. All tests have failed to prove that they have. The crippled child who has a personality handicap was not born that way. He was deprived of emotional satisfactions and made that way.

The parents of a handicapped child face problems which are difficult to surmount. The crippled child is more difficult to accept. Every parent wants a normal child. Giving birth to a child who deviates from normality is a frustration. It is also a blow to parental pride and hope. It takes superb ego strength to surmount this disappointment. To raise the handicapped child infinitely more wisdom, skill and parental security are required. All of these factors tend to impede the parents' capacity to develop a strong affectionate relationship with their child.

Many parents cannot accept a handicapped child emotionally without the help of professionally trained workers. It is understandable why they cannot. In addition to disappointment, often they are afraid of the responsibilities that his care entails. They are also frightened because they know the attitude of society toward the crippled child and those who produce him. Often they are angered and grief-stricken as well. With frustration, anger is inevitable; it is also natural, understandable and a feeling that needs the acceptance of professional people within hospitals and clinics.

The handicapped child feels the impact of his parents' feelings toward him and the problems that his birth has created. He reacts to his parents' feelings toward him. Many times he senses their frustration and feels that he is a disappointment to them. His adjustment to his limitations will depend upon the interplay between his defect and the parental and social attitudes that he experiences.

Children respond to physical handicaps in many different ways. Some feel unloved and withdraw into a world of fantasy. They never learn to use the powers that they have. Some compensate for their difficulties and fight to overcome their limitations. Denial of their limitation is another way in which some children solve their problem. Some feel pity for themselves. They demand solicitude without any feeling of responsibility toward others. Some have grown discouraged concerning their capacity for social relationships and deny their need for love. They often try to hurt others as they have been hurt. Others unconsciously seek punishment because their hostility makes them feel guilty. Then there are others who find substitute modes of expression. If they are unable to enunciate clearly, for instance, they find ways to express themselves in writing, painting, etc.

The handicapped child needs guidance that will help him toward a realization of the powers which he possesses and help him to accept his limitations with emotional tranquility. He needs this kind of guidance so that he may become self-reliant and find his place within his society. His adjustment will be determined by his courage, self-evaluation and judgment. The child with a handicap needs guidance that helps him feel competent, self-satisfied and acceptable to others. The nurse should find out what he can do. Then she should give him every opportunity to develop whatever capacities he possesses. Children over and over again measure up to what is expected of them. *Success is the result of the faith that others have in them.* Many of these children learn to do because they have confidence in their teachers. They trust their judgment and absorb the deep faith that their elders have in them.

Many parents require help in acquiring faith in their children's capacity for constructive adjustment. They do not know what the handicapped child can accomplish. They have had no experience that can guide their teaching. The nurse who has faith in the handicapped child's capacity for wholesome adjustment can help him succeed. She can also help his parents in periods of discouragement. If she understands their feelings of disappointment, guilt, frustration or resentment against the tremendous responsibility that they are forced to carry she can be of real service to them. Helping them to feel that they are not alone with this problem is of immeasurable value to many parents. Discovering that someone understands their frustration and feelings of being overburdened prevents guilt feelings. It also often helps them formulate more constructive attitudes toward their child. The nurse can help also by giving parents concrete help that makes them more effective teachers. Commending a mother's success in teaching gives her hope and increased self-confidence. These feelings often swing the pendulum toward adjustment because they are essential for adaptation to difficult problems. The crippled child does not want or need pity; he craves understanding and guidance which helps him become secure in his relationships with others. He wants to develop his capacities for self-direction and competence. There exists an emotional attitude toward the crippled child, a pity and a fear of him which sometimes make it practically impossible for him to acquire a wholesome attitude toward himself and toward life. Pity toward a handicapped child engenders in him a sense of self-pity. He may react as if he expected everyone in his world to wait upon him and give him special privileges. Or he may feel the hostility beneath the pity and react as if those in his world were his bitterest enemies. Understanding carries no taint of pity. It recognizes and accepts his differences and permits a wholesome relationship toward him as a person. The person with understanding accepts the implications of his handicap. He directs his energy toward finding ways to help the child find substitute activities which foster security, self-esteem and the development of social interest.

In working with a child who is crippled, the nurse needs to be aware of her feelings toward him and his parents. If she feels pity, fear or repugnance, it is better that she tell her supervisor so that the child may have the benefit of a relationship with a truly accepting person. Feelings of pity, fear or aversion are not unusual; nor are they anything of which the nurse needs to feel ashamed. All people have them until they face them. When they discover that their fears are unrealistic and realize how unwholesome these attitudes and feelings are for the child, they are able to accept them in a more wholehearted fashion.

Many a nurse who has grown accustomed to the quiet, listless and apathetic children among those chronically ill or is prepared to meet the nursing challenge in the care of the critically ill feels utterly lost when she enters a ward of convalescent or orthopedically handicapped children. There she finds an amount of surplus energy with which she is unprepared to cope. Many times she resorts to a type of discipline to which she as a child and as a student nurse may possibly have been expected to submit. She lays down rules. She is restrictive beyond actual necessity and resorts to "don't" instead of "do." The results are usually disastrous. The older boys lead the younger ones on to pranks. The nurse is often totally distracted, and ward order is reduced to chaos.

Restrictive discipline produces no growth; it brings order out of chaos but none of the qualities that a child needs to become self-directing. The child who is subjected to rigid, autocratic discipline becomes an obstructive factor in a social situation instead of a co-operative one. He submits because he must, but with no spirit of co-operation.

Situations like the above arise because the nurse has not been sensitive to the children's need for constructive, satisfying relationships and

activity. The majority of convalescent and orthopedically handicapped children are bursting with
energy. They cannot be expected to
lie quietly in bed with nothing to
do. Autocratic discipline increases
their tension, and the need for activity is intensified, not lessened.
They want adventure, fun, opportunities to practice their skills and to
learn. The pediatric ward is for
children. The nurse needs to help
them know that this is true. The
older children can be won readily by
a nurse who enlists their help and
shows them that she actually needs
that help. They will revel in responsibility because it gives them a feeling
of satisfaction and importance. It
wins them to the side of law and order
rather than to opposition. If the
nurse finds the ring-leader, wins his
co-operation by acknowledging his
powers and encourages him to work
with her, she will be on her way to
establishing peace and comfort for
her patients. Commands should be
kept to a minimum. Nonessentials
should be ignored. Making an issue
of a triviality incenses the child
equally as much as it irritates the
adult.

SITUATIONS
FOR FURTHER STUDY

1. Of what value is an activity
program in a pediatric ward?

2. Observe one of your patients
and describe his response to the activity program of the ward. Of what
value was it to him personally?

3. Observe a group meal period
in the ward. Describe the children's
response to it. What do you think
they gained from the experience?
What did you learn from the experience?

4. Describe a situation in which
you prepared and supported a child
through a painful treatment. Include in your description the methods you used to prepare and support
the child and the child's response
to your care.

5. Of what value are visiting
hours to children and parents? Observe 2 children during visiting hour
and describe what you saw, heard
and felt. What did you observe that
gave you a better understanding of
these children?

6. Collect data from the mother
of a newly admitted preschool child.
Of what value was this information
to you? What was the mother's
response to your inquiries?

7. Observe a child being admitted to the hospital and describe
what you saw, heard and felt. How
were the child and his parents
helped to meet the situation? Discuss ways in which they might have
been given more help.

8. Do you agree that children
should be prepared for hospitalization? Support your decision with
the reasons why you agree or dis-
agree.

9. Why do parents need help at
the time their children are being
admitted to the hospital?

10. Establish a relationship with
a newly admitted child and describe
the total experience.

11. How may the nurse help to
give a child a sense of security?
Describe a situation in which you
alleviated a child's anxiety.

12. What are the various ways in
which children may reflect a sense
of insecurity? Observe children in
the ward. Describe behavior that
reflected insecurity in 2 children.

What do you think made them anxious?

13. Prepare a child for operation. Describe your approach, your technic and the child's response to the experience. Accompany the child to the operating room and describe the child's response to each phase of the situation. What were his needs during the experience?

14. Describe a child who is handicapped with a physical deformity. How do you think he feels about his handicap? What evidence do you have to substantiate your answer to the above question? Describe a situation in which you taught the child to be more independent. What was the child's response to his accomplishment?

BIBLIOGRAPHY

Blake, Florence: Factors influencing the child's adjustment to new situations which bring separation from family and home, p. 263, in The Child, His Parents and the Nurse, Philadelphia, Lippincott, 1954.

Dudley, Nancy: Linda Goes to the Hospital, New York, Coward-McCann, 1953.

Frank, Ruth: The frightened child, Am. J. Nursing 51:326, 1951.

Jessner, Lucie, and Kaplan, Samuel: Observations on the emotional reactions of children to tonsillectomy and adenoidectomy, p. 97, in Problems of Infancy and Childhood, New York, Macy, 1949.

Hanson, Margaret B., and Shaw, Mary M.: Mealtime in the pediatric department, Am. J. Nursing 49:212, 1949.

Killilea, Marie: Karen, New York, Prentice-Hall, 1952.

Podolsky, Edward: How the child reacts to his physical defects, Ment. Hyg. 37:581, 1953.

Prugh, D.: Study of emotional reactions of children and families to hospitalization and illness, Am. J. Orthopsychiat. 23:70, 1953.

Ross, Helen: The handicapped child and his family, The Crippled Child 30:10, 1953.

Sever, Josephine A.: Johnny Goes to the Hospital, New York, Houghton, 1953.

Spence, Sir James: The doctor, the nurse and the sick child, Am. J. Nursing 51:14, 1951.

Stevens, Marion: Parents are welcome on the pediatric ward, Am. J. Nursing 49:233, 1949.

Vander Veer, Adrian: The psychopathology of physical illness and hospital residence, p. 50, in Personality Development and Its Implications for Nursing and Nursing Education, Springfield, Ill., Dept. of Public Health, 1949.

Wallace, Mildred V.: Feeding the hospitalized child, J. Am. Dietet. A. 29:449, 1953.

Wallace, M., and Feinauer, V.: Understanding a sick child's behavior, Am. J. Nursing 48:517, 1948.

Ware, E. Louise: Mental hygiene of the orthopedically handicapped child, (pamphlet), New York Assoc. for the Aid of Crippled Children, 1947.

————: Parents of the orthopedically handicapped child, (pamphlet), New York Assoc. for the Aid of Crippled Children, 1950.

Wessel, Morris A.: The pediatric nurse and human relations, Am. J. Nursing 47:213, 1947.

Wilkins, Gladys: The role of the nurse in the admission of preschool children to hospitals, (unpublished master's paper), Dept. of Nursing Education, Univ. of Chicago, 1950.

Emotional problems associated with handicapping conditions in children, (pamphlet), Washington, D. C., Superintendent of Documents, U. S. Government Printing Office, 1952.

FILM

Robertson, James: A Two-Year Old Goes to Hospital, New York, New York Film Library, 1953.

Pediatric Therapy

◇◇◇

FLUID ADMINISTRATION
DRUG ADMINISTRATION

SITUATIONS FOR FURTHER STUDY

In her care of sick children the pediatric nurse participates in many varieties of treatment. While she rarely has the responsibility for determining the type of therapy to be used or the exact details of dosage, her care of the child will be enhanced if she comprehends the general principles that she is serving and is successful in helping the child understand and accept it. Some of the medications and technics have rather limited usage and are described with the particular diseases to which they most commonly apply. It is the purpose of the authors in this chapter to consider therapeutic measures which have common application to many sorts of illness in childhood.

In dealing with child patients, the factor of size always must be considered in regulating doses of medicine, amounts of fluid to be administered, and in determining the variations that are necessary in certain technical procedures. With adult patients it is possible to use fairly standard dosages and technics, for the differences in size among patients is not very great. A large fraction of the nurse's adult clientele will weigh between 100 and 200 pounds, and all but the very unusual will be encompassed by the range from 75 to 300 pounds. The maximum discrepancy here is 4-fold. But in her pediatric experience, commonly her patients will range over a 30-fold difference in weight, from 5 to 150 pounds. If we include small premature infants and obese adolescents, the discrepancy may be as much as 100-fold. In some instances dosages may be computed on the basis of age, which is a rough guide. However, in most instances the calculations are more nearly accurate when they are referred to weight. Sometimes a more precise method of comparison through calculation of the surface area of the individual is used but it has not found general favor because of its complexity. Size differences also dictate variations in certain technical procedures, such as transfusions, where the diameter and the accessibility of veins create special problems in the very small child.

FLUID ADMINISTRATION

PHYSIOLOGIC CONSIDERATIONS

Water. A continuous supply of water is a more urgent requirement for life than a supply of food. Martyrs have been known to starve themselves for a month or more and still survive, but life will not go on for more than a few days if the body is denied water. The essential processes of the body not only require water for their continuing operation but also they gradually exhaust the internal supply. During healthy existence there is a continuous loss of water in stools and urine, from the evaporation of sweat from the surface of the body, and with the air exhaled from the lungs. Disease not only aggravates these losses through such changes as fever, diarrhea, vomiting and increased urine output, but also it may increase the water requirement by speeding up some of the body processes through increased metabolic rate. At the same time the individual may be unable or unwilling to ingest even his normal quota of fluid. If the process continues, he uses up the reserve fluid stored in his tissues and begins to show the symptoms of dehydration—dry mouth, thick secretions, hollow eyes, loosening skin, concentrated urine and loss of weight.

The child, and more particularly the infant, reaches a stage of dehydration faster than the adult. In part this is due to the fact that he is less able to recognize and satisfy his needs for water, and in part it is because the smaller he is, the greater is the proportional quantity of water in his body and the more rapid is the rate at which it is used. This rapid use of water becomes apparent when we remember that it is not difficult for some adults to get along indefinitely on a pint and a half of fluid per day. Yet the newborn infant, who may weigh only one-twentieth as much, usually cannot manage on much less than a pint of fluid per day.

When viewed under a microscope the various organs and tissues of the body are seen to be composed of tiny units, the cells. It is upon the activity of these small units that the body depends for its vital activities. Although cells differ widely in their appearances, in the functions they serve and in their chemical contents, they have certain general properties in common. Each is surrounded by a semipermeable membrane which ordinarily retains the protein and other large constituents of the cell. Water, oxygen, nutrient materials and certain salts and minerals can enter through this membrane, while the waste products and substances which the cell is designed to produce diffuse out through it into the surrounding space. Cells in general are distinguished chemically from the surrounding tissue fluids by their heavy content of protein and by the predominance of potassium and phosphate salts.

INTRACELLULAR WATER. In both adults and infants about 45 per cent of the body weight represents the water contained within these vital units. It is called the intracellular water. To function properly, each cell must be supplied not only with the oxygen and the nutriment that it requires, but its water and salt contents must be kept from varying beyond certain narrow limits. The body tends to defend the integrity of the cells during health and disease.

The blood vascular system, consisting of arteries, veins and capillaries, is a closed system of tubes reaching to all the recesses of the body which serves as an avenue of fluid communication among the various organs. The arterial side of the vascular tree carries oxygen and nutriments to the cells; the venous side removes their wastes and the soluble substances which they have fabricated for general use by the body.

PLASMA. The fluid portion of the blood *(plasma)* contains protein which cannot pass out of the walls of the vessels, and water and mineral salts which can freely leave the vascular bed and enter the surrounding tissues. To function properly the fluid volume of the vascular bed must be kept within certain limits. If it becomes too small, due to loss of blood or to extreme dehydration, shock will result; if it becomes too large, the heart may be unable to move it along at the normal rate, and fluid will ooze from the vascular bed to produce edema of the subcutaneous tissues or, more seriously, of the lungs. In health both the adult and the infant have about 5 per cent of their total body weight as plasma or intravascular fluid. In addition to its characteristic content of proteins, the plasma has mineral salts in concentrations which are quite different from those of the intracellular water, since the predominating components are sodium and chloride. As in the case of the intracellular fluid, many mechanisms in the body tend to keep the composition of the plasma within a narrow range.

INTERSTITIAL FLUID. Around the cells and between the blood vessels there is a third type of fluid—the interstitial fluid—which has a composition very similar to that of plasma except that it is practically devoid of protein. Interstitial fluid represents the reservoir within the body which responds most easily to the shifting conditions of disease. When it increases, edema results; during dehydration it is depleted in preference to the plasma or intracellular water supply. Unlike the latter two fluid compartments, its relative magnitude is greater in infants than in adults. The adult carries about 15 per cent of his total body weight as interstitial fluid; the small infant begins life with 25 per cent of his body weight in this form but approaches the adult proportions as he passes beyond the age of 2 years.

Electrolytes. Changes in the fluid content of the body during disease are relatively easy to visualize and understand. The infant with diarrhea and vomiting obviously is losing more fluid than he can take in. The consequent loss of weight due to exhaustion of his interstitial fluid is readily apparent. Conversely, the edema of the child with anuria and a persisting intake of fluid is easy to comprehend.

Unfortunately, however, these changes involve not only shifts of water alone but much more complex alterations in the concentrations of the various mineral salts (electrolytes) within the fluid compartments. The complexities of these changes are not entirely understood by biochemists. Without special knowledge of chemistry, it is difficult for the nurse to understand the details of such changes. However, a few of the mechanisms which operate should be understood in general terms.

As the body must take in water continually to replace the losses through normal metabolism and excretion, so too it must have access to a continuing supply of minerals, such as sodium, potassium, calcium, magnesium, etc., and of their salts, the chlorides, bicarbonates, phosphates and sulfates. Under normal circumstances there is an ample supply of these materials in the food from which the body can select to replace losses through metabolism, excretion or normal wear and tear. In the various fluid compartments mentioned above the concentrations of each of these substances (called ions) is kept within definite limits. The kidney plays the most important role in regulating these concentrations, for it has the ability to hoard or discard them selectively, depending upon the needs of the moment.

Acid-base Balance. The relative concentrations of the various ions within the tissue fluids influence the acidity of these fluids. During health the plasma maintains a very constant slightly alkaline reaction. In chemical terms this is measured and expressed by the concentration of hydrogen ions or pH. An exactly neutral fluid has a pH value of 7.0; an acid fluid has a pH value which is below 7.0 and an alkaline fluid has a value which is greater than 7.0. The normal range for body fluids is from 7.35 to 7.45. Life is seriously threatened when the pH value of the plasma falls below 7.0 or rises above 7.7.

In maintaining the acid-base balance of the blood and tissue fluids, the kidneys and the lungs play major roles. The kidney helps to maintain normal equilibrium by its differential excretion of unwanted ions and other substances and by its ability to form ammonia, which greatly enhances its capacity to excrete the acid products of metabolism. The lungs assist in maintaining equilibrium by varying the rate at which carbon dioxide is blown off, hoarding this slightly acid substance when the plasma is getting too alkaline, and blowing it off at a faster rate when the plasma is getting too acid. During health normal body activities result in the production of an excess of acid substances which must be excreted. Thus the usual productions of the body metabolism (urine, sweat and expired air) are essentially acid in character in order to maintain the balance.

Disease (with a few notable exceptions) tends to aggravate the production of acid substances and places an increased demand upon the lungs and the kidneys. This demand must be met if the acid-base balance is to be maintained. Ordinarily, these organs are equal to the task because of their great reserve capacities. When a study of the chemical constituents of the blood reveals that kidneys and lungs are being placed under stress but are meeting the challenge successfully and preventing the blood pH from shifting out of the normal range, a condition of compensated acidosis or alkalosis is said to exist. When the stress has become so great that they can no longer prevent the blood pH from descending below 7.35, uncompensated acidosis is present. If the pH rises above 7.45 the condition is called uncompensated alkalosis. (It should be emphasized that in clinical usage the terms acidosis and alkalosis refer to deviations from the normal range of blood pH and are not determined by reference to chemical neutrality. Even in severe clinical acidosis with pH values of 7.0 to 7.2 the plasma is still chemically slightly alkaline.)

In clinical pediatrics most of the disturbances of acid-base balance are due to metabolic disorders. Under such circumstances the blood concentration of bicarbonate usually indicates the severity of the process. When facilities for more nearly complete chemical determinations are not available, the values of the CO_2 content or CO_2 combining power of the plasma are commonly used to guide treatment. These levels (which are essentially the same as the plasma or serum bicarbonate) decrease during acidosis so that in a rough way, a mild acidosis is usually present when the values are 2/3 of the normal, and a severe acidosis is present when they have fallen to 1/3 normal. In alkalosis the levels rise, and an increase by ¼ ordinarily indicates mild alkalosis; an increase by ½, a severe disturbance. Convenient as these relations are, they do not always indicate the chemical changes accurately. In certain types of acid-base disturbances which originate in respiratory abnormalities, the relationship is actually reversed. For illustration of these statements see the table below. Additional discussion of acid-base changes will be found with the specific disease entities and in Chapter 19.

EXAMPLES OF ACID-BASE DISTURBANCE

	pH	CO_2 CONTENT (MEQ./L.)*	CO_2 COMBINING POWER (VOLS. PER 100 CC.)	CHLORIDE (MEQ./L.)
Normal infant	7.35-7.45	22	49	98-106
Normal child	Same	25-30	55-65	Same
Mild metabolic acidosis (diarrhea)	7.25	18	40	112
Severe metabolic acidosis (diabetes)	7.10	9	20	95
Mild metabolic alkalosis (pyloric stenosis)	7.50	35	75	90

* This abbreviation is read milliequivalents per liter. It means that the serum contains so many thousandths of a chemical equivalent in each liter. The concept of a chemical equivalent cannot be described in simple terms.

Calories. During the course of disease there is usually an increased need for calories because the metabolic rate has been increased by fever; but at the same time several factors commonly conspire to reduce the child's ability to ingest and digest food—vomiting, loss of appetite, weakness, disturbed digestive processes. Consequently, his caloric requirements are usually unmet during the acute stage of an illness, and he must live on reserve stores within his tissues. To an imperfect degree some of his caloric deficit may be met by including calories in the form of glucose in the oral or parenterally administered fluids which are given to combat the more immediate danger of excessive fluid depletion. Calories given in this form also spare body protein and combat the tendency toward the accumulation of some of the organic substances (ketone bodies, acetone and diacetic acid) which play an important part in the causation of acidosis. When fluids can be given only by the parenteral route, the ability to provide calories from glucose or plasma is limited by the amounts of plasma and the concentration of glucose which can be administered safely.

REPLACEMENT THERAPY

Fluids by Mouth. During many illnesses the loss of fluid and electrolytes is slight, and the child is able to replenish his deficit gradually by taking *fluids by mouth*. The daily amount of fluid required varies with the degree of disturbance and with the size of the child. For infants the daily intake must exceed the normal requirement of 125 cc./Kg. of body weight if they are to catch up. Older children require less per unit of weight so that intakes of 1,500 to 3,000 cc. per day are ordinarily sufficient. It can be assumed that the electrolytes will be restored if mineral-containing fluids, such as milk, fruit juices and soups, are included as part of the intake. Enough fluid to produce a copious flow of urine is desirable in order to give the kidneys the optimum chance to correct minor changes in the electrolyte composition of the plasma and hence of the interstitial and the intracellular fluids. If the volume of urine is small, the opportunity for renal correction is handicapped.

Parenteral Administration. When illness is complicated by vomiting, by loss of consciousness, by refusal to eat, by the necessity of resting the gastro-intestinal tract, or by a severe loss of water and electrolytes which requires rapid correction, fluids must be restored by routes other than the oral one. Such *parenteral administration* may be given under the skin, i.e., directly into the interstitial fluid compartment from whence it will be taken up by the blood and distributed in time to the other tissues of the body; or it may be given directly into the vascular system by injection into a vein. A third route which is used occasionally is the injection of fluid into the peritoneal cavity, from whence it is absorbed in a fashion similar to that which follows subcutaneous injection.

Fluids which are to be given parenterally must meet certain requirements. They must be prepared sterilely and must be protected from bacterial contamination until the injection has been completed. Otherwise, the direct insertion of bacteria into one of the fluid spaces may result in local or generalized infection. Parenteral fluids must have a nearly neutral chemical reaction or they will be irritating and painful to the subcutaneous tissues or to the veins into which they are injected. In exceptional circumstances this requirement is broken with respect to intravenous injections, but it cannot be broken for subcutaneous injections. A third requirement of parenteral fluids is that they have approximately the same osmotic activity as the interstitial fluid (isotonicity). Osmotic activity is the capacity of a fluid to attract water from or dispense water to the surrounding medium. It is determined by the concentration of ions and molecules. An isotonic solution of sodium chloride (commonly called normal saline) is a 0.9 per cent solution; glucose is isotonic in concentration which lies between 5 and 10 per cent and in practice is used in either of these dilutions. Other fluid mixtures, too, must be constructed so as to meet the requirement of isotonicity in order to avoid undesirable shifts in the distribution of water in the tissues into which they are injected. *Distilled water is never an acceptable fluid for either intravenous or subcutaneous use.* (Given intravenously it may cause hemolysis of the red blood cells which results in a serious or even fatal reaction. Given subcutaneously it is quite painful and may damage the tissues into which it is injected.)

Subcutaneous Infusion (Clysis). When fluids are given by subcutaneous infusion or clysis the total quantity used is adjusted according to the size of the child and his needs. The rate at which the fluid is administered usually is governed by the speed of absorption from the subcutaneous space, the flow being adjusted so that painful swelling of the tissues is avoided. There is little likelihood that too rapid injection of fluid will cause any disturbance other than local discomfort when subcutaneous fluid is used, for the blood stream accepts what it needs at the moment and leaves the remainder unabsorbed. In some instances an enzyme (hyaluronidase) is added to increase the rate of absorption. Then care is required in adjusting the rate of flow.

Intravenous Infusion (Transfusion). When fluids are given by intravenous infusion or transfusion the total quantity administered and the rate of injection must be calculated very carefully. Such fluid is passing into a closed space which is distensible within certain limits, but if it is overloaded it may lead to serious or even fatal embarrassment of the circulation. The normal intravascular space may be visualized as a partially inflated balloon. During a dehydrating illness the balloon collapses somewhat, due to loss of its fluid content. Filling it with fluid to distend it back to normal size is desirable in order to promote good circulation; however, if it is overdistended and tense the circulation will be hampered, and if pushed to the bursting point life will cease. Fluids which contain only water and nonprotein solutes are relatively safe because they can ooze through the walls of the blood vessels at a fairly rapid rate and relieve the mounting internal pressure if necessary. However, there is a limit to the speed at which they can diffuse out of the vascular bed. For nonprotein-containing fluids it is probably safe to administer 30 cc./Kg. at one time to an infant. When continuous infusion of such materials is being given, the daily volume should not exceed 150 cc./Kg./day.

Caution is imperative when protein-containing fluids (blood or plasma) are being used, for these substances cannot ooze out, and whatever increase in distension of the vascular space is produced will remain for a period of hours or days. The hazard is particularly great in infants. As a general rule, it is unwise to give more than 20 cc. per kilogram of body weight to an infant in a single dose. It is usually wise to allow 12 to 24 hours to elapse before the procedure is repeated. (The technic of exchange transfusion, which will be described in Chapter 7, involves simultaneous withdrawal of blood so that these rules do not apply to it.)

Nursing Care

Oral Fluids. A skillful nurse can play an important therapeutic role by encouraging the child to accept an adequate amount of fluid by mouth. In doing so she may be able to help him avoid the discomfort of parenterally administered fluids. She will be more successful if she can adopt an attitude of patient and pleasant encouragement than if she displays demanding exasperation at the child's failure to co-operate. Too much urging may result only in overfilling the child's stomach with the induction of vomiting. In most instances some latitude of choice in the selection of the particular fluid to be given is permitted. Offering the older child a choice or trying the infant on several types of liquid may provide the solution to an obstinate refusal.

Accurate record-keeping is always important in order that the necessity for parenteral fluids can be judged by the physician in charge. Estimates of the volume of vomited fluids should be subtracted from the intake administered. Truth and accuracy in such records promote the best interests of the patient. Observation of the frequency and the volume of urine production of a child who is in need of fluid therapy is also important. If urine is being produced freely, it probably means that the kidneys are able to perform their corrective work; if urine is scanty or absent, the fluid intake is probably insufficient.

Venipuncture. Measurement of the chemical constituents of the blood is usually desirable in the presence of important degrees of dehydration. With older children the technic of obtaining blood is the same as that used in the adult. However, infants and small children seldom have a vein of adequate size in the antecubital fossa, so that blood must be obtained from the external jugular vein, the internal jugular vein, the femoral vein, or in rare instances from the superior longitudinal sinus. Since failures are frequent and the risk of reinjection of blood into the vein is a real one, only sterile syringes should be used in venipunctures on infants and small children. When the specimen has to be obtained under oil, sterilely prepared mineral oil is required. In spite of the small size of the child, a No. 20 gauge needle is usually necessary. Blood will flow slowly through a No. 22 needle, but the risk of clotting is increased.

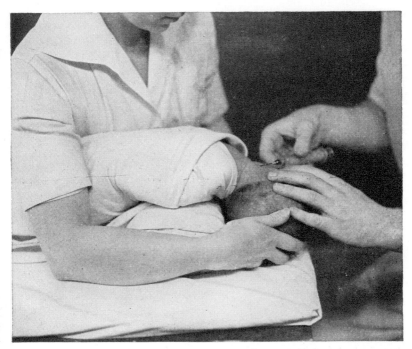

FIG. 6. Method of using the external jugular vein for venipuncture.

Positioning of the infant for these procedures is important in order to afford the operator the best chance to obtain his specimen rapidly and with minimum discomfort to the child. Positioning of the infant for puncture of the external or internal jugular vein is illustrated in Figure 6. The restraint most commonly employed is designated as *mummying*. A child is "mummied" by securing a sheet or a receiving blanket about the body in such a manner that the arms are held to the sides, and flexion of the lower extremities is relatively difficult (Fig. 7). The upper edge of the wrapping should be low enough to leave the tops of

the shoulders out. The head is turned to the side so that the chin touches the shoulder. Then the neck is extended over the edge of a table or a small pillow so that the sternocleidomastoid muscle is well stretched. The nurse holding the infant must control the head and keep it in position without hampering the operator's approach to the vein. When the external jugular vein is used it will become visible during crying and will collapse when the infant inhales. Blood flows most readily if the infant continues to cry during the procedure. The internal jugular vein is not visible beneath the muscle and must be approached

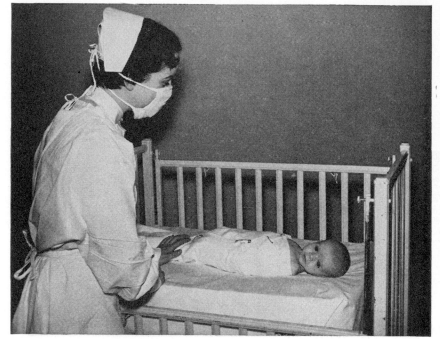

Fig. 7. An infant "mummied" for puncture of the external and the internal jugular veins.

blindly. If it is punctured accurately, rapid and easy removal of blood is achieved.

For puncture of the femoral vein the infant's groin is exposed, and the leg is extended on the abdomen and held firmly. The operator palpates the femoral artery as it emerges from the abdomen and punctures the vein which runs along its inner surface. The infant is usually wrapped so as to restrain the arms. Then the legs are abducted on either side of a corner of the table and held with the knees flexed over the table edge (Fig. 8).

Puncture of the longitudinal sinus of the skull for blood samples is done only in cases of emergency. The fontanelle must be open in order to afford access to the sinus coursing in the leaves of the dura mater. A special short needle is used and is inserted exactly in the mid-line, first through the skin and then through the dura. The infant is wrapped as for other procedures, and the nurse holds the head firmly with the face straight upward, the operator usually standing behind the infant's head. This procedure looks and is easy to perform, but the hazards of thrombosis of or hemorrhage from the cranial sinus are too great to permit its common usage.

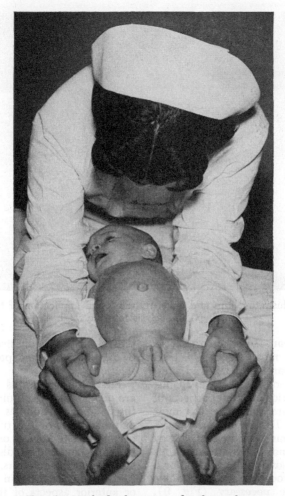

FIG. 8. Method of restraint for femoral puncture. The arms are restrained at the sides with a diaper. The child's body is placed diagonally across the table. Her legs are held in flexion over the edge of the table. The nurse immobilizes the trunk with her forearms.

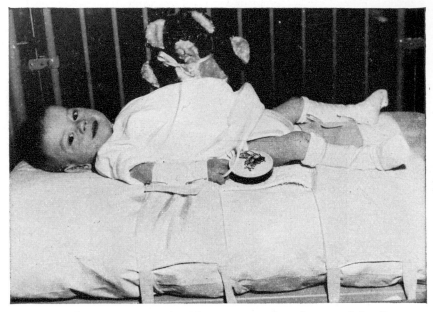

Fig. 9. Illustrating arm and ankle restraints and application of the diaper for hypodermoclysis into the thigh.

Subcutaneous Infusion or Clysis. This is the most frequently used method of parenteral fluid administration. Several sites are available, but the anterior or lateral aspects of the thighs are generally the most serviceable. The child must be restrained on his back in such a way that he will not be able to reach his legs and remove the needles. For a prolonged procedure arm and ankle restraints are necessary (Fig. 9). The equipment for a subcutaneous infusion or hypodermoclysis, as it is sometimes called, consists of a graduated bottle, tubing, a Y-glass connector, 2 adaptors, 2 needles of gauge No. 19 to 21 and 2½ to 3 in. long, 2 stop cocks, cotton and iodine, Merthiolate or Zephiran for cleansing the skin, restraints, safety pins, 4 strips of adhesive tape ½ by 3 in., an irrigating pole and the solution.

First, the apparatus and tubing are filled with the fluid to be infused, and air bubbles are washed or milked out of the tubing. Then clamps are tightened on each rubber tube, and the needles are firmly attached to the adaptors. After careful cleansing of the skin of the outer or anterior aspects of the thighs, a needle is inserted into each thigh. After insertion of the needles, the tubing is secured to the thighs with adhesive tape. Then the clamps are opened so as to allow a flow of fluid which will not result in uncomfortable distention of the tissues.

The precautions to be observed are that careful sterile technic should be used throughout and maintained until the apparatus is finally removed; that the needle points should lie between the skin and the muscle layers of the leg and not within the substance of either; that the needles should not be near the course of the femoral or the saphenous vessels along the inner aspect of the thigh; and that restraint should be maintained adequately so that the needles do not come out before the treatment is concluded.

Other places into which clyses may be given are the pectoral region and the back. If the pectoral region is used, the arms must be pinioned behind the back to prevent removal of the needles. The needles are inserted below and lateral to the nipples, and fluid is permitted to distend the loose space of the axilla. Frequently, the back is used as a site for single injections of fluid into premature or small infants, in which case a large syringe is used rather than the cumbersome apparatus mentioned above. Sometimes the back is used in older children when the thighs are not accessible. A child who is restrained on his face must be watched carefully to prevent suffocation.

The nurse can do a great deal to mitigate the discomforts of subcutaneous infusion by explaining the nature of the procedure to the older child, by restraining him with gentleness, by regulating the flow of solution and by providing the child with distractions, verbal solace and sympathetic understanding. The manner in which a child is restrained determines his feelings toward the measure and toward the person who carries it out. Young-

sters can tolerate restraint if it is done with the feeling that it is a protective measure rather than a punishing one. The young child knows that he cannot restrain himself during painful procedures. He welcomes aid in holding himself still if it is done with a helping attitude made manifest in the nurse's approach and method of procedure. When it is obvious that the child needs help in immobilizing himself for either a subcutaneous or an intravenous infusion, it is best to carry out the necessary procedure as quickly as possible so that the least amount of his energy is expended. An explanation like the following one given prior to application of restraint communicates understanding and interprets the reasons for the nurse's actions: "Timmy, it is hard for children to be still when they are getting a treatment. I know they need help. I'm going to put this restraint on to help you lie still. Then you will be able to remember to help us by lying still."

The child should not be left alone during painful and restricting procedures. He needs comforting with words, stories, songs and caresses. If a pacifier is not contraindicated medically, the infant will welcome it because it provides a tensional outlet and therefore gives comfort. Close observation is necessary to prevent the solution from running too rapidly; blanching of the skin from internal pressure is to be avoided. At the completion of the procedure, the needles are removed, and the injection sites are covered with small dressings. Undoubtedly, the young child will need to be held when the treatment is over.

Intravenous Infusion or Transfusion. OLDER CHILDREN. The same sort of apparatus and method of immobilization which is used for the adult is satisfactory for the older child who is able to co-operate and has a good vein in the antecubital region. The arm is immobilized by taping it to a padded splint or a sandbag. With adequate taping the child will not have to concentrate on maintaining a fixed position while the fluid runs in. Pressure on the arm proximal to the point of needle insertion must be avoided or flow through the vein may be hampered. Veins on the back of the hand, the flexor surfaces of the wrist or the medial side of the ankle may be used in similar fashion.

When fluids are injected directly into the venous system, careful observation of the patient, the apparatus and the rate at which the solution is flowing into the vein is essential. Between the graduated funnel and the needle adaptor a glass-enclosed dropper is inserted so that the speed of flow can be watched and measured from moment to moment. By counting the number of drops per minute the nurse can make a quick estimate of the rate of flow. She must also watch the rate at which the level is descending in the graduated cylinder and adjust the screw clamp or the height of the graduate accordingly. Ordinarily, the doctor will designate the speed of infusion which he desires. If the level is descending too rapidly, the drop rate must be slowed down; if it is descending too slowly, the rate must be increased. If an infusion is turned off completely, even for a few minutes only, it may be impossible to start the flow again because of the formation of clots in the needle. If the nurse finds that the infusion will no longer run or that so much has gone in that she thinks it should be turned off, she should consult the doctor at once. Air bubbles must not be permitted to enter the vein. Bubbles above the dropper are of no consequence, but any in the tubing or adaptor below the dropper are potentially dangerous and should be called to the doctor's attention. Pain accompanied by swelling at the point of insertion of the needle usually means that the needle point has slipped out of the vein and that it needs to be reinserted.

When blood is being administered, the nurse has additional responsibilities. The rate of flow must be adjusted to the speed determined by the doctor. If the child complains of generalized discomfort, chilly sensations or backache, it may be a forewarning that he is going to have a transfusion reaction. The young child, who cannot verbalize the above discomfort, will manifest his feelings in his behavior. He grows restless and cries, and close observation probably will show changes in color, in respiration and heart rate. Whenever any of these symptoms are noted, the flow should be stopped, and the doctor should be notified.

INFANTS. The smaller the child the more difficult and potentially dangerous is the technic of intravenous fluid therapy. Special problems are created by the infant because he is harder to immobilize, his veins are smaller and less accessible, and often there is a very narrow margin between a safe speed of

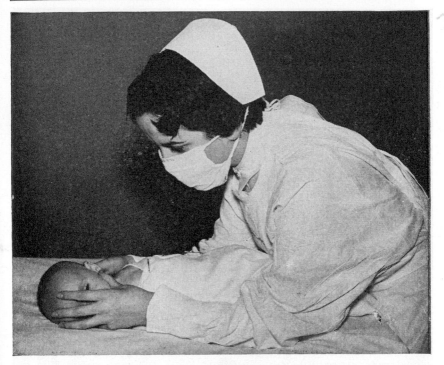

Fig. 10. Method of holding an infant for scalp vein technic. The nurse cups her hands over the occiput and the face, and holds the infant's head rotated at 90° and immobilizes his trunk with her forearms.

infusion and one that will keep the channels open.

In addition to the veins commonly used for infusions in the older child, the infant presents relatively large channels over the temporal region of his scalp which offer the best opportunity for successful entry. When such veins are to be used, first the scalp is shaved, and the infant is mummied as in the procedure of venipuncture of the neck veins. The nurse or other assistant then holds the head firmly turned to one side (Fig. 10). By pressing the head steadily and firmly against the table top it is possible to prevent slight movements of the head which may disturb the operator's aim or dislodge the carefully placed needle point. Care must be taken to allow the infant ample breathing space while he is being restrained. Sometimes it is possible to tape a needle in place and permit the slow continuous infusion of fluid into a scalp vein from the same type of apparatus as described above. Usually the needle which must be used is so small that prolonged flow cannot be expected, and a system of pumping syringes is arranged in the tubing so

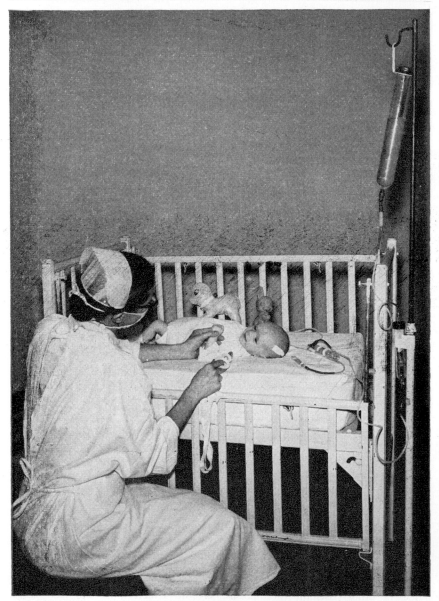

FIG. 11. Equipment for a continuous infusion into a scalp vein. A tongue depressor is taped to the polyethylene tubing which encloses the connecting needle to keep it straight to avoid puncture.

that a third person can slowly pump the fluid or blood through the small needle. (No. 22 to No. 27 gauge.) Thus a single dose of fluid may be injected in a period of 20 to 30 minutes if the volume restrictions previously outlined are observed carefully. There is a psychological danger of giving too much when the team is flushed with the success of completing a difficult maneuver. Other veins may be used in this same fashion, but the difficulty of immobilizing a hand or a foot is somewhat greater and calls for a strong and steady grip.

When it is anticipated that prolonged intravenous fluid administration will be necessary for the infant, often continuous intravenous infusion is used (Fig. 11). The scalp vein technic is satisfactory in instances where it is possible to maintain good immobilization of the head over a long period of time, or, as illustrated in the figure, when a length of polyethylene tubing is used to connect the scalp needle with the adaptor and the needle from the infusion set. More often a vein at the ankle or in the antecubital fossa is exposed by surgical dissection. Then a length of ureteral catheter or plastic tubing is inserted and tied into the vein. A tightly fitting needle adaptor then connects the vein catheter to the conventional type of intravenous infusion apparatus used for older children.

When the above technic is used, the flow rate must be carefully regulated and recorded. Prolonged stoppage of flow will necessitate a repetition of the tedious surgical dissection which is not only a nuisance but

results in the loss of one of a limited number of serviceable veins. On the other hand, permitting the fluids to enter the vascular system too rapidly may result in serious overloading or even fatal heart failure. The nurse who is charged with watching a continuous infusion in a small infant has a very important responsibility which demands accurate recording of the fluid level, frequent observation of the rate at which the fluid is dropping, and prompt notification of the doctor when the rate cannot be adjusted in a satisfactory manner.

Sometimes intravenous infusions or transfusions are given to infants through an adaptor temporarily tied into an exposed vein, usually at the ankle. The quantity of fluid and the rate of injection must be watched in this technic also, but the responsibility is primarily that of the operator who controls both.

Continuous intravenous therapy causes the child great discomfort because the immobilization often blocks all avenues for discharge of tension. Prolonged restraint evokes feelings of anger unless the child is old enough to understand the reasons why intravenous therapy is essential. Whenever possible, the infant's legs should be free for activity. Loneliness combined with immobilization cannot be tolerated by the infant and the young child. They either fight and utilize vital energy or withdraw from a world which must seem hostile and foreboding. Therefore, constant attention from the mother or a substitute must be provided to safeguard physical and emotional health.

DRUG ADMINISTRATION

GENERAL CONSIDERATIONS

It is the physican's responsibility to determine what kind and what amount of drugs are to be used in the treatment of a child. Determination of the proper dose of drugs is the legal and moral responsibility of the doctor and is usually converted into a written order so that there will be no misunderstanding. The dose of a number of drugs is calculated routinely on the basis of body weight rather than on age, although the age and the weight are related to each other in childhood. For example, in childhood the sulfonamides usually are given on the basis of weight, regardless of age. In some instances, the dosage varies with both age and weight.

All the drugs in common use are well borne by children when given in the proper dosage and dilution. Children are more susceptible to morphine and its related alkaloids than adults are, and a relatively smaller amount is prescribed. Certain drugs, for example, chlortetracycline (Aureomycin) and salicylates, although otherwise well borne, act as irritants in the alimentary tract and so disturb digestion. Salicylates preferably should be in a soluble form and well diluted. Choral, when given orally, is best given in milk. Because of its irritant effect it is often given by rectum.

It is well to remember that certain drugs have a therapeutic limit beyond which they cannot be increased with safety. This limit is manifest by clinical signs peculiar to each drug. To this group belong all the drugs that are known (and labeled) as poisons. The important drugs of this class are belladonna or atropine, digitalis, morphine and its derivatives, and thyroid extract. The signs of excessive dosage of these drugs are the same in children as in adults.

It is impossible to place too much emphasis on the grave responsibility which the nurse carries when administering drugs to any patient. However, when dealing with a child, that responsibility is all the greater because of the fact that drugs are being administered to a child. He is often unable to communicate verbally signs of distress that indicate he has been given too much drug or has an idiosyncracy to it. The young child cannot say, "Have you not made a mistake? I never have received this amount of medication before." He has to rely upon the nurse's accuracy and on her ability to detect undesirable effects from the drugs that need to be reported to the physician.

When the nurse is familiar with the dosage of a given drug and believes that an order is erroneous, she should call it to the doctor's attention before proceeding to the administration. Occasional errors and misunderstandings will creep into the best systems of order controls. The alertness of the nurse in discovering them may spare her patient a serious episode. It is better to question and be embarrassed about being wrong than to miss an opportunity to rectify an error. In pediatric care this is especially important because many drugs are not used in standard dosage and must be regulated according to the size of the child, as has been mentioned previously.

There are further responsibilities that the nurse has in relation to the administration of medicines. From her knowledge of pharmacology, the nurse should have some general understanding of what the treatment is intended to accomplish and what an appropriate dose of the drug should be. Some of the drugs commonly used in pediatric practice will be considered below. Others will be described in relation to specific diseases. The nurse also needs to find ways in which to make the unpalatable and the more uncomfortable medications more acceptable to the child. Medications are treatment. Giving them in a way that establishes and maintains a constructive relationship with the child is nursing care and is as important psychologically as the drug is important therapeutically.

Oral Medicines. In administering medications to an infant, the nurse's chief responsibility lies in getting the prescribed amount into his stomach with the least possible discomfort to him. Many medicines can be made more palatable by mixing them with a small amount of syrup. They can be given from the tip of a coffee spoon or with a medicine dropper. The baby's head and shoulders should be elevated as a few drops of the medicine are placed well onto his tongue. Giving medicine slowly enough to be swallowed and to prevent choking is a measure of great importance. If too much is given at one time, the infant will spit it out or choke. Choking is uncomfortable and negatively conditions him to the experience of taking medicines.

The nurse's approach in administering medications to the toddler will determine his capacity for co-operation. The toddler has a mind of his own and he expresses his feelings with avidity. He not only knows what he likes and dislikes but he often resists vehemently everything that does not meet with his approval. He may say, "No! I don't want it," or he may attempt to push it away or close his mouth in an effort to control the nurse. This developmental phase of growth needs to be anticipated, understood and accepted with poise. Medicines like treatments are necessary for his recovery. Therefore, they must be taken even though he thoroughly dislikes them and feels resistant toward the entire procedure. Explanations, coaxing, bribing and pleading for co-operation are of no value. They make the child feel that he has a deciding vote as to whether or not the medicine should be taken. He does not have the judgment necessary to realize its importance. The nurse must possess the judgment and present the medication in a way that helps the child to participate in his own treatment.

The nurse's task is to help the child learn that medicines are important and must be taken even though they taste a bit disagreeable momentarily. She does this when she puts the matter up to him calmly, confidently and with faith in his ability to learn to participate. "Johnny, it is time to take your medicine now," tells the child what is expected. An attitude of expectancy and faith supports the child's ego. It helps him to know that co-operation is expected. It also helps him to learn to control his natural resistance and to participate in the experience. An attitude of expectancy requires self-confidence and freedom from anxiety. If the nurse is fearful of her capacity to gain the child's co-operation, she will reflect it in her approach, her voice and the manner in which she handles the child. Her anxiety will be communicated to him. As a result he will be less able to co-operate.

When a child seems to lack the power to come to a decision himself and shows it with mounting anxiety, he is evidencing his need for supportive help. Force in giving medicines is never justifiable because it conveys hostility instead of helpfulness. Besides, it accomplishes nothing because the child always can have the last word. Usually he can vomit the medicine that has been forced upon him; and he will if he feels dominated instead of supported. Instead of force, the nurse should communicate her understanding and provide the strength that he does not have within himself. The ideas that follow communicate understanding: "I know that you don't want to take the medicine, Johnny. It is hard for children to take medicine that tastes bitter. I am going to hold you and help you to take it." After the nurse has helped the child to take it, saying something like the following prepares the child for further learning: "Someday, you will be able to take the medicine by yourself. I know you will learn to do it all by yourself." Each bit of co-operation should be commended. Gradually, the child will take in the nurse's strength and make it a part of himself. When he succeeds in taking it independently, he will want recognition of his accomplishment with words something like those which

follow: "I knew you would learn to take it by yourself. I'm proud of you, Johnny."

The above procedure takes more time initially than forcing but it safeguards the nurse-child relationship, which is essential in helping the child to get well and to master the hospitalization experience. This means that time must be given for administering the first doses of medicine when dealing with a child who has not learned how to co-operate and participate in his own treatment. He needs help in understanding that medicines will help him get well. This idea is best conveyed with deed rather than with words. The helpful, poised approach communicates this idea to the young child more effectively than words.

The administration of medicines calls for the greatest understanding and patience on the part of the nurse. It is a situation in which the nurse with limited understanding of children can easily become irritated. If irritation creeps into her voice or manner, the situation is lost, because the child gets scared and is left unsupported. A nurse who understands can be patient and serene even in the face of verbal or behavioral resistance. Here, again, the importance of the voice needs to be re-emphasized as well as the need for an attitude of expectancy and faith in the child's capacity to co-operate. The preschool child may wish to hold the glass himself. Or he may respond favorably when he is given the opportunity to choose between a spoon, a straw or a glass. Often with this simple device, the medicine is taken willingly. In the sick child's shaking hand, a few drops of the solution may be spilled, but the progress made in developing a constructive relationship between child and nurse outweighs any loss of medicine that first time that it is given. A good relationship solves the problem in regard to all medicines that are to follow. The simple device of holding the glass or offering a choice may not solve the problem. Sometimes another child's encouragement will help. Often watching other children take medicines stimulates a child's interest in learning to take his.

There is no one absolute technic that can be given to nurses for winning a child's co-operation. Each child is different, and he manifests his uniqueness at medicine time just as he does at every other time. If the nurse thinks of children as learning and growing rather than behaving, she will find that she approaches situations with a more understanding and less critical attitude. As a result she will be motivated to study her patients and to find ways of teaching which help the child to learn and desire to co-operate in the process of getting well.

Injected Medicines. The psychological principles of giving subcutaneous and intramuscular injections of medicines are the same as those cited for administration of oral medications. The child's need for preparation, support and permission to vent his feelings in relation to painful treatments has been discussed already. Method of restraint has been cited also. Intramuscular injections are painful; they are also frightening to the vast majority of children. The sick child's threshold of pain and fear is lower than that existent in the well child. Therefore, every possible measure must be taken to eliminate emotional trauma.

Previous mastery of the technic of giving injections of medicine gives the nurse the confidence and the poise that are required in working with children. The nurse needs not only skill but also good equipment, which includes sharp needles of appropriate length and gauge (1½ in. long, gauge No. 22 for the older child; 1 in. No. 22 gauge for the infant). Antiseptic treatment of the skin at the site of injection with aqueous Merthiolate, alcohol or green soap and saline must precede the injection. Maximum effect of the drug is obtained and discomfort is minimized when the tissue at the site of injection is held firmly, when the site of injection is varied and when the syringe and the needle are held in a perpendicular position and inserted to the hilt quickly and deftly. After testing has been done to make sure that the needle is in the muscle rather than in a vein, the medication can be injected rapidly. Care must be taken to get the medicine into the muscle. If the drug is injected into the subcutaneous tissues, discomfort results; absorption into the blood stream is less rapid; and there is greater danger of abscess formation. The nurse, who is skillful and plans her approach to the child thoughtfully, can do a great deal to minimize the emotional trauma which so often becomes a part of intramuscular treatments. The first injection is of great importance because it patterns the child's feelings and behavior for subsequent treatments. If the child's first experience with intramuscular injections is emotionally traumatic, his days will be heavily weighted with anxiety, for he will dread medicine time thereafter. The infant has fewer fears than the preschool child. He is less sensitive to pain and can be pacified easily at the completion of the procedure. Holding him a few minutes usually eases his discomfort.

Toddlers and preschool children have the greatest difficulties in accepting prolonged treatments with intramuscular medicinal therapy. Preschool children are in a period when fears are characteristically more numerous, pronounced and difficult to handle. Understanding the reason for intramuscular therapy and for being subjected to pain is impossible at this age level. However, the child can understand that it is medicine that is given in his buttocks or his arm, and that it will hurt like the sting of a bee or a mosquito. A preschool child can help also by choosing the site of injection if it is a single dose and by cleansing the area if it is accessible to him. Every effort to avoid forcibly restraining the child should be made. When two nurses are available, restraint is usually unnecessary. One nurse can distract and support; the other one can give the injection swiftly and skillfully as a means of lessening anxiety arising during a period of fearful waiting. After the drug has been administered, the child should be guided into doing something to alleviate his tension. Giving him a cotton pledget to rub the area provides a way to help him feel effective and as though he were an important participant. The nurse should remain with him until his equilibrium becomes re-established. A few minutes of play after he has dissipated his feelings serves to communicate the nurse's acceptance of his individual way of responding to a difficult and painful experience.

The school-age child and the adolescent can understand explanations and will become less fearful when they are helped to comprehend the nature of the medicine and the treatment. The approach to them should be direct and matter-of-fact. It should communicate the nurse's awareness of the youngster's capacity for control and co-operation.

CHEMOTHERAPY

Sulfonamides. The sulfonamides are a group of chemically related substances that have the property of interfering with the operation of essential enzyme systems of bacteria. In general, they do not kill the bacteria but render them more susceptible to the usual defense mechanisms of the body. Treatment must be continued over a period of several days as a minimum because the germs are not completely destroyed early in therapy. As with any other chemotherapeutic agent, the bacterial strains may become resistant to a particular sulfonamide and learn how to exist in spite of its presence. This circumstance can be discovered by appropriate laboratory studies of the sensitivity of organisms that are infecting a given patient. Historically, the earliest sulfonamides discovered were sulfanilamide, sulfapyridine and sulfathiazole. These particular sulfonamides are not often used any more because they have undesirable toxic reactions.

The more commonly used substances at present are sulfadiazine, sulfamerazine and gantrisin. To be

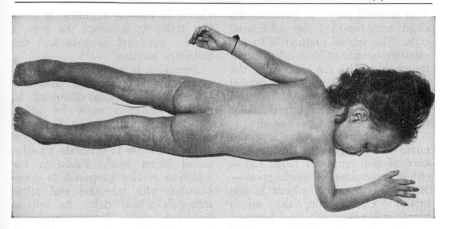

Fig. 12. A sulfonamide reaction.

effective these substances must be given in such a way as to maintain a minimum concentration in the blood, the urine or the spinal fluid, depending upon the variety of disease under treatment. Usually doses are repeated every 4, 6 or 8 hours. Under most circumstances an adequate level can be maintained if 0.1 Gm. of the sulfonamide per kilogram of body weight is given during each 24-hour period. Infants require somewhat more per unit of weight, and under special circumstances the level of dosage may be increased temporarily above this level. Excretion of these drugs is accomplished mainly by the kidneys, and unless an adequate flow of urine is being maintained, the drug may accumulate in the blood to undesirable levels because the expected fraction is not draining away in the urine. In addition to the dangers from the toxic effects of high blood levels, sulfonamides that are being excreted in highly concentrated and acid urine have a tendency to crystallize

in the tiny tubules of the kidney. In mild concentration such crystals can be detected only by microscopic examination of the urine; in moderate concentration they irritate the tubules and produce bloody urine; in heavy concentration they may completely plug the tubules so that urine cannot be excreted from a part or even the whole of the kidney.

During the administration of sulfonamides the nurse then has two responsibilities: (1) to see that an adequate volume of fluid is consumed (usually at least 1,000 cc. per day for a child of 2 years); and (2) to watch carefully for the appearance of red or chocolate-brown urine which indicates renal irritation from the drug. In addition to maintaining a large urine output and consequently a dilute urine, sometimes two other measures are used to decrease the tendency toward crystalluria. One measure is to administer alkali in the form of sodium bicarbonate or sodium lactate in order to maintain an alkaline or neutral urine.

This method may fail because the child resists taking the additional pills. The second method is to administer several sulfonamides simultaneously. With the total dose the same, the tendency toward crystal formation in the urine is reduced when two or more slightly different compounds are being excreted.

Other adverse reactions that the nurse can observe are the appearance of skin eruptions (Fig. 12)— either generalized or single spots— or the occurrence of ulcers in the mouth. Occasionally, the white blood cell count becomes lowered during sulfonamide therapy, but this reaction can be detected only by microscopic examination of the blood. Unexplained fever in some instances may be due to the sulfonamide.

In the treatment of gastro-intestinal disorders, two sulfonamides— sulfaguanidine and sulfasuxidine— are used frequently. These particular sulfonamides are so poorly absorbed that the dangers of renal irritation or other toxic reaction do not exist. Of course, they are unsuited for the treatment of any disease which requires the distribution of drug to other parts of the body than the intestinal tract.

Penicillin, one of the first antibiotics discovered, probably is used the most commonly. This distinction is merited because of the wide variety of infections against which it is effective and because of the relative infrequency of sensitivity reactions. It is universally effective against beta-hemolytic streptococcus infections and is usually effective against pneumococcus, gonococcus, meningococcus and some staphylococcus infections. It is the drug of choice in treating syphilis. It lacks the ability to influence the growth of the intestinal bacteria and the influenza bacillus.

Penicillin is most reliable when given by intramuscular injection. Crystalline penicillin dissolved in aqueous solution must be given either frequently (every 3 hours) or in very large dosage (2 or 3 times a day) in order to maintain an adequate blood level. Penicillin for injection is also prepared in combination with procaine and other materials which delay its release from the tissues. Procaine-penicillin in the usual pediatric dosage of 300,000 units continues to release an effective amount of drug for about 24 hours. Other preparations delay the release of drug for periods as long as 2 weeks. In this latter type of penicillin the quantity available to the body at any one time is relatively small so that the effectiveness of the drug may be insufficient to combat an acute infection.

Penicillin in pill and liquid form is also available. This method of administration is less reliable than the injection method, because absorption is more variable. Orally administered penicillin should be given on an empty stomach in order to provide optimum absorption. At least one half hour before the next meal should be allowed. Doses must be given 4 or 5 times a day. The quantity must be at least double the minimum dose used for parenteral administration.

Exact dosage with penicillin is not a consideration so long as enough is given. None of the toxic effects of penicillin are due to excessive blood levels. They occur only in a certain few individuals who have acquired sensitivity to the drug. Hives, peeling skin, swollen fingers and toes and painful muscles and joints are the common manifestations of penicillin sensitivity which may not appear until days or even weeks after the last administration of the drug. In general, until a given individual has demonstrated sensitivity to the drug, no restrictions on the quantity administered need be imposed for any reason except expense. In sensitive individuals (fortunately a rather rare occurrence among children) no penicillin at all can be used safely.

Streptomycin and Dihydrostreptomycin. These two closely related antibiotics are useful primarily for their ability to combat infections with the tubercle bacillus, secondarily for their effectiveness against influenza bacilli and some of the organisms commonly found in the intestinal tract. They are also effective against many of the organisms that are susceptible to penicillin. Were it not for two serious disadvantages these drugs would compete with penicillin for preference in antibiotic therapy. One disadvantage is the toxic effects upon the eighth cranial nerve which follow prolonged usage. The other disadvantage is the apparent ease with which many strains of bacteria become resistant to the effects of streptomycin and dihydrostreptomycin.

Streptomycin administered by mouth has no effect except upon bacteria within the intestinal tract, for it is not well absorbed. It is used in this form to treat some types of diarrhea and to sterilize the intestinal tract before operative procedures. No toxic effects result from oral administration.

For general treatment streptomycin must be injected intramuscularly. The daily dose for infants is usually about 40 mgm. per kilogram of body weight. Older children receive amounts of 0.5 to 1.0 Gm. per day. If treatment is not continued beyond a period of one week the likelihood of toxic reactions is small. With many acute infections such brief treatment is adequate. In severe tuberculosis treatment must be continued over periods of several months. The hazards of loss of equilibrium must be faced if streptomycin is used, or loss of hearing when dihydrostreptomycin is the drug selected. Since the total quantity of drug used seems to be the main factor that determines the appearance of toxic symptoms it is hoped that by using the two drugs simultaneously the incidence of the two types of eighth nerve damage will be reduced.

The emergence of resistant strains of tubercle bacilli can be prevented in most instances by giving large doses of para-aminosalicylic acid or promizole to the child during prolonged streptomycin treatment.

Chlortetracycline (Aureomycin), Oxytetracycline (Terramycin) and Chloramphenicol. These three antibiotics are sometimes called the broad spectrum antibiotics because they combat most of the bacteria that respond to penicillin plus those that respond to streptomycin (with the notable exception of the tubercle bacillus), and in addition have activity against some of the infections of rickettsial and viral origin. There are minor differences among them in the ranges of bacterial susceptibility. They are generally given by mouth in 3 or 4 doses per day, totaling from 20 to 40 mgm. per kilogram of body weight. In severe infections they may be given intravenously in doses as high as 100 or even 200 mgm. per kilogram. The oral preparations are quite bitter and must be offered either in capsule form or in some carefully disguised syrup.

Adverse reactions to these drugs are mainly gastro-intestinal. Chlortetracycline (Aureomycin) is likely to stimulate vomiting which may be too troublesome to permit its continuation. Oxytetracycline (Terramycin) is more likely to activate a mild diarrhea that seldom interferes with a short course of therapy. Because occasionally it has been responsible for fatal aplastic anemia, chloramphenicol ordinarily is reserved for those serious infections such as typhoid fever and influenza bacillus meningitis in which it appears to have special virtue. Sometimes prolonged or repeated use of these drugs is followed by an annoying, long-lasting but not serious diarrhea in infants and young children. Erythromycin and tetracycline (achromycin) are two antibiotics that have somewhat the same range of usefulness as chlortetracycline but have been released too recently to have found their places in therapy.

Other Antibiotics. There are many other antibiotics which have occasional or limited usefulness. In addition, new preparations are being tested constantly. A complete listing is beyond the scope of this text. Bacitracin and polymyxin (aerosporin) are powerful but too toxic to the kidneys and in general are used only for local application in the form of ointments. Neomycin

and magnamycin are also too toxic for general use. Viomycin is under test as a substitute for streptomycin in the treatment of tuberculosis.

ACTH AND CORTISONE

Physiology. In health the pituitary gland produces small amounts of a substance called adrenocorticotrophic hormone (ACTH) which enters the blood stream, circulates through the body and eventually reaches its target organ, the adrenal cortex. There ACTH stimulates the production of steroid hormones among which are cortisone (compound E) and hydrocortisone (compound F). These substances enter the blood stream from the adrenal cortex and exert a remarkably widespread and varied influence upon the internal workings of the body. Many of these effects are as yet incompletely understood. Information comes from a number of types of study. Deficient production of the steroid hormones can be observed in persons with Addison's disease in which the adrenal cortex is destroyed by disease, or in persons who have had their adrenals removed for the control of advanced cancer. A rare disorder known as Cushing's syndrome affords opportunity to observe the effects of excessive production of ACTH by the pituitary gland with consequent increased production of cortisone by the adrenal cortices.

Since 1949 first ACTH and then cortisone has become available for clinical use, and their effects upon the body in both health and disease have been studied widely. In most respects they have the same sort of action. It must be remembered that ACTH cannot influence an individual whose adrenal cortices are unable to respond.

The nurse who cares for a child under treatment with these substances will have the responsibility for observing the favorable effects that reverse the course of disease, but in addition she should be alert to the appearance of undesirable effects from the therapy itself. The nature of the favorable effects will depend upon the disease under treatment. Some of the undesirable effects are described below.

INCREASE IN WEIGHT. Prolonged administration of large doses of these substances may produce side effects which decrease their therapeutic usefulness. Increase in weight is a side effect which is due to several factors. The steroid hormones produce a retention of salt, sodium in particular, within the body which holds water in the tissues. In addition, the child deposits fat, usually in a peculiar distribution which is more obvious about the face, the shoulders and the hips. A round moonlike face and hunched shoulders are characteristic. At the same time the child's appetite usually increases, often becoming voracious. The changes in the body and the facial contours are not often of critical significance, but in certain diseases the retention of salt and fluids may be dangerous. In rheumatic fever, for instance, excessive increase in blood volume must be prevented because of the danger of heart failure.

INCREASED EXCRETION OF POTASSIUM. The retention of sodium in the tissues may be accompanied by an increased excretion of potassium. The substances produced by the adrenal cortex increase the renal tubular resorption of sodium and the excretion of potassium in the urine. Increased excretion of potassium also results because some of the excess sodium passes into the cells to replace the potassium that has been lost. Cellular potassium deficits, hypopotassemia, hypochloremia and alkalosis may result. The effects of potassium loss are not immediately visible to the nurse and can be determined only by chemical analysis of the blood or by periodic electrocardiograms, which are sensitive indicators of potassium deficiency in the myocardium. If tissue depletion of potassium proceeds too far, very serious muscular and circulatory disturbances appear quite suddenly.

HYPERTENSION, CONVULSIONS or PSYCHOTIC BEHAVIOR and INCREASED SUSCEPTIBILITY TO INFECTION. These other undesirable effects may result from prolonged or high-dosage administration of cortical steroids or ACTH. The appearance of convulsions or manifestations of psychotic behavior demands cessation of treatment, for they may be very difficult to control. Fortunately, these symptoms rarely occur. Children who are receiving these substances have an *increased susceptibility to infection* and sometimes display very poor resistance to even the most trivial childhood diseases.

HIRSUTISM, ACNE, GLYCOSURIA AND WOUND HEALING. Other effects which may be attributed to treatment with ACTH or cortisone are hirsutism, the increased growth of hair on the face and the body, acne and glycosuria. Wound healing may be delayed.

Nursing Care. When patients are receiving ACTH and cortisone certain nursing measures are necessary to detect early signs of untoward reaction to the drug. Daily weights and blood pressure readings twice daily should be taken in order to discover early changes in the weight and the blood pressure level. Intake and output of urine must be recorded carefully. In some instances 24-hour urine collections will be indicated. Children should be protected from exposure to contagious diseases and to the common communicable diseases such as colds, sore throats and bronchitis. When patients under hormone therapy are placed among other children it is common practice to give them some type of antibiotics as protection even before they show any evidence of infections.

When ACTH and cortisone were first used, all patients receiving either of the drugs were placed on low-salt or salt-free diets to balance extrarenal losses, and potassium chloride was administered by mouth. The administration of potassium chloride continues to be indicated, but unless the child is receiving ACTH or cortisone in large doses over a long period of time, salt-free or low-salt diets are not required.

When a low-salt or salt-free diet is prescribed the nurse has the problem of helping the child accept it. The child, who has been accustomed to seasoned food, may be reluctant to accept a bland, unseasoned diet. He may feel deprived or rejected because the food he has been accustomed to was deeply meaningful. The older child usually responds to interest in his feelings about the new diet and explanations concerning his need for it. The younger child, who reacts as though he felt deprived or rejected, needs help and encouragement from both his mother and his nurse. Knowledge of his likes and dislikes is important. The elimination of those foods he dislikes often helps him to feel that he is receiving personal consideration. Substitute pleasures can also be provided. If the nurse extends herself and provides pleasurable shared experiences, the child will be much more likely to take his changed diet in his stride. Effort expended in serving his tray attractively is also of value.

The nurse, who understands the therapeutic value of salt-free or low-salt diet, will convey her feelings and attitudes in her approach to the child. She will approach him expecting that he has the capacity to adapt himself to a new dietary regimen. She will know that he may feel disappointed and want food that is different from what he has been served. She will understand his feelings and help him to accept his diet just as she helps him adapt to other therapeutic requirements which are necessary to restore him to health.

The school-age child and adolescent can utilize the knowledge that the nurse and the dietitian impart in helping in the process of planning their menus. If the child is going home on a special diet, his parents will need help in understanding his dietary requirements and the reasons for them. This can be a co-operative project involving all those who are participating in the therapeutic regimen. The school-age child and the adolescent, who have an opportunity to participate in plans for their care, will co-operate infinitely more effectively.

Technic of Administration. Unlike other drugs there is little difference in the amounts of these substances which are administered to children of different sizes. Usually the initial daily dose is fairly large (50 to 200 mgm.) in order to obtain an initial response. As symptoms are brought under control the dose is decreased to a point at which it will just control the undesirable features of the disease. The determination of appropriate dosage is an individual matter which must be varied according to the child and the nature of his disease.

ACTH must be given by injection. The intramuscular route is used ordinarily, but the substance may also be given intravenously. It disappears rapidly from the circulation, so that the total daily dose is usually given in 4 aliquots about 6 hours apart. Slowly released ACTH is also available in the form of gels which need to be given only once a day.

Cortisone (and hydrocortisone) is ordinarily given in pill form by mouth. Depending upon the total dose administered, 2, 3 or 4 portions may be spaced through the 24-hour period.

Diseases That Respond to ACTH and Cortisone. These substances have been found to exert an ameliorating influence upon an amazingly large and diverse number of disorders. In many instances their effect seems to be one of suppressing the symptoms of the disease rather than that of producing a permanent cure. When the drugs are stopped the disease usually returns to its expected state after a variable interval. Thus their greatest usefulness lies in tiding children over the severe symptoms of an illness which is ordinarily self-limited. In addition, they prolong life and ameliorate discomfort for those whose difficulties are inevitably progressive.

No complete list of the conditions which are favorably affected is possible because the substances are not yet completely tested. The group of collagen diseases which includes rheumatoid arthritis, rheumatic fever, and some rarer disturbances, is influenced favorably. Many allergic disorders, such as hay fever, asthma, and drug sensitivities, are also responsive. Some of the inflammations of the eye and the skin, ulcerative colitis, nephrosis, leukemia, purpura and hemolytic anemia are also benefited temporarily or permanently. Further discussion will be found under the consideration of the individual disease states.

SITUATIONS FOR FURTHER STUDY

1. What understanding does the nurse need when nursing a child who requires intravenous therapy?

2. What observational skills does the nurse require when nursing a child requiring intravenous therapy to replace fluids, calories and electrolytes lost during the acute stages of diarrhea?

3. What are the symptoms of dehydration? Why is dehydration serious for an infant?

4. Describe the ways in which you helped a child to co-operate with you in meeting his oral fluid requirements?

5. Observe an infant of from 1 to 2 years of age and describe his reaction to restraint.

6. How do you imagine a 1-year-old child feels when he is com-

pletely immobilized and having fluid administered via a scalp vein? Describe a child for whom you are caring who is receiving fluids via the scalp vein. What substitute satisfactions were you able to provide for him? What was his response to you, his doctor, his mother and the treatments he was receiving?

7. What are the nurse's responsibilities in administering medications?

8. Describe a situation in which you helped a child to co-operate in the process of taking his medicine. What were the factors that helped you to be successful? How did the child respond to his accomplishment?

9. How is the therapeutic usefulness of ACTH increased? How can the nurse help to minimize or prevent the nontherapeutic effects of the hormone?

10. Describe a child receiving ACTH therapy. What was his reaction to the drug? How did he respond to the nursing care which he required during the time he was receiving ACTH therapy?

BIBLIOGRAPHY

Blecha, Elmira: Low sodium diets, Am. J. Nursing 51:464, 1951.

Greenman, Lawrence: Sodium restriction during ACTH therapy, Am. J. Nursing 53:444, 1953.

Lowe, C. U.: Principles of parenteral fluid therapy, Am. J. Nursing 53:963, 1953.

Wallinger, E. M.: Intramuscular injections for children, Am. J. Nursing 48:112, 1948.

Wilkins, Gladys: The patient, the nurse, and the low sodium diet, Am. J. Nursing 53:445, 1953.

Wilson, L. D.: ACTH and cortisone in clinical practice, Am. J. Nursing 50:649, 1950.

Unit Four

NURSING IN THE CARE OF THE
SICK INFANT AND CHILD

Care of the Newborn

IMMEDIATE CARE OF THE NEWBORN
EARLY ADJUSTMENT TO LIFE OUTSIDE
   THE UTERUS
NORMAL ASPECTS OF THE NEWBORN

SIGNIFICANT DISORDERS OF THE
   NEWBORN
PREMATURITY
SITUATIONS FOR FURTHER STUDY

To his parents the newborn infant is the culmination of plans, hopes and fears experienced during the long period of gestation. Understandably, parents are likely to be in a state of emotional instability and suppressed excitement during the early days of the infant's life. Parents of first-born children are apt to find that their relief over the successful conclusion of labor and delivery is soon followed by concern over the normality of their child and over their ability to give him the proper care. Every aspect of his physique and behavior will be subjected to their anxious scrutiny. It is important that those who are assisting with the early care of the infant be able to help parents to discriminate between aberrations that are of temporary or trivial significance and those that may have far-reaching consequences to the infant. In the discussion below, the more or less normal peculiarities of the newborn infant are separated from the important diseases and abnormalities that may affect him.

IMMEDIATE CARE OF THE NEWBORN

After the cord is cut, the baby should be received into a warm blanket and placed immediately upon a table or in a crib where resuscitative measures can be carried out if needed. Mucus should be aspirated gently from the pharynx. If respiration is not initiated spontaneously within a minute or two, resuscitative measures should be commenced. These are described later in this chapter under Asphyxia.

Whenever the circumstances of delivery will permit, ligation of the cord is delayed until it has stopped pulsating so that the infant will receive as much of the blood contained in the placenta as possible. Permanent ligation or clamping should be secure, and the cord stump should be covered with a sterile dressing.

Most states have laws requiring the instillation of silver nitrate into the conjunctival sacs at birth in order to prevent gonorrheal opthalmia. The eyelids are cleansed gently with cotton, then separated, and a few drops of a 1 per cent solution of silver nitrate are instilled. After a minute or two the lids should be separated again and the silver nitrate flushed out with normal saline solution. Some states now permit the use of penicillin in place of silver nitrate, since it is equally effective and much less irritating. A solution of penicillin containing 2,500 units per cc. is instilled daily for 4 days.

Before the baby leaves the delivery room, some means of identification should be provided. This may be in the form of a necklace or a bracelet of lettered beads, a tape with a number, or a military type of "dog tag" fastened around the wrist. Many hospitals also make simultaneous records of the infant's foot and palm prints and of the mother's finger prints in order to have conclusive proof of identity.

The preliminary appraisal of the infant should include observation of the color of his skin and mucous membranes and of the character of his respirations. The general behavior and degree of activity should be noted, and a cursory examination for the presence of abnormalities should be made. The length and the weight should be recorded; preferably, the head and the chest circumferences should be measured as well.

When the infant is born in a hospital, usually the foregoing procedures will be the responsibility of the delivery-room staff. They should be completed with minimum exposure of the infant before he is sent to the nursery.

EARLY ADJUSTMENT TO LIFE OUTSIDE THE UTERUS

At birth suddenly the newborn infant is required to take over a number of important functions which his mother previously performed for him, i.e., carrying oxygen to his tissues through the activity of heart and lungs, ingesting his food, regulating his body temperature, defending himself against infection, and eliminating his wastes through his kidneys and bowels. In addition, he must attract attention to his wants and discomfitures through the medium of his cry. Several of these functions depend upon the integrity of his brain and central nervous system. The persons in attendance upon the newborn must assist him to carry out many of these vital activities. Even with minimal aid, more than 90 per cent of newborns make a rapid and satisfactory adjustment. The small fraction who have difficulty in so adapting require special attention, particularly during the first day or two of life. From the tables in Chapter 2, it can be seen that of all infants who fail to survive the first year, well over half of them die in the first month of life, and nearly a third die during the first day. Careful observation of *all* infants during the early days will speed the recognition of those who are going to have difficulty.

GENERAL ASPECTS OF ADJUSTMENT

Activity varies a great deal among newborns. For a period of a few hours to 2 or 3 days, many will be quite sleepy and inactive, due presumably to the effects of maternal medication during labor or to the compression of the brain during its passage through the birth canal. Such inactivity need occasion no alarm if the respirations and the color are normal, if the infant arouses at least momentarily on mild stimulation, and if the cry and the sucking response are present. After the period of somnolence is over, the newborn still sleeps much of the day, but in a tentative sort of way with spontaneous movements of the extremities, fitful turning and prompt awakening after mild stimulation. In small or slender infants, rapid and vigorous response to mild disturbances may appear during the first few days.

Tissue Oxygenation. This is gauged by the color of the skin and by the type of respiratory behavior. Normal skin color ranges from a delicate pink to a ruddy red. It is most constant on the trunk and the face. The hands, the feet and the upper lip are not always reliable indicators, since they may have a dusky hue during repose but become pink when the sluggish circulation is stimulated by crying or increased activity. Infants who are having difficulty in oxygenating their tissues respond instead with an increase in the depth and the extent of cyanosis during crying. In deeply pigmented infants observation of the skin coloration is more difficult. Reliance must be placed upon the appearance of the mucous membranes.

The newborn breathes with shallow, rapid respirations. The rate varies from 30 to 80 per minute, and the rhythm may be irregular. The abdomen usually moves more than the chest, bulging with inspiration and falling with expiration. The excursions of the chest are effortless when the infant is resting; during crying they become slower and deeper. Rapid, labored or grunting respirations indicate imperfect aeration of the lungs, particularly if they are accompanied by retraction of the chest wall during inspiration and by cyanosis of the skin or the mucous membranes.

The pulse rate is not easily determined in the newborn. By auscultation of the chest the rate in a healthy infant is found to be from 120 to 160 per minute.

Body Temperature. The body temperature of the newborn falls immediately after birth to around 96° F. in spite of efforts to maintain warmth. During the first half day it climbs slowly to a range of 98° to 99° F. where it stabilizes in the full-term infant. Deviations beyond this range may indicate improper environmental temperature, insufficient fluid intake or early illness.

Ingestion of fluids and food can be commenced very soon after birth. The healthy newborn is able to suck and swallow as soon as he has recovered from the immediate effects of delivery. Early feedings must be given cautiously to forestall overloading of his stomach, vomiting, and aspiration into the trachea. Usually it takes about a week before he is able to consume the requisite amount of food and fluid for his body needs. A fuller discussion of feeding is given in Chapters 20 to 23. Persistent nausea, vomiting or choking during feeding should serve as a warning that there may be an anomaly of the upper gastro-intestinal tract.

Weight Loss. A weight loss of from 5 to 10 per cent of the initial weight is common during the first 10 days of life. The newborn's weight curve is bound to dip during the first few days because of his inability to consume his full complement of food. Some infants who have an excess quantity of tissue fluid at birth, lose weight rapidly during the first 48 hours of life, as the kidneys excrete large amounts of urine. Obviously, such infants cannot be expected to regain their birth weights as rapidly as the average.

Elimination of urine and stool often takes place at the time of delivery. During the first 2 or 3 days, urine production may be scanty, and the urine highly concentrated. A record should be made of the time of the first voiding. It may not appear for 12 to 24 hours after delivery, occasionally even later. The first stools passed are composed of meconium, a tarry green substance which is replaced after 2 or 3 days by transitional stools. Failure to pass meconium during the first day may indicate an intestinal abnormality, particularly if there is associated abdominal distention or vomiting. The first passage of stool should be recorded as well as the frequency and the type of stool passage thereafter. The number of stools passed per day varies considerably from one infant to another. The consistency of the stool is determined in part by the type of feeding, a subject which is discussed more fully in Chapter 21.

Susceptibility to Infection. This condition exists during the early months of the infant's life. He comes suddenly from a completely sterile environment into a world teeming with bacteria. Eventually, he will be able to defend himself against most of these organisms.

Until the infant has built up his own defenses against infection, measures must be taken at home and by the hospital to minimize the opportunities for harmful bacteria to enter his food or the air that he breathes, or to infect his skin. In the home, his contacts should be reduced by excluding unnecessary visitors. His formulas should be prepared with sterile technic. His skin, clothing, bedding, and the hands which attend him always should be clean. Members of the household who harbor infections should be kept at a distance. The same sort of precautions should be exercised in the hospital with even greater strictness because the number of persons involved in his care is much greater, and many babies are being cared for in one unit. In the hospital, individual equipment and meticulous aseptic technic are essential to protect him from infection.

Crying. The infant's cry has meaning and needs to be heeded because it is his only way of communicating discomfort from hunger, distention, loneliness, an uncomfortable position, chilliness, excess warmth, functional insufficiency or disease. The newborn infant is a helpless creature who is completely dependent upon those in his environment for the satisfaction of his needs. A crying baby is in need of care. He has no inner resources to withstand the frustration, the anxiety and the tension which come when his requirements remain unfulfilled. To ignore his response to physical or emotional need is to neglect a phase of nursing that is of great importance to his physical and emotional health.

NORMAL ASPECTS OF THE NEWBORN

POSTURE

Before birth the infant's body is packed into the egg-shaped confines of the uterus. During pregnancy the mother or the obstetrician will often note changes in the baby's position. But after birth many newborns show the effects of habitual intra-uterine postures. With a little gentle manipulation the infant can be restored to such a position, and, even though it be a bizarre one, he generally prefers it. Thus, babies delivered by cephalic presentation usually keep their knees doubled up on the abdomen, and indeed it may be impossible to extend their legs fully. Often the lower legs bow outward, and the soles of the feet turn toward each other as a consequence of the squatting position *in utero*. In contrast, a breech-delivered baby has legs that are fully extended and is more likely to be knock-kneed than bowlegged. Infants delivered from brow or face presentations prefer to lie with heads extended backward rather than in the more universally acceptable position of flexion upon the chest. These postural peculiarities gradually correct themselves as muscles and ligaments lengthen and the curvature of bones is slowly corrected during growth. Treatment is seldom required unless there has been interference with the growth of bone or marked displacement of bony structures, such as occurs in clubbed feet.

Tonic Neck Reflex. Two postural reflexes are peculiar to the first few weeks of life. The tonic neck reflex may be observed in the sleeping position of the newborn—head turned to one side with the arm and the leg on that side drawn up and the arm and the leg on the opposite side extended. At times the position of the extremities can be seen to reverse if the head is turned to the opposite side, either actively or passively.

Moro Reflex. The moro reflex or startle response is elicited when the infant is awakened suddenly or is caused to fall a short distance onto a bed or a table. It consists of an embracing motion of the arms and general tensing of musculature, usually with an accompanying cry. Both these reflexes are evolutionary heirlooms that have no importance to the modern infant.

SKIN

The skin of the newborn varies considerably from one baby to another in respect to its color, texture and general toughness. Many have skin that is poorly supplied with natural oils, making it easily irritated and prone to infection. Hospital routines for initial care differ. Some leave most of the vernix caseosa on at birth to act as a temporary protective vanishing cream. Others bathe the infant completely and then anoint him thoroughly with a bland oil or an ointment with antibacterial properties. For some infants, water acts as an irritant if applied too frequently. Those whose skin is dry, or parchmentlike, or peeling, or those who have cracks and fissures or deep folds which cannot be kept dry, profit from liberal applications of oil and a minimum use of water.

Mongolian Spots. These irregular areas of greenish-blue pigmentation are concentrated over the lower back. They are present universally in infants of Asian extraction, are frequent among Negroes and the Mediterranean races, and are rarely found on Caucasian infants. They disappear by school age. They have no relation to mongolian idiocy.

Pigmented Nevi. Pigmented nevi, or moles, either brown or black in color, may be found at birth. The larger ones may be cosmetically undesirable, but otherwise they have no significance. Large, flat areas of brown pigment are called *café au lait spots.*

Cutis Marmorata. This term describes a faint purple marblelike pattern of the skin capillaries in small infants visible during periods of inactivity or chilling. It is a normal phenomenon which is abolished by an increase in the circulation through the skin. The coldness and the occasional blueness of the normal infant's hands and feet has been described already.

Telangiectasia or widening of the skin capillaries is extremely common at the nape of the neck, less common over the forehead, the eyelids and along the mid-line of the scalp and the trunk. These flat, dark-red or purple areas of skin have sharp but irregular borders. Sometimes they are called "stork bites." They fade out but do not disappear entirely as the infant's skin becomes thicker during normal growth. Occasionally, a similar area of skin will precede the development of a *strawberry hemangioma.* This is a raised, bright-red collection of small blood vessels which is seldom present at birth but appears during the second or third week of life. Such tumors almost invariably break up and disappear spontaneously before the fourth year of life. No treatment is required.

Forceps Marks. These marks may be identified over the face at the time of birth but invariably disappear within a day or two.

Bruises. After difficult deliveries sometimes bruises are present on the face and the scalp. They are common about the buttocks and the external genitalia of breech-delivered infants. Even large bruises clear up within a few days, leaving no scar.

Milia are small white lumps about the size of a pinhead, seen usually on the face. They are small collections of the secretions of sebaceous glands trapped beneath the surface of the skin. They eventually establish an opening to the surface and disappear.

Blebs. Sometimes a similar collection of material is found in larger blebs in the skin folds of the neck, the axilla or the groin. They too disappear rapidly once the superficial skin is broken.

Hives are seen occasionally on the second or the third day of life. They are small raised white spots surrounded by an area of erythema. They look much like small insect bites. Although they probably are due to some allergic response derived from the mother, they have no known relation to allergy in later life.

HEAD AND NECK

Pressure applied to the head before and during labor may produce a number of temporary changes which disappear shortly after birth without affecting the infant's welfare.

Molding of the skull with overriding of the bones along the suture lines results when the head is pushed through a tight birth canal. The skulls of most infants delivered by cephalic presentation show some such overlapping of the bones with elongation of the occipital portion of the skull. These irregularities disappear during the early weeks of life. Breech-delivered infants usually have heads that are flattened in the occipital region. Cesarean-delivered infants, of course, have symmetrically round or slightly square heads.

Caput Succedaneum. This is a poorly defined area of edema of the scalp which indicates the first portion of the head to pass through the uterine cervix. A caput usually is gone by the third day.

Craniotabes is a term used to describe areas of softening of the flat cranial bones. It is most common along the suture edges but sometimes is present in the center of the bone. The condition results from a combination of intra-uterine pressure and minor disturbances of the mother's calcium metabolism. The areas calcify rapidly after birth and seldom can be identified after 2 months.

Cephalhematoma. This is a collection of blood beneath the fibrous investment of one of the flat cranial bones, usually the parietal (Fig. 13). It is most common in first-born infants whose heads have been subjected to prolonged compression during labor. Often inconspicuous at first, the swelling enlarges rapidly during the first 2 or 3 days, produc-

ing a smooth, fluctuant, prominent mass, the margins of which are limited by the edges of the cranial bone involved. Some of the smaller hematomas absorb rapidly. The larger ones usually calcify gradually, be-

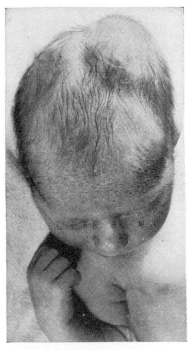

Fig. 13. Cephalhematoma of left parietal bone. (Davis, M., and Sheckler, C.: DeLee's Obstetrics for Nurses, Philadelphia, Saunders)

ginning at the base and eventually converting the swelling into a firm bony lump which remains until it is gradually engulfed by the increasing size of the skull. Cephalhematomas produce no inward pressure on the brain and are innocuous except for their peculiar appearance. Aspiration of the contents of the swelling is unwise because of the danger of infection.

Petechiae are tiny hemorrhages into the skin which are sometimes seen sprinkled over the face, the scalp and the neck. They result from the sudden compression of the chest and the abdomen during delivery. They clear up within a few days.

Subconjunctival Hemorrhage. This flame-shaped collection of blood on the white portion of the eyeball results from the same mechanism. It usually takes a week or slightly longer to disappear.

· **Facial Paralysis** (Fig. 14). This may result from intra-uterine pressure upon the facial nerve as it runs through the cheek. When the infant cries, the paralyzed side of the mouth fails to retract backward

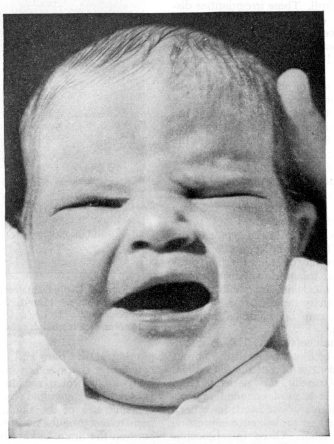

Fig. 14. Facial paralysis in a newborn baby, in this instance resulting from a spontaneous delivery.

and upward as it should. The nerve usually recovers its function during the first 6 to 8 weeks of life. Infrequently, the paralysis is permanent.

Hematoma of the Sternocleidomastoid muscle. This is a small firm lump in the belly of the muscle which results from tearing of muscle fibers when traction is exerted upon the head (or shoulders in a breech delivery). The lump disappears slowly, and unless excessive fibrosis takes place during healing, it does not interfere with the function of the muscle.

EYES

Chemical Conjunctivitis. Irritation by the silver nitrate instilled into the eyes at birth may result in a chemical conjunctivitis. On the second day of life the eyes are red, swollen shut, with pus exuding from between the lids. If there is any suspicion that the process might be infectious, the pus should be examined for the presence of bacteria. The eyes should be cleansed gently or irrigated with warm saline solution. In spite of the initial severity, the inflammation subsides within a few days, leaving no harmful effects upon the eyes.

Obstruction of the Nasolacrymal Duct. This condition may be recognized toward the end of the newborn period by excessive tearing and the accumulation of small amounts of pus in the eye without inflammation of the globe itself. In most instances the duct opens up spontaneously during the first few months of life, requiring no special treatment.

MOUTH

Several features of the normal newborn's mouth may occasion unnecessary concern. Frequently, the gums are rough, almost serrated. The frenulum of the upper lip may extend down, partially cleaving the upper gums. Posteriorly, the gums are usually very white. On either side of the mid-line of the hard palate a raised white plaque, called an epithelial pearl, may be seen. Concern over tongue-tie is usually unjustified. The newborn's tongue is normally short and broad with the frenulum extending out to the tip. It cannot be protruded much beyond the gum margin until its shape is changed by elongating growth in later months.

Thrush (Fig. 15) is a trivial infection of the mouth, caused by a fungus which usually is derived from the mother's vaginal secretions during birth. The tongue and the mucous membranes are diffusely red and speckled with closely adherent white patches. The infection is easily cured by a few applications of aqueous gentian violet solution or 1:1,000 Merthiolate solution.

UMBILICUS

Granuloma. After the cord separates, healing usually takes place promptly at the navel. Occasionally, a small piece of granulation tissue remains uncovered by epithelium and grows to form a granuloma; the weeping surface produces a chronic discharge. The granulations may be cauterized with a silver nitrate stick which terminates the discharge by drying up the weeping surface.

Umbilical Hernia. This is the result of a defect in the anterior abdominal wall through which a loop of intestine may bulge out under the skin when the infant cries or strains. Although unsightly and often worrisome to the mother, such hernias produce no important symptoms. All but the larger ones close over spontaneously by the second or the third year as the abdominal muscles strengthen when the child begins to stand. Application of abdominal binders or adhesive strapping have little effect in hastening the closure of the defect.

MALE GENITALIA

Hydroceles. The testes are normally descended at birth but may be placed high in the inguinal canal. Frequently, they are surrounded by small collections of fluid called hydroceles. These latter absorb during the early months.

Circumcision. The prepuce is usually long and tightly adherent to the glans. Since there are no

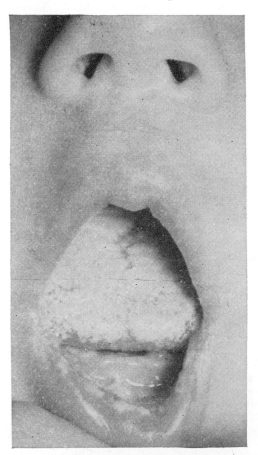

FIG. 15. Thrush. (Potter, E. L.: Pathology of the Fetus and the Newborn, Chicago, Yr. Bk. Pub.)

significant medical reasons for or against circumcision, the choice should be left to the parents. If the operation is to be done, it should be completed during the newborn period. If it is not done, the mother should be instructed in gradual stretching of the prepuce to permit its retraction behind the glans for proper cleansing. She should be warned that a tight prepuce must be restored promptly to its original position lest it become trapped behind the coronal ridge, swell progressively and lead to a paraphimosis which may have to be relieved surgically.

Hormonal Effects

During the latter part of pregnancy, hormones are transmitted from the mother to the infant. Both male and female infants may show enlargement of the breasts with secretion of "witches milk" which may persist for a period of 4 to 6 weeks. In addition, female infants commonly have marked enlargement and swelling of the external genitalia. Occasionally, there is a small discharge of blood simulating menstruation. No treatment is indicated except ordinary cleanliness.

SIGNIFICANT DISORDERS OF THE NEWBORN

Congenital Malformations

Between 2 and 3 per cent of all infants are born with significant defects in the formation of their bodies. Such malformations are assuming increasing importance as the infectious causes of infant deaths are being brought under control. Today in areas where the infant mortality rate is low, from one

eighth to one quarter of the infant deaths under a year of age can be ascribed to a congenital malformation. A few types of malformation are known to be determined hereditarily; and a few are known to result from radiation therapy to the mother's abdomen or rubella during the first trimester of pregnancy. But the bulk of these disorders are due to undetermined factors and constitute a challenge to medical progress. While congenital malformations can be produced in the young of certain experimental animals by depriving the pregnant mother of various vitamins or of an adequate concentration of oxygen in the air which she breathes, there is no evidence to show that malformations of the human infant are produced in this way.

Some abnormalities, particularly those involving the skeleton and the central nervous system, are immediately obvious at birth. Examples are cleft lip, spina bifida, hydrocephalus, microcephaly, extra digits and clubbed feet. Other abnormalities are present at birth but require careful examination by a physician to disclose their presence (mongolism, congenital heart disease, polycystic kidneys, for example). A third variety, although present at birth, is overlooked during early life because no clue suggests its presence until months or even years have elapsed. As examples of these silent abnormalities, hydronephrosis, cretinism, Meckel's diverticulum and certain types of mental deficiency may be cited. Discussion of the common malformations is to be found in the chapters dealing with particular organ systems.

DISORDERS THAT DEPEND UPON THE MOTHER'S CONDITION DURING PREGNANCY

Syphilis may be transmitted from the mother to her unborn child (Chap. 18). Other infectious diseases are rarely passed from mother to child before birth.

Diabetes in the mother increases the hazard to her infant, especially if the disease is of long duration or poorly controlled. Infants of diabetic mothers usually are oversized for the gestational age, edematous, and bothered by excessive secretions of mucus from the pharynx and the stomach. Repeated aspiration and careful observation are necessary to prevent interference with the respiratory exchange. Symptoms of low blood sugar, such as irritability or convulsions, are seen occasionally on the first or the second day of life. Some of these babies require temporary care in an incubator to supply additional warmth and oxygen. Infants of diabetic mothers who are delivered by cesarean section run a greater risk of resorption atelectasis than do normal infants delivered by the same route. They also run an increased risk of being born with a congenital abnormality.

Anoxia occurs when the infant's vital organs, the brain in particular, have their oxygen supply seriously reduced. It may occur before birth if the mother suffers from some severe illness, such as extreme anemia, heart failure, shock or pneumonia which prevents her circulation from supplying the placenta with adequate amounts of oxygenated blood. It may occur also from compression of the umbilical cord within the uterus, or from premature separation of the placenta from the inner wall of the uterus (abruptio placentae). Anoxia is a serious circumstance to the infant, and when it is recognized, usually steps are taken to deliver him rapidly. At birth the infant is usually limp and unresponsive, and measures to support him are of vital importance. He has difficulty establishing his respirations and maintaining his body temperature. External warmth, oxygen and the resuscitative measures described under Asphyxia (page 217) usually are required. Infants may recover quickly and completely from brief periods of anoxia; but after prolonged oxygen lack, the brain is damaged to such an extent that respiration either cannot be established at all or can be maintained for a few hours only after birth. It is believed that some of the central nervous system disturbances that appear in later life (cerebral palsy, for instance) may be the aftermath of nonfatal periods of anoxia experienced during or just prior to birth.

Erythroblastosis fetalis is an acute hemolytic anemia occurring at birth in an infant whose mother has become sensitized to his red blood cells. Most often the disease depends upon sensitization to the Rh factor; infrequently, it may concern the A and B substances of the blood cells or other antigens. Only Rh-negative women, i.e. those who lack the Rh factor in their red blood cells, are capable of becoming sensitized to it. About 15 per cent of all Caucasian women are Rh-negative. (Only a very small percentage of Negro and Asian women lack the Rh substance.) If an Rh-negative woman marries an Rh-positive man, some or all of the infants of such a marriage will be Rh-positive. During such a pregnancy, blood from the Rh-positive fetus may find its way back across the placental circulation into the mother's blood stream where it can stimulate the mother's body to form antibodies against the Rh factor. These antibodies are capable of clumping and destroying Rh-positive cells. If they pass back through the placenta into the infant's blood in sufficient quantity, the symptoms of erythroblastosis result. Actually, the disease never appears in the first Rh-positive child of an Rh-negative woman. It seems as though additional stimulation of antibody formation by a second Rh-positive child is required before the mother can form antibodies in sufficient amount to damage the child. Also, it should be emphasized that most Rh-negative women never become sensitized, even though they bear several Rh-positive children. The popular misconception that every Rh-negative woman is threatened with erythroblastotic babies is far from true. However, once a given mother has born an infant with the disease, there is a very strong probability that future Rh-positive infants will be affected similarly.

The cardinal symptoms of erythroblastosis are jaundice and anemia, which are present at birth or appear during the first 36 hours. *Any infant who is found to be jaundiced on the first or the second day of life should be brought to the doctor's attention because he requires thorough investigation.* In severe cases the mother delivers a stillborn fetus or one suffering from *hydrops fetalis,* which is characterized by extensive edema, marked anemia, jaundice, and enlargement of the liver and the spleen. Similar findings of lesser intensity are present in infants afflicted with milder forms of the disease. If no treatment is given, both the anemia and the jaundice are likely to increase in severity during the first few days of life. Sometimes hemorrhages into the skin are present, and occasionally a fatal pulmonary hemorrhage occurs on the fourth day.

Infants who are severely jaundiced run the risk of serious damage to the brain (kernicterus). The symptoms of this complication appear from the third day on and consist of vomiting, spasticity, convulsions and inability to feed. Kernicterus is often fatal shortly after its appearance. Survivors suffer from severe forms of mental retardation with spastic paralysis.

Mild forms of erythroblastosis produce no symptoms except slight jaundice and anemia—indeed, cases may be overlooked entirely unless special laboratory tests are performed. The effect of the antibodies obtained from the mother is temporary. If the infant survives the tenth day of life without evidence of complications, his outlook is good. Except for anemia which is corrected easily by transfusion, erythroblastotic infants suffer no additional consequences of the disease after this time.

The treatment of erythroblastosis consists in the transfusion of Rh-negative blood to combat the anemia. The Rh-negative cells will persist in the infant's circulation since they are unaffected by the antibodies received from the mother. While repeated simple transfusions are often effective, the more elaborate technic of exchange transfusion is to be preferred. Through a catheter inserted into the umbilical, or some other large vein, small amounts of the infant's blood are withdrawn, and an equal amount of the Rh-negative donor's blood is injected. The procedure is continued until most of the circulating blood of the infant has been replaced. This technic not only provides new red cells, but also removes the harmful maternal antibodies and the products of the destruction of the infant's red cells which produce jaundice. Even moribund infants are sometimes salvaged by the prompt application of this treatment.

Exchange transfusion requires considerable preparation and is frequently an emergency procedure. Hence, it is desirable that the birth of an erythroblastotic infant be anticipated so that preparations may be made in advance. This can be done if all pregnant women are Rh-typed and if Rh antibodies are sought periodically during pregnancy in the blood of those who might be expected to produce an erythroblastotic baby.

The nursing care of an infant with erythroblastosis consists of careful observation and supportive measures which provide protection during the period when he is receiving medical treatment. Babies born with erythroblastosis frequently require measures to combat shock. When the birth of an infant with erythroblastosis is anticipated, an incubator and oxygen should be in readiness to maintain the infant's temperature and to combat cyanosis. These babies are lethargic, due

to generalized weakness and anemia. Frequent change in position prevents atelectasis and intercurrent infections.

Usually, the infant's strength to suckle is greatly reduced, indicating a need for a method of feeding that will conserve his energy. A nipple with enlarged holes or a medicine dropper may be required for feeding a weakened infant. With all methods of feeding, patience in feeding the infant slowly enough to prevent aspiration is necessary.

In caring for an infant with erythroblastosis, the nurse must be constantly on the alert to detect untoward symptoms. The nurse must not only assist with the replacement transfusion but also she must observe the infant's response during the procedure and in the period after it is completed. Untoward symptoms that need to be brought to the attention of the doctor include increasing weakness and jaundice, edema, pigmentation of the urine, increased respirations, cyanosis of the face or the nailbeds and convulsions that result when the basal nuclei of the brain become damaged.

Hemorrhagic Disease of the Newborn. This is a condition in which spontaneous bleeding occurs during the first week of life. Hemorrhages may occur into the skin, from the orifices of the body, or from the umbilicus. Blood passed in the stool is called *melena*. Large hemorrhages or very numerous small ones occasionally threaten life from the loss of blood.

The disturbance is due to a failure of the blood to clot properly, which in turn is caused by an insufficient production of prothrombin, one of the main activators of the clotting mechanism. The body requires vitamin K in order to manufacture prothrombin. Before birth the infant obtains vitamin K from his mother; after birth it comes from his food or from the synthetic activity of the bacteria which invade his intestinal tract shortly after his birth. All infants have relatively low levels of prothrombin in the blood during the first few days of life. Premature infants and full-term infants whose mothers have not provided them with adequate amounts of vitamin K may suffer decreases of prothrombin to such low levels that hemorrhage occurs.

Treatment consists in supplying vitamin K by intramuscular injection, following which the infant begins to produce prothrombin at an adequate rate within an hour or two. In severe cases where significant blood loss has occurred, transfusion is desirable to supply red blood cells and to correct the prothrombin deficiency at once. Prevention of hemorrhagic disease is advocated by some. Routine vitamin K injections are given either to the mothers a few hours before delivery or to the infants immediately after birth.

Disorders Due to Trauma at Birth

Intracranial Injury. This is the most common and serious form of birth trauma. Since the head is the largest portion of the infant body which must traverse the birth canal, it is most likely to be damaged when delivery is difficult. Sudden, violent alterations in the shape of the skull, such as occur with precipitate delivery or difficult forceps or breech extractions, are more likely to result in injury than is the gradual molding of a slowly progressing labor. Temporary or permanent damage is suffered by various portions of the brain if their blood supply is compromised by edema or hemorrhage from large blood vessels that have torn or have burst in response to the unusual stresses. Large hemorrhages occur most commonly from the veins coursing in the membrane that separates the two halves of the brain (falx cerebri) or in the membrane that divides the cerebellum from the cerebrum (tentorium cerebelli). In premature infants the delicate vessels of the choroid plexus may burst, resulting in a hemorrhage into the ventricular system of the brain.

Following intracranial injury, the infant is abnormally sleepy, difficult to arouse, does not demonstrate the Moro reflex and may be unable to suck or to swallow. If intracranial pressure is high, his respirations are slow, irregular and periodic; his heart beats slowly; his fontanelle bulges; and his eyes turn inward. There may be generalized spasticity of the muscles with backward arching of the head and the neck and extension of the legs. Evidence of irritation of the cerebral cortex may be present in the form of generalized convulsions or convulsive twitchings of muscle groups. The body temperature may be elevated or may hover at subnormal levels. In mild cases the symptoms are limited to general listlessness, poor appetite and occasional vomiting.

The prognosis following intracranial injury varies considerably, depending upon the extent and the location of the damage. When large or vital areas of the brain are affected, the immediate mortality is high, and infants who survive are likely to show spastic paralysis or mental retardation in later years. When the brain damage is less extensive, recovery may ensue with reasonably normal mental development. Neurologic complications, such as hemiplegia, convergent squint or convulsive attacks may appear later. In some cases recovery is complete without any residua.

Treatment is unsatisfactory, for there is seldom any opportunity to stop the bleeding or control the increased pressure within the skull. While waiting hopefully for the symptoms to subside spontaneously, general supportive measures are used. If there are convulsions, phenobarbital is indicated. Vitamin K usually is given in order to minimize bleeding. Unresponsive infants are not fed or handled any more than necessary, and measures to supply warmth or decrease elevated temperature are instituted. Sometimes it is possible to relieve intracranial pressure by withdrawing bloody fluid from the spinal canal or from the surface of the brain by tapping the dura at the lateral angle of the fontanelle. The latter procedure may be repeated effectively if the bleeding has become localized to a walled-off area over the surface of the brain (subdural hematoma). The best management of intracranial injury is to prevent it through judicious obstetric management of the mother. Under ideal circumstances it is possible to reduce the infant deaths from this cause to less than 1 per thousand live-born babies.

Fractures sometimes occur during birth. The clavicle suffers most frequently. It is broken by direct pressure of the finger during extraction of the shoulder. No special management is required, for this bone heals rapidly with the formation of a callus but without producing much pain or disability. Occasionally, linear fractures of the skull are discovered in infants whose birth has not been unusually difficult. Unless there is associated intracranial hemorrhage, such cracks are of trivial importance and heal quickly. Rarely, the humerus is broken during efforts to sweep the arm down over the face during breech delivery; or the femur may be fractured during version and extraction. Breaks of an extremity are usually apparent from the abnormal angulation that they produce. They heal well when immobilized in corrected position.

Brachial Palsy. This is a partial paralysis of one arm which results from excessive stretching of the nerve fibers that run from the neck through the shoulder and toward the arm. The trauma is produced by the forcible pulling of the shoulder away from the head during obstetric maneuvers. The most common type of paralysis involves the muscles of the upper arm and spares those of the hand and the fingers. The arm is held at the side with the elbow extended and the hand rotated inward. In mild cases when the injury is the result of stretching of nerve fibers that have not broken, recovery is rapid and may be complete within 3 weeks. More commonly, the fibers are stretched to such an extent that they break within their sheaths. Recovery from paralysis then depends upon the regeneration of nerves which are guided back to the appropriate muscles by the intact sheaths. Regeneration usually takes from 2 to 3 months. During the waiting period, the muscles of the shoulder should be manipulated gently and given massage to prevent contractures from forming. When recovery fails to take place within 3 months it probably indicates that the nerve roots have been torn loose from their connections with the spinal cord and that recovery will not occur unless the pathways can be restored surgically—a very difficult feat.

ASPHYXIA OR RESPIRATORY FAILURE

Initiation of Respiration in the Normal Infant. Once the newborn infant is separated from his mother he takes over the responsibility for oxygenating his blood through the activity of his own lungs. Under optimal circumstances the baby is born with a small amount of thin fluid in his respiratory passages. Perhaps even before his body is delivered, the stimulus of chilling or of manipulation, or the chemical changes taking place in his blood as the flow from the placenta is diminished, will activate the respiratory center in his brain. Thus a series of reflex muscular activities is set in motion, and they cause him to gasp and emit a cry—a most welcome sound in the delivery room! During the first few cries, most of the amniotic fluid in his lungs is expelled and the air sacs become distended with air. Thus, oxygen is brought in contact with the lung capillaries. Adjustments are made in the fetal blood circulation which throw a larger proportion of blood through the lungs. The respiratory center in the brain gives periodic signals that remind him to breathe, and within a few seconds the infant is ready to oxygenate his own tissues and participate in his own survival.

Causes of Asphyxia. Taking over the responsibility for oxygenating his own blood through the activity of his own lungs is a critical step for the newborn infant, for if he fails to discharge this duty within a matter of a few minutes, he will either die or suffer irreparable damage. Infants who have difficulty in making this transition are said to suffer from asphyxia. The term is admittedly a broad one which encompasses respiratory failure from a number of causes. The asphyxiated infant presents an emergency which must be dealt with before there is time for more than a cursory examination. Frequently, the exact reason for this difficulty is not immediately apparent.

The normal sequence of events cited above may be impeded if (1) the respiratory movements are adequate but the air passages are obstructed, (2) the respiratory center fails to emit the proper signals to the muscles that move the chest and the diapraghm, (3) the respiratory movements and the airway are adequate but intrinsic factors in the lungs or the chest interfere with proper expansion of the lungs, or (4) respiratory movements, airway, lungs and chest are all normal but oxygenation of the blood is incomplete because of an abnormality of the heart or its major vessels.

OBSTRUCTION OF THE AIR PASSAGES. In actual practice attention is first directed to the infant's *airway*. Even before the first breath is taken, the secretions of the mouth and the nose should be sucked out gently to prevent them from being drawn back into the lungs. Thick mucus may block branches of the bronchial tree and prevent full expansion of the lungs. Inhaled meconium is an even worse offender, since it is very irritating and difficult to remove. During suction of the mouth the infant should be held inverted to promote drainage from the trachea. If these measures are deemed insufficient to clear the airway, an operator skilled in the use of the tracheal catheter or the infant bronchoscope should be called to deal with the secretions below the larynx. On rare occasions the airway may be blocked by congenital abnormalities of the larynx or by compression of the trachea by an anomalous structure within the chest.

INACTIVITY OF THE RESPIRATORY CENTER. This condition is the most hazardous aspect of asphyxia. Under normal conditions, a fall in the oxygen content of the blood triggers the center to send out its signals. But the center will fail to respond if the oxygen concentration falls too low or if it is already damaged by prenatal anoxia, by intracranial injury, or by the injudicious administration of sedatives or anesthetics to the mother during the course of delivery.

If the infant has made no effort to breathe during the first minute after birth, resuscitative measures are begun. Frequently, a torpid respiratory center can be aroused by physical stimulation of the infant's skin through rubbing, slapping or blowing upon it. Usually, oxygen is administered so that the maximum benefit will be derived from any respiratory effort, no matter how feeble. If a tracheal catheter is in place, oxygen can be carried directly

into the lungs. Caution is needed in regulating the pressure so that the delicate lungs are not damaged by overdistention. Similar care must be exercised if any of the methods of artificial insufflation are used, i.e. mouth-to-mouth breathing, inflation of the lungs through a catheter, mechanical respirators or other devices. There is considerable difference of opinion about the actual effectiveness of these methods.

Drugs are sometimes but not dependably effective in stimulating respiration. Caffeine is the most dependable; epinephrine, Coramine, alpha-lobeline and Metrazol are also used. Recently an antagonist for the morphine group of drugs (nalline) has appeared which seems to be effective in infants who are narcotized by overdosage of the mother.

INTRINSIC DISORDERS OF THE LUNG. *Atelectasis.* Chief among the intrinsic disorders of the lung which produce asphyxia is atelectasis. This term indicates that areas of the lung are collapsed without air in the alveoli (air sacs) and consequently are useless for respiratory exchange. At birth the lungs are normally collapsed and devoid of air, but with the first breath many air sacs inflate, and with each succeeding breath more areas are opened until expansion is complete. Atelectasis may be due to the initial failure of the air sacs to open up. This in turn may depend upon incomplete development of the lung, or feeble respiratory movements, or blockage by mucus in the small ducts leading to the air sacs. The anterior and superior portions of the lung open most easily so that atelectatic areas usually are found posteriorly at the base of the lung.

The symptoms depend upon the extent of the collapse. Small areas of atelectasis are often discovered accidentally when a chest roentgenogram is taken for some other purpose. No discernible symptoms may be present. Moderate degrees of atelectasis produce mild cyanosis but little distress. When extensive portions of the lung are involved there is cyanosis, labored or grunting respirations, weakness and ultimately exhaustion. Treatment consists of continuous administration of oxygen and saturation of the inspired air with water vapor. Oxygen is given so that those areas of lung that are open will have the maximum effect in oxygenating the blood passing through. The moist atmosphere is desirable in order to liquefy secretions and make it easier for the infant to cough them up. Frequent changes of position offer the best opportunity for the collapsed areas to open. Since there is danger that the inactive portions of lung will become infected secondarily, often some type of antibiotic is administered.

Resorption Atelectasis. A peculiar type of atelectasis is seen in some premature and some cesarean-delivered infants. It is called resorption atelectasis because the lungs seem to expand fairly well at first and then collapse again in spite of vigorous respiratory efforts on the part of the infant. This disorder usually ends fatally within the first 48 hours. The lungs examined after death reveal a peculiar hyaline membrane lining the walls of some of the alveoli. The origin of the membrane is not known.

The course of atelectasis depends upon the infant's general condition and the extent of the collapse. Vigorous infants with mild or moderate degrees of collapse usually improve slowly but progressively and seldom have symptoms that extend into the second week. They suffer no permanent damage to the lung. Feeble, weak, or anoxic infants have a poorer chance of survival. Among premature infants the outlook depends in part upon the birth weight —the smaller the infant the poorer his prognosis. Infants of 1,000 Gm. birth weight or less usually succumb because their lungs have not yet reached a stage of development that will support extra-uterine life.

Malformations, Interstitial Emphysema and Pneumothorax. Other varieties of intrinsic disease of the chest or the lung include malformations, interstitial emphysema and pneumothorax. The lung may be completely absent on one side; or the diaphragm may be defective, permitting the intestines to invade the chest; or one or both lungs may be seeded with cysts containing air. Interstitial emphysema results when air is admitted into the space between the air sacs from a tear in the lining of one of them. If a large amount of air becomes trapped in this way, there will be insufficient room within the chest to permit expansion of the alveoli. Pneumothorax in the newborn is an extension of the process just mentioned. Air passes into the pleural space and collapses the lung, rendering it temporarily useless.

CONGENITAL MALFORMATIONS OF THE HEART AND THE GREAT VESSELS. These abnormalities are considered in Chapter 10.

Nursing Care. Infants who suffer from anoxia or asphyxia require careful observation and skilled nursing care. Often they are weak and close to the point of exhaustion. They need alert nurses who can detect signs of increasing distress. Airways must be kept free of secretions, and oxygen must be administered constantly until cyanosis is gone and recovery seems to be well established. Feeding or even administration of fluids is often deferred for the first 2 days, since by the end of that time either death or definite improvement is likely to occur. Infants who are still having respiratory difficulty after this period need to be fed by dropper or by gavage. Handling should be reduced to a minimum. Preventing distention is important, for it impedes normal expansion of the lungs. In most instances additional warmth should be supplied. Nursing measures to prevent infection are imperative, because a mild upper respiratory infection may cause death.

POSTNATAL INFECTIONS

During the latter portion of the pregnancy the mother transmits to her infant antibodies against some of the infectious diseases to which she has become immune. Passive immunity of this sort protects the infant for a variable time after birth—about 6 months in the case of measles, probably less than 3 months for chickenpox, and not at all for whooping cough. Unfortunately, such a protective mechanism exists for only a few diseases. To most of the infectious ills of man, the newborn is highly susceptible. In fact, he may even become infected by those bacteria that normally dwell in his intestines (colon bacilli) or on his skin (staphylococci). The special measures which are designed to shield him from infection have been discussed earlier in this chapter. When these safeguards fail, the character of the ensuing infection has special implications for the newborn.

Sepsis occurs when bacteria gain access to and multiply in the blood stream. Thus, organisms are transported to all parts of the body and may set up secondary areas of infection almost anywhere. The portal of invasion is not always apparent. Sometimes the route passes from an infected umbilicus through the umbilical vessels to the liver and thence to the general circulation. At other times invasion appears to take place through normal skin or through the mucous membrane of the intestinal or respiratory tract.

The symptoms of sepsis are not uniform. In some cases there is a dramatic rise in temperature, rapid weight loss, convulsions, jaundice and hemorrhagic phenomena. Abscesses appear in the skin, or pus is coughed up from the lungs. To an experienced eye, the nature of the disease is obvious at once. In other cases the onset is more insidious. The temperature may remain normal or fall to subnormal levels. Sudden weight loss in spite of a reasonable food intake may be the only warning of trouble. Usually those caring for the infant sense that something is amiss, but the true state of affairs may not be uncovered until a systematic search for infection is made by taking cultures of the blood, the spinal fluid and the secretions of the nose and the throat.

In all cases cultures are most important, for treatment rests mainly upon the use of antibiotics, the rational use of which depends upon isolating the invading bacterium and determining its sensitivity to the drugs that are available. In addition to specific antibacterial therapy, transfusions and oxygen are commonly needed.

The prognosis of sepsis depends to a great extent upon the speed of recognition of the disease and the accuracy of antibiotic administration. Even with good care the mortality is high. If meningitis occurs, complications such as hydrocephalus, convulsions or mental retardation must be feared as sequels, even when a bacteriologic cure is obtained.

Pneumonia in the newborn is always a serious disease. The added burden of infection is frequently more than the lungs can tolerate, for even in the healthy newborn they are tenuously prepared for their new function of respiration. Furthermore, the bacteria responsible for pneumonia of the newborn are less likely to respond to the common antibiotics. Instead of pneumococci and streptococci, the infant is more likely to be infected by staphylococci, colon bacilli, or other varieties of intestinal organisms. Pneumonia occasionally begins before birth when there is prolonged rupture of the membranes with infection of the amniotic fluid. When present at birth it is difficult to differentiate from atelectasis.

Epidemic diarrhea of the newborn is, as the name implies, a highly contagious disease which sweeps rapidly through nurseries into which it is introduced. The course is usually severe, and the mortality may run as high as 25 to 50 per cent of those affected. A single causative agent has not been clearly identified. The disease is presumed to gain access to the nursery either by breaks in technic during formula preparation or by spread from infected mothers or personnel who do not recognize disease in themselves.

The management of epidemic diarrhea is similar to that described for diarrhea in the older infants (Chap. 25). Extreme isolation precautions must be invoked to limit the spread of the epidemic. Admission of infants to the nursery is discontinued, and unaffected infants and their mothers are dispersed to their homes as rapidly as possible. Personnel responsible for the care of infants outside the area should not be permitted to enter it.

Impetigo and furunculosis of the skin occur more easily in the newborn than in the older child, because the resistance to skin bacteria is lower. These disorders are described in Chapter 13. The reputation of impetigo as a scourge of newborn nurseries probably is unwarranted today when the disease can be controlled rapidly with antibiotics.

Tetanus of the newborn is practically unknown in the United States but still occurs in countries where hygienic care of the umbilicus is so poor that tetanus spores may gain access to and grow in its recesses. The disease is described in Chapter 18.

Gonorrheal conjunctivitis (ophthalmia neonatorum) is losing its importance as a cause of congenital blindness, due in part to the impact of state laws that require prophylactic treatment of all infants at birth and in part to the advent of penicillin which provides an effective cure of the infection in both the mother and the child. The disease is acquired during birth by contamination of the infant's eyes with the infected secretions of the mother's vagina. The symptoms are similar to those of chemical conjunctivitis of the newborn but become evident on the second or the third day of life rather than in the first 12 to 24 hours. Prompt differentiation is important, for a delay in the treatment of gonorrheal conjunctivitis may permit ulceration and scarring of the cornea to occur. False security sometimes arises from the knowledge that silver nitrate presumably has been instilled in the birth-room. The technic of instillation of the drops into the eyes of a newborn infant is sufficiently difficult, however, that drops sometimes fail to get into the sacs. When the disease is suspected, smears and cultures of the pus should be made, but treatment usually is initiated before the laboratory results are known. Penicillin given by injections and by direct instillation into the conjunctival sacs at frequent intervals results in prompt healing.

Tuberculosis is practically unknown during the newborn period, but it must be kept in mind as a disease to which the small infant is highly susceptible. It is hazardous for him to go home into an environment in which he will come in contact with someone harboring an active form of tuberculosis. Special efforts should be made to see that not only his mother but all other members of his family as well are free from the disease.

PREMATURITY

DEFINITION

A premature infant is one who is born before the conclusion of the normal period of gestation. Ideally, the determination of prematurity should be based upon the length of time that elapses between conception and birth. Methods for estimating the date of conception are so notoriously inaccurate that a less debatable standard of classification—the birth weight—has been adopted universally. By international agreement a premature infant is now defined as one which weighs less than 2,500 grams (5½ lbs.) at birth. In setting this standard it is admitted that some infants who are actually premature by gestational age (less than 37 weeks) will be classified erroneously as mature; and, conversely, that some infants who are small for reasons other than short gestation periods will be labeled wrongly as premature.

CAUSES

A physiologic reason for prematurity is apparent in only about half the cases. Abnormal conditions in the mother are the most frequent explanation—toxemia of pregnancy, uterine bleeding, early rupture of the membranes, chronic heart, kidney or thyroid disease, diabetes, syphilis, tuberculosis, acute infections, accidents, or abdominal operations. When there is more than one fetus in the uterus, the excessive size sets off premature labor approximately 3 times out of 10. Some varieties of severe malformation of the fetus are responsible for premature labor.

Research to discover other causes of prematurity is urgently needed, for the majority of premature infants are born to women who show no symptoms of physical illness. Studies that have been done already disclose the fact that good prenatal care which included an adequate protein intake decreases the incidence of toxemia and prematurity.

INCIDENCE

Accepting the definition of prematurity stated above, most obstetric services find that from 5 to 8 per cent of their liveborn babies arrive prematurely. Because certain races normally have small infants, the incidence of prematurity is higher in population groups that have a large proportion of Negro or Asiatic mothers.

PREVENTION

The medical profession is attempting to prevent prematurity through improved services to all prenatal patients. Care that protects the infant as well as the mother is being provided for prenatal patients with placenta praevia and premature rupture of the membranes. Mothers with placenta praevia are hospitalized where bed rest and transfusions can be provided. Instead of inducing labor when membranes rupture spontaneously, some obstetricians are prescribing antibiotics, bed rest and careful perineal care. With special care obstetricians are finding that the pregnancy continues for days and in some instances to term.

HANDICAPS AND CARE REQUIRED TO COMBAT THEM

It is to be expected that an infant born before he has completed the biologic steps desirable for extrauterine life will have a more difficult time making the adjustment than will the infant who is appropriately mature. This hypothesis is confirmed by mortality figures which show that the premature's chances of failing to survive are 10 to 15 times as great as the risk run by a full-term child. Of all the infant deaths occurring in the first month of life, more than half are in babies who were born prematurely. The handicaps that the premature must surmount in order to survive differ in kind, number and severity, depending upon the degree of his immaturity. The smaller the infant is at birth, the more arduous his struggle for survival. After a general survey of the problems that all prematures face and the care that these handicaps necessitate, the characteristics, the prognosis and the additional nursing care for infants with different degrees of immaturity will be considered in more detail.

Prenatal Disturbance. The same prenatal disturbance that produced the premature birth may constitute a serious handicap. An infant hastily delivered because of his mother's toxemia of pregnancy may be ill from the effects of the maternal disease; one who was extracted because of maternal bleeding may have suffered anoxic damage to the brain as described previously. Syphilis in the mother may mean both premature birth and an infection for the infant. Erythroblastosis or severe anomalies may pose insuperable handicaps for the premature infant.

Difficulty in Establishing Respiration. There are many reasons why difficulty in establishing respiration is by all odds the most common single cause of death among premature infants. In the very immature infant the fault lies within the lungs themselves, for important structural changes take place during the second half of pregnancy which enlarge the potential air sacs and bring them into closer approximation to the lung capillaries. Failure of this change to proceed to a critical point in the development of the lung accounts for most of the deaths attributed to "previability." In addition, the small premature is handicapped by weakness of the muscles that move his chest wall and by the plasticity of the bony framework which permits it to retract during inspiration, cutting down the effective expansion of the lungs within. Frequently, the stimulation of the respiratory center in the brain is irregular. An added hazard of the first few days is resorption atelectasis, a peculiar variety of lung disorder which has been mentioned above and is primarily a disease of premature infants.

Even when the respiratory apparatus permits survival, symptoms of respiratory difficulty are apparent. The small premature infant is likely to show irregular, periodic breathing interspersed with long moments of apnea. Mild cyanosis is intermittently present.

Since the administration of oxygen relieves cyanosis and increases the rate and the regularity of respirations in the premature infant, it has become standard practice to keep all small infants in an oxygen-rich, highly humidified atmosphere until they have demonstrated respiratory competence. The water content of the air-and-oxygen mixture should be kept as high as possible, for if the secretions within the bronchial tree are allowed to dry out, they will block the exchange of air and produce additional areas of atelectasis. In many nurseries devices are now used to create a mist or fog within the incubator in which the smaller infants are housed.

The question of respiratory adequacy usually is settled within the first 2 or 3 days of life. If the infant survives this period he may still have some unexpanded areas of lung, but unless he is handicapped further by infection, the areas of atelectasis will be of decreasing importance to him. As with most other handicaps, the frequency and the severity of atelectasis are greater the less mature the infant is at birth.

Body Temperature. The premature infant has difficulty in regulating his body temperature, for it responds rather promptly to changes in the temperature of the surrounding environment. When placed in cold or drafty surroundings he has trouble conserving his body heat. As a result, his temperature may fall to subnormal levels. The factors that interfere with his efforts to hold or produce body heat are the relatively large surface area in proportion to his body size, the lack of an insulating layer of fat beneath his skin, poor reflex control of his skin capillaries, and the smallness and the inactivity of his muscles—the main source from which body heat is obtained. When the premature is placed in a hot environment, poor control over his skin capillaries and the lack of an adequate sweating mechanism prevent him from losing heat, and his body temperature rises accordingly.

Some type of mechanical incubator is highly desirable if not essential to the small premature infant in order to keep him at a stable temperature and to supply adequately humidified air. Now it is recognized that environmental temperature should be adjusted so that his body temperature ranges between 35.5° and 36.5° C. (96° to 98° F.) rather than attempting to push it up to the accepted normal range for older infants. At such lower levels stability is more easily obtained. The premature nursery should be kept warm (80° F.) and free of drafts. In hot climates and seasons, air-conditioning is desirable. The humidity of the air should be kept between 55 and 65 per cent. Premature infants dehydrate easily. In humidified nurseries it has been found that initial loss of weight is less, the regaining of birth weight is more rapid, body temperature stabilizes more easily, and the incidence of respiratory infections and gastrointestinal disturbances is lower.

Poor Resistance to Infection. The premature infant's resistance to infection is notoriously poor. He receives less than the usual quantity of protective substances from his mother's blood and is denied the benefits of her early milk (colostrum). In addition, his ability to manufacture his own body proteins, including antibodies, is below par.

Protective measures to prevent infection are imperative because even trivial infections may be devastating to him. The organization of the nursery facilities should be such that prematures are kept in a unit separated from other children and even from the nursery for full-term newborn infants. None but a minimum number of essential personnel should be permitted within the unit. Strict isolation and aseptic precautions should be observed. The mere suggestion of an infection in one of the personnel should be considered as an adequate reason for excluding that individual from the unit until recovery is complete. Prematures born outside of the hospital and those who develop infections should be kept in a separate area. Modern incubators provide additional safeguards within the nursery. Some are so designed that the infant's complete care can be carried out without removing him from the enclosed space of the incubator. It is desirable to sterilize the clothing that comes in direct contact with the infant's skin and the cotton and oil that is used for cleansing. The nurse needs to be constantly alert to observe symptoms which might indicate the onset of any type of skin, respiratory or gastro-intestinal infection. In some nurseries it is standard practice to administer antibiotics to all small prematures until they have made a promising start and whenever any suspicion of infection arises.

Biochemical Handicaps. A large number of biochemical handicaps of the premature infant can be enumerated. These arise in part from his extremely rapid growth rate, in part from the immaturity of organs such as the liver and the kidneys, and in part from his failure to linger within the uterus long enough to acquire his full complement of certain essential materials.

The premature infant grows more rapidly than the full-term infant and requires a relatively large amount of food to supply building materials and energy. No other human being grows as rapidly as the premature infant. It is not uncommon for him to double his initial birth weight in the brief span of 2 months! In order to do this, if calculated in terms of calories per unit of weight, his requirements are from 30 to 50 per cent greater than those of the full-term infant.

The immaturity of the premature infant's digestive and nervous systems complicates the technic of meeting his food requirements. The limited capacity of his stomach must not be exceeded, for vomiting and aspiration of food into his lungs are to be avoided at all costs. The mere ability to suck and to swallow is sometimes lacking or too exhausting for him to perform frequently. Special methods must be used to convey food into his stomach. The ability of his intestinal tract to digest the food brought to it is also limited, particularly in respect to fat which he tolerates poorly. Care must be taken to see that too much is not forced upon him, for if his tolerance for digestion is exceeded diarrhea may result.

Immaturity of the liver accounts in part for the premature's poor resistance to infection (he forms antibody protein poorly); for his tendency to bleed (he forms prothrombin poorly); for his tendency to become edematous (his total serum protein concentration is low); and for his susceptibility to jaundice (his liver cannot adequately clear the blood of the pigments which result from the normal postnatal destruction of circulating red blood cells). Immaturity of the kidneys contrib-

utes to his limited tolerance for salt, to his tendency to become edematous and to the mild state of acidosis in which the premature normally lives.

The premature infant is born before he has fortified himself with his full quota of vitamins A, C, D and K and of the minerals phosphorus, calcium and iron, yet the rapidity of his immediate postnatal growth demands an unusual supply of these substances. During the last 2 months of pregnancy the full-term infant draws upon his mother for stores of vitamins and minerals and therefore is protected temporarily from the vitamin-deficiency diseases. To forestall the vitamin-deficiency diseases in the premature, such as rickets, scurvy and hemorrhagic disease of the newborn, prophylactic quantities of the corresponding vitamins usually are given in double the dosage recommended for the full-term infant. Calcium and phosphorus are present in milk in abundance to satisfy the needs of prematures. Iron is not supplied in adequate amounts by most feedings. Even when the diet is supplemented with medicinal iron, absorption is poor during the first 6 to 8 weeks of life. However, it is commonly added in the hope of preventing as far as possible the anemia that regularly develops in the growing premature.

Retrolental Fibroplasia. Since 1940 a disease peculiar to premature infants has been recognized with alarmingly increasing frequency. In its fully developed form retrolental fibroplasia involves both eyes and produces complete or nearly complete blindness due to separation and fibrosis of the retina. It now constitutes the chief cause of neo-natal blindness and is the object of intensive study by many institutions that care for prematures.

The main peculiarities of the disease are that it apparently did not exist before 1935; that it attacks the most immature infants more frequently than the larger prematures; that its incidence is extremely variable among different populations of prematures; and that its effects are not immediately apparent but are discovered only after weeks or months have elapsed. If the eyes of all premature infants are examined at regular intervals with the aid of an ophthalmoscope, the early pathologic changes may be observed some time before the infant reaches a weight of 1,500 to 1,800 Gm. These consist of dilatation of retinal veins, hemorrhage and exudate into the retina and areas of separation of the retina from the inner surface of the eyeball. In some infants these changes regress, but in others there is progressive detachment of the retina until it is brought forward into an irregular, useless fibrotic mass retaining perhaps some light perception but no useful vision. The matted retina can be seen through the pupil as a greenish opacity. Unless routine ophthalmoscopic examination of eyes is made, loss of vision may be easily overlooked in small infants until they are 3 to 4 months of age.

The cause of retrolental fibroplasia is still unsettled in spite of the fact that many theories have been advanced and some have been tested. Currently, suspicion is directed at excessive oxygen administration and the sudden increases in circulating blood volume which may be produced by transfusion or by the administration of too much salt in the feeding.

Nursing Care of the Premature. In spite of the many hazards that beset prematurely born infants, from 75 to 85 per cent of them will survive if given reasonably adequate care. Better obstetric practices, new medical discoveries and improved mechanical aids are all contributing to better care for these infants. But the benefits of such advances are easily erased if the daily nursing care of the infant is slighted. Many a prematurely born child owes his life in a very real sense to the devotion, the skill and the judgment of the nurses who ministered to his early needs. The requirements of care differ with the initial size of the premature and will be considered separately for each of the main subdivisions by weight.

PREMATURES OF 400 TO 1,000 GM. (14 oz. to 2 lbs. 3 oz.). With good luck and meticulous care about 10 per cent of these infants can be reared. Fetuses of less than 400 Gm. are classified as abortions. They never develop effective respirations and die within a short time after birth. Infants of birth weights between 400 and 1,000 Gm. are called previable and generally are not expected to survive but some show unusual strength and survive despite their initial handicaps. Infants of such small size are infrequent. They comprise about 0.5 per cent of all live births and about 7 per cent of premature births.

Many external evidences of immaturity are present in this group of premature infants whose gestation period ranges from 20 to 28 weeks and length measures from 28 to 35 cm. (11 to 14 in.). The head is proportionately quite large, with high forehead and small facial features. The eyes are tiny, scarcely visible; the ears are soft and poorly developed; the chin recedes. The extremities are spindly with tiny muscles and soft rudimentary nails on the fingers and the toes. The skin may be covered with lanugo hair. The subcutaneous tissues are usually full, giving the appearance of plumpness. But if the infant survives a few days the skin hangs loosely on his body, demonstrating that the original appearance was due to edema rather than subcutaneous fat. Nipples and genitalia are small, and in male infants the testes are often undescended. Activity of the infant is limited to the respiratory efforts, which may be weak and unpredictable. The soft chest wall retracts excessively during inspiration, and the mouth often opens in a gulping fashion. The sucking, swallowing and gag reflexes are usually absent in these very immature infants. They seldom cry. Cyanosis may be present constantly or during periods of prolonged apnea.

If he can weather the first 48 hours of life, the previable infant has a chance of ultimate survival. Deaths are usually due to failure to establish respirations, and less commonly to intracranial hemorrhage.

The first objectives of nursing care are to maintain a stable, appropriate body temperature, to conserve body heat and muscular energy, and to support the respiratory effort by the administration of humidified oxygen supplemented by stimulation as indicated. The infant should be placed at once in an incubator, pref-

erably one that has been preheated to 90° to 95° F. Oxygen in a concentration of 40 to 50 per cent or higher should be provided in the highest concentration of water vapor that can be obtained with the available apparatus. Then the infant should be disturbed only for necessary suction aspiration of secretions from the mouth and the nose and for the injection of vitamin K and antibiotics as prescribed. Stimulants or periodic brief inhalations of a 5 per cent carbon dioxide in oxygen mixture may be required if the respiratory effort fails.

Constant nursing care during the first 24 hours after birth is essential. Respirations, color, activity, temperature, cry, condition of the skin and the cord, the bladder and bowel function should be observed. A bulb syringe or a suction set consisting of a mouthpiece, 4 inches of rubber tubing, a Murphy drip bulb and a No. 8 or 10 catheter should be in readiness in the infant's unit (Fig. 16). When cyanosis and difficult breathing occur the nurse should pass the catheter through the mouth and into the back of the throat to remove by suction the mucus obstruction. This should be done *before* carbon dioxide 5 per cent in oxygen is administered. Carbon dioxide stimulates respiration. If it is given before mucus is withdrawn by suction, the infant may aspirate as he inhales.

When mechanical incubators are not available for the care of a small premature, other means of supplying external heat must be provided. Stabilization of body temperature may be attempted by wrapping the infant in a close-fitting parka made of outing flannel or of alternate layers of cotton and gauze (Fig. 17). A bed constructed within a box or large basket and heated by hot water bottles or electric lamp may serve to keep the immediate environmental temperature suitable. A thermometer should be placed between the blankets and the infant as an aid in controlling the temperature. Bottles should be filled with water at a temperature of from 100° to 105° F. When the water is changed, it should be done at the bedside to avoid a prolonged drop in environmental temperature. The room should be kept at a temperature of 85° to 90° F. The infant's temperature will stabilize more readily when environmental temperature is elevated than when he is heavily clothed and covered with additional blankets. His temperature should be taken every 2 to 3 hours until stabilization is acquired; thereafter, twice

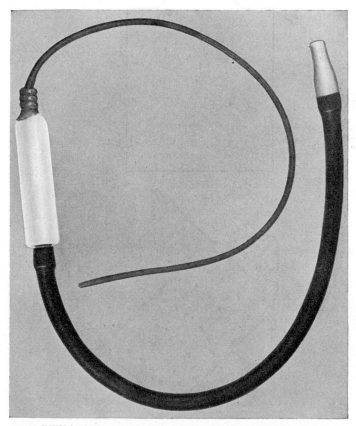

Fig. 16. A mouth suction set for aspirating secretions from the upper respiratory tract.

daily is sufficient. Administration of oxygen through a mask is serviceable but gives poor humidification and variable control of concentration.

Administration of food or fluid to these delicate infants usually is deferred for a day or two until they have had a chance to establish their respirations and to lose the edema fluid with which they were born. Since early feedings will have to be small in volume, additional fluid may be given by subcutaneous injection. Glucose solutions are generally preferred to salt-containing fluids that may result in a return of edema.

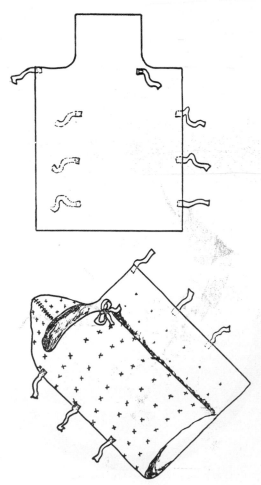

FIG. 17. Illustrating method of making jacket for a premature infant.

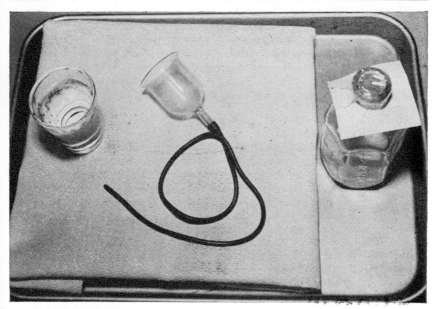

FIG. 18. Equipment for gavage. The bottle to the right contains the milk mixture. The medicine glass contains sterile water for catheter lubrication and testing for anatomic position.

In the absence of the normal reflexes of feeding, the first food must be administered by gavage. This process of tube feeding is also least tiring to the infant. The technic is as follows:

Equipment for gavage (Fig. 18) consists of a sterile catheter (No. 8 or 10F), a medicine glass containing sterile water, a glass syringe barrel, and the prescribed food. The infant is placed on his back for the treatment. The distance from the tip of the nose to the ensiform process should be marked on the catheter with an indelible pencil before preparation of the equipment. This distance corresponds to that from the lips to the lower part of the esophagus immediately above the cardiac orifice. This site for the end of the catheter is preferable in the case of the prematurely born infant in order to avoid vomiting. The catheter should be connected to the syringe barrel, lubricated with sterile water and passed into the esophagus through the mouth. When the marked portion of the catheter reaches the lips, the mouth of the syringe barrel is placed in the medicine glass of water to test the position of the catheter. The tube is not likely to enter the larynx and the trachea, but if it should, air will bubble through the water in the glass on expiration by the baby. In addition, the baby would become cyanotic, and if he were sufficiently vigorous he would have a spasm of coughing at the time the tube was inserted. After the tube has been passed properly, the syringe barrel is held stable in one hand, and the food is poured into the barrel with the other. After the food is poured, the barrel may be elevated sufficiently to allow the food to run slowly into the stomach. After the food has run in, the tube should be removed, *first having been tightly pinched or bent onto itself.* Because the infant tends to gasp as the tube is removed, every precaution. must be taken to prevent aspiration of milk that may have remained in the tube. At the end of the feeding, the infant should be turned on his right side to lessen stomach-emptying time. If a tendency to regurgitation exists, the infant's head and thorax should be elevated slightly.

The type of food, the amount, the frequency and the method of feeding are prescribed in accordance with the infant's weight, physical response to ingestion of food and to his ability to suckle. Although breast milk is used sometimes as a feeding for small prematures, artificial formulas consisting of half-skimmed milk with added salt-free carbohydrate are generally preferred. The quantity of feeding must be restricted to a few cubic centimeters at a time until the infant's capacity is learned. Overloading his stomach must be avoided at all costs, for a single episode of vomiting and aspiration is likely to prove fatal. Not only is regurgitation to be avoided, but also abdominal distention. Distention is a cause of cyanotic attacks because it interferes with respiration, which is chiefly diaphragmatic. Gavage feed-

ings may be given as often as every 2 hours. The amounts given are increased gradually until the food intake reaches 120 to 140 calories per kilogram (55 to 65 calories per pound) of body weight. Water-miscible preparations of vitamins A, B, C and D which may be added to the gavage feedings are available. When the infant begins to suck on the gavage tube, cautious trials may be made with feedings from a dropper.

Carefully given medicine-dropper feedings protect the premature infant and increase his pleasure in the feeding experience. A medicine glass containing the prescribed feeding should be kept warm throughout the procedure. After the infant's diaper has been changed and the nurse's hands thoroughly washed, the nurse should support his head and shoulders with one hand and open his mouth by applying gentle pressure to the chin. Milk is dropped from a medicine dropper, sheathed in rubber tubing, well back onto the tongue, a drop at a time until the infant's ability to swallow has been ascertained. The feeding should not be hurried or forced. Gentle pressure on the back of the tongue may be used to stimulate swallowing. Food should not be left in the mouth at the conclusion of the feeding. The infant may be supported partially erect for a while in order to permit bubbling. Then he should be placed on his right side with head slightly elevated to facilitate gastric emptying.

During the initial medicine-dropper feedings, the nurse should observe him for signs of fatigue. If the feeding experience brings cyanosis and increased lassitude instead of pleasure, resumption of gavage feedings is indicated until he demonstrates increased capacity to participate with comfort.

The necessary early caution in feeding, combined with the loss of edema fluid, results in a rather sizeable loss of weight during the first 2 weeks. Ordinarily, it takes from 3 to 5 weeks at least for the previable infant to regain his initial weight and make a steady daily increment. Three months or more may elapse before such an infant reaches the premature graduation weight of 2,500 grams.

The prognosis of the previable infant is difficult to estimate. Too few of those who survive are observed in follow-up studies, and as a result any accurate estimate of the long-range prognosis is impossible. Previable infants who survive generally have rather large heads with narrow faces and slender body habitus. Their early growth and development is likely to be at least 3 months retarded for their chronologic age. Most of them catch up gradually, and some at least reach adult life with perfectly normal mental competence. The risk of retrolental fibroplasia is a significant one in these small infants. Current theories about its causation make it prudent to delay transfusion as long as possible, even in the face of fairly marked anemia. Medicinal iron usually is given at 4 to 6 weeks of age. Administration must be started cautiously in order to avoid vomiting or diarrhea.

PREMATURES OF 1,000 TO 1,500 GM. (2 lbs. 3 oz. to 3 lbs. 5 oz.). Since most of these infants have reached a stage of pulmonary maturity that can support life, the anticipated survival rate is distinctly better—from 40 to 50 per cent. Most of the deaths will occur in the first 48 hours of life from resorption atelectasis, pulmonary hemorrhage, or the effects of anoxia or intracranial injury. The number of infants born with weights in this range is slightly greater than the number of previable infants—a little over 0.5 per cent of total live births and about 10 per cent of all premature births. The gestational age ranges from 28 to 32 weeks, and the infants measure from 35 to 40 cm. (14 to 16 in.) in length.

The physical features are similar to those of the previable infant but less extreme in their divergence from the normal-term infant. Periodic and ineffectual respiratory effort is common but not universal. Temperature regulation is poor. The sucking, swallowing and gag reflexes may be present at birth, but gavage feeding is still required as an introductory measure.

The early nursing care is identical with that of the previable infant but is required for a shorter period of time. Many infants in this group will be able to dispense with gavage feedings, oxygen administration and the mechanical incubator within the first weeks of life. Initial weight losses are usually marked, but the food intake can be increased at a more rapid pace and the birth weight is often regained by 3 to 4 weeks of age, and steady weight progress is made thereafter.

Prematures in this group can tolerate more handling after their initial adjustment to extra-uterine life has been made. The exposure incident to a daily soap-and-water bath should be avoided in most instances, at least for the first week or two. Warmed oil baths may be given every other day until the infant reaches the weight of 5½ pounds. On alternate days care should be given to the head and the genitalia as the entire body and behavior are observed to appraise his general condition. During the period of adjustment daily weighing also should be eliminated. When he is weighed, exposure should be prevented. The scale should be balanced with a diaper or paper that completely covers the scale pan, and with whatever clothing is being used. The infant should be covered with a blanket while being carried to the scales. Before the infant is weighed, he should be dressed in the clothing provided. This method prevents undue exposure and lessens the amount of handling.

These infants, too, will bear the marks of their prematurity for many months after birth—large, narrow heads, important degrees of anemia, retardation of growth and development by at least 2 months. Their chances for eventually having normal mentality and size are good. The risk of developing retrolental fibroplasia is still considerable.

PREMATURES OF 1,500 TO 2,000 GM. (3 lbs. 5 oz. to 4 lbs. 6 oz.). The added maturity greatly improves the rate of survival in this group of infants, so that 75 to 80 per cent may be expected to live. The gestational ages approximate 32 to 35 weeks, and the length at birth varies from 40 to 43 cm. (15½ to 16½ in.). About twice as many infants are born with weights in this range as in the preceding group—somewhat over 1 per cent of total live births and about 20 per cent of all prematures.

The physical characteristics of extreme prematurity are less marked. Heads are not as large relatively, edema is less common, and some of the infants show a modest amount of subcutaneous fat. Although initial respiratory difficulty will create a problem for some of them, routine use of oxygen and high humidity is no longer necessary. The ability to stabilize body temperature is much better, so that most of these infants can be transferred rapidly to a heated crib or an ordinary crib in an evenly warmed room. The sucking, gag and swallowing reflexes are regularly present unless the infant is abnormal in some manner apart from his prematurity. Feeding by gavage is generally unnecessary.

Medicine-dropper feedings may be necessary temporarily for some of these babies, but the majority of them soon indicate their ability and eagerness for sucking activity. The more vigorous infants in this group may be fed from a bottle with a soft-rubber nipple after the initial dropper feeding. The nipple should be chosen with care. It should not have holes that are too large or too small. When the nipple holes are too small, the infant becomes unduly fatigued; when they are too large the baby is forced beyond his capacity and he is deprived of the pleasure and the exercise that sucking supplies.

As soon as the infant's physical condition permits, he should be fed according to his manifest hunger needs and held throughout the feedings. Like the full-term infant, he, too, needs freedom from frustration, as well as cuddling associated with his feedings. From the moment of birth the nurse should be sensitive to the discomforts and the hazards that the prematurely born infant is experiencing, both physically and emotionally. Nursing measures that preserve life and provide gratification should be carried out. He needs a soothing, warm and tranquil environment; he requires interest in him as an individual and care that takes into account his emotional as well as his physical needs. It is possible to gratify an infant when he signals his distress, be it from insufficient sucking, hunger or sheer loneliness and a need for closeness, without exposing him to infection, overfeeding or fatigue.

Within this group steady weight gains are generally established by 2 to 3 weeks of age, and growth and development proceed at a rate that is about 1 to 2 months behind the average for the chronologic age. The risk of retrolental fibroplasia is greatly diminished but not entirely absent.

PREMATURES OF 2,000 TO 2,500 GM. (4 lbs. 6 oz. to 5 lbs. 8 oz.). The degree of prematurity is mild in this group of infants, and a proportional reduction in the handicaps permits from 90 to 95 per cent or even more of them to survive. The bulk of the premature infants fall within this weight range—about 4 per cent of the total births and from 60 to 65 per cent of all the premature births. The gestational ages approximate 35 to 38 weeks, and the infants measure from 43 to 47 cm. (16½ to 18 in.) in length.

Apart from smallness, the physical characteristics and care differ little from those of full-term infants. Slenderness and hyperactivity are common. Mechanical apparatus for the regulation of body temperatures or for the administration of oxygen and humidified air is seldom required. Bottle feeding may be commenced at once, and the infants can be picked up and held during feeding. Some of the larger and more vigorous members of this group can be cared for in the regular nursery or may visit their mothers. Most of them will begin to gain weight steadily after 10 days to 2 weeks. Few of them will have to remain within the confines of the premature nursery for more than a month. Immediate direct breast-feeding is feasible for some of the larger infants; eventual nursing can be carried out for most of them. Mothers should be encouraged to keep their supplies of breast milk flowing by regular emptying of the breast with manual expression or by the use of a breast pump. The main reason for segregating these large prematures from the full-term infants is to shield them from infection and to give them the benefit of skilled assistance in their early feedings.

Growth and development proceed at a pace which is only temporarily behind that of other infants of the same age. Nearly all of them will catch up within the first 6 months of life. Retrolental fibroplasia is seldom found in infants of this degree of maturity.

Preparation of the Mother for the Care of Her Prematurely Born Child. Preparing the mother for the care of her prematurely born infant should begin in the immediate postpartum period and continue until she has developed confidence in her ability to understand and meet his needs. To alleviate the mother's anxiety the nurse must be able to understand the emotional problems common to those who give birth to prematurely born infants. Also, she must satisfy the mother's need to learn about her infant and offer reassurance which will help her to assume the responsibilities entailed in his care after he leaves the hospital. The necessity for frequent, cautious feeding, for the administration of vitamins, for avoidance of infection and for periodic medical examination can be emphasized in a way that not only ensures protective care of the infant but also conveys the nurse's confidence in the mother's ability to meet his needs as well. A practical demonstration with opportunity to practice various aspects of the infant's care should be offered to the mother toward the end of his stay.

Many mothers of prematurely born infants need the help of the visiting nurse during the period when they are becoming adjusted to their maternal role. Ideally, the nurse should visit the home before the infant leaves the hospital. In such a visit the nurse can center her interest in the mother in an attempt to understand her problems as she anticipates taking over the care of her baby. Also, she can appraise the physical surroundings, the available equipment, and the mother's readiness to give her infant care. She will need to discover the supportive supervision that the mother will require in the period when she begins to take over the responsibility of his care. She will need to return later after the baby has been discharged

to render assistance in accordance with her individual requirements.

The mother of a premature infant often requires extended counseling and support to alleviate anxiety and to help her to understand his changing needs. Her attitude toward the infant is easily distorted by the anxieties that assail her at various stages of his early life. At first she is concerned about whether or not he will survive. Then she worries about his prospects for achieving ultimate normal development. At the time of departure from the hospital she is likely to be anxious about the special precautions and requirements of his care and perhaps be dubious about her ability to carry them out as expertly as the nurse. She often believes that he will need the same protective care that he required when he was smaller and one among many in a hospital nursery. The infant's early behavior at home is not always reassuring, for often he is emotionally unstable, requires frequent, self-regulated feedings and much more attention and holding than the average full-term infant who has just emerged from the hospital. This is especially true if he has been in a busy nursery and subjected to rigid schedules which have not taken his individual requirements into consideration. In so far as she can honestly do so, the nurse should offer reassurance and encouragement rather than criticism and hints at additional topics for concern.

After the mother has weathered the first months at home, she will need help to direct her attention to the infant's needs to become gradually prepared for the socialization process. She may need help in recognizing her infant's developing powers and signs of readiness to explore, to begin learning to tolerate small doses of frustration and to develop increasing amounts of independence. Like any other child, he must learn to deal with disappointment and frustration and gradually learn to adapt himself to social living. If his mother shields him from such experiences for too long a period he is likely to be an unhappy child, poorly prepared for neighborhood and school life.

Certain personality characteristics have been observed in infants born prematurely. Investigators who have studied children who were born prematurely found that they showed a tendency to prolonged thumb-sucking, maternal overdependence, negativism, emotional instability, difficulty in establishing bowel and bladder control and in mastering correct pronunciation.

Investigators have ascribed the premature behavior syndrome to certain physical and environmental factors. The prematurely born infant's nervous system is less mature than is that of the full-term infant. He is exposed to extra-uterine existence before he is ready to adapt himself to it. As a result he experiences more frustration and untimely stimulation than the full-term infant. In addition, he must begin life with the care of many people rather than with the care that only a well-prepared mother can give. Often he also experiences inconsistency in care as well. Early in life he requires extra protection and solicitude. Many mothers have difficulty in accepting the fact that the original delicate condition which required special protective measures

was a temporary phenomenon. They overprotect and infantilize their children after they have approached the status normal for their age. However, simultaneously in their eagerness for them to stand well with other children of their age, they expect performance that is beyond their capacity to achieve. Under such circumstances disturbances in the mother-child relationship are inevitable.

Assisting mothers in observing their infants' individual readiness for experiences which help them to adapt to the social customs of their society can help to prevent the premature behavior syndrome that Shirley describes. The behavior expected should conform to the infant's biologic age rather than to his extra-uterine chronologic age. Over-expectancy produces tension within the child; therefore, learning becomes more difficult. Permitting the infant the gratification that comes when his signal of need is met early in life and observing clues that indicate his preparedness for less dependent care and more self-directed activity is the kind of guidance that any young child requires, be he premature, physically handicapped or normal. Both infantilization and unreasonable expectation which forces the child to accomplish developmental tasks that he is unready for deprive the child and stunt personality development.

SITUATIONS FOR FURTHER STUDY

1. What are some of the characteristic fears of the new mother? How can the nurse help to alleviate them?

2. What adjustments must the newborn infant make to extra-uterine life?

3. What are the physical and emotional needs of the infant during the neonatal period?

4. What are the dangers of anoxia? How can the nurse function to prevent it?

5. How may disease or a congenital anomaly frustrate a newborn infant's emotional needs?

6. Select a newborn infant in the pediatric ward, observe him and describe the way his physical condition frustrates his emotional needs. How could you lessen his frustration? Describe the nursing care that you think he needs.

7. From observation of a prematurely born infant of from 800 to 1,000 Gm. in weight, list the characteristics that differentiate him from a full-term infant. As a result of these physiologic characteristics, what are his nursing needs? How would his nursing care differ from that required by a premature infant of 2,000 Gm. in weight?

8. Should you be given the responsibility of caring for a prematurely born infant in the home, what adaptations would you have to make to include principles of nursing care?

9. Study mortality-rate statistics of infants born prematurely. At what period of life do most deaths occur? By what measures could this rate be reduced?

10. How do you think a mother would feel giving birth to a premature infant? What emotional problems might parents of a pre-maturely born infant have? How might the nurse help parents with their problems?

BIBLIOGRAPHY

Blake, F. G.: Nursing care during the adjustment period (birth to 3 months): Its influence on the child's feelings about the world, chap. 3, p. 53, in The Child, His Parents and the Nurse, Philadelphia, Lippincott, 1954.

Blodi, F. C., and Parke, Priscilla: Retrolental fibroplasia, Am. J. Nursing 53:718, 1953.

Dunham, E. C.: Premature infants; A manual for physicians, Washington, U. S. Gov't Printing Office, 1948.

Grece, D. S.: Talipes equinovarus, Am. J. Nursing 51:707, 1951.

Greene, D. M.: Caring for the premature baby, Am. J. Nursing 50:458, 1950.

Hess, Julius, and Lundeen, Evelyn: The Premature Infant, ed. 2, Philadelphia, Lippincott, 1949.

Parmelee, A. H.: Management of the Newborn, Chicago, Yr. Bk. Pub., 1952.

Potter, Edith: Pathology of the Fetus and the Newborn, Chicago, Yr. Bk. Pub., 1952.

Prugh, D. G.: Emotional problems of the premature infant's parents, Nursing Outlook 1:461, 1953.

Shirley, Mary: A behavior syndrome characterizing prematurely-born children, Child Develop. 10:115, 1939.

Vaughn, V. C.: Treatment of erythroblastosis fetalis, Am. J. Nursing 52:320, 1952.

$\mathcal{D}$iseases of the $\mathcal{D}$igestive $\mathcal{S}$ystem

CLEFT LIP AND PALATE

The deformity of cleft lip (harelip) or cleft palate or both combined is a congenital malformation resulting from failure of growth and union of the bony and soft tissues on either or both sides of the mid-line of the palate and the upper jaw. Failure of union on one side results in a single fissure; bilateral failure results in a double fissure. The fissure may extend partly through the lip or the palate or completely through both. A deformity of either the lip or the palate interferes with suckling.

The only treatment is surgical repair (Fig. 19). If suckling is impossible, early operation is desirable in those instances in which it seems probable that the ability to suckle will be restored thereby. Only operations on the lip and the anterior portion of the palate are undertaken at such an early age. If the lip is not repaired within a short time after birth for the purpose of permitting suckling, the repair should be undertaken when the baby is between 1 and 3 months of age. Some surgeons prefer to wait until the third month of life to repair the lip because they believe that the baby is in a better nutritional state for operation. If the palate has a wide anterior cleft, it also is repaired anteriorly at 1 month; otherwise, it is repaired later. Usually, the palate is not repaired until the child is at least 2 years old and preferably at 3 years or later. Such delay in the operation permits better results because the structures have completed a larger fraction of their total growth. The operation usually performed at present is two-stage; it

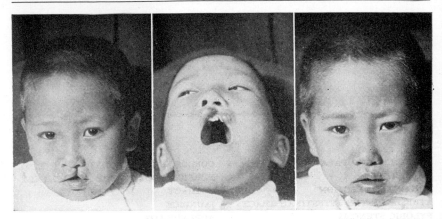

FIG. 19. *(Left)* Incomplete cleft lip. *(Center)* Complete cleft palate. *(Right)* Cleft lip repaired.

lengthens the palate and does not pull the upper teeth closer together. With such an operation the subsequent speech results are better than with former operative procedures.

NURSING CARE OF THE INFANT WITH CLEFT LIP

The artificial feeding of infants who cannot feed at the breast may be successful when carried out in the usual manner, if the hole in the nipple is larger than customary and the nipple is soft. A "lamb's nipple" often serves better than those in common use; they are longer and softer. Otherwise, feeding may be by means of a medicine dropper, a bulb or a spoon. When an infant with a cleft lip sucks, he is likely to swallow excessive amounts of air; more frequent bubbling is necessary to prevent regurgitation.

To accustom the infant to the postoperative method of feeding, he should be fed with a rubber-tipped medicine dropper a day or two before operation. Insertion of the dropper into the corner of his mouth will prevent interference with the suture line and will prevent much suction on the repaired lip. Feedings should be given slowly and at a rate suitable to the capacity of the individual infant, the milk mixture being kept warm continually throughout the procedure.

The nurse should observe the infant for signs of respiratory or gastro-intestinal disease during the preoperative period, for it is imperative that surgery be performed when the infant is in the best possible physical condition. Protective isolation precautions are helpful in preventing cross-infection. Arm restraint immediately after the operation is necessary, and the effect is less distressing to the infant if he has become accustomed to it before. If the infant is old enough to turn himself onto his abdomen and face, a jacket restraint to keep him on his side or back will also be necessary.

After operative repair of the lip, the infant needs observation and meticulous care. Water may be given as soon as he is awake and able to swallow. Milk feedings are resumed within 3 to 4 hours post-operatively. The infant with a cleft lip repair requires slow, careful feeding and adequate bubbling, to prevent regurgitation. After feeding he should be placed on his side to prevent aspiration of any regurgitated milk or mucus that may accumulate. Support with a rolled bed pad will be necessary to keep him in this position. A sterile bulb syringe should be in readiness to aspirate mucus from the mouth. Arm and body restraints should be in readiness for application immediately after his return to the ward. Tongue-depressor arm restraints will prevent the infant from getting his hands to his mouth but will not prevent him from rubbing his face with his upper arms. For this reason, the cuffs should be pinned securely to the shirt. Every 4 hours he should be given relief from his restraint. His arms should be massaged and exercised one at a time. Restraints should not be removed for weighing, nor should both be removed at one time during the morning bath. The infant's position should be changed frequently to prevent both hypostatic pneumonia and discomfort. Crying causes tension on the suture line. His need for emotional satisfactions are no different from the normal infant. The infant who has had a surgical repair of the lip cannot suckle; therefore, he needs extra cuddling to keep him free from anxiety and tension.

A tray containing sterile swabs, hydrogen peroxide or saline, forceps in alcohol, and a paper bag should be in readiness when the infant returns from the operating room. Careful and frequent cleansing of the entire suture line to promote healing is a major responsibility of the nurse. Should there be sloughing of the sutures, the vermillion border of the lip becomes uneven and additional repair makes a good cosmetic effect impossible. Cleansing of the suture line should be done after feeding and as often as serum collects. When a crust forms, scar formation is more prominent. Tightly twisted tooth pick swabs moistened in hydrogen peroxide or saline are used to remove serum and milk. Cleansing should be done gently to avoid injury, and excess solution should be removed with dry swabs. All sutures need care, including those on the inner surface of the lip.

During the first 48 hours after operation, difficulty in breathing may be encountered. When bilateral clefts have been repaired, the infant must become accustomed to nasal breathing, a type not required before. In some instances a sterile airway made of a small piece of ¼-inch rubber tubing is sutured to the corner of the infant's mouth before he leaves the operating room. If no airway has been inserted and difficult breathing is observed, downward pressure on the chin to open the mouth will bring relief. If a Logan bar has been applied to prevent suture tension, care should be taken to keep the adhesive strapping dry and clean. Moisture loosens it, and then its effectiveness is negligible.

After sutures have been removed and the wound is entirely healed (2 to 3 weeks), bottle or breast feedings may be resumed. If the mother still has breast milk, she should be encouraged to maintain her supply during the period in which the infant is having surgical repair. The use of pumped milk during the postoperative period is an added advantage to the infant.

NURSING CARE OF THE CHILD WITH CLEFT PALATE

When a cleft lip has been repaired successfully in a baby who has an associated cleft palate, the improved appearance has a remarkable psychological effect on the parents. It gives them hope and helps the mother to face the future care that the infant with cleft palate requires. Before the infant leaves the hospital, the mother should be assisted in learning how to feed her infant effectively and how to prevent respiratory infection. Many infants with cleft palates can learn to suckle from a bottle if the nipple bulb is soft and long and if the holes are large enough. If the usual method of feeding can be used, the mother is less inclined to feel that her child is abnormal. It may even prevent her from assuming an overprotective role, an attitude that eventually would influence the child's feelings toward himself. Should the cleft be so large that feeding from a bottle is impossible, the use of a special cleft palate nipple with a rubber flange to close off the cleft may be helpful in teaching the baby to swallow more effectively. When these babies are fed too rapidly, air is swallowed, and regurgitation— perhaps even aspiration — results. Holding him in a sitting position helps to prevent the food from going into his nostrils.

Respiratory infections are fre-quent. Milk often flows over the delicate mucous membranes of the upper respiratory tract, making them more susceptible to infection. Ear infections are frequent, and degrees of deafness often complicate the adjustment of the child born with a cleft palate. Some degree of overprotectiveness is essential in preventing infection during the period before an operation can repair the cleft, but instructions can be given to the mother in such a way as to prevent an oversolicitous manner.

Ideally, the child should enter the hospital several days prior to surgical treatment for cleft palate. During the preoperative period he should be helped in his adjustment to the hospital and to the treatment that he will require after repair has been performed. He should have an opportunity to become adjusted to the nurse who will have to anticipate his needs when he is unable to make his wants known. The nurse in that period can prepare him psychologically for the operation by telling him in words he can understand where he is going, who will take him, how the anesthetic will be given, and that she will be there when he returns to his own bed. Arm restraints should be applied at intervals during this period so that he may become accustomed to the feeling of them and get to know the reasons for their use. Mouth irrigations, an important phase in postoperative care, should be introduced and the child's co-operation obtained by making them interesting and fun for him. The first time the equipment is presented, time should be allowed for acceptance of it. He will enjoy filling and emptying the syringe. Little by little he can be taught its use. Thus fear and resistance can be prevented during the postoperative period, and effectiveness of the irrigation will be ensured. The child needs to be in good physical condition at the time operation is performed. During the preoperative period, careful observation to detect signs of infection should be made. The nurse will have to assist the doctor in taking nose and throat cultures. The child's co-operation can be gained through thoughtful explanation and an attitude that anticipates co-operation. Isolation technic, using a mask, is generally recommended to protect the child from respiratory infection. On the day before operation, frequent feedings of sweetened fluids should be encouraged as a shock-preventive measure.

In the immediate postoperative period careful observation is necessary to prevent aspiration of mucus and blood, to detect signs of shock or hemorrhage and to prevent injury to his mouth. When the child returns from the operating room, he should be placed on his abdomen. In this position, the danger of aspiration can be prevented. Vital signs should be taken every ½ hour until the child is fully conscious and his vital signs are within normal limits. Arm restraints should be ready for immediate application. For the child under 2 years of age, tongue depressor arm restraints will prevent him from putting his hands to his mouth, but they will not immobilize the elbows of the older child. Tying his wrists to the crib sides limits position change, antagonizes him and deprives him of all opportunities for independent play.

Basswood splints that have been padded with sheet wadding can be used to immobilize his elbows. They should be long enough to extend from the axilla to the wrist and should be kept in place with an Ace bandage. These splints can be removed easily at bathtime and for periods of play when the nurse is with him to help him to remember to keep his fingers away from his mouth.

A tray containing a bowl of sterile saline solution, a sterile rubber ear bulb and an emesis basin should be at the bedside for postoperative mouth irrigations. The mouth irrigation can be done most effectively with the child in a sitting position with his head tilted downward. Slight pressure on the bulb will produce a gentle stream of solution, which should be directed over the suture line. Teaching the child to allow the solution to run out of his mouth into the emesis basin should be done in the preoperative period when he is having his first experiences with the irrigation equipment. Every hour for the first 6 hours the suture line should be moistened with saline to give the child comfort and promote healing.

When nausea and vomiting have ceased, the child's need for fluid and nourishment must be considered. Fluids are given by cup or from the side of a spoon; they are never given from a straw, a nipple or a syringe. For the first 3 days, clear fluids with additional carbohydrates are given at 2-hour intervals. After this period milk, eggnogs and creamed soups can supplement the diet. Sips of water should be given after the feedings to cleanse the mouth. Most children will accept their food and irrigations more readily if their arms are unrestrained and if they are allowed to hold the glass for drinking and the basin for the irrigation. A fluid diet is continued until all sutures are removed. The child should be weighed periodically to make sure that his nutrition is being maintained.

Children begin early to be aware of their handicap and realize that they have difficulty in making themselves understood. When their speech defect is pronounced, other children laugh at them. Some teachers have difficulty in understanding them and fail to give them opportunity to express themselves because they often appear to be stupid. As a result of these attitudes toward them, these children often withdraw, become shy and retiring as they see that their effort to become understood is futile. They develop a sense of inferiority and often grow overly dependent upon their mothers.

When the above children are admitted to the hospital for operation they will need additional help to feel comfortable in the ward. Opportunities for social relationships should be provided as soon as the child's physical condition permits. These children need opportunities for creative expression from which they can gain recognition and satisfaction. If a psychologist or a social worker is available on the hospital staff, the parents should be referred to him in the hope of helping them to gain increased understanding of their child's psychological needs.

After the initial postoperative period, adjustment to a liquid diet is a difficult task for the child. His appetite increases, and he often begs for the food that he sees being served to other children. Substitute satisfactions are essential to prevent feelings of deprivation. If his mother cannot be with him, play and a satisfying relationship with his nurse is necessary to minimize the discomfort that he experiences from the operative manipulation on his mouth, from restraint and from the limited diet that he is served.

Many times the child who has had his cleft palate repaired is discharged from the hospital before all the sutures are removed. In these instances the mother will require help in learning about his dietary requirements. In the home greater difficulty will be encountered in restricting the child to the prescribed fluid diet, since food will be more accessible and the temptation greater.

When speech clinic facilities are available, arrangements for the child's referral should be made. If the cleft palate was repaired before speech patterns were set, much can be accomplished with skillful guidance and training. Parents may need help in understanding the value of speech therapy for the child's future adjustment.

In the hospital the nurse may see children who have not had cleft palate repairs and speech therapy early enough to prevent them from acquiring speech defects which make them feel different from other children. Often these children's emotional and social growth has become stunted because they have met rejection in their homes and in their social worlds.

STOMATITIS

Inflammation of the mucous membranes of the mouth may result from a variety of causes. It may be a part of a general disease, such as measles or chickenpox; it may be due to trauma from the teeth or too vigorous attempts to cleanse the mouth; it may result from injury by heat or chemicals or the allergic response to drugs such as sulfadiazine or penicillin; or it may be due to infection with bacteria (streptococci), with viruses (herpes), with spirochetes (Vincent's infection) or with a fungus (thrush). Deficiency of vitamins of the B complex such as niacin and riboflavin may also be responsible. A few of the characteristic forms of stomatitis will be described.

Geographic Tongue

This condition is produced by a wandering eruption on the tongue which in appearance gives some suggestion of a map. The condition is symptomless and of no importance other than that its recognition permits reassurance of worried parents. The condition is common, and the cause is unknown. The lesion consists of a broad irregular line which travels slowly across the tongue. As the line progresses, desquamation occurs in the older parts of the lesion, leaving a bright red tongue surface. New areas of epithelial thickening appear in the older parts of the desquamated surface, and these in turn progress across the tongue in the same manner. The configuration of gray and red epithelium changes constantly. No treatment is required.

Catarrhal Stomatitis

This disease is characterized by a general reddening of the mucous membranes with a tendency to easy bleeding. There is pain and an increased flow of saliva. The discomfort may produce restlessness and usually interferes with the taking of food. Slight fever may be observed. Uncomplicated catarrhal stomatitis is of short duration and requires no treatment. Mechanical cleansing of the mouth should be avoided.

Aphthous Stomatitis
(Canker Sores)

In this painful but afebrile disorder of the mouth one or more ulcers appear suddenly. They presumably originate as small blisters of the membranes which break rapidly. Their cause is uncertain. Discomfort usually lasts about a week, after which the lesions heal without a scar. Gentian violet or tincture of benzoin may be applied locally.

Herpetic Stomatitis

This is a common disorder of children of preschool age. It is a specific infection with the virus of herpes simplex, which in the older child or adult produces a few fever blisters on the lips or may be responsible for some canker sores.

The disease is more important in infants and young children who are having their first encounter with the virus. A diffuse reddening and swelling of the gums and the mucous membranes usually is followed by superficial ulcerations. Fever and local soreness may be marked, and the lymph nodes of the jaw may enlarge. The child usually salivates more than he does when well. The discomfort from eating ordinarily limits food intake to milk or a few other bland substances. Temporary underfeeding may result. Fortunately, the disease is self-limited so that healing can be predicted in approximately 10 to 14 days. Local treatment is ineffectual. Chlortetracycline (Aureomycin) or oxytetracycline (Terramycin) sometimes appears to shorten the period of symptoms.

THRUSH

Thrush of the mouth is found almost exclusively in small infants. It is due to the implantation and the growth of a yeast fungus called *Monilia albicans* or *Candida albicans*. The lesions begin as small slightly raised areas which become larger and confluent. The mycelia of the fungus grow down between the epithelial cells, making the plaque difficult to remove. Symptoms are absent except in very extensive infections. Usually the disease is acquired at birth from the mother's vaginal secretions which sometimes are infected with the fungus responsible for thrush. Later contact with the mother or spread from another infected infant through contaminated objects in the nursery or even by the medium of fungus spores floating in the air are additional means by which infection may be acquired.

Treatment is usually effective within a few days. The most common method is application of a 1 per cent aqueous solution of gentian violet to the lesions. Merthiolate in a 1:1,000 dilution or ferric chloride in a 2 per cent solution are also effective.

VINCENT'S INFECTION

When infection with the organisms described by Vincent is present mainly in the mouth, the disease is also called trench mouth or ulcerative stomatitis; when it involves the tonsils or the pharynx extensively it may be called ulceromembranous tonsillitis or Vincent's angina. Two causative agents are found—one a large fusiform bacillus, the other a spirochete. The same organisms may be found in mouths that have no apparent infection, and now it is believed that niacin deficiency or the presence of a debilitating illness is necessary before the organisms can produce their destructive effects upon the membranes.

The early symptoms are offensive breath, increased salivation and local tenderness of the inflamed areas, whether it be gums or pharynx. Later there may be swelling and pain in the lymph nodes of the neck or the jaw. Lesions usually begin about the dental margins or opposite the teeth on the buccal mucous membrane. An ulceration appears which becomes covered with a dirty grayish or yellow membrane which bleeds when it is removed. In severe or neglected cases the teeth may loosen and fall out, or extensive areas of necrosis (noma) may result.

Treatment consists of the administration of niacin in therapeutic doses and the local application of oxidizing agents such as hydrogen peroxide, sodium perborate or potassium chlorate. Penicillin given intramuscularly is regularly effective in producing rapid healing of the lesions.

ATRESIA OF THE INTESTINAL TRACT

ATRESIA OF THE ESOPHAGUS

Failure of the embryonic development of the esophagus to result in a continuous tube connecting the pharynx with the stomach is a serious but rather uncommon congenital malformation. Several variations of this condition are known. The most common one consists of a blindly ending pouch at the upper end of the esophagus and an errant lower segment which runs upward from the stomach and opens through a fistula into the trachea near its bifurcation. At the time of birth, air enters the stomach by way of the trachea, the fistula and the lower segment of the esophagus. Attempts to swallow liquids or even the normal secretions of the mouth result in rapid filling of the blind pouch and overflow of liquid into the larynx and the trachea. The infant chokes, coughs and turns blue whenever attempts are made to feed him. Unless the situation is corrected quickly he will contract bronchitis or pneumonia from the repeated aspiration of food and secretions. Rarely, the esophagus is fully open but communicates with the trachea by an abnormal fistula. The same sort of symptoms result, and the treatment is identical.

Diagnosis of atresia is made by stoppage of a catheter at the site of atresia or by a roentgenogram with iodized oil in the esophagus; barium never should be used for this purpose because of the danger of pneumonia from its aspiration.

Treatment and Nursing Care. Only prompt surgical treatment offers any hope of correcting the defect and saving life. Surgical treatment consists of ligation of the fistula and end-to-end anastamosis of the upper and the lower segments of the esophagus. This pro-

cedure is successful in some instances. Occasionally, a stricture develops subsequently at the site of anastamosis; the stricture usually is overcome satisfactorily by dilatation. In a few instances anastomosis is not possible at the primary operation because of shortness of the lower segment or the wide separation of the two segments. In such cases the fistula is ligated, the upper segment of the esophagus is brought to the surface, and gastrostomy is done. Subsequent feeding is by way of the gastrostomy.

If the esophagus has been brought to the surface, the exposed portion should be protected by a sterilized gauze dressing held securely in place by a knit binder of the type used as an abdominal binder. After the first few months, when salivary glands become more active, frequent change of dressing is necessary. Saline solution should be used to cleanse the area, and the surrounding skin should be kept scrupulously clean. Frequent change of position is desirable to help prevent respiratory infection. Back supports are useful in maintaining the position and in preventing asymmetry of the head and the face that results from the infant's turning his head away from the esophageal opening.

If gastrostomy has been done, feedings are begun several hours postoperatively. A tray is required, containing the warmed formula, a funnel, and an empty feeding bottle and a nipple. Before compression of the gastrostomy tube is released, the funnel should be attached and partially filled with the formula. Further to prevent air from entering the stomach, the funnel always must contain fluid. Elevation of the funnel should be sufficient to allow the food to run in slowly. When the milk is at the level of the end of the funnel, the tube should be folded onto itself and compressed with a rubber band or a clamp. While the milk is running into the stomach, the infant should be given an empty bottle with a nipple to suck. The nipple provides normal sucking activity, exercises the muscles of the jaw and relaxes the musculature. When opportunity for sucking is not provided, the infant will suck his fists to satisfy his needs. It has been observed that unless the infant is comfortable and happy, the formula fails to run into the stomach. When the feeding is completed, the infant should be picked up for a period of attention. Normal babies have pleasure associated with their feedings. Babies with gastrostromy usually require long periods of hospitalization, and unless attention is paid to their psychological needs, they do not thrive.

The skin round the gastrostomy tube should be kept clean and protected with zinc oxide or aluminum paste. The adhesive strips that hold the tube in place should not adhere to the gauze dressings that encircle the tube. Reinforcing the inner side with an additional piece of adhesive makes the necessary dressing change possible without removing the adhesive tape. Such removal frequently displaces the tube.

ATRESIA OF THE DUODENUM

Strictly speaking, this term should be applied to the failure of the duodenum to open into a continuous tube, connecting the stomach with the upper small intestine. Also, it is used to describe obstruction in the duodenum due to valves or diaphragms within the lumen or from bands, kinks and abnormal pressure from without. The symptoms of all these conditions begin immediately after birth and consist of persistent nausea with vomiting of bile-stained fluid. Diagnosis may be confirmed by x-ray examination, which will show that neither air nor barium passes out of the duodenum. Treatment is by surgical relief through release of the obstructing mechanism or by an anastomosis which bypasses the area of atresia.

ATRESIA OF THE SMALL INTESTINE

Single or multiple regions of the small intestine which have failed to canalize properly in their development are not very uncommon. The symptoms and the treatment are like those of duodenal atresia. The lower they are along the course of the intestinal tract, the later the symptoms will occur and the greater the accompanying degree of abdominal distention.

ATRESIA OF THE RECTUM AND THE ANUS

Abnormal development of the lower intestinal tract may be apparent on inspection of the infant if no anal opening is found or if the initial attempt to take the baby's temperature reveals a shallow blind pouch instead of a normal anus (Fig. 20). At other times the failure of the infant to produce meconium and the progressive distention of his abdomen lead to the discovery of an incomplete canalization of the rectum in spite of an externally normal anus.

In the normal embryologic development of the lower bowel, a blind

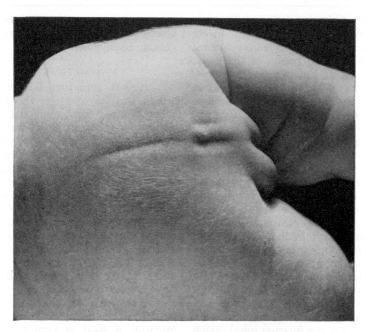

FIG. 20. Imperforate anus. (Potter, E. L.: Pathology of the Fetus and the Newborn, Chicago, Yr. Bk. Pub.)

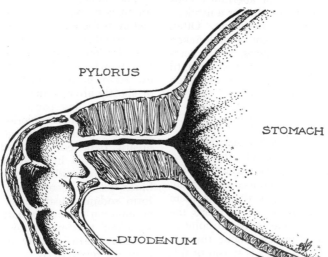

PYLORUS

STOMACH

--DUODENUM

FIG. 21. Showing hypertrophied circular muscle of the pylorus in pyloric stenosis.

pouch within the abdomen descends toward the perineum and meets another pouch which is invaginating the skin in the region of the anus. The ends of the two pouches fuse, and the septum between them breaks through to form a continuous passageway. The mildest form of atresia is that in which the development is complete, except for the disappearance of the membrane between the two pouches. This situation is relieved easily by splitting the membrane with a small knife introduced into the anus. Even if the two pouches have not quite met, the surgeon may be able to join them from below and make a proper anastamosis at once. The opening must be dilated periodically for several months afterward to prevent its constriction during scar-tissue formation. More serious abnormalities result when the internal blind pouch lies at some distance from the skin of the perineum or aberrantly joins the vagina, the urethra or a fistulous opening into the perineum. Often primary union cannot be undertaken in these circumstances, and a temporary colostomy is necessary until a later, more extensive operation can be performed.

PYLORIC STENOSIS

Pyloric stenosis is a narrowing or tight constriction of the lumen through the pyloric orifice of the stomach which produces obstruction, more often partial than complete (Fig. 21). Two factors cause the constriction. One is hypertrophy of the circular muscle about the pylorus; and the other is spasm of this muscle. Although both factors are presumably present in all cases, the symptoms in one case may be due chiefly to spasm and in another chiefly to hypertrophy.

SYMPTOMS

The first symptom is vomiting, which has its onset in the first 2 months after birth, but not commonly in the first 2 weeks. The vomiting increases in severity. It becomes forceful, and the vomitus may be projected several feet. Often the vomitus is expelled also through the nose. It may contain mucus but never bile. Emesis occurs during or soon after feeding and is not associated with nausea. Because of food loss the babies are always hungry. They lose weight and usually are constipated and have scanty urine. The color of the stools depends on the amount of food passing the pylorus; when the amount of food is very small the stools become dark.

The general appearance of the infant is normal at first. Later emaciation is the chief feature. No fever is present except sometimes from dehydration, and no pain except that which may be associated with excessive gastric peristalsis during or shortly after feedings.

The vomiting causes loss of hydrochloric acid and chloride. In time, the body stores of chloride become greatly depleted. The sodium that remains when hydrochloric acid is formed from sodium chloride combines with plasma carbonic acid to form sodium bicarbonate. The accumulation of bicarbonate may be sufficient to cause serious or fatal alkalosis. This variety of alkalosis may be relieved by parenteral administration of chloride (Ringer's or salt solution).

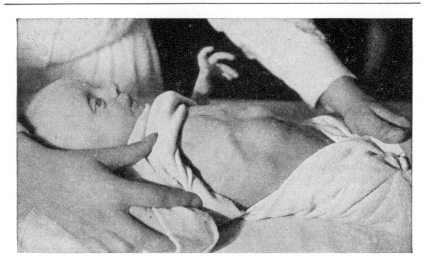

Fig. 22. Showing peristaltic waves in a case of pyloric stenosis.

Diagnosis

The vomiting and the age at which it begins are important. Vomiting may occur with each feeding, or several feedings may be retained for a time and all be vomited together. Observation of the peristaltic activity of the stomach after feeding is an important point in diagnosis. When the waves are visible, a rounded tumor appears from under the ribs on the left and slowly passes to the right (Fig. 22). Usually it is followed by other similar tumors with a depression traveling along between them. Palpation of the hypertrophied muscle at the pylorus is also an aid. It is about the size and the shape of an olive and is not always found easily. It should be sought half-way between the ensiform process and the umbilicus and about 1 inch to the right of the mid-line. Roentgenographic study is usually unnecessary, but, if made, it shows partial or complete failure of material to pass the pylorus.

Prognosis

In the case of infants under observation from the beginning of symptoms, there should be no mortality. Unfortunately, many infants come under care only after they have been weaned and fed a variety of formulas with indifferent success. Such infants, after a few weeks of inadequate treatment, are sometimes in poor condition, and operative and other risks are increased. Once recovery has occurred, by any method of treatment, it is complete and permanent.

Treatment

The treatment is either medical or surgical. Approximately half of the infants with pyloric obstruction can be treated successfully by medical means. For the remainder operation is indicated. The chief considerations that determine the treatment to be adopted are as follows:

In the case of a breast-fed infant with stenosis of such a degree that he is not gaining weight, or is actually losing it, usually an operation is performed without delay if atropine used as described subsequently, does not give prompt relief. Thus, the mother's milk supply can be maintained, and the infant can be returned to the breast within a short time after operation.

In the case of an artificially fed infant, usually a fair trial of medical treatment is made, but unless such treatment is successful within a short time, the infant is operated on. The symptoms of pyloric stenosis tend to decrease after the age of 3 or 4 months. If an infant has been treated with more or less success up to this age, usually medical treatment is continued. As time passes, little diminution of hypertrophy occurs, but the lumen enlarges with growth.

Medical Treatment. This includes several or all of the following procedures: gastric lavage, refeeding after vomiting, thickening the formula with cereal, administration of atropine derivatives or sedatives or both.

Atropine is given to abolish the spasm of the pyloric sphincter. A 1:1,000 solution of atropine sulfate (½ gr. to the ounce) is used. The solution should not be kept longer than 2 weeks. The dose is given in a small amount of water 20 minutes before each feeding. The dose at the start is one drop of the solution. The amount is increased rapidly until flushing of the skin occurs, and then this amount, or an amount slightly smaller, is given before each feeding. Doses above 3 or 4 drops usually are to be avoided. Eumydrine, an atropine derivative with less marked side effects, is used in an initial dose of 0.05 mgm. once a day, increasing to a maximum of 0.5 mgm. per day. Phenobarbital may be used in individual doses of 15 mgm. 2 or 3 times daily.

If thickened feedings are to be used, the formula should be one suitable for the age of the infant, but thickened with cereal. The method of preparation is discussed elsewhere. Food thus thickened is not vomited as easily as customary formulas. In those instances in which it may seem desirable not to use a thickened feeding, the formula should be one that produces very fine curds in the stomach.

Refeeding is often of value. If a portion of the food is vomited within an hour after feeding, approximately this same amount of additional food may be given. The entire feeding may be retained under these conditions.

Surgical Treatment. The surgical treatment of choice for pyloric stenosis is known as the Rammstedt or Fredet-Rammstedt operation. It consists of an incision through the hypertrophied circular muscle down to, but not through, the mucosa and parallel with the pyloric lumen. This procedure allows the pylorus to expand so that food will pass. The operation is over quickly, and the baby is little disturbed by it.

If the baby is emaciated or dehydrated when he comes under care, the treatment described under "Malnutrition" is indicated both before and after operation. Such treatment includes transfusions and parenteral administration of fluids, especially saline solution.

PREOPERATIVE NURSING CARE

To prevent vomiting, sometimes gastric lavage is ordered preceding the feeding. Gastric lavage in a baby is carried out in the same manner as in an adult, with a few minor differences. The infant may be recumbent or held in the lap of an assistant. In either case, restraint by means of wrapping in a sheet usually is necessary. A catheter (size 10 or 12 French) connected to a funnel by about 2 feet of rubber tubing is moistened in sterile water and passed rapidly into the stomach. Passage into the larynx is practically impossible. If by chance the catheter should go into the larynx or the trachea, breathing would stop, and cyanosis from suspended respiration would develop rapidly. As evidence that the tube is in the stomach, the infant is able to breathe (not through the tube), and usually gastric contents will appear in the funnel. In infants, when the tube has been inserted 9 inches from the gums or the teeth it reaches well into the stomach. Coughing, gagging and redness of the face caused by passage of the tube cease quickly if the tube is held without motion. After syphoning off the stomach contents, an amount of fluid somewhat less than the gastric capacity is allowed to run in. An initial failure to flow, due to a column of air in the tube, can be corrected by "milking" the tube gently.

The stomach is emptied by lowering the funnel and the tube below the level of the child. The process is repeated until the water returns clear. Usually from 1 pint to 1 quart of fluid is required. Suitable amounts for each washing are: 1 week, 1 ounce; 1 month, 2 ounces; 6 months or more, 4 to 6 ounces. For removal, the tube is pinched tightly in order that fluid may not leak into the pharynx and cause choking. Gastric lavage is seldom required more than twice daily. The fluid commonly used for lavage is either sterile water or normal saline.

Atropine is a toxic drug when given in overdosage. It should be diluted with water and given with a medicine dropper. When the dosage has been increased cautiously until flushing occurs, the flushing appears soon after the drug has been given and disappears after a short time. The effect is transitory and harmless. The flushing is the most obvious sign that the tolerance without harmful effect has been reached. In some instances, atropine in a flushing dose causes moderate fever. High fever should be reported.

A thickened feeding should be so thick that it will not drop from an inverted spoon. A baby may be fed with a spoon, or the food may be placed in a large "Hygeia" nipple, the tip of which has been cut off so as to leave a large hole. The nipple is placed in the infant's mouth, and the food is pressed into the end of the nipple by a spoon or a spatula.

When unthickened feedings are ordered, the formula should be given with such care that the likelihood of vomiting is decreased. Infants with pyloric stenosis tend to suck their hands and get a great deal of air into the stomach. Bubbling before the infant begins to eat is often necessary. Because he is hungry he tends to eat his food rapidly, and the food must be given slowly if vomiting is to be prevented.

When vomiting occurs, the infant's face, head and folds of the neck will require bathing. Charting accurately the approximate amount vomited, the type and the color, and its relation to feeding aids in diagnosis. Refeeding the infant an equivalent of the amount vomited should be done when it is directed.

Impairment of nutrition causes lowered resistance to infection, and every means possible should be used to prevent the infant from developing intercurrent infection. Technic to protect the baby from infections in the wards should be carried out. Position should be changed frequently. If the infant has a lowered body temperature, extra warmth should be added to keep his temperature stable and in a normal range. Lamps attached to a bed cradle can be placed over the infant to give this additional warmth. Supportive treatment, such as blood transfusions and fluids parenterally, is given the infant to supplement his food and fluid intake. Urine output should be noted, and accurate charting of the stools is important.

POSTOPERATIVE NURSING CARE

When the infant returns from the operating room, he should be placed on his side to prevent aspiration of vomitus. Additional warmth will be needed to prevent shock. The quality of the pulse, the type of respiration, and the color of the infant's skin should be noted frequently. If shock does occur, the foot of the bed should be elevated, and addi-

tional warmth should be supplied. Position must be changed, but it should be done gently to prevent vomiting.

Customs differ as to when the first feedings are given after operation. If the pyloric mucosa has not been punctured at operation, no strong contraindication exists to feeding small amounts soon after operation when a local anesthetic has been used or as soon as recovery occurs from general anesthesia. However, peristalsis is impaired by the operation, and some vomiting is usual when food is given early. Because of impaired peristalsis and resultant vomiting, it is customary in some hospitals to leave a nasal tube in the stomach for about 24 hours and to defer feeding for the same length of time, maintaining body fluids by parenteral administration. While the nasal tube is in place, the infant's arms should be restrained to prevent removal of the tube. When feedings are resumed, they are ordered in small amounts. Hunger is observed soon after operation, and to prevent vomiting from hurried feedings, the food should be given by medicine dropper. During the early period when vomiting is so frequent, it is best to feed the baby in bed with his head slighty elevated. When the feedings are increased and tolerance is noted, they may be given by nipple and bottle, with the infant in the nurse's lap where he can be cuddled and bubbled more effectively. The amount of food is increased as the infant shows greater tolerance for it. His behavior before and after feeding is a guide to his tolerance and food needs.

If the infant received breast feedings prior to operation, the feeding of human milk should be resumed subsequent to operation. At first, he can be fed expressed milk in order to regulate the quantity, but within 2 or 3 days he can be placed directly at the breast and allowed to suckle for the usual length of time. During the period when the milk is being expressed, the breasts should be emptied completely in order to maintain the supply.

Until the stitches have been removed, protection of the dressing will help prevent wound infection. Applying the diaper low, below the dressing, prevents wound contamination.

VOLVULUS

Early in fetal life a large portion of the intestinal tract lies in the umbilical sac outside the abdomen and in a position reversed from that which is normal later; that is, the ascending colon is on the left. With continued fetal development the intestine gradually is withdrawn into the abdomen with concurrent rotation to the newly and permanently normal position. After withdrawal and rotation, the mesentery attaches to the posterior wall of the abdomen, and the transverse colon becomes attached to the stomach by the gastrocolic ligament.

In a few instances, rotation of the bowel is faulty, in that it is incomplete or absent. In such circumstances, the mesentery cannot attach in the normal places or in the normal manner. The abnormal attachment may give rise to peritoneal bands which may cause obstruction subsequently by pressure on the bowel at some point or by entangling a loop of bowel. A bowel with incomplete mesenteric attachment is not well anchored and at any time may become twisted in such a manner as to cause obstruction and to cut off the blood supply of a portion of itself. Volvulus is the term applied when obstruction occurs from twisting of the intestine. Volvulus from abnormal rotation may occur at any time in the first few years but is much more common in early infancy. The only treatment is prompt surgical attention, with cutting of constricting bands or with the untwisting of a twisted intestinal loop. Often some anchoring of unattached bowel is indicated.

MECKEL'S DIVERTICULUM

Approximately 2 to 3 per cent of all children have a vestigial remnant of the omphalomesenteric duct remaining as a small pouch off the ileum about 18 inches from its junction with the colon. Usually this structure, called a Meckel's diverticulum, gives no symptoms. In some children there is aberrantly placed gastric mucous membrane within the pouch which secretes acid gastric juice. This juice is irritating to the wall of the ileum and may produce ulceration and bleeding. The usual symptoms are painless passage of tarry or grossly bloody stools. Diagnosis is made from suspicion when no other explanation of the bleeding can be found. It cannot be confirmed without an exploratory abdominal operation. Surgical removal of the diverticulum is simple and curative. The postoperative care is the same as that for any abdominal operation.

MEGACOLON

Megacolon is most commonly a primary congenital abnormality

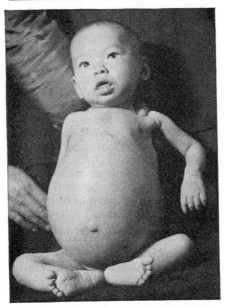

Fig. 23. A baby with Hirsch-sprung's disease.

(Hirschsprung's disease). The essential lesion is partial obstruction in the distal portion of the colon, which causes obstinate constipation, enlargement of the abdomen and dilatation and hypertrophy of the colon. When the bowel is examined at operation or at autopsy no gross explanation for the obstruction can be found. The fault appears to lie in an abnormality of the innervation of the intrinsic musculature of the bowel wall, which under normal circumstances produces the co-ordinated peristaltic movements that propel feces and gas downward toward the anus. In Hirschsprung's disease one or more segments of the colon do not participate properly in co-ordinated peristaltic activity, either because the essential ganglion cells are absent from the muscles or because

there is a disturbance of the balance between the activities of the sympathetic and the parasympathetic nerve fibers. Stool reaching such an area is not passed along normally, and the bowel proximal to it eventually hypertrophies in its attempt to force the accumulating mass through the malfunctioning segment of bowel. Often such an area can be identified by a small barium enema and careful study of the activity of the area between the rectum and the sigmoid colon.

Megacolon may also occur as a disorder secondary to anatomic (rectal stricture or rectovaginal fistula with a small opening) and psychogenic obstruction. Of course, in these instances successful treatment will depend upon the ability to provide an adequate channel by surgical measures or to correct the emotional disturbance that leads to spastic withholding of stool.

SYMPTOMS

The symptoms of megacolon are manifest early in infancy. Constipation that persists in spite of treatment, and progressive enlargement of the abdomen are the first symptoms (Fig. 23). Periodically, the distention may be so great as to cause discomfort, vomiting and interference with respirations. The absorption of toxic materials retained in the bowel may produce nausea, lethargy or even collapse when the obstipation has been prolonged. Unless close attention is given to bowel evacuation, the accumulation of dry fecal masses may lead to inflammation or even ulceration of the bowel so that once the obstruction is relieved, diarrhea ensues. The effort of the colon to pass the fecal mass along is often apparent by peristaltic activity which is visible through the abdominal wall. Malnutrition may be present as a consequence of vomiting or food refusal. In some of the milder cases spontaneous recovery may take place. Children who continue with the disorder unrelieved may have a serious social problem because of inability to control the escape of gas under pressure. An occasional child who reaches adolescence will learn how to evacuate his bowel successfully by the use of his abdominal muscles.

Diagnosis

Diagnosis is seldom difficult. The combination of gross enlargement of the abdomen, visible peristalsis and obstinate constipation with passage of stools of excessive size is regularly present in all cases. A roentgen study of the colon is indicated in order to confirm the diagnosis and to identify, if possible, the main area of disturbed peristalsis. This procedure should be undertaken cautiously in instances where the obstruction can be identified as anatomic or functional in the lower rectum, for the addition of barium to the retained fecal mass above such an obstruction may turn a partial intestinal obstruction into a complete one.

Treatment and Nursing Care

These may be considered under three general headings—emergency relief of fecal impaction, long-term medical management and surgical treatment.

Intestinal obstruction from fecal impaction requires prompt relief. Various types of enemas are used to soften the impacted mass and increase the effectiveness of bowel contractions. Because of the large size of the colon, the enemas are only partially returned. It is possible to produce water intoxication in these patients if excessive amounts are run in without being recovered. Normal saline solution is probably safer to use than plain water. In neglected cases the danger of perforating a colonic ulcer must be considered. Digital removal of stool from the rectum is often the safest and most effective method of relieving fecal impactions.

Long-term medical management may be successful in keeping the child in good health and maintaining an adequate rate of colonic evacuation. An attempt is made to keep the stools soft by offering a low-residue diet or by the continuous administration of mineral oil. Mild laxatives may be given periodically. Many children will require regular cleansing of the colon with enemas or colonic irrigations administered through a large tube passed well up into the descending colon. Drugs that alter the activity of the sympathetic and the parasympathetic nervous systems are sometimes useful in effecting more or less regular bowel evacuations. These include Prostigmin, Urecholine, atropine, Syntropan, Mecholyl Chloride and others. Dosage must be initiated cautiously, for all of these drugs have toxic effects that must be recognized promptly. Children who can be managed successfully by medical treatment require careful attention to general hygiene and diet.

A number of surgical approaches may be considered when medical management is deemed unsatisfactory. The practice of sectioning the sympathetic nerve connections to the colon has not given very satisfactory results, since constipation usually is ameliorated but not cured. In cases where an area of constriction can be demonstrated by barium enema, sometimes a complete cure may be effected by removal of the constricted area and anastamosis of the bowel. This procedure offers the best chance of a completely satisfactory cure. It is not usually undertaken in children under the age of two. When medical management is failing and the preferred surgical approach cannot be done, colostomy or even complete resection of the colon may be performed. The postoperative care will depend upon the variety of procedure that is done.

Procedure for Cleansing Enema for an Infant. The equipment consists of an irrigating can and pole, rubber tubing, glass connector, stopcock, catheter No. 10 to 12 French, lubricant, treatment rubber and towel, rubber-covered pillow, bedpan and cover, kidney basin, enema solution (105° F.) and oiled cotton for cleansing after the enema has been expelled. For a soapsuds enema, 2 drams of soap jelly to 1 pint of water is used; for a saline enema, 1 dram of salt to a pint. When giving a cleansing enema to an infant, not more than 300 ml. of solution should be used unless specific instructions have been given. After protecting the bed with the treatment rubber and towel and removing the diaper, the pillow is placed under the infant's back. Since retention of fluid is impossible for the infant, the bedpan padded with a diaper is placed under the buttocks. After the catheter is lubricated and the air is expelled, it is inserted from 2 to 4 inches into the rectum. Hanging the can not higher than 18 inches above the infant's hips allows the fluid to run in slowly. When the tube has been removed, the abdomen may be massaged gently until the solution has been expelled, if there are no contraindications. After expulsion, the buttocks should be cleansed and the diaper reapplied. In charting the procedure, the results should be noted.

Procedure for an Enema for a Child. A rectal tube No. 14 to 16 French is used. Securing the child's co-operation is essential. To minimize untoward psychological effects of an enema, the child needs to feel that it is given to help him. He needs to know why the enema is given and that it will be given slowly, carefully and in accordance with his directions. Co-operation usually is acquired when the nurse allows the child to help him in controlling the speed of flow and the time the tube shall be withdrawn. When the child complains of pain or pressure, the tubing should be clamped off until the distress has subsided. A child will retain the solution if he understands why it is necessary to do so and if he is supported during the period he must tolerate some degree of discomfort. Pressure over the anus after the tube has been removed may facilitate retention until the feces have been softened sufficiently to make passage possible.

Procedure for an Oil-Retention Enema. The equipment consists of a funnel, rubber tubing, glass connector, catheter No. 12 to 14

French, lubricant, bedpan and vegetable oil, from 60 to 150 ml., at 100° F. In some instances it may be necessary to inject the oil slowly into the rectum with a syringe. Pressure over the anus or adhesive strapping will prevent the oil from being expelled. After the oil has been retained for 30 minutes, a cleansing enema should be given.

INTESTINAL HERNIA

A hernia of the intestine is the protrusion of a part of the bowel through an abnormal opening in the containing walls of the abdomen. Hernia may be either congenital or acquired. The majority of acquired hernias in childhood depend on congenital abnormalities. The management of a hernia in a young child is the same, whether congenital or acquired, and no further distinction between these two types need be made. The most frequent locations for hernia are at the umbilicus and through the inguinal canals. Hernias through the diaphragm are uncommon, and those at other sites are rare.

INGUINAL HERNIA

In the male the testis descends from the abdominal cavity into the scrotum, carrying with it the parietal peritoneum, thus forming a tube from the abdomen to the scrotum. Normally, this tube closes completely. When it has partially or completely failed to close, descent of the intestine into it is possible, thus producing hernia. In girls, the round ligament extends from the uterus through the inguinal canal to its attachment in the abdominal wall. In fetal life, the ligaments are surrounded by a peritoneal process which later obliterates. Weakness of the tissues about the round ligament, together with increased abdominal pressure, sometimes permits inguinal hernias in girls. However, about 90 per cent of the inguinal hernias of children occur in the male. An inguinal hernia in an infant causes no symptoms unless it becomes strangulated, and this event is uncommon. Strangulation results when a portion of bowel becomes so tightly caught in the hernial sac that its blood supply is cut off. Severe symptoms of pain, intestinal obstruction and inability to reduce the mass occur. If unrelieved, gangrene of the bowel will result. Immediate operation is demanded.

Usually, an inguinal hernia is reduced easily. When the inguinal rings are small, reduction cannot be accomplished by pressure alone upon the herniated bowel, because the hernia then mushrooms against the external inguinal ring. In addition to moderate pressure, it is necessary to make lateral pressure on the bowel with the fingers at the base of the mass in order to elongate the bowel at this point. Sometimes reduction is made easier by having the child lie with the buttocks elevated.

If the hernia can be kept constantly reduced by means of a truss, the defect in the abdominal wall will close in many instances. Use of a truss for a year or more may be necessary. If the truss fails to hold the hernia or to permit ultimate cure, surgical repair is indicated. Even the youngest of infants stands a hernia operation well if he is in good condition.

Nursing Care. A type of truss commonly used for infants is made

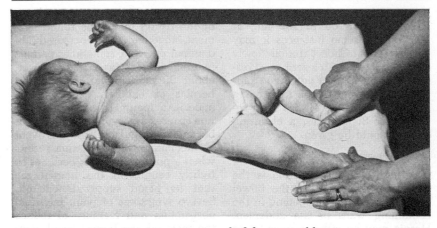

FIG. 24. A yarn truss applied for inguinal hernia.

from a skein of yarn. Such a truss is illustrated in Figure 24. One fourth or less of a skein is rewound into a smaller skein. The size should be such that when the two sides are brought together into a single unit, it will be long enough to pass entirely around the infant's waist with an additional loop passing from the waistline in front down under the crotch and up to the waistline in back. To apply it, first the yarn is passed around the waist snugly. Then one end is passed through the loop of the other end to make a slip knot, which is adjusted to lie directly over the site of the hernia and press against it. Then the free end is carried down through the crotch and attached to the segment that passes across the back.

The advantage of the yarn truss is that in addition to being effective, it is soft, washable and easily adjusted to any size of infant. Satisfactory pneumatic trusses may be purchased. The truss treatment of hernia in an infant should begin as

soon as the hernia is discovered and continue until no evidence of the hernia can be found.

When a hernia is corrected surgically the postoperative care is directed at keeping the wound clean until healing has taken place. Diapers are left open to prevent wound contamination. Infants may be picked up for feedings and to relieve distress. Older children may be permitted activity as soon as they feel able to play. Unless bowel resection is required, feedings can be resumed a few hours after operation.

UMBILICAL HERNIA

Umbilical hernia consists of a protrusion of a portion of the intestine or omentum through the umbilical ring, producing a bulge under the skin at the navel (Fig. 25). The size of the tumor varies but seldom exceeds that of a golf ball. Umbilical hernias are usually not apparent at birth but appear within the early months of life and enlarge during the acts of crying or strain-

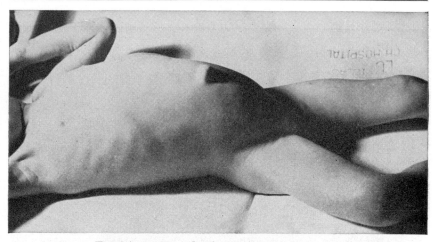

Fig. 25. An example of a small umbilical hernia.

ing. They are reduced easily, and strangulation is practically unknown. All but the largest hernias will heal spontaneously at least by the time the child begins to develop strong abdominal muscles—between 3 and 4 years of age. The traditional treatment of strapping or binding the abdomen of such an infant is generally unnecessary, although it improves the cosmetic appearance. Hernias that are large and fail to close spontaneously may be repaired surgically in later childhood.

INTUSSUSCEPTION

Intussusception is the invagination of a portion of the bowel into the portion immediately distal to it. This telescoping effect is illustrated in Figure 26. It probably is caused by hyperactive peristalsis in the proximal portion of the bowel with relative inactivity of the distal segment. Although it may occur at any level of the small or the large intestine, nearly always it is dis-

covered at the junction of the ileum and the colon. As the bowel invaginates it carries along its mesentery. Thus the blood supply is cut off, and if the condition continues, the bowel will become gangrenous. Death may result if the condition is not recognized and corrected. Most of those who develop intussusception are infants and usually they are robust boys who have been thriving.

Symptoms

The disease may begin suddenly with a shriek of pain and rapidly appearing symptoms of intestinal obstruction—vomiting, constipation, abdominal pain and eventually prostration and shock. At times the origin of symptoms is more insidious, with indefinite discomfort, poor appetite and unexplained vomiting. Despite the constipation characteristic of obstruction, small bloody stools containing mucus and little or no fecal matter may be passed. The tumor mass that results from intus-

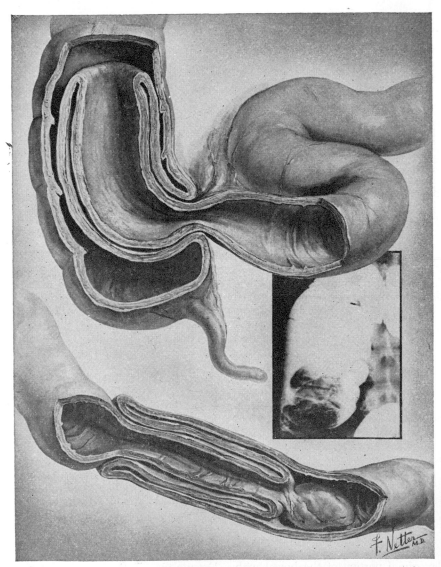

Fig. 26. Intussusception. *(Top)* Ileocolic variety. *(Insert)* Roentgen appearance. *(Bottom)* Ileoileal variety. (Ciba Collection of Medical Illustrations)

susception may be palpated through the abdominal wall or may be detected with the finger on rectal examination if it has progressed far enough down the colon.

TREATMENT

Intussusception requires immediate relief, for the mortality rises sharply with increasing duration of symptoms. In rare instances the intussusception will reduce spontaneously, but this is not an outcome that can be awaited with safety. In some instances the barium enema given to confirm the diagnosis will exert enough retrograde pressure to reduce the telescoped bowel, and the fluoroscopic examination or films will demonstrate that complete relief has been achieved. Usually, however, prompt surgical exploration is indicated in order to reduce the intussusception before irreversible gangrene of the bowel has occurred. In the latter instance, resection of bowel is necessary—a procedure which is poorly tolerated by a seriously ill infant.

NURSING CARE

The postoperative symptomatic care of the infant is not unlike that given after other types of abdominal operation. If simple reduction of the bowel is accomplished, feedings may be started shortly after peristaltic activity is audible in the abdomen. If resection of gangrenous bowel is necessary, constant gastric suction and parenteral administration of fluids are required for several days. During this period an infant may find some measure of solace in being permitted to suck on a pacifier or a nipple stuffed with cotton.

CORROSIVE ESOPHAGITIS

Sometimes corrosive chemicals, particularly lye, are swallowed by young children. Such chemicals destroy tissues with which they come in contact. Usually the alimentary tissues from the lips all the way to the stomach are affected, even though only one swallow is taken. The primary symptoms of such a burn include pain, prostration and inability to swallow. The inflammation may cause sufficient edema to obstruct respiration, a condition requiring tracheotomy. If the child survives, the acute symptoms subside, and progress seems to be satisfactory until evidences of esophageal obstruction appear within a month or two. The obstruction is due to contracture of scar tissue and may become so severe that no food or liquid can pass into the stomach.

Emergency treatment in the beginning includes neutralization of the swallowed chemical and relief of pain with sedatives. The antidote should be given much diluted, for neutralization generates considerable heat; thus an antidote given in a concentrated state may do as much harm as the original corrosive. The extra fluid used in dilution absorbs the heat of neutralization so that the tissue will not be damaged further. Gastric lavage is contraindicated. Olive or other food oil may be useful in helping alleviate pain. Until ability to swallow returns, food and fluid must be given parenterally.

Stricture may be prevented by passage of appropriate-sized catheters at intervals beginning within 48 hours of the accident. After stricture has occurred, usually it is possible to dilate it, but the process is slow. If the opening is insufficient to permit the passage of food, the child must be fed through a gastrostomy until dilatation is accomplished. Often retrograde dilatation is advantageous; it may be accomplished through the gastrostomy opening.

FOREIGN BODY IN THE ALIMENTARY TRACT

It is common for young children to place foreign bodies in the mouth. Small foreign bodies may be swallowed and cause no difficulty. Foreign bodies that reach the stomach usually are passed through the remainder of the tract without symptoms. If they are opaque, their progression should be observed with roentgenograms. Long bodies may be expected to cause some trouble in the sharp curves of the duodenum, and therefore should be removed through the esophagus with the help of an esophagoscope, or surgically through the abdominal wall. Large foreign bodies may become lodged in the pharynx or the esophagus.

A foreign body in the pharynx may cause gagging, choking and perhaps obstruction to respiration to an alarming degree. Except in definite emergency, attempts at removal with the fingers should not be made.

A foreign body in the esophagus may cause only moderate discomfort and difficulty in swallowing. Liquid foods may pass easily. Prompt removal is important, particularly in the case of sharp-edged objects, because of the probability of perforation and ulceration and extension of the inflammation to the mediastinum or the respiratory tract.

BEZOAR

Most foreign bodies that reach the stomach pass on without trouble. Certain types of indigestible material, when swallowed in large amounts, tend to accumulate in masses so large that passage beyond the stomach becomes impossible. Any such mass is known as a bezoar. The most commonly encountered bezoar is composed of hair, which usually has been pulled from the head and swallowed over a long period. The hair becomes matted in a large ball or mass. The symptoms are vague, and health and nutrition suffer little. A tumor is felt, and a filling defect is shown by x-ray studies with barium. The only treatment is surgical removal, a relatively simple procedure.

JAUNDICE

Jaundice is a symptom of various conditions. However, in all circumstances it results from one or more of 3 fundamental causes: excessive destruction of blood, impaired function of the liver and obstruction to excretion of bile. The pigment is bilirubin, a product of hemoglobin breakdown. Some hemoglobin destruction occurs normally and constantly; this function is carried on by the reticuloendothelial system. The bilirubin so formed is in combination with an albumin fraction of blood protein. On passage through the liver, bilirubin is freed from the protein combination and is excreted by way of the bile ducts along with bile salts and cholesterol. Bilirubin and cholesterol are waste products, whereas the bile salts, produced in the liver, aid in absorption of fat and the fat-soluble vitamins. Bilirubin is converted in the intestine to urobilinogen, some of which is excreted as such, some oxidized to urobilin, the coloring matter of the stool, and some is reabsorbed into the portal circulation, returned to the liver, converted to bilirubin and excreted.

When the destruction of blood within the body is excessive, combined bilirubin is formed at such a rate that the liver is unable to deal with the excess. Even though a larger quantity of bilirubin than normal is converted and excreted, the circulating level may increase and produce jaundice. The stools are not acholic, and urobilinogen is increased in the urine. Such a condition exists in icterus neonatorum, transfusion with incompatible blood and hemolytic anemias of various sorts.

When jaundice is related to impaired liver function, in the early stages of disease the liver is still able to free bilirubin from its combined form but is unable to excrete it in normal amounts. Thus retention of bilirubin occurs, producing jaundice. If liver damage progresses, the liver loses some of its ability to free bilirubin from its combined form, and both types of bilirubin accumulate in the blood. This situation occurs in hepatitis, in certain infections outside the liver and when the liver has been poisoned by phosphorus or chloroform.

When obstruction to the excretion of bile occurs, bilirubin is freed from its combined form, accumulates in the liver and overflows into the blood. The stools are acholic. Bilirubin appears in the urine, and urobilinogen disappears. If the obstruction is unrelieved, enough damage eventually occurs to impair the liver's ability to free bilirubin from the combined form, and both types of bilirubin accumulate in the plasma. Gallstones in the larger ducts, strictures of the ducts and tumors compressing the ducts are causes of obstruction which are seldom seen in childhood. Congenital atresia of the bile ducts belongs in this category.

The degree of jaundice may be stated in arbitrary units called the icterus index, which is the amount of yellow color in blood serum as determined by comparison with a dichromate standard solution. The Van den Bergh reaction offers a more precise aid to diagnosis, since it indicates both the total amount of bilirubin circulating in the plasma and the relative amounts of the free and combined forms. In the chemical determination the protein-bilirubin combination is dissolved by treatment with alcohol. Before this is done the amount of free bilirubin is first determined (direct reaction). This indicates the amount that is circulating because of obstruction. Then the serum is treated with alcohol, and the additional amount of bilirubin released from combination with protein is measured (indirect reaction). As stated above, this represents the amount produced by hemolysis under uncomplicated circumstances.

Jaundice is only a symptom. The treatment required depends upon a knowledge of the underlying causative mechanism.

OBSTRUCTION OF THE BILE DUCTS

Obstruction of the bile ducts of the newborn may be caused by congenital stenosis or atresia, or absence of any part of the duct system; it may be caused also by a plug in the larger ducts of thick viscous biliary secretion somewhat similar to the material that obstructs the pancreatic duct in cystic fibrosis of the pancreas.

When the bile ducts are obstructed, bile does not enter the intestinal tract; it accumulates in the liver. Bile pigments enter the blood and are carried to all parts of the body with resulting jaundice, which increases in intensity. Usually, obvious jaundice from obstruction does not appear until the age of 2 weeks, often after icterus neonatorum has disappeared.

Continued unrelieved obstructive jaundice ultimately leads to death. A baby so affected may live for as long as several years. During the early weeks or months, nutrition and general health seem to be little affected, but soon evidences of illness appear. Because of absence of bile from the intestinal tract, absorption of fat and the fat-soluble vitamins is poor. Deficiencies of vitamins A, D and K result unless special precautions are taken. Absorption of calcium is impaired. Eventually, cirrhotic changes occur in the liver, and liver function becomes impaired.

When a baby with obstructive jaundice comes under care, a dietary regimen adapted to his condition and physiologic capacity is established. The diet is low in fat and generous in protein; the remaining energy needed is supplied by carbohydrate. The fat-soluble vitamins are supplied in water-miscible form.

Obstruction from congenital malformation cannot be distinguished clinically from obstruction by a mucus plug unless some intermittency can be observed. Jaundice from atresia progresses steadily; that from a mucus plug may do likewise. If the degree of jaundice varies or if bile pigments appear in the stool from time to time, obstruction from a mucus plug becomes a likely diagnosis. In those instances in which a mucus plug is suspected, trial at dislodging it can be made by depositing in the duodenum by way of a catheter a hypertonic (25 per cent) solution of magnesium sulfate. This procedure has been successful in a few instances. In all other instances of obstructive jaundice, surgical exploration is indicated.

A suitable elective age for operation is 1 month or as soon thereafter as the baby comes under care. The operation is undertaken as an exploratory procedure. In approximately 20 per cent of the cases drainage of bile into the intestine can be established. The remainder are "inoperable." In those instances in which early operation is successful, recovery is complete.

Usually at least some preoperative preparation is necessary. If vitamin K has become deficient, the prothrombin level of the blood may be low, and hemorrhage may result, either spontaneously or from surgical manipulation. The prothrombin level is brought within the normal range by giving vitamin K parenterally. Often a short period of good nutritional care, including hydration, is given before operation.

Nursing Care. Postoperatively, shock-preventive measures should be instituted. Rate and quality of respiration should be noted. Pulse rates in infants fluctuate so rapidly that they are not accurate guides to the infant's condition. Before and after operation these infants tend to be lethargic and slow in physical movements, and therefore they need help in adjustment of their position. They should be moved carefully to prevent wound injury. Frequent inspection of the abdominal wound should be made, for these babies have impaired healing power, and evisceration and bleeding may occur. An abdominal binder fastened tightly for support is desirable. Distention due to accumulation of peritoneal fluid or paralytic ileus is a possible complication, and observation to detect its onset is an important nursing responsibility. Gastric suction often is begun immediately after operation and is continued until peristalsis is heard. Elbow restraints to prevent the infant from removing the tube should be applied at the time the tube is inserted. Irrigations of the tube with small amounts of warm saline keep it patent.

Until adequate feeding can be resumed, fluids are administered parenterally. When feedings are begun, they should be given slowly from a medicine dropper. These infants may be picked up for feeding and bubbling, but it must be done with care.

If an anastamosis has been performed successfully, change in the color of the stools will be noted postoperatively, and their description should be charted accurately.

Infectious Hepatitis

Infectious hepatitis is the most common cause of jaundice in children beyond the period of infancy. The infectious agent (a virus) is acquired by alimentary contact from an infected individual, or from direct injection into the body of human blood, plasma, or of vaccines made from plasma.

Symptoms may appear within 2 to 6 weeks after natural exposure but do not begin until 2 to 4 months when the infection is the result of a contaminated injection. The predominant symptom is jaundice; in mild cases it is the only symptom. More commonly there is nausea, loss of appetite, abdominal pain and vomiting at the beginning of the illness. In severe or protracted cases there may be prostration, loss of weight and permanent liver damage from cirrhosis. The urine is darkly colored from the presence of bile pigments, and the stool is light or completely white because of their absence.

Treatment is symptomatic with a high-carbohydrate, low-fat and high-protein diet. Supplements of vitamin B complex and methionine are usually given. In children the prognosis for complete recovery without liver damage is nearly always excellent.

APPENDICITIS

Appendicitis is less frequent in children than in adults. It is uncommon under 5 years and rare under 2. In all instances the fundamental cause is the same, namely, obstruction of the lumen of the appendix. Obstruction may be due to a variety of causes.

Symptoms

In the adult, the usual findings are sudden onset of nausea, vomiting, localized tenderness, leukocytosis, fever and constipation. In the older child the symptoms may be entirely similar to those of the adult; but children in general, and the younger victims in particular, often present an insidious onset with symptoms that are difficult to evaluate. The classical localization of tenderness in the right lower quadrant of the abdomen may be obscured by poor co-operation or by general hypersensitivity. Pain may be referred elsewhere or may be overshadowed by crying and restlessness. Vomiting is frequently present but is not a very helpful symptom since it is a common aspect of so many childhood ailments. Very often the diagnosis of appendicitis in a child remains in doubt until he has been observed and examined repeatedly over a period of several hours.

A number of conditions may be confused with appendicitis and lead to unnecessary abdominal exploration. The early symptoms of infectious hepatitis or gastro-enteritis often suggest appendicitis. The mesenteric lymph nodes in children sometimes enlarge and become painful during the course of acute tonsillitis. Irritation of the peritoneum may occur in rheumatic fever. Pain may be referred to the abdomen in right-sided pneumonia, in pyelitis and occasionally in meningitis. Some of the most disconcerting patients are the small number of children who suffer from recurring bouts of afebrile abdominal pain which on repeated or close examination give inconsistent or bizarre findings. Many of these children suffer from hysterical or psychosomatic disorders which are more likely to be aggravated than helped by a fruitless operation.

PROGNOSIS

The prognosis of appendicitis in children is generally good when the disease is recognized and treated. Delay in making the diagnosis or unusually rapid progression of the infection in a young child may increase the hazard to recovery, for diffuse peritonitis may occur within a short time of the initial symptoms.

TREATMENT

Once the diagnosis is made, treatment is by surgical exploration and removal of the infected appendix. Preceding the operation the child should be kept at bed rest. If postponement is necessary for some reason, an icebag will help to relieve pain and decrease peristaltic activity of the bowel. Enemas are permissible but cathartics are unwise. If operation is contemplated within a short time, usually fluids and feedings are withheld. The sulfonamides, penicillin and streptomycin are of great value in preventing or minimizing peritonitis. Postoperative care of children is usually simple, for they seldom suffer from paralytic ileus.

INTESTINAL PARASITIC WORMS

Intestinal worms have been blamed erroneously for a wide variety of symptoms such as nose-picking, restless sleep, grinding the teeth while asleep, circles under the eyes, and convulsions. Most of these symptoms are related to emotional disturbances in the child and have nothing to do with intestinal parasites. Children who do harbor worms usually have no symptoms. An accurate estimate of the frequency of worm infestation is possible only by intensive and repeated study of stools and anal swabs. Such studies usually demonstrate a remarkably high prevalence of pinworm and roundworm infestations not only in the southern climates but also in the northern cities of the United States.

PINWORM (THREADWORMS, SEAT-WORMS, ENTEROBIUS VERMICULARIS, OXYURIS VERMICULARIS)

This is by far the most common variety of intestinal parasite. The worms are small white threads from ⅛ to ½ inch in length which are seen most commonly about the anus after the child has been asleep for an hour or two. Sometimes they are found on the surface of a stool. Infestation occurs when eggs are swallowed. The eggs hatch within the intestinal tract, and the gravid female worms inhabit the cecum until ready to lay their eggs. They then crawl out the anus, usually after the child has gone to sleep. They either lay their eggs shortly after emerging or are broken open and scatter the eggs about the child's perineum and into his clothing. The eggs survive for several days and are the source from which the same or another individual in the environment may acquire a new infestation. The period between ingestion of the egg and appearance of the gravid female at the anus is about 6 to 8 weeks.

Symptoms of pinworm infestation may be entirely lacking, and the condition may be discovered only by finding the worms. When infestation is heavy there may be itching about the anus or about the vagina in the female. The scratching that results traps new eggs under the finger nails and affords an easy means of their transfer back to the mouth.

Diagnosis is usually made by finding and recognizing the worms as they emerge from the anus. The eggs may be found by swabbing the anal region with scotch tape and examining it under a microscope. Since the females do not lay eggs within the intestinal tract, eggs are not found in the stools.

Treatment attempts to intoxicate the worms so that they will leave the intestine before completing their maturation, and attempts to eliminate the eggs deposited in the environment before they can cause another infestation. Gentian violet in enteric coated tablets is the standard vermifuge for pinworms. It may cause nausea and mild abdominal pain and must be used over a 10-day period to be effective. Several newer drugs have been tried with variable success. Sometimes worms are removed by repeated administration of enemas, but this is a disturbing procedure and probably no more effective than oral medication. Underclothing, night clothing and bed linen should be boiled at least twice a week in order to destroy eggs deposited therein. Careful cleansing of the perineum, the hands and the nails should be carried out several times a day. Application of a soothing ointment, such as ammoniated mercury or blue ointment, may allay the itching and reduce the viability of the eggs that have been deposited. All individuals in the family who have any suspicion of being infested must be treated simultaneously if success is to be attained.

ROUNDWORM (ASCARIS LUMBRICOIDES)

The adult roundworm is a large (6 to 15 in.) white or pink parasite about the diameter of a lead pencil. It lives for periods up to 6 months in the intestinal tract during which time the females lay enormous numbers of eggs that are discharged in the patient's stools. The eggs require from 2 to 4 weeks and a moist, shaded environment to develop into an infective stage. The infestation is passed from one individual to another only in regions where flush toilets are absent and defecation is performed in outhouses or on the open ground.

An egg that has developed to the stage of infectivity and is ingested follows a somewhat complicated development within the child. It is transformed first into a larval stage within the intestine. The larva is able to migrate through the intestinal wall; it gains access to the portal venous system and the general circulation and then reaches the lungs, where it breaks out of the blood stream into the alveoli. From the lungs the larvae are coughed up and swallowed to complete their growth into adult worms in the intestinal tract. The full development requires from 4 to 6 weeks.

Symptoms. Roundworms produce no symptoms except when present in unusual number so as to block the intestinal tract, or through unusual migrations as into the bile duct.

Treatment. A number of highly toxic drugs are used to expel the worms from the intestine. These include hexylresorcinol, santonin and oil of chenopodium. The former is preferred in treatment because of its lesser degree of toxicity.

HOOKWORM
(UNCINARIA AMERICANA)

The hookworm is a small (¼ to ½ inch) worm that lives in the upper intestinal tract where it is attached firmly by a mouth with teethlike parts through which it derives nourishment by sucking blood from the intestinal wall. The females lay large numbers of eggs which are passed in the patient's stools. The eggs require warm sandy soil for their development into larvae within about 2 weeks. Larvae may be ingested, or more commonly they penetrate through the skin of a child who is going barefoot. They enter the blood stream and circulate to the lungs where they enter the alveoli, are coughed up and swallowed and complete their development in the upper intestinal tract. Hookworm disease is limited to the southeastern portion of the United States and depends for its spread upon outdoor toilets and barefootedness.

Symptoms. The symptoms of hookworm disease depend upon the number of worms present in the individual. When the number is large, the loss of blood to the worms may be sufficient to cause anemia. Chronic infestations also produce anorexia, malnutrition and chronic fatigue. A sensitized child may develop itching at the site of entrance of larvae into the skin of his feet.

Diagnosis is made by finding the ova in the stools.

Treatment is effected by vermifuges such as tetrachlorethylene or hexylresorcinol. In chronic cases careful attention to the diet is required to restore nutrition.

BEEF TAPEWORM
(TAENIA SAGINATA)

The beef tapeworm requires an intermediate host, the cow, for its passage from one individual to another. It is acquired by eating infested beef which has not been cooked sufficiently to kill the larvae present within the meat. A larva so ingested develops in the upper intestinal tract into an adult worm with a tenacious head which attaches itself to the intestinal wall. It grows by progressive segmentation until it reaches considerable length—10 to 20 feet or more. Segments of the worm may break off and be noticed in the stool, or the end of the worm may protrude from the anus. There are no symptoms.

Treatment attempts to intoxicate the worm so that it will release its hold upon the intestinal wall and pass out of the tract. Oleoresin of aspidium, hexylresorcinal and atabrine are used. It is important to save all segments of the worm which are passed, for the head must be identified in order to be sure that treatment is complete. If some of the worm is broken off and the head left behind, it will continue to grow.

Dwarf Tapeworm
(Hymenolepis Nana)

This is a common but unimportant tapeworm that lives only a few weeks. It requires no intermediate host and may be passed from man to man. Treatment is the same as that for the beef tapeworm. No symptoms occur.

Trichina
(Trichinella Spiralis)

This is a fairly common infestation obtained from the ingestion of uncooked pork in which the encysted larvae of the worm reside. Digestion in the stomach of the patient frees the larva from its thick capsule and permits it to develop in 3 to 5 days in the intestine into the

adult form. Adults then burrow into the intestinal wall and release larvae which enter the blood stream and take up residence in the skeletal muscles. Infestation by a few trichinae may pass entirely unnoticed, but heavy infestation may produce severe or even fatal disease.

Symptoms of a heavy infestation may begin within a few days of the ingestion of the contaminated pork. The activity of the developing worms in the intestinal mucosa may produce diarrhea and fever. Marked constitutional symptoms of fever, pains in the muscles, swelling of the eyes and myocarditis may accompany the invasion of larvae into skeletal and heart muscle during the first 3 to 6 weeks. There is no effective treatment.

CHRONIC ULCERATIVE COLITIS

Chronic ulcerative colitis is an inflammation of the colon of unknown cause. In some instances the disease is related to psychosomatic factors. It runs a chronic course but has periods of remission and acute phases of progression. The onset may be insidious, or it may be more acute, like that of dysentery. It is much more common in adults than in children, and in general is much more severe in adults.

Symptoms

The child comes under care with persistent or recurrent diarrhea. The stools contain mucus, and in the acute phases there are small amounts of blood also. Fever is present in exacerbations, and often abdominal pain and tenesmus as well. Because of chronic diarrhea nutrition suffers, with loss of weight, progressive anemia, hypoproteinemia and often evidence of vitamin deficiency.

DIAGNOSIS

Diagnosis is made from the history of persistent diarrhea, failure to find causative organisms in the stools, and the finding of inflammation and ulceration on proctoscopic examination. As the condition becomes chronic, the changes in the colon are such as to cause haustra to disappear, as determined by x-ray examination with barium enema, and the colon becomes a smoothly outlined tube.

TREATMENT

No specific treatment exists. Special attention to psychogenic factors, such as emotional and environmental stresses, produces relief in many instances. Usually, psychiatric therapy is indicated. Attainment and maintenance of a good nutritive state help greatly in producing remission. The diet should be one of low-residue and high-energy value. Occasional transfusions may be in-

dicated for anemia. Paregoric is useful during periods of more acute diarrhea. The sulfonamide drugs have a beneficial effect on the symptoms, but diarrhea usually recurs when their use is stopped. The adrenocorticotropic hormone often produces striking remission, although subsequent relapse is common. Radical surgery, which is indicated for most adults, is seldom necessary for children. Surgical treatment consists of ileostomy as the first step, with subsequent removal of the colon as the second step.

RECTAL PROLAPSE

Sometimes a distinction is made between anal and rectal prolapse. In anal prolapse, the mucous membrane immediately proximal to the anus is extruded. In rectal prolapse the large tumor is composed also of bowel wall (Fig. 27). A combination of relaxed sphincter, large hard stools and straining at stool is likely to cause moderate prolapse in children otherwise normal. Rectal prolapse is associated with weakness of

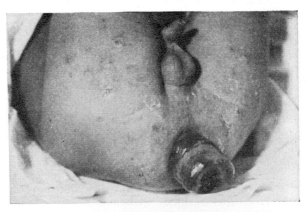

FIG. 27. Prolapse of the rectum, with beginning gangrene of the distal ½ inch of mucosa.

the muscles of the pelvic floor. Any condition such as severe malnutrition, which brings about muscle weakness is thus a predisposing cause. The immediate cause is straining, due either to diarrhea or constipation. It occurs only at defecation and is common in only the first 2 or 3 years.

TREATMENT

The prolapsed part should be replaced and, as far as possible, kept replaced. During defecation, the buttocks should be held firmly, either manually or by adhesive strips. A tight pad or bandage may be used. Constipation or diarrhea should be managed in such a way that straining is avoided. Usually no other measures are necessary. Surgical treatment is unsatisfactory.

FECAL INCONTINENCE

Fecal incontinence or encopresis results from a number of organic causes such as spina bifida, myelitis, coma and mental deficiency. These disorders are not amenable to treatment. Occasionally, a child is incontinent of feces for no organic reason, the symptom arising from unfavorable emotional and environmental conditions in the home. It occurs mainly in emotionally disturbed children. It may or may not be accompanied by enuresis. If the symptom persists beyond 3 or 4 years of age, the services of a child psychiatrist are indicated.

SITUATIONS FOR FURTHER STUDY

1. A 3-week-old infant has been discharged from the hospital after repair of a cleft lip. A cleft palate anomaly remains to be repaired later. If you were to supervise this infant's care at home, what guidance would the mother require? How would you assist the mother in preparing the child for hospitalization and operation?

2. Investigate community facilities available for speech training of children with cleft palate repairs. Visit a speech clinic to observe methods of speech training and to learn ways in which a nurse can help parents to continue speech training in the home.

3. In a young infant what symptoms would suggest a strangulated hernia?

4. What are the emotional needs of a baby with cleft lip? With pyloric stenosis? How can they be satisfied in the hospital?

BIBLIOGRAPHY

Battersby, J. S., and Greve, M. L.: Modern treatment of atresia of the esophagus, Am. J. Nursing **50:**158, 1950.

Lemmer, K. E., and Watson, S. R.: Inguinal hernia, Am. J. Nursing **53:**1,471, 1953.

Sterling, D. G., and Richmond, J. B.: Psychogenic megacolon manifested by fecal soiling, Pediatrics **10:**474, 1952.

Sperling, M.: Psychoanalytic study of ulcerative colitis in children, Psychoanalyt. Quart. **15:**302, 1946.

The child with a cleft palate, (pamphlet), Washington, U. S. Govt. Printing Office, 1953.

Diseases of the Respiratory System

◇◇◇

THE COMMON COLD	CONGENITAL LARYNGEAL STRIDOR
CHRONIC RHINITIS	CROUP
PARANASAL SINUSITIS	FOREIGN BODIES IN THE RESPIRATORY
EPISTAXIS	TRACT
TONSILS AND ADENOIDS	ACUTE LARYNGOTRACHEOBRONCHITIS
ACUTE TONSILLITIS	BRONCHITIS
PHARYNGITIS	ASTHMA
RETROPHARYNGEAL ABSCESS	PNEUMONIA
OTITIS MEDIA	PLEURISY
DEAFNESS	SITUATIONS FOR FURTHER STUDY

THE COMMON COLD (ACUTE CORYZA, ACUTE RHINITIS)

ETIOLOGY

The common cold is initiated by a specific virus. The virus produces inflammation which makes the mucous membranes vulnerable to secondary invasion by pyogenic bacteria. The pyogenic bacteria are of many varieties and they are responsible for the purulent stage of a cold and for the various complications. The virus is transmitted easily. All persons are not susceptible at all times. Many things may lower resistance temporarily, but even when it is lowered a cold does not result unless the virus is present or is acquired at the same time.

SERIOUSNESS

A cold is of such common occurrence that detailed description of the symptoms is scarcely necessary. The infection by the secondary invasion of pyogenic bacteria may remain limited to the nose and the throat, or it may extend to the ears or the bronchi. From otitis may result mastoiditis; from bronchitis, pneumonia. These more serious consequences are more frequent among infants than older children, while among adults they are relatively uncommon. This infection is especially serious in institutions where babies already in a poor state of health are housed. The babies of a hospital ward, because of the illness or condition for which they are in the hospital, are usually very susceptible to respiratory infection. At times epidemics may sweep through a ward, leaving a trail of otitis and pneumonia. In infancy, the poorer the nutrition and the lower the resistance, the more likely is the result to be serious. In the case of prematurely born infants, respiratory infections are serious affairs which not infrequently result in death.

PREVENTION

For outdoor play children should be dressed warmly enough but not overdressed. If they are overdressed with heavy outdoor clothing, they cannot run about. Instead, their activities are sedentary; they sit on the edge of the porch or on the edge of the sandbox and become thoroughly chilled. Too frequently the process of dressing for outdoor play is a prolonged one. Often the child's clothing is scattered about the house; it takes time to assemble it, and the child becomes annoyed by the delay. He becomes irate and overheated and, when he finally gets outside, he becomes chilled in a very short time. Children's clothing for outdoor play should be kept ready to put on. If the child is taught to come home when his feet are wet and cold, instead of being warned to keep out of puddles and snowbanks, the incidence of colds would be reduced. Puddles of water and banks of snow offer too many opportunities for pleasurable activities not to be tempting to children. Threatening them with the consequences of wet feet only prevents them from returning home for a hot bath and a change of clothing; it does not prevent the occurrence of a common cold.

Children who are too closely supervised in the home environment do not have sufficient opportunity to develop natural resistance to the cold virus. They may escape colds in the preschool period, but when they join a group of children at school, the frequency of infection increases.

No nurse with a cold should be allowed—nor should she permit herself—to attend an infant. An infant with a cold should be isolated from other infants. The great frequency of respiratory infections at certain seasons of the year calls for judicious use of common facilities in hospitals and institutions which care for infants and children. Whenever possible, infants or children who are known to be infected should be kept isolated from those who are well. Isolation procedures are particularly important to protect malnourished or debilitated children or those who are to undergo surgical procedures or are convalescing therefrom.

Some children develop colds with considerable frequency, others have them rarely. The essential difference between these two groups of children is not known. Attempts to prevent colds usually concentrate upon maintenance of good nutrition and the removal of infected tonsils and adenoids. Often there appears to be little relation between these aspects of health and the frequency with which individual children acquire colds.

Immunization against colds has not proved to be feasible. The active immunity produced by the cold itself is brief—probably no more than 1 or 2 months. Vaccines are prepared from various secondarily invading bacteria, but their effect is dubious. Ultraviolet light therapy is not effective in reducing the incidence of colds.

TREATMENT AND NURSING CARE

In the treatment and the nursing of uncomplicated coryza in infancy, the most important measure is to keep the nose clean in order that the infant may breathe and suckle. Babies cannot suckle satisfactorily unless they breathe through the nose. Nasal breathing is more comfortable for the older child also, but it is not so important for him as for the infant. Freeing of the nose for breathing can be accomplished in the early stage by dropping into the nose a very small amount of a solution of ephedrine (½ or 1 per cent) or Neosynephrine Hydrochloride (¼ per cent), which decreases the swelling of the mucous membrane and permits drainage. Drops of the solution should be put into the infant's nostrils from 5 to 10 minutes before his food is given to him.

When dropping solutions into the nose for the purpose of treatment, the head should be held backward until it is below the level of the shoulders. After 3 or 4 days, when the discharge has become purulent, suction may be used for the removal of the secretions.

Solutions containing oil should not be used in the nose, since they are known to pass unchecked through the larynx and into the trachea. Their accumulation in the lung may be responsible for lipid pneumonia.

When the nasal secretion is profuse and irritating, the nostrils and the upper lip should be protected with cold cream or petrolatum. If symptoms are acute, and if the infant is irritable and uninterested in his food, no attempt should be made to encourage him to take the usual amount of food. When fever accompanies the cold, infants often reduce their own diet, a procedure that tends to prevent gastro-intestinal disturbances. Water should be en-

couraged between feedings. The infant's position should be changed frequently. Unless he is elevated on a back rest, he should be kept off his back in order to prevent the nasal secretions from dropping into the pharynx and lodging in the eustachian tube. His room should be well ventilated but free from drafts. Increasing the humidity of the infant's room often proves to be valuable.

There is no essential difference in the treatment and the nursing care of the older child. Nose drops will be accepted more readily if the need for proper position is explained to him and if he is given opportunity to press the dropper bulb that releases the solution into the nostrils. Rest in bed is necessary as long as fever persists and should be continued for 48 hours longer. When the child's temperature becomes normal, he will feel much improved. Unless interesting play materials are provided for him, bed rest will be difficult to maintain in the home. In the home, cribsides are not high enough to prevent the child from leaving his bed to go where playthings are accessible. In order to prevent the spread of infection into the eustachian tube, children should be taught a safe method of clearing their nasal passages. They never should be directed to "blow hard." Instead, they should be taught to keep their mouths open while they ease the secretion from both nostrils at the same time.

Sedative or antipyretic drugs are often used to decrease discomfort in both infancy and childhood. In infancy they also decrease restlessness. Those used include aspirin, codeine and the barbiturates. Although sulfonamides and antibiotics are widely used in the treatment of colds, they probably should be reserved for use in complications or to terminate a protracted infection. In premature or debilitated infants the immediate administration of antibiotics is rational.

CHRONIC RHINITIS

Causative Factors

Chronic rhinitis may be due to any one of a number of causes. In infancy, it may be a manifestation of inherited syphilis. At any age, but especially in infancy, it may be the result of nasal diphtheria. Phlyctenular disease of the eye always is accompanied by a chronic nasal discharge. A foreign body in the nose gives rise to a chronic purulent discharge from the same side as that in which the foreign body is located. Allergy to pollens is a cause of chronic discharge in hay fever. Allergy to other materials, such as feathers and animal hair, often causes chronic rhinitis that is not seasonal. All the causes enumerated are relatively uncommon as compared with chronic pyogenic infection unassociated with any of the conditions mentioned. Chronic rhinitis of this character usually is caused and maintained by an abnormality in and about the nose. Such causative factors may be enlarged adenoids, hypertrophy of the turbinate bones, marked deviations of the septum and disease of the paranasal sinuses.

Treatment

When examining a child with chronic rhinitis, the causative factors enumerated should be considered as possible agents, and those not responsible excluded by appropriate tests and special examinations. The treatment depends altogether on the nature of the cause. When the rhinitis is due primarily to pyogenic organisms, any associated abnormal conditions should be corrected in so far as this is possible. Diseased tonsils and adenoids should be removed, and sinusitis, if present, should receive appropriate treatment.

PARANASAL SINUSITIS

The paranasal sinuses are cavities, normally filled with air, which are outlying portions of and communicate with the nasal chambers. Clinically, they are of little importance until they become diseased. The sinuses are only partially developed at birth and do not attain their maximum size until maturity. The maxillary and the ethmoidal sinuses are sufficiently developed at birth to be of clinical importance. The sphenoidal sinuses have relatively little development before 5 years. The frontal sinuses develop later than the others and are not of clinical importance until the latter part of childhood.

Etiology

The paranasal sinuses are invaded by every generalized intranasal infection, such as the common cold. If the mucosa of the upper respiratory tract is normal, and if no anatomic anomalies are present, any such infection usually will subside completely. However, if for any reason drainage from the sinuses is impeded, or if the mucosa loses its ability to combat the invasion, the inflammatory process in the sinuses may persist and become firmly established. Adenoids or deviated nasal septum may produce obstruction and thus serve as a causative agent in continued sinus inflammation. This statement is borne out by the clinical observation that in infants and children the sinus disease disappears spontaneously in a considerable proportion of cases when such obstructions have been removed. Repeated or persistent infections may lead to alteration in the mucosa: it loses its ciliated structure, and polypoid degeneration occurs. These changes favor persistence of the infectious process. In the adult, periapical dental abscesses are occasionally a cause of maxillary sinusitis; in the child, such an association is not frequent. Swimming is reputed to be a frequent cause of sinus infection.

SYMPTOMS

Sinus disease may present itself in a variety of forms. It may be acute or chronic, and it may involve any or all of the sinuses present. Most instances are characterized by the presence of exudate, which may be serous, mucoid or purulent. In some cases the changes are chiefly hypertrophic. The symptoms of sinus disease vary with the acuteness of the infection, its extent and distribution, and the adequacy of the drainage of the exudate. If the drainage is blocked, the retention will lead to local pain and to absorption of toxic products with resultant generalized effects. Chronic sinusitis may be associated with low-grade intermittent fever. The accompanying symptoms seem to be irrelevant, but they suggest continued absorption of toxic products.

Anorexia, lassitude and weakness, with vague muscle stiffness and pain, are present, especially in the early morning. Pallor may be marked, out of proportion to the decrease of hemoglobin, and the ears often appear waxy and translucent. During certain stages of the attacks mental acuity may seem to be impaired.

COMPLICATIONS

Many types of disease, both local and remote, have been attributed to sinus infection. In some conditions the causal relationship is definite; in others, it is largely circumstantial. The incidence of these complications is not constant; many children have sinus infections of considerable severity without exhibiting any recognizable effect outside the area involved by the process. Furthermore, when complications do arise, their nature may be different in a series of persons whose local infectious processes seem to be similar in nature and extent.

These accompaniments of sinus infection differ in some respects in infants from those in older children. In infants, sinusitis may produce serious disturbances of the gastrointestinal tract and of the water balance (see Diarrhea). The subacute and chronic forms may lead to emesis, food refusal and frequent, acid, excoriating stools. When these symptoms serve as a signal for therapeutic underfeeding in an attempt to correct the symptoms by diet, the nutrition necessarily suffers, often sufficiently to produce a most severe degree of malnutrition.

In the older child, the list of conditions which have been attributed to the systemic effects of sinusitis includes practically all the conditions which may arise secondary to absorption of toxic material from a suppurative focus, as well as disease of the lower respiratory tract. The role of sinusitis in causing these conditions is considered in the discussion of the various diseases. The list includes chronic deforming arthritis, nephritis, rheumatic fever, chorea, carditis, bronchiectasis and certain other conditions possibly not so definitely related.

DIAGNOSIS

Although the existence of sinusitis may be suspected from the history, the diagnosis is made on the basis of objective findings. It is made ultimately by finding evidences of inflammation in the sinuses, although it can be fairly substantiated by collateral related findings. In the presence of chronic sinusitis, the lymphoid tissue of the oropharynx is usually hyperplastic and somewhat reddened. The inflammation is most marked laterally (lateral pharyngitis) in the case of maxillary and ethmoid disease, and centrally in adenoid and sphenoid disease. The tonsils, if present, usually show some evidence of inflammation. The soft palate may appear reddened and slightly granular. Pus may or may not be seen in the posterior pharynx. Often the discharge is swallowed by the child without his being conscious of its presence. Regional lymph glands usually are enlarged and may be tender.

Examination of the nose by both the anterior and the posterior nasoscope may reveal the presence and the location of nasal discharge. During acute sinusitis, no discharge may be visible because of acute retention. When chronic maxillary sinusitis is suspected, aspiration of the sinus is considered useful as a diagnostic procedure. Roentgenograms of the sinuses are made frequently as a routine procedure. In the diagnosis of sinus disease they have not been infallible, and mistakes in both directions have been made. However, they are usually reliable, and when operative procedures are contemplated they provide information about the size, the location and the degree of development of the sinuses. Transillumination as a diagnostic aid in children has not proved to be wholly reliable and satisfactory.

PREVENTION

Prevention of chronic sinus infection is dependent on the correction of anatomic obstructions, good nutrition and avoidance of the common cold. Removal of adenoids is a simple and effective measure. When we have learned to control the common cold, we shall have accomplished much in the prevention of sinus disease.

TREATMENT

In the treatment of sinusitis in children, conservative measures to the extent that they prove to be adequate should be employed. One of the primary requirements of treatment is drainage of the sinuses. Often this may be accomplished by intranasal medication. Ephedrine or Neosynephrine solutions applied frequently during the day by dropping, spraying or nasal packing cause a decrease in swelling of the mucous membrane of the nasal cavities, thus freeing the natural opening of the sinuses.

In the presence of sinusitis the tonsils and the adenoids, especially the latter, are likely to be hypertrophied and chronically infected. Their presence often serves to continue and aggravate the sinus infections. Removal of the tonsils and the adenoids is followed in a considerable proportion of instances in childhood by gradual disappearance of sinusitis.

When the maxillary sinuses are inflamed and contain pus that does not drain adequately with the conservative treatment mentioned, they may be washed out at intervals, or the opening from the nose into the sinuses may be enlarged. In the great majority of cases in childhood, more radical procedures than these are neither necessary nor indicated.

EPISTAXIS
(NASAL HEMORRHAGE)

Epistaxis may occur as a symptom of heart disease, typhoid fever, whooping cough and diseases of the blood, such as purpura and leukemia. It may be due also to inflammation within the nose. Frequently recurring nasal hemorrhage in the absence of systemic disease is usually due to an ulceration in the anterior part of the septum. Very commonly, hemorrhage results from injury, either an external blow, as from a fall, or an internal trauma, as from picking the nose.

In the common variety of nasal hemorrhage, the bleeding is from the anterior and inferior portion of the nasal septum. Such a hemorrhage is controlled easily. If the child remains quiet, the hemorrhage may stop spontaneously in a few minutes. Pressure on the bleeding point by pinching the nose is ac-

complished easily and usually is effective. In case the hemorrhage persists, it always can be stopped by packing into the anterior part of the nose a small piece of cotton or strip of cloth, either plain or moistened with thromboplastin or a vasoconstrictor such as epinephrine or ephedrine. In case of the more severe and less common type of hemorrhage from some other part of the nose, posterior packing may be necessary.

TONSILS AND ADENOIDS

The term *tonsils,* when used without qualification, usually refers to the faucial tonsils which are located anteriorly in the oropharynx, one on each side. The term *adenoids* refers to a mass of lymphoid tissue of the same general structure as the faucial tonsils located in the nasopharynx posteriorly. Adenoids are known also as the pharyngeal tonsil. The lingual tonsil is located at the base of the tongue. The tubal tonsils are situated near the eustachian tube, one on each side of the pharynx. All these lymphoid tissues as a group are referred to as Waldeyer's ring.

Acute inflammation of any of these lymphoid tissues may be catarrhal, follicular or membranous, depending on the severity and the type of infection. The lingual, the pharyngeal or the faucial tonsils may be involved separately, or all may be affected at the same time. Similarly, any of these tissues may be the site of chronic infection or may be abnormally hypertrophied.

Relatively normal faucial tonsils vary considerably in size, the pillars are not adherent, the crypt mouths are open and show no inflammatory products on pressure, and the color of the tonsil is the same as that of the mouth.

Chronic disease or abnormality of the faucial tonsils may manifest itself in several ways. The tonsils may be large and ragged from hypertrophy. They may be small and fibrous, and, in addition, they may be buried between adherent pillars. The crypts on pressure may exude pus or cheesy material. The surface of the tonsil may be redder than normal and have the appearance of being subacutely inflamed. Enlargement of the cervical lymph glands is corroborative evidence of chronic tonsillar inflammation.

Chronic infection of the lymphoid tissues of the pharynx may be a factor in the occurrence of rheumatic fever, pyelitis, arthritis, otitis media, partial deafness, cervical adenitis, recurrent colds and infections of the nasopharynx, unexplained fever, periodic gastro-intestinal and metabolic upsets, and other conditions.

TONSILLECTOMY

The finding of definite chronic disease in the tonsil is an excellent indication for tonsillectomy. Repeatedly recurring acute disease and hypertrophy to the extent of interference with breathing are equally good indications for tonsil removal. In such of the conditions listed in the preceding paragraph where it seems to be certain that the underlying cause is a chronic focus of infection, it is justifiable and proper to remove the tonsils, on the assumption that they are harboring infection, even though little or no evidence of infection exists.

While there is no question about the benefits of tonsillectomy for properly selected children, it does not necessarily follow that all children are better off without their tonsils and adenoids. So long as these structures remain healthy they provide a first line of defense against respiratory infection. They also probably limit the spread of such diseases so long as they function normally. The decision to remove tonsils and adenoids must also take into consideration the risks of anesthesia, silent bleeding in the small infant, and the psychic trauma to a young child who is unable to comprehend what is being done to him. During the period of the year when poliomyelitis is prevalent, tonsillectomy should be avoided, because there is good reason to believe that a child with a recent tonsillectomy wound runs a greater risk of the bulbar type of poliomyelitis if exposed to the virus.

When tonsillectomy and adenoidectomy are indicated, the nurse in the doctor's office or in the clinic should assist the mother in learning how to prepare her child for his hospital experience. Frequently, erroneous information is given children prior to hospitalization. One constantly sees the result of it in the admitting room and in the hospital wards. It increases the adjustment problems for the child; it complicates his postoperative nursing care; and it indicates to him a lack of parental honesty. The period of hospitalization before surgery frequently is too brief for the nurse to establish the type of relationship that gives the child a sense of security and confidence in her. Preparation that relieves fear and anxiety should be given by someone in whom the child has faith, security and confidence; therefore, it is the parent who should prepare the child for his new experience. However, the nurse should function by helping the parents to gain insight into the necessity for preparation and by imparting the knowledge that serves as a basis for truthful child-teaching. In instances where the mother has not prepared the child, the nurse will need to do it for her. This is essential because the child should know what he will experience before and after operation.

Postoperative Nursing Care

When the child returns from the operating room, he should be placed in a prone position with a pillow under his chest and abdomen to facilitate drainage and to prevent aspiration of blood or secretions. When the child becomes fully conscious, he can be turned on his back and supported in a sitting position. Fluids should be given cautiously until vomiting ceases; then they can be increased as rapidly as they are tolerated. Cold and sweetened synthetic fruit juices and milk drinks usually are tolerated a few hours postoperatively. The child's pulse rate and behavior should be observed at frequent intervals to detect early signs of bleeding. Restlessness, frequent swallowing, clearing the throat and vomiting often accompany bleeding. Apparatus for suction and materials necessary for checking hemorrhage should be in readiness for use in case of need. In some instances, throat icebags relieve the pain; in others, they tend to annoy and to increase restlessness. Aspirin may be indicated for relief of discomfort.

Before the child leaves the hospital the mother should be instructed to provide soft, warm, nonirritating foods for her child until the soreness of the throat has subsided. Also, she should understand the necessity for keeping him in bed for a few days and for providing daily rest periods for a short time subsequently. Earache, not accompanied by fever, sometimes occurs after tonsillectomy, and the mother should be forewarned of this to prevent anxiety should it occur. Also, she should be told of the importance of any mild or sudden bleeding during the convalescent period.

ACUTE TONSILLITIS

Acute faucial tonsillitis is caused most commonly by streptococci but may be caused by any of several pyogenic bacteria. It is less common in the infant than in the older child.

Symptoms

Tonsillitis commonly has an acute onset with fever, headache and malaise. The onset may be accompanied in the older child by a chill and in the younger on rare occasions by a convulsion. Pain on swallowing usually is present. Gastro-intestinal symptoms, chiefly vomiting and diarrhea, are frequent and are more pronounced in the younger child. The lymph glands receiving the drainage from the inflamed area, the submaxillary and the cervical glands, are frequently enlarged and tender. Though tonsillitis usually causes marked constitutional symptoms, some children may have an acute infection with only few and mild subjective symptoms. Sometimes acute and sharply localized abdominal pain accompanies tonsillitis, presumably caused by inflammation of the mesenteric lymph glands. The symptoms may be of such a nature as to lead to the suspicion, or even the diagnosis, of an acute abdominal condition, such as appendicitis.

COMPLICATIONS

The most common complications of acute tonsillitis are otitis media and cervical adenitis. Under modern treatment, adenitis seldom progresses to the point of suppuration. If the initial infection is caused by a hemolytic streptococcus there may be recurrent fever and mild adenitis over a period of weeks or months, due either to incomplete treatment or to the relatively feeble resistance of a young child. Peritonsillar abscess is seen occasionally in an older child following tonsillitis. The relation between acute tonsillitis and a number of systemic diseases is considered under the discussion of the etiology of rheumatic fever, nephritis, arthritis, purpura and scarlet fever.

TREATMENT

Chemotherapy is usually effective. The choice of drug should be determined from a knowledge of the causative agent, but often this is not done because of the lack of adequate facilities. Most infections will respond promptly to penicillin; a little more slowly to the sulfonamides. Oxytetracycline (Terramycin) and chlortetracycline (Aureomycin) are required sometimes when the infecting agent does not respond. Aspirin is useful to relieve fever, headache and general malaise. Gargles, compresses, sprays and local applications to the tonsils have very limited usefulness for children. The diet should be light and nonirritating, and the fluid intake should be kept high.

PHARYNGITIS

Inflammation of the pharynx is relatively common. It is a part of what is frequently spoken of as upper respiratory infection. Also, it may precede other evidences of associated respiratory inflammation, such as rhinitis or laryngitis.

SYMPTOMS

The pharynx appears red and dry. Pain on swallowing and nonproductive cough may be present. When the infection is acute, fever, and often headache, may be present. In infancy, the fever may be high, and convulsions and gastro-intestinal symptoms may occur.

TREATMENT

The treatment does not differ from that for acute tonsillitis.

RETROPHARYNGEAL ABSCESS

A retropharyngeal abscess arises from suppuration in the lymph glands back of the posterior pharyngeal wall. Infection in these glands is preceded by infection elsewhere in the upper respiratory tract. Often the primary infection is a common cold. Retropharyngeal glands are present at birth and tend to atrophy and disappear after a few years. For this reason, retropharyngeal abscess occurs most frequently under 3 years of age.

SYMPTOMS

As the abscess develops, the child becomes restless and is found to have fever, which, though variable, is often high. Prostration frequently is out of proportion to the obvious physical findings. Swallowing is painful, and attempts to swallow may give rise to choking. Sometimes the taking of food is impossible. The head may be held retracted toward the affected side, the abscess usually having a unilateral origin. A swelling may be visible externally on the affected side. When the swelling in the pharynx increases sufficiently, obstruction to breathing occurs, and stridor and dyspnea result. Respiratory obstruction may be great enough to threaten life unless promptly relieved.

DIAGNOSIS

Examination of the throat is difficult because of the small size of the child, difficulty in opening the mouth, and often the presence of frothy mucus in the pharynx. Usually the diagnosis must be verified by palpation. By palpation the presence of swelling is determined. It may have a boggy feeling, and sometimes fluctuation will be observed. The use of a laryngoscope usually is of considerable assistance in the diagnosis because of the better opportunity for adequate inspection.

The condition must be distinguished from peritonsillar abscess and from abscess resulting from tuberculosis of the cervical vertebrae. Peritonsillar abscess (quinsy) is an abscess about the tonsil resulting from tonsillar inflammation and is located farther forward than a retropharyngeal abscess. It is rare in childhood. A tuberculous abscess is a cold abscess, i.e., not associated with acute inflammation. There may be little or no fever and no prostration except that which might be associated with respiratory obstruction. A roentgenogram will show erosion of the underlying vertebrae.

TREATMENT

The treatment of retropharyngeal abscess is incision and drainage, always without an anesthestic. If respiratory obstruction is present, an anesthetic prevents the use of accessory muscles of respiration. As a consequence, respiration may cease from obstruction as soon as the anesthetic is given and before the abscess can be drained. An anesthetic will abolish the cough reflex, and, as a result, pus may be aspirated. The incision should be small, and, if necessary, the opening should be enlarged by inserting closed scissors or forceps and then spreading and withdrawing them. Incision through a laryngoscope has several advantages. A better view of the incision site is obtained. The head is held downward while the abscess is lanced, and suction for removal of pus can be applied immediately through the laryngoscope. After operation the wound should be spread each day until drainage ceases. After drainage the healing may be prompt. In other instances, inflammation with its accompanying fever and prostration may not subside completely for several weeks.

NURSING CARE

Immediately after incision specific nursing care consists of maintaining the child in a position suitable for mouth drainage. He may be placed in a prone position with the foot of his bed elevated, or a pillow may be placed under his chest and abdomen to facilitate drainage. A "mummy" restraint is required when the incision is made and when the abscess is spread daily. After operation, the taking of fluids should be encouraged as rapidly as ability to swallow develops. Observation to detect signs of hemorrhage should be made as long as the infection continues.

OTITIS MEDIA
Acute Otitis Media

Etiology. The middle ear is a small air-containing cavity interposed between the drum, which separates it from the external ear, and the inner ear which is set into the temporal bone and contains the organs of hearing and equilibrium. The ear drum is a sensitive curtain hung between the air of the external and the middle ear. It transmits the minute changes of pressure created by the sound waves through a chain of small bones (the ossicles) to the oval window of the inner ear. The middle ear communicates through a long narrow channel (eustachian tube) with the pharynx. During health the eustachian tube is closed most of the time by its external muscular coating, but opens briefly during the acts of swallowing, yawning and crying to permit rapid equalization of air pressure between the middle ear and the pharynx. (Except during violent nose-blowing, the pressure in the pharynx is automatically the same as that of the air on the external surface of the ear drum.) The symptoms of mild pain in the ear and blurred hearing which are experienced during air travel are due to imperfect equalization of air pressures on the two sides of the drum. The middle ear also communicates with the mastoid antrum and its ramified system of air cells within the temporal bone.

Infection of the middle ear almost invariably arises from the pharynx by way of the eustachian tube. Consequently, the bacteria usually involved are the same ones responsible for pharyngitis and tonsillitis—hemolytic streptococci, pneumococci and influenza bacilli. A wide variety of other organisms may be implicated under the special circumstances of specific diseases, such as diphtheria and tuberculosis, or during debilitating illness or prolonged treatment with antibiotics which sometimes changes the flora of the respiratory tract.

The mechanical changes that occur during otitis media usually begin with obstruction of the mouth of the eustachian tube due to swelling of the mucous membrane. Complete or partial obstruction prevents air exchange between the pharynx and the middle ear, and the air within the middle ear is slowly absorbed. The ear drum bulges inward due to the unopposed external air pressure, and tension of the drum results in pain and blurring of hearing. If the obstruction persists, the air in the middle ear is replaced by fluid which may produce outward bulging of the drum. If the fluid is not infected, the process is called catarrhal otitis media. When infection has spread up the tube to the middle ear the accumulation of fluid is more rapid, and the drum bulges outward tensely, becomes exquisitely painful and not infrequently ruptures, permitting the accumulation of pus in the middle ear to discharge into the external canal.

Infants are more prone to middle ear infection than are older children or adults. The eustachian tube is shorter, wider and straighter in the infant (Fig. 28) so that infected material is carried more readily from the pharynx to the middle ear. Infected adenoid masses in the vicinity of the mouth of the eustachian tube are often responsible for recurring blockage of the tube or otitis media.

Symptoms. The child who is old enough to communicate complains of pain in the ear and blurred hearing. The severity of the pain depends upon the rapidity with which fluid accumulates in the middle ear. Fever, headache and vomiting are also present in variable degree. Smaller children and infants cannot localize their symptoms. The source of their fever, irritability, discomfort and vomiting may be disclosed only through a comprehensive physical examination. In small infants there may be convulsions, diarrhea, refusal of food and rolling of the head from side to side.

Complications. With almost any acute inflammation of the middle ear there is some extension of the infection into the mastoid antrum and air cells. When treatment is delayed or ineffectual, mastoiditis may occur. From the mastoid area there may be spread of the infection to the venous sinuses within the skull (sinus thrombosis and septicemia) or to the meninges (meningitis) or to the brain (brain abscess). These complications are now rare since the antibiotics have made treatment simple and usually successful.

Prevention. The prevention of otitis depends upon the rapid and accurate treatment of pharyngitis and tonsillitis in most instances. Some children who are unusually prone to otitis media benefit from the removal of hypertrophied or infected adenoid tissue.

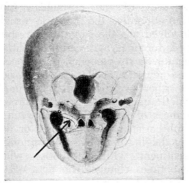

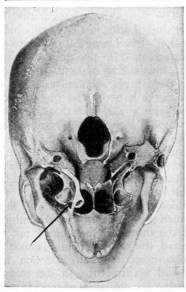

FIG. 28. Schematic representation of the eustachian tube in the infant and the adult, showing relative position and direction.

Treatment and Nursing Care. Antibiotics are indicated to combat the infection. At the beginning of treatment the appropriate drug may not be known, because the bacteria responsible for the infection have not yet been determined. Penicillin is effective in most instances and usually is given initially. Oxytetracycline (Terramycin), chlortetracycline (Aureomycin) or sulfonamides may be used when the response to penicillin is inadequate or when bacteriologic study indicates that they will be more effective.

Often symptomatic relief of pain may be obtained by giving nose drops to shrink the nasal mucous membranes and promote drainage from the blocked eustachian tube. Neosynephrine (0.25 per cent) or ephedrine (2 per cent) may be used every 2 to 3 hours until relief is obtained. Sometimes drops containing phenol and glycerine are instilled into the external ear. Their effect is variable and they have the disadvantage of preventing accurate observation of changes in the ear drum. Occasionally, when the drum is extremely tense, incision (myringotomy) may be indicated to relieve pain and promote drainage. Aspirin and sedatives with the barbiturate drugs will give temporary relief of pain until the other measures have had time to take effect.

When there is drainage from the middle ear, the ear canal must be kept clean. The nurse's hands should be washed thoroughly before cleansing the canal to prevent mixed infection of the middle ear. Sterilized cotton should be made into pledgets and used to cleanse the canal of all drainage. Hydrogen peroxide is useful in preventing the exudate from caking. In cleansing the ear canal of the young child, the ear lobe should be pulled down and back to straighten the canal; in the older child, the ear lobe should be pulled up and back. Ear wicks should be small and inserted lightly; packing them in tightly prevents free drainage and may cause extension of the infection into the mastoid process. When drainage is profuse, zinc oxide ointment or petrolatum should be applied to the external auricle to prevent excoriation of the skin. If the infant puts his hands to the infected ear and the drainage is profuse, elbow restraints should be applied. This is necessary to prevent the infant from getting the drainage into his eyes and mouth. The character and the amount of the drainage should be recorded.

If after myringotomy the drainage ceases or becomes thicker and the child's temperature rises after a period of remaining normal, the nurse should be alert for signs of complications.

CHRONIC OTITIS MEDIA

In some instances, the ear discharge persists and becomes chronic. If the condition is untreated, the discharge may continue for years. The usual result of chronic discharge is impairment of hearing, even to almost complete loss in some instances. A less common result is, soon or late, an inflammatory invasion of the surrounding temporal bone, with perhaps serious results such as meningitis or brain abscess. Sometimes chronic ear discharge will cease when adenoids have been removed and the nose and the throat are brought to a relatively normal state. In other instances, it is necessary to give postauricular drainage to such inflammation as exists in the mastoid process. Tuberculosis of the middle ear is also a cause of persistent discharge.

MASTOIDITIS

Mastoiditis is a term used, somewhat colloquially, to designate inflammation of and in the mastoid process of the skull. It occurs almost exclusively as a complication of otitis media. It is the most frequent complication of otitis media. Indeed, it is probable that some inflammation and pus are present in the mastoid antrum in every case of otitis media, since the middle ear and the antrum are connected directly. However, unless more than this minimum inflammation is present in the antrum, mastoiditis cannot be diagnosed, and such inflammation as is present is of no great clinical significance. In the majority of instances, it clears up with adequate drainage from the middle ear. Instances in which the inflammation becomes more severe and invasive are clinically important. In many cases of more severe inflammation, especially in infants and young children, the communication between the antrum and the middle ear becomes closed because of inflammatory edema. When the pus has no outlet for drainage, the symptoms become more severe, and the consequences more serious.

Modern treatment with antibiotics has greatly reduced the incidence of mastoiditis in children. Occasionally, it appears when treatment of otitis media has been too long delayed or when the presence of unusually thick pus hampers drainage from the mastoid cells back into the middle ear.

Symptoms. Mastoiditis occurs at all ages, even in earliest infancy. In most instances, fever is present, and often it is high. Sometimes the temperature is constantly at a high level, while at others it fluctuates widely at short intervals. Tenderness over the mastoid process is frequent, especially in older children. Often when tenderness cannot be elicited on pressure, it becomes manifest when the area is tapped with a finger or a percussion hammer. In some instances, the inflammation extends exteriorly through the bone. External extension produces back of the ear a swelling which lifts the external ear away from the skull and pushes it forward. The swelling may be caused by edema alone, or pus may break through the periosteum to form a superficial abscess. All these symptoms and signs are inconstant. In infancy the local symptoms of mastoiditis may be slight, but serious constitutional symptoms of vomiting, diarrhea and malnutrition may be present.

Treatment. When chemotherapy has failed to improve the patient's condition, it may be necessary to establish drainage from the infected cells by mastoidectomy. This operation consists of removing the bone overlying the mastoid cells or antrum to permit direct drainage to the exterior.

Nursing Care. Elbow restraints are required postoperatively. The child's ear is painful, the dressing is annoying, and children recovering from anesthesia are likely to pull at the dressing and remove it. Resistance to restraints can be overcome by telling the preschool child in the preoperative periods that restraints will be necessary after operation until he is awake enough to remember to keep his hands away from the dressing. When the pain subsides and he is awake sufficiently, restraints usually can be removed without danger. Fluids may be given after nausea has ceased; solid foods may be introduced rapidly after tolerance to fluids is shown. The nurse needs to remember that she must talk loudly to the child with bilateral mastoidectomy. His dressings are large, and his hearing is impaired. Unless she makes herself understood, the child will have difficulty in co-operating. In addition, he will feel closed off from people when he needs to feel closest to them. High temperature and pulse rate, increased restlessness, neck stiffness, convulsions, nausea, vomiting, aphasia and visual disturbances are symptoms which may indicate such complications as sinus thrombosis, meningitis, brain abscess or incomplete drainage.

DEAFNESS

Bilateral complete deafness is a very serious handicap to a child. It is due most commonly to congenital abnormalities of the external or the internal ear, of the auditory nerve, or of the auditory centers within the brain. It sometimes results from the effects of disease such as congenital syphilis, erythroblastosis fetalis, meningococcus meningitis, mumps, encephalitis or extensive infection of the middle ear. Complete deafness in early infancy may go unrecognized until the child's failure to develop speech and to relate himself normally to his parents or other children stimulates an investigation of the acuity of his hearing. Loss of hearing should be suspected in infancy if the child fails to blink at loud noises. A similarly objective test must be used in the preschool child in order to distinguish between an inability to hear and an unwillingness to pay attention. Children who grow up without the ability to hear require special training in order to develop speech and to learn lipreading. Without such help the child becomes socially isolated and is unable to pursue a normal school career.

Complete deafness that is unilateral may be caused by the same disorders enumerated above. It is a relatively minor handicap if hearing is normal in the other ear.

Bilateral partial deafness may be responsible for poor school performance or for various types of behavior disorders. It is most commonly the result of chronic or recurring infections of the middle ear or blockage of the eustachian tube. It may be the forerunner of more serious hearing loss in later life. The detection of impaired hearing is an important responsibility of school health personnel and always should be a part of health examinations. Thorough treatment of acute otitis media can be expected to prevent hearing loss in most instances. When the defect is due to eustachian tube blockage without infection, the services of a skilled otologist are required to determine what measures are needed to maintain the patency of the tube.

CONGENITAL LARYNGEAL STRIDOR

Congenital laryngeal stridor is a noise produced on inspiration because of obstruction to air flow. It is due to any one of several laryngeal conditions, all of which are the result of immaturity of the larynx or persistence of fetal characteristics. The larynx may be soft and collapsible, large tissue folds may be present between the larynx and the epiglottis, the epiglottis may be soft and flaccid. In any of these conditions the parts are brought together on inspiration to cause obstruction and noise; they are pushed apart on expiration, and no symptoms are present. During inspiration also the soft parts of the chest are pulled in.

The noisy breathing appears in the first few days after birth and persists from 1 to 2 years, by which time the larynx has grown and matured sufficiently to permit normal breathing. The stridor is worse during periods of crying and excitement. At such times cyanosis is likely to appear. During quiescent periods no cyanosis is present, and the baby appears in no distress. Rarely, if at all, is congenital stridor dangerous to life, though there are occasions when the appearance and the behavior of the baby are alarming to the parents. By means of laryngoscopy the diagnosis can be confirmed and a more serious abnormality excluded. No treatment is indicated.

CROUP

Croup is a general term for inflammations of the larynx that cause hoarseness, barking cough or obstruction to breathing, or combinations of these. The term *membra-*nous croup has been used as a synonym of laryngeal diphtheria. In many young children, catarrhal inflammation of the larynx causes spasmodic contraction of the larynx, which results in respiratory difficulty. This latter condition at present is commonly referred to as croup and is the condition discussed here. It is known by a variety of names: for example, catarrhal croup, spasmodic croup and spasmodic laryngitis.

Symptoms

Croup is a mild, acute infection, of low communicability, occurring chiefly in children under 5 years of age. It is associated with little, and often no, fever. There is a laryngeal cough, hard and barking, usually spoken of as croupy. Attacks of spasm of the larynx occur chiefly, and often only, at night. They may last from ½ hour to between 2 and 3 hours. They may recur once or twice the same night. The attacks recur on the second, and often on the third, night, after which time spontaneous recovery from the infection occurs. Except for hoarseness and occasional croupy cough, the child seems to be completely well between the attacks of spasm.

During a spasmodic attack, there is very difficult inspiration and an inspiratory stridor. Expiration is little disturbed, and there is no expiratory stridor. The child sits up in bed, brings the accessory muscles of respiration into use, and on inspiration there is retraction of the soft tissues above the clavicle and between the ribs and retraction of the ribs at the attachment of the diaphragm. In a severe attack, the whole picture is very alarming because of the appearance of impending asphyxia. However, croup rarely results seriously.

DIAGNOSIS

The diagnosis of croup usually is not difficult. Diphtheria may be excluded by examining the larynx and finding an absence of membrane. The obstruction due to diphtheria is both inspiratory and expiratory; it gradually increases in severity and does not occur in spasmodic attacks, although occasionally in diphtheria, spasm is superimposed on the typical clinical picture. Streptococcic laryngitis may cause swelling and membrane formation which give symptoms similar to those described for diphtheria. In laryngospasm of tetany, other signs of tetany usually are present, and the chemical changes in the blood are diagnostic.

TREATMENT AND NURSING CARE

Treatment and nursing care of croup are directed chiefly toward relief of laryngeal spasm. Breathing warm moist air often gives complete relief. Various volatile drugs, such as benzoin, may be employed along with "steam," but the essential part, and usually the only necessary part, of the inhalation is the warm-water vapor. Various methods may be used to supply warm moist air. The

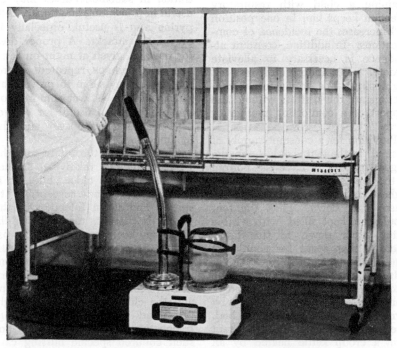

FIG. 29. A croup tent and a croup "kettle." A wire screen protects the child from being burned.

most satisfactory is a "croup tent" kept filled with moist air by a "croup kettle." Croup tents may be made by draping a sheet and a bath blanket over the crib. The spout of the croup kettle should point upward and away from the child to prevent the condensing steam from dropping and scalding him. Unless the child can have a nurse with him constantly, a jacket restraint must be used to prevent the child from moving toward the apparatus and being burned. An alternative is to provide a wire screen to be attached to the bed between the child and the steam outlet (Fig. 29). When constant nursing is available, it should be provided, because restraining a child with respiratory infection keeps him in one position and increases the incidence of complications. In addition, constant attendance is necessary to alleviate anxiety. Respiratory distress is frightening. The young infant cannot tolerate this distress without the support of a comforting mother or nurse.

Provision for a constant supply of fresh air to the tent should be made. A good plan is to have the bottom of the tent at the same level as the highest portion of the child's face when lying down. Then the tent should be kept filled with visible water vapor down to this level. There is then space for ventilation beneath the tent.

In the home, croup tents may be made by draping a sheet and a blanket over the crib or the baby carriage or over an umbrella in bed. The steam may be led into the tent from a croup kettle heated by an alcohol lamp or a gas or electric

plate. A lead-in pipe may be improvised from rolled paper or cardboard. Sometimes in institutions rooms are equipped specially with steam outlets, and steam is delivered in such quantity that a tent is unnecessary.

Several antispasmodic drugs are useful in preventing or relieving the muscle spasm of the larynx. If ipecac is used, the preparation known as syrup of ipecac is the one commonly employed. For a child of several years or older in the midst of an attack, the syrup may be given in teaspoonful doses every 15 minutes until emesis occurs, or until 3 doses have been given. Administration in subemetic doses may be useful in preventing an attack. Antipyrine also is useful, especially in preventing attacks. A proper dose for the age, given at night on retiring, and perhaps repeated during the night, may serve to prevent an attack entirely. A wet compress on the neck is often useful for control of both laryngeal spasm and the inflammation.

The larynx of the infant and the young child is relatively smaller than that of the older child. It is more flexible and susceptible to spasm, and when infection of the larynx is present, respiratory difficulty may become marked and prostrating. In caring for the child with croup, the nurse should be constantly alert for signs of respiratory embarrassment. If cyanosis develops and the child becomes increasingly prostrated from labored breathing, tracheotomy may be indicated. For such children specific nursing care is required.

FOREIGN BODIES IN THE RESPIRATORY TRACT

Foreign bodies of small size and wide variety may be aspirated into the lower respiratory tract, especially by children. These may remain in the pharynx or pass into the bronchi. Seldom do they lodge in the trachea. In the larynx they are the cause of immediate and acute distress with violent coughing and with stridor due to obstruction or to spasm of the larynx. If the foreign body remains fixed in one place in the larynx, coughing subsides, but usually an inflammation occurs, the edema of which obstructs respiration, and operative relief becomes imperative.

When a foreign body passes into a bronchus, the effects vary with the size and the nature of the foreign material. If the bronchus is completely occluded, the air in the lung beyond the obstruction is absorbed, and the lung collapses. If a large or primary bronchus is affected, the resultant pulmonary collapse may give rise to alarming symptoms, including cyanosis and dyspnea. A foreign body of any variety in a bronchus causes inflammation; but certain kinds, especially nuts, more easily induce inflammatory changes which are of a serious type. In a child who survives the immediate effects of a foreign body, the late result is likely to be a lung abscess or chronic pneumonia and bronchiectasis, unless the foreign body is removed early. The primary indication in treatment is removal of the offending material by laryngoscope or bronchoscope, as the need may be.

NURSING CARE

After the foreign body has been removed by laryngoscope or bronchoscope, the child should be placed in a ventilated "croup tent" that is kept filled with warm, moist air. The child should be observed closely for signs of respiratory difficulty. Trauma during laryngoscopic or bronchoscopic examination may produce edema of the larynx with accompanying respiratory embarrassment. Increased, labored respirations, crowing, hoarseness, retraction of the soft parts of the chest on inspiration, cyanosis and restlessness are danger signals that should be reported immediately. If respiratory embarrassment occurs, tracheotomy may be necessary.

CARE OF THE CHILD WITH A TRACHEOTOMY

After tracheotomy, the child should be placed in a warm bed in a room at 80° F. to prevent chilling. Respiratory difficulty exhausts a child, and often after tracheotomy he is prostrated. Elbow restraints should be applied immediately to prevent the child from removing the tracheotomy tube.

Normally, air is filtered, warmed and moistened in the upper respiratory tract before it is breathed into the lungs. After tracheotomy, nursing measures must provide warm, moist and filtered air for the child to breathe. Care in a "croup tent" will provide warm, moist air. Two thicknesses of gauze saturated with normal saline solution placed over the opening of the tracheotomy tube will filter and moisten the inspired air. The gauze should be changed as it becomes dry and soiled with drainage.

A tray with the following sterile equipment should be at the child's bedside: duplicate tracheotomy tubes, with tapes attached, obturator, scissors, 2 curved clamps, pipe cleaners, medicine dropper, gauze dressings, tongue depressors, applicators and a catheter No. 8 or 10 F. which has additional holes near the tip to facilitate aspiration. Other necessary equipment includes 2 covered jars of sterile normal saline solution, a jar of hydrogen peroxide, a jar of sterile petrolatum and suction apparatus.

Constant nursing care is required for the infant or child after tracheotomy has been done. He cannot cry or call, and respiratory embarrassment results when aspiration does not keep the tracheotomy tube free from mucus and drainage. The child must become accustomed to breathing through the tube. In the adjustment period, the nurse should be in constant attendance to soothe the infant and allay the anxiety of the older child. During the first 48 hours after tracheotomy, the tube must be cleaned frequently by aspiration. The frequency is dependent on the amount of drainage and the needs of the individual child. Inspired mucus or drainage causes pneumonia; aspiration must keep it removed from the respiratory tract. Before aspiration, a few drops of normal saline solution should be put into the tracheotomy tube with a medicine dropper. The drops of normal saline moisten dried mucus, stimulate coughing, loosen the mucus and make it easier to aspirate. Aspiration tends to produce excitement, fear and coughing. Un-

til the child learns that the procedure brings him relief, reassurance is necessary. After the lock of the tube has been turned upward toward the face, the inner canula should be removed and placed in the jar of hydrogen peroxide. To aspirate, the catheter should be compressed and inserted through the outer canula opening until it reaches approximately the end of the tube. Then compression on the tube should be released to aspirate the secretions. The catheter should be removed, flushed with normal saline solution and reinserted until all drainage has been removed. After aspirating, the inner canula should be cleansed with pipe cleaners and hydrogen peroxide and, before it is reinserted into the outer canula, it should be examined carefully to ensure complete cleanliness. If aspiration and cleansing of the inner canula does not relieve the child's respiratory difficulty, the physician should be notified at once.

The dressing around the tracheotomy tube should be changed as frequently as necessary. Applicators dipped in hydrogen peroxide should be used to cleanse the area round the incision, and a tongue depressor should be used to coat the area with sterile petrolatum. A gauze square cut to the center should be placed round the tube and under the tapes that hold the tube in position. Any bleeding from or signs of infection in the wound should be reported. Before the dressing is changed and before aspirating the tube, the nurse's hands should be washed thoroughly. If the tube should be coughed or pulled out, the nurse should establish an airway by spreading the incision with a curved clamp.

Fluids and food may be given the child as he tolerates them. In the early period after tracheotomy, the child may be fearful of swallowing lest he have pain. However, as he finds that it causes him no discomfort, he will begin to take fluids and food more eagerly. Any coughing associated with swallowing should be reported.

When drainage and respiratory difficulty have ceased, a cork plug is inserted in the inner canula to obstruct the tube partially. Gradually, the opening is obstructed completely, and breathing takes place entirely outside the tube, the trachea being much larger than the tube. If no respiratory embarrassment occurs during the ensuing 24 hours, the tracheotomy tube is removed, and the wound is closed and covered with a sterile dressing. The tray containing the duplicate tracheotomy tube and obturator should be kept at the bedside until respiratory difficulty has subsided completely. Continued observation is imperative always during this period.

ACUTE LARYNGOTRACHEO-BRONCHITIS

ETIOLOGY

The causative organism is variable and sometimes not determined. Hemolytic streptococci, influenza bacilli and pneumococci at times appear to be responsible, but frequently no bacteria other than those normally expected in the pharynx can be isolated. Often, infection with a virus has been suspected but never proved. The disease appears to depend more upon the low re-

sistance of the individual child than upon the specific infecting agent. It is much more common in infancy and early childhood than at later ages.

SYMPTOMS

The symptoms depend in part on the severity of the infection, but in larger measure on the character of the exudate. The temperature tends to be high. The inflamed tissues are edematous, but the edema does not cause special difficulty except as it may affect the vocal cords and the region immediately below them and produce obstruction to respiration. In all instances the inflammatory exudate is a major cause of symptoms. It is so thick and viscous that it cannot be coughed up. The normal reflex for cough is incited by movement of foreign material in the respiratory tract. If the material is exudate that is too thick to move, no cough occurs. Thus the cough reflex may be abolished. Respiratory obstruction may occur from accumulation of the exudate. A large bronchus may become plugged with exudate, and so atelectasis of that part of the lung supplied by the bronchus results. Air passing partial obstruction causes stridor. Dyspnea and cyanosis also result from respiratory obstruction. The mortality is high. Death may be due to respiratory obstruction, to secondary pneumonia, to general sepsis or to exhaustion.

TREATMENT

Immediate treatment includes full dosage with one of the broad-spectrum antibiotics such as Oxytetracycline (Terramycin), chlortetracycline (Aureomycin) or chloramphenicol and placement of the child in an atmosphere saturated with water vapor. How much additional treatment is given will depend upon individual circumstances and often requires astute clinical judgment. The administration of oxygen may give immediate relief of cyanosis and dyspnea, but unless the oxygen is well humidified, ultimately it may aggravate the disease by drying out the thick secretions and making it more difficult for the child to cough them up from the respiratory tract. When obstruction at the larynx is severe, tracheotomy must be done. Sometimes the decision to do a tracheotomy is delayed too long; at other times the tracheotomy increases the inspissation of mucus in the bronchial tree and leads to generalized obstruction of bronchioles. Sedatives must be used with caution, and atropine derivatives are contraindicated. When the child is struggling to maintain his respirations, food and oral fluids are best avoided and hydration preserved through subcutaneous infusions.

Nursing Care

Careful observation is essential in all cases of acute laryngotracheobronchitis. A close watch must be kept for evidence of increasing respiratory obstruction or fatigue. Advancing cyanosis, restlessness, tachycardia, or pyrexia are danger signals which should be called to the attention of the physician. If a tracheotomy has been done, the care of the patient is similar to that described in the preceding section. Even when the tube is in place, continued watchfulness must be maintained to detect evidence of obstruc-

tion at the end of the tube or deeper in the branches of the bronchial tree. General reassurance and adept attention to the patient's needs without disturbing him unnecessarily are important factors in maintaining comfort and preserving his strength. Often the nursing care is rendered under uncomfortable conditions because of the absolute necessity of maintaining a very humid environment around the patient.

BRONCHITIS

Acute Bronchitis

Etiology and Symptoms. Acute bronchitis is one of the common illnesses of infancy and childhood. It is somewhat more frequent before 2 or 3 years of age than after. It may be primary or secondary. When primary, it has much the same causes as the common cold; when secondary, it is a complication of other diseases.

The mild and common variety of acute bronchitis usually has a gradual onset. For the first 2 or 3 days the temperature may be from 100° to 102° F., after which time it becomes approximately normal. Prostration is not great and is of short duration. The appetite is decreased, and lassitude and headache are present. During the first few days the cough is dry and nonproductive. The usual resonance to percussion over the chest remains unchanged. Auscultation reveals rales which are variously described as dry, sonorous and whistling. Moisture gradually appears in the bronchi, and after a few days the rales become bubbling. The cough becomes looser and productive. Cough is often started by change in position. It is increased in the morning on awakening and on first lying down at night. The cough is variable in severity in different cases. In some instances, repeated paroxysms of cough disturb sleep through the night. In the average child bronchitis may be expected to last from 7 to 10 days.

In the more severe type of bronchitis the smaller bronchi are affected. This type is more common in infants than in older children. The rales are smaller, and fever and prostration are greater than in cases of bronchitis of the larger tubes. Pneumonia is much more likely to result. The cough is tight, and dyspnea and cyanosis may be present. In infants, diarrhea and vomiting are common.

In many instances, bronchitis in infancy and early childhood is associated with asthmatic symptoms. In these cases, wheezing respiration is prominent, and difficulty in getting sufficient air into and out of the lungs may be experienced. The asthma disappears along with the symptoms of bronchitis.

Treatment and Nursing Care. Children with bronchitis should be kept in bed while fever is present. In mild bronchitis this period will be only a few days. They should be kept in the house in inclement weather for a week. The clothing need be no different from that worn by the children when they are in health, either day or night. It is desirable to have sufficient clothing to maintain a more or less normal skin temperature.

In the acute stage of bronchitis, inhalations of "steam" with or without the addition of benzoin or creosote are useful. These may be given for periods of from 15 to 30 minutes

every 3 to 6 hours, or as ordered. The air of the room should be kept fresh but warm and preferably moist. A good room temperature is from 68° to 70° F.

Drugs other than those used for chemotherapy accomplish little except symptomatically. If cough is distressing, a sedative is indicated. Expectorant mixtures are commonly employed, but their usefulness is doubtful. Chemotherapy is indicated when bronchitis is severe, but usually not when the illness is mild, especially in the older child.

OBSTRUCTIVE BRONCHITIS OF INFANCY (CAPILLARY BRONCHITIS, BRONCHIOLITIS)

Etiology and Symptoms. Sometimes infants are afflicted with a type of diffuse bronchitis which blocks the egress of air from the air sacs and results in overdistention of the lungs, dyspnea, cyanosis and exhaustion. The disorder has no specific bacterial etiology. It may result from any process that produces widespread inflammation of the bronchial mucous membrane in a small infant. The swollen mucosa and the sticky exudate within the lumen of the tiny bronchioles may permit air to enter the alveoli during inspiration, but the orifice closes and traps air within the lung tissue during expiration. Each breath thus adds more to the volume of air within the lung without permitting an equivalent amount to escape. As the lungs become progressively distended many of the alveoli lose their normal function of aerating the blood since they are unable to exchange the air from which oxygen has already been absorbed. Small areas of pneumonia may also be present within the lungs.

The infant with obstructive bronchitis displays an overdistended chest which collapses poorly on expiration and retracts during inspiration. The respiratory effort is labored, rapid and shallow. As the process advances, varying degrees of cyanosis appear. The infant is restless, has a hacking cough and eats and sleeps poorly. Fever may be absent, intermediate or high. In fatal cases the child dies from exhaustion and inability to oxygenate his blood. Usually the severe stage of the disease is limited to a period of two or three days.

Treatment and Nursing Care. Antibiotic therapy is usually given at once, although its effectiveness is variable. In some instances the response is prompt; in others the drug selected has no effect. Measures similar to those used in laryngotracheobronchitis should be employed to keep the bronchial secretions fluid and as mobile as possible. The air should be completely saturated with moisture, and oxygen must be used cautiously because of its drying effect. Infants often get some relief from being placed on their abdomens, since this fosters better drainage of secretions from the trachea and permits the weight of the back to assist in compressing the distended lungs during expiration. The fluid intake should be maintained by subcutaneous infusion if necessary. Feedings may be omitted temporarily if the infant finds the process of eating too tiring.

Chronic Bronchitis

Bronchitis that lingers or recurs over a period of several weeks usu-ally is associated with persisting infection of the paranasal sinuses or adenoids. The symptoms are cough which is worse at night and on arising, and a sensation of tickling in the throat or the trachea. Fever is usually lacking. Treatment must be directed at the focus of infection in the upper respiratory tract. Chronic bronchitis also accompanies other conditions such as cystic fibrosis of the pancreas, asthma and bronchiectasis. The possibility of tuberculosis or heart disease must be entertained when other explanations are lacking.

Bronchiectasis

Bronchiectasis is an extreme form of chronic bronchitis in which branches of the bronchial tree are enlarged or sacculated as a result of the distorting effects of infection which has penetrated beyond the mucous membrane.

Etiology. Certain of the contagious diseases—whooping cough, measles and influenza—are sometimes complicated by a type of pneumonia that damages the structure of the bronchial wall and fosters prolonged infection. Long-standing sinusitis or foreign bodies that have lodged in the bronchi may also be responsible for perpetuating the infection that results in bronchiectasis. No specific bacteria are responsible.

Symptoms. The chief symptom of bronchiectasis is chronic cough that produces purulent sputum. Fever is not usually present except during bouts of superimposed pneumonia or acute sinusitis. If the disease is extensive the breath may be malodorous, the child's nutrition poor, and there may be enlargement of the ends of the fingers and the toes (clubbing). Usually there is some degree of nasal obstruction due to the chronic sinus infection which is a common companion of bronchiectasis.

Diagnosis. The disease should be suspected when there is a history of chronic cough and sputum production over a period of months or years. Ordinary chest roentgenograms do not provide conclusive evidence of the deformity of the bronchial tree. Films taken after the instillation of an opaque oil such as Lipiodol are required to outline accurately the location and the extent of the disease (Fig. 30).

Prognosis and Treatment. With the possible exception of mild bronchiectasis in which the dilatation is slight, the disease tends to progress very slowly because the abnormal structures never can quite clear themselves of the infected secretions. Medical treatment attempts to clear up sinus infection when present and to provide regular systematic drainage of secretions from the bronchial tree by postural drainage. In the latter procedure the child is placed head down over the side of the bed and kept in this position for increasing periods of time several times a day to let the

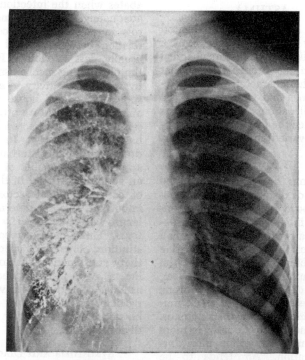

Fig. 30. Bronchiectasis of the lower lobe of the left lung shown by "mapping" the left lung.

infected portions of lung completely discharge their contents by gravity. Antibiotic therapy and periodic aspiration through a bronchoscope may supplement this procedure. Sometimes antibiotics are given in the form of an aerosol which the child inhales for a quarter or a half hour 2 or 3 times a day. When it is apparent that medical measures are not stemming the progress of the disease, surgical removal of the diseased lobe or lobes of lung must be considered. If the disease involves only the lower portion of one lung, successful operation usually results in a permanent cure.

ASTHMA

Asthma is really a complicated pulmonary symptom rather than a specific disease. The mechanical changes in the bronchial tree that lead to the characteristic obstruction, dyspnea and wheezing are the same in all patients, but the factors that produce the mechanical disturbances are varied and often complex.

ETIOLOGY

The lungs are afflicted by the same sort of disturbance as that described above for obstructive bronchitis of infancy. There is widespread narrowing of the small branches of the bronchial tree due to a combination of spasm of the circular muscles surrounding them, of edema of the mucous membrane which lines them, and of thick mucus contained within their lumens. The obstruction to air flow is more marked during expiration than during inspiration. Air tends to be trapped in the alveoli, producing overdistention of the lung and re-

quiring the child to make a forcible effort during expiration in order to push air through the narrowed bronchioles. The result is an overdistended (emphysematous) chest with rapid, shallow inspirations and prolonged wheezing expirations.

Children who have asthma are generally considered to be allergic subjects. This implies a constitutional predisposition toward abnormal sensitization and in many instances the trait is clearly inherited. Among infants and young children the appearance of asthma is usually restricted to periods when there is obvious acute infection of the respiratory tract and the symptom abates when the infection is treated adequately. Infection may play a role in older children too, but the relation between it and asthma is usually less obvious. Frequently, the obstructing mechanism is set off by specific sensitivity to an inhalant such as ragweed, house dust or an animal dander. More often, specific sensitivites are suspected but cannot be identified clearly. In some children emotional disturbances alone appear to be capable of setting off an attack of asthma; in the majority of cases emotional factors play an important role in determining the length and the severity of symptoms. Thus, one can recognize constitution, infection, specific sensitivity and emotional factors as playing a part in the production of asthma. The degree to which each participates is a matter that must be determined by study of the individual child.

SYMPTOMS AND DIAGNOSIS

A typical asthmatic attack usually occurs in a school-age child abruptly at night and without antecedent illness. There is no fever. The child develops a hacking cough and has difficulty sleeping because of the necessity for making a conscious effort to breathe. He finds that he must push during expiration and that he is more comfortable if he is propped up in bed. Characteristically, he is quiet, less upset than his parents are about the symptoms and tends to resist efforts to assist him. He seems to prefer to be left alone to cope as well as he can with the necessary task of breathing. Mild cyanosis may be present. Asphyxiating asthma is rare in children, except in those who have repeated attacks over a long period of time. After the symptom has persisted for a day or two the child may produce thick tenacious secretions during coughing spells. The symptoms tend to become worse at night and to clear somewhat in the daytime. Sleep and the ingestion of food may be seriously curtailed during prolonged attacks. Single attacks may be as brief as an hour or may last for several days to be followed by an additional period of bronchitis.

The diagnosis is made by observation or from the accurate description of an attack by the parent. It is confirmed by physical examination and analysis of the character of the respirations. Prompt relief following the injection of adrenalin helps to substantiate the diagnosis. Determination of the precipitating factors for the individual child is usually a difficult and protracted process which may involve allergic technics or the services of a child psychiatrist, or both.

TREATMENT OF THE ACUTE ATTACK

Adrenalin administered by injection or by inhalation usually gives relief for a brief period of time. Ephedrine and aminophyllin operate more slowly but have a longer-lasting effect. Treatment is usually more effective if used early after the appearance of symptoms. Sedation with barbiturates is helpful in reducing the child's anxiety and encouraging sleep. If the attack is prolonged or severe, removal to a hospital is usually desirable. For reasons which probably are grounded in the relief of emotional tension, treatment of asthma in a hospital setting is rapidly effective in nearly all instances, even though the same measures have been tried previously at home without too much result. Unusually severe attacks of asthma may require oxygen administration or the use of ACTH or cortisone.

PREVENTION OF FUTURE ATTACKS

To forestall future attacks of asthma it is necessary to understand the importance of the various factors that precipitate attacks in the individual child. Sometimes the task is relatively simple. If attacks occur only at certain seasons in the year, pollen sensitivity is likely to be responsible, and the offending agent can be discovered by allergic skin testing. Treatment then depends upon the individual's avoiding the pollen in question, or if this is not feasible, in receiving desensitizing injections over a period of several weeks. When asthmatic attacks are clearly related to the onset of respiratory infections, the attention must be directed toward clearing up sources of chronic infection in the nose and the throat if such can be identified. When the child is losing an excessive amount of sleep or is unable to attend school because of recurring respiratory infections with asthma, sometimes it is desirable to keep him on small doses of sulfonamides or oral penicillin throughout the winter months as prophylaxis against reinfection—a technic which is commonly used for the child with rheumatic fever.

When the factors which precipitate asthma are not so obvious, prolonged allergic or psychiatric study may be required to bring the symptoms under control. Since both of these technics are likely to be long, arduous and upsetting to both the child and the parents, generally they are reserved for children whose asthma is frequent, disabling or so severe that permanent damage to the structure of the lung is threatened if they continue. Severe prolonged asthma almost always stems from an emotional conflict between the child and some member of his immediate family. The most careful and extensive program of desensitization, drug management or change of climate may be unavailing if no consideration is given to the psychological implications of the disorder.

PNEUMONIA
(PNEUMONITIS)

Pneumonia or pneumonitis is an inflammation of the lung. It may be caused by any pyogenic bacterium or, in some instances, by a virus. It may occur as a primary disease or it may be a secondary or complicating infection in association with some other illness. As a primary infection with pneumococci, the inflammation may be massive in one lobe of a lung and involve all the alveoli of the lobe. In such case the disease is designated as lobar pneumonia. Pneumonia may be disseminated in various parts of the lungs, not be confined to a lobe or not involve a whole lobe completely, and in such case the disease is designated as lobular pneumonia or bronchopneumonia. Regardless of the cause or the type of pneumonia, the function of the lungs is affected in a characteristic manner.

In pneumonia, the affected portions of the lungs are not aerated because the air spaces (alveoli) are filled with exudate. This factor, together with the shallow breathing of this disease, causes poor oxygenation of the blood. Blood that passes through the affected portion remains unaerated and venous in character, and later mingles with the blood from the aerated portions of the lungs. Blood passing through the aerated portions cannot be oxygenated sufficiently, even with oxygen therapy, to compensate for the lack of oxygenation in the affected portion. Thus the oxygen saturation of arterial blood is always reduced in pneumonia. The average reduction in lobar pneumonia is approximately 15 per cent. It is greater in bronchopneumonia. Symptoms of anoxia (oxygen want due to defective oxygenation) appear when the blood has reached about 85 per cent oxygen saturation. The mortality rate increases as the saturation decreases. The rate is high with saturation less than 80 per cent.

The shallow breathing of pneumonia is caused in part by the inflammation of the lung, a reflex mechanism. Often, in addition, the breathing is shallow because of pain on breathing, as when pleurisy is present. This effect on the breathing is increased by the effect of anoxia on the respiratory center; the greater the anoxia the more shallow the breathing.

Anoxia produces cyanosis, dyspnea and cerebral symptoms, including delirium and inability to sleep. These symptoms increase as anoxia increases. Anoxia is also a cause of failure of circulation. The cardiovascular system is affected adversely by lack of oxygen. It suffers also because of excessive loss of carbon dioxide produced by dyspnea. When carbon dioxide of the blood is lowered, hemoglobin gives up its oxygen less easily, thus increasing the effect of anoxia.

Pneumonia occurring as a complication of some other illness is called secondary pneumonia and is of the lobular pneumonic or bronchopneumonic type, regardless of the age of the child. It may be caused by almost any pyogenic bacterium. Primary pneumonia (caused by pneumococci) is of the lobar type in the older child and the adult, but in the infant it is of the lobular type. Lobular pneumonia or bronchopneumonia of the primary type behaves differently from that of the secondary type. However, primary pneumonia of infants resembles secondary pneumonia in many of its symptoms and signs, and by many authors these two conditions are classified in the one group of lobular pneumonia or bronchopneumonia. One reason for considering these two conditions together is that clinically in the early stages of the disease it is not always possible to distinguish one from the other. Some authors choose to classify pneumonia according to the infecting organism. Each classification has its advantages. It is chosen here to discuss pneumonia from the standpoint of its clinical appearance.

PRIMARY BACTERIAL PNEUMONIA

As a primary disease pneumonia is likely to appear suddenly, without warning, or with only mild preceding symptoms, such as those accompanying a common cold. It classifies easily as a communicable disease, although predisposing factors are important. Anything that lowers resistance, such as a chill, predisposes to pneumonia when pneumococci are present. In most instances, primary pneumonia is not caused by organisms commonly found in the mouth. A few types of pneumococci are found only with pneumonia.

Primary pneumonia of infants is a disseminated inflammation in the lungs in contrast with lobar pneumonia, the primary pneumonia of the older child, which is localized and sharply limited in extent. The same conditions of infection produce these two quite different types of lesion. Presumably the difference is due to immunologic changes with age. The infantile type is found chiefly in the first two years after birth, and after this time with decreasing frequency. Lobar pneumonia is seldom observed in the first year, but it occurs with increasing frequency with advancing age and becomes the predominant type after 3 or 4 years of age.

Primary Pneumonia in Infants. SYMPTOMS. The onset of primary pneumonia in infancy is likely to be sudden, with fever and prostration. Vomiting is frequent, and convulsions may occur at onset. The temperature is high and usually irregular, with fluctuations of from 3° to 4° F. The respirations are rapid, from 60 to 70 or more to the minute, and associated with effort and with retraction of the soft parts of the chest on inspiration. The alae of the nose move laterally with each inspiration. The pulse rate increases to 160 or more and is likely to be irregular. Cough is frequent, persistent and annoying. Moderate diarrhea usually is present. Leukocytosis is high (20,000 to 50,000). Blood culture grows the pneumococcus occasionally and with greater frequency than in lobar pneumonia. In the milder illnesses and without chemotherapy, improvement occurs in approximately a week. In the more severe illnesses, improvement, if it occurs, may not be observed for as much as 2 weeks or even longer.

Certain exceptions to the clinical course as described are to be encountered. On rare occasions a hyperacute form occurs, with stormy onset, high temperature and extreme prostration. Death may occur in from 12 to 48 hours after the onset and before any physical signs have developed in the chest. In some instances of primary pneumonia in infancy severe enough to cause death, the temperature may remain low. This type of illness occurs especially in young, delicate and malnourished infants. Also in delicate infants, pneumonia, although it may have the usual course at first, may spread from one area to another, thus prolonging the illness, increasing prostration, causing emaciation and usually terminating in death. This course is not so likely with the use of modern chemotherapy.

DIAGNOSIS. The correct diagnosis is often suspected by an experienced person merely from observation of the infant's respiratory behavior. Physical examination of the chest discloses areas of moist rales in the involved portions of lung. When the patches of consolidation are large enough there may be typical changes in the quality of the breath sounds heard through a stethoscope. Roentgen examination is frequently conclusive, but if the consolidated areas are small, interpretation of the shadows which they cast is sometimes difficult. The etiologic diagnosis is important as a guide to proper antibiotic therapy. Cultures of the nose, the throat, or sputum when it is available, always should be made. Blood cultures may yield the invading organism in some instances. Once isolated, the organism should be tested for sensitivity to the various antibiotics in order to speed selection of the most effective drug.

COMPLICATIONS AND PROGNOSIS. Otitis media and fibrinous pleurisy are common complications of pneumonia; usually they are not serious and they respond to the treatment being given for the pneumonia itself. Rarely, an infant develops meningitis, peritonitis or empyema. These serious complications increase the mortality of the disease and require special measures of treatment as described under the sections that deal with them.

Primary pneumonia of infancy is a serious disease if it remains untreated or is treated inadequately. Before modern antibiotic treatment was available the mortality rates ranged as high as 30 to 50 per cent. The outlook is very much better today, but pneumonia in the small infant is not a disease to be regarded lightly.

TREATMENT AND NURSING CARE. Most of the cases of primary pneumonia in infancy are caused by pneumococci or hemolytic streptococci. These organisms respond promptly to penicillin, which should be given intramuscularly in full dosage. Other types of antibiotic may be necessary when the pneumonia is shown to be due to organisms other than the above or when a resistant strain is encountered. Ordinarily, if treatment is effective the infant's temperature will approach normal levels within 24 hours. A delay in response beyond 48 hours should raise the suspicion that the wrong antibiotic has been selected. Immediate testing of the sensitivity of organisms isolated from infants with pneumonia will greatly assist in directing the choice of drug.

Oxygen is administered when there is cyanosis or other evidence of anoxia. Methods of administration and nursing care are described in the next chapter.

In a large measure the nursing care of the infant with pneumonia is symptomatic and geared to his individual requirements. He requires rest and relief of his physical and psychological discomforts. Nursing procedures should be organized in such a way as to disturb the infant as little as possible. Frequently, feedings are omitted until the expected improvement from antibiotic therapy has taken place. Usually fluids are administered by mouth when possible; by subcutaneous infusion when necessary. The infant's position may influence his comfort to some extent. He may be more

comfortable in a semierect posture or when lying with the affected lung down.

Abdominal distention from paralytic ileus is a common and distressing aspect of pneumonia in infants. It is both painful and embarrassing to the respiratory effort and should be relieved by enemas or by the external application of turpentine stupes. Turpentine and sweet oil are used in a proportion of 3 cc. of turpentine to 30 cc. of sweet oil. The two ingredients should be mixed thoroughly, and the mixture should be applied to the skin of the abdomen with cotton balls before and during the procedure. The warmth of the wet flannel stupes should be tested on the back of the hand before they are applied to the abdomen. Oiled silk and dry flannel should be applied over the wet stupes. The wet flannels should be changed every 3 minutes for a period of from 15 to 20 minutes. During the procedure a rectal tube should be kept in place to facilitate the passage of flatus. Children burn easily, and the condition of the skin should be observed very carefully each time the procedure is repeated. Oiling the skin after the stupe has been completed tends to keep the skin in good condition.

Temperatures up to 104° F. usually require no special measures for their control. Excessive fever is best controlled by hydrotherapy. Hydrotherapy is useful also for restlessness, nervousness and insomnia. Since pneumonia is a communicable disease, isolation precautions must be taken.

Lobar Pneumonia. SYMPTOMS AND DIAGNOSIS. Lobar pneumonia is abrupt in its onset, any preceding indisposition being not more than a few hours in duration. Vomiting is frequent among the symptoms of onset, and, especially in young children, diarrhea is common. The temperature elevation is rapid, sometimes rapid enough to cause a chill or a convulsion, although chills are much more frequent in adults than in children. The temperature rises to 104° or more and remains elevated continuously with relatively little remission throughout the course of the marked symptoms. Along with the temperature rise, the pulse and the respiration rates increase, the respiration out of proportion to the other two. The nasal alae move laterally with each inspiration. Very quickly after the onset the child appears to be acutely ill, becomes apathetic and weak and loses his appetite. Restlessness and marked thirst are common. Cough appears a day or two after onset and persists, although seldom is it annoying.

When specific or chemotherapy is not used, the disease runs a rather typical course. Although the child may be somewhat more comfortable after 4 or 5 days, little change in the symptoms is to be observed until the crisis, which may be expected about the sixth or the seventh day. Sometimes the temperature drops temporarily and briefly the day preceding the crisis. This drop has been termed the pseudocrisis. The crisis represents termination of the acute symptoms. The temperature drops rapidly to normal, as do also the pulse and the respiration rates. The child becomes comfortable, loses his apathy, regains his appetite and recovers rapidly and completely. The physical signs of lobar pneu-

monia consist chiefly of those produced by a massive area of consolidation in a lung. With typical involvement of an entire lobe, dullness on percussion and tubular breathing on auscultation over the affected lobe are easy to determine. Rales are seldom prominent. After the crisis, however, when the exudate is liquefying, rales are characteristically present. Early in the illness the consolidation may involve only part of a lobe, perhaps only the periphery. In such case, when no continuity of consolidated lung between the stethoscope and a large bronchus exists, tubular breathing is not heard. Without a roentgenogram the diagnosis of pneumonia or at least its localization may be difficult.

The diagnosis of lobar pneumonia is accomplished in the same way as that described for primary pneumonia of infants. Typical findings of lobar pneumonia almost always mean that the infecting agent is a pneumococcus. Sometimes roentgen examination will disclose a shadow which cannot be detected by physical examination; conversely, the physical findings may precede the appearance of consolidation which is visible in the roentgenogram.

PROGNOSIS. Uncomplicated lobar pneumonia in the child of 3 years or over carries a very good prognosis. Even before antibiotics were available the mortality was as low as 3 to 5 per cent. Today the response to therapy is almost invariably prompt, and few children succumb unless the disease is complicated by myocarditis, empyema or meningitis.

TREATMENT AND NURSING CARE. This differs in no essential point from that given for primary pneumonia of infants.

SECONDARY BACTERIAL PNEUMONIA (BRONCHOPNEUMONIA, LOBULAR PNEUMONIA)

Secondary pneumonia is lobular, or bronchopneumonia and is similar in many respects to primary pneumonia of infants. It may occur at any age as a complication of any acute illness. It is a more frequent complication in infancy than in late childhood. It is especially frequent as a complication of measles, pertussis, diphtheria, influenza and bronchitis.

Etiology. Any one or several of a variety of organisms may be found associated with the disease as the cause. In a large measure, secondary pneumonia is caused by the ordinary bacteria of the pharynx and the upper respiratory tract which gain entrance to the lungs by aspiration or during inspiration. Hemolytic streptococcic pneumonia, such as occurs in measles, must be considered as communicable.

Symptoms. The onset of secondary pneumonia is usually gradual, with subsequent increase in the severity of the illness. The amount of fever varies with the severity of the illness and the general condition of the child. In general, it tends to be high and irregular or intermittent in type. Prostration is present. The symptoms and signs are the same as those described for primary pneumonia of infants. Clinically, secondary pneumonia differs from primary pneumonia chiefly in its persistence. In the absence of modern chemotherapy, the course of secondary pneumonia tends to be protracted and, as a rule, lasts for a period of from 3 to 6 weeks. Sometimes during this period new areas of inflammation develop while older ones may be subsiding. The symptoms end by lysis in nearly all instances of spontaneous recovery. Recovery is slow, and relapses are relatively frequent. Pleurisy is seldom a striking feature in secondary pneumonia, except when streptococci are the cause. Occasionally, streptococcic empyema occurs.

Prognosis. Secondary pneumonia is a much more serious disease than primary pneumonia. Several factors contribute to its relatively bad prognosis. Many of the victims are already weak and poorly nourished from the effects of a protracted illness or from convalescence following a surgical procedure. Their resistance is consequently poor. If the original illness is characterized by vomiting or immobility, some of the pulmonary changes may actually be due to lipid pneumonia from aspiration of milk or to atelectasis from failure to clear the secretions from the bronchi. The type of secondary pneumonia which follows acute contagious diseases, such as pertussis, measles and influenza, may respond adequately to antibiotic therapy but may invade the structure of the lung to set the stage for bronchiectasis as described in a preceding section. The bacterial etiology of secondary pneumonia is often mixed or composed of organisms which are less easily influenced by the available antibiotics.

Treatment and Nursing Care. The same measures are required as in the case of primary pneumonia. Some prevention of secondary pneumonia is possible if its occurrence is anticipated. Chronically ill or immobile patients should be isolated from contact with respiratory infections among the patients around them. They should have their positions changed frequently to avoid imperfect ventilation of portions of the lung. Sometimes prophylactic administration of antibiotics is warranted when the risk of secondary pneumonia is great.

SPECIAL TYPES OF PNEUMONIA

Staphylococcus Pneumonia. Pneumonia that is due to infection with the staphylococcus is mainly a disease of small infants. Occasionally, it is seen as a complication of staphylococcus bacteremia in the older child or the adult. The disease is characterized by a tendency to form multiple abscesses throughout the lungs. Even in small infants the contents of these abscesses may be apparent in purulent sputum or vomitus. Abscesses that form on the surface of the lung often create an empyema or pneumothorax by discharging their contents into the pleural cavity and at the same time establishing a communication between the pleural cavity and the bronchial tree. The diagnosis is made by culture of sputum and by the discovery of characteristic abscess shadows in the roentgenogram of the chest. Treatment is complicated by the fact that increasing numbers of staphylococci are becoming resistant to the older antibiotic drugs such as penicillin. The newer antibiotics, such as erythromycin or chloromycetin, are more regularly effective than penicillin, but the sensitivity of each individual strain must be tested in order to guide treatment. When empyema is present, the mechanical principles described in the next section should be used. Untreated, staphylococcus pneumonia is almost universally fatal. Even with early and adequate treatment by antibiotic drugs the mortality is likely to approach 25 per cent. Small infants may die before the nature of the disease is recognized.

Primary Atypical Pneumonia. This is a type of pneumonia, presumably caused by a virus, which produces symptoms of cough, fever and general malaise. Its course is likely to be protracted to 2 or 3 weeks in length, but the child is seldom alarmingly ill, and the prognosis is universally good. Diagnosis is made by exclusion of bacterial pneumonia and by the discovery of various types of pulmonary consolidation in the roentgenogram of the chest, often in the absence of physical signs in the chest. The treatment is entirely symptomatic. Chlortetracycline (Aureomycin) has been considered effective in shortening the course of the illness, but its worth is debated. There are no complications of this type of pneumonia.

Kerosene Pneumonia. Small children in the toddling age occasionally swallow kerosene which is carelessly left around the home. Frequently, an extensive pneumonia ensues due to the irritant effect of kerosene which has been aspirated or is being excreted from the body by way of the lungs. Immediately after ingestion of kerosene the child may feel well except for nausea. Respiratory symptoms and fever appear during the first 48 hours and pursue a variable course, depending upon the amount of kerosene taken. In mild cases there may be little or no pulmonary irritation and no fever. When large amounts are taken and retained, hyperpyrexia, dyspnea and convulsions may ensue. The roentgenogram of the chest usually demonstrates large areas of pulmonary consolidation extending out from the central portion of the lung fields. In the absence of hyperpyrexia and convulsions, the child usually recovers completely after a few days of dyspnea and cough. Diagnosis can be made from the characteristic odor of kerosene. Early treatment probably demands gastric lavage to recover as much of the kerosene as possible from the stomach. Treatment of the pneumonia, once it is present, is mainly symptomatic and directed at control of hyperpyrexia.

Lipid Pneumonia. Lipid pneumonia is pneumonitis produced by oils or fatty material aspirated into the lung. It occurs chiefly in small, weak infants, seldom in older children, unless the cough reflex is diminished. The aspirated fat may be nose drops, cod-liver oil, mineral oil or fat from the milk formula that has been vomited. Fats of animal origin have more severe effects than those of vegetable origin. A very few fats have no ill effect; for example, the poppyseed oil used in the preparation of iodized oil.

Lipid pneumonia tends to occur in the posterior dependent portions of the lung, more often on the right side. The onset is insidious, often without symptoms. In such instances it is diagnosed by x-ray examination. Small infants develop dry, nonproductive cough and rapid respirations. They usually show impairment of growth. Older children also have chronic cough and, in addition, are subject to repeated attacks of bronchitis. Occasionally, bronchiectasis results. Evidences of inflammation, such as fever and leukocytosis, vary according to the amount of associated infection. Often no infection is present.

Diagnosis is made chiefly by exclusion. Always more of a lesion is present than is indicated by physical examination. The distribution of the lesion on x-ray examination and its chronicity are helpful in diagnosis.

No special treatment exists. The milder forms may persist for as long as a year before recovery occurs. Severe forms produced by some of the animal fats may become complicated by abscess or bronchiectasis and persist for a much longer time.

Prevention is highly important. Oily nose drops should not be used in infancy. The giving of oils to young or weak infants must be done with caution, care being taken to see that they are swallowed.

PLEURISY

Pleurisy is an inflammation of the linings of the pleural cavity, i.e. the inside of the chest wall and the outer surface of the lung. It usually produces pain in the chest on respiration. Sometimes the pain is referred to the shoulder or to the abdomen. If the accumulation of inflammatory exudate is large, there may be embarrassment of the respirations and cyanosis.

The accumulation of exudates within the pleural space is seen in a wide variety of conditions. The term pleural effusion is used when the exudate is bacteriologically sterile. Effusion may be seen during nephrosis and with heart failure. It is rarely found in other conditions such as nephritis and over the lesions of pulmonary metastatic tumors. A variety of pleural effusion which is not really sterile is seen with early tuberculosis. During the course of pneumonia, fibrin is often deposited upon the surface of the lungs and produces pleural pain with pneumonia caused by staphylococci or hemolytic streptococci, or when adequate treatment of pneumococcus pneumonia is delayed, significant collections of infected purulent exudate may accumulate in the pleural space, forming an empyema that requires special attention.

EMPYEMA

Genesis. The onset of empyema after pneumonia usually is not very obvious. Pneumonia may end by crisis, and then the temperature gradually rises again; or the temperature may not fall at the time recovery from pneumonia is to be expected. At first the pus in the pleural sac is thin. It increases in amount and allows the lung on the affected side to collapse increasingly. Finally, it causes the heart to be displaced toward the opposite side of the chest. As the fluid increases in quantity, increasing cardiac and respiratory difficulty occurs. The child lies on the affected side. Withdrawal of the pus by aspiration is desirable to relieve these symptoms. In the course of several days, in the case of pneumococcic infection, the pus becomes thick, often so thick that it is not easily withdrawn through a needle.

Diagnosis. Increased dullness on percussion and altered breath sounds on auscultation are present in empyema. These should lead one to suspect that empyema is present. Roentgenograms are very helpful

and often make the diagnosis almost certain. The diagnosis is made definitely by removal of pus through an aspirating needle. Aspiration should be made at the point of maximum dullness, wherever it may be.

Course and Prognosis. Pus present in the pleural cavity in large quantity is not likely to be absorbed, although in some instances it may be. Rarely, it may drain spontaneously by making a way for itself through the soft tissues at some point between the ribs or through the lung tissue into a bronchus. Thus, in some cases empyema may terminate by spontaneous recovery. On the other hand, death may occur from wasting which accompanies chronic infection, from the spread of infection to the pericardium, or from compression of lung space to the point of insufficiency. Continuance of underlying pneumonia also may be a cause of death. The mortality rate from empyema is much higher in infancy than in later childhood. Also, it is higher in those cases in which radical surgical treatment is undertaken early than when very early treatment is more conservative. This is especially true in infancy and in those cases of pneumococcic empyema in which the pus has not yet become thick.

Treatment and Nursing Care. The chemotherapy that has been used through the course of preceding pneumonia should be continued. Otherwise, the early treatment, especially in infancy, should consist of nothing more radical than withdrawal of pus by aspiration. In many instances such treatment will be followed by absorption of the remaining pus and complete recovery. Recovery may be hastened by injecting from 50,000 to 100,000 units of penicillin in saline into the pleural cavity once or twice daily after aspiration. When empyema persists despite these measures, surgical drainage is indicated. Surgical drainage through the chest wall is greatly preferable to spontaneous drainage through a bronchus, since the latter may lead to chronic pneumonia and bronchiectasis.

Sometimes pus is not generally distributed throughout the pleural cavity but is encapsulated between the parietal and visceral layers of pleura. In such case also the treatment is the same as that already discussed. If the empyema is wholly interlobar, conservative treatment without operation is usually indicated.

THORACENTESIS may be done for diagnosis, for relief of dyspnea caused by pressure of fluid, for the obtaining of exudate for culture or for the instilling of penicillin into the pleural cavity. Sterile equipment required for thoracentesis consists of: 50-cc. syringe, 2-cc. syringe, hypodermic needles, 3-way stopcock with short piece of rubber tubing attached, aspirating needles, Novocaine 1 per cent, curved clamp, lumbar puncture drape sheet, cotton balls, small gauze squares, graduated receptacle, gloves and medication as ordered by the physician. Unsterile equipment consists of a skin preparation tray, culture media, test tubes and adhesive plaster. Epinephrine should be ready for use in case of need.

One of several positions may be required for successful thoracentesis. The child may be placed in a sitting position with his arms and trunk brought forward, or he may be placed on his unaffected side in a semirecumbent position. Whatever the position, care must be taken to ensure maximum comfort for the child. An overbed table and pillow to lean on may lessen exertion and provide a degree of comfort when a sitting position is desired for an older child. One nurse will be required to hold the child in the desired position, to prepare him for the procedure, to give him emotional support and to observe his response to treatment. A second nurse will be needed to assist with the skin preparation and to collect specimens of aspirated fluid. During the procedure the nurse should watch for changes in the child's respiration and pulse rates, for changes in his color and for any increase in coughing.

After the treatment the child should be kept warm and observed for changes in his general condition. Charting should include a description and the amount of the aspirated fluid, amount and kind of medication instilled, any symptoms of shock or syncope and the child's physical and psychological response to the treatment.

SITUATIONS FOR FURTHER STUDY

1. What help do parents need to prevent common colds in their children during the period of infancy and childhood?

2. What feelings do you think a hospitalized infant experiences when he is hospitalized for laryngotracheobronchitis? How can a nurse eliminate feelings of anxiety? Why is constant attendance of a mother or a nurse essential in his care?

3. In what diseases might a tracheotomy be necessary? How would the nursing care of those patients differ from the care necessary for a child who had had a tracheotomy after a foreign body had been removed from the respiratory tract?

4. A 3-year-old child with papilloma of the larynx required a tracheotomy. After the child had been hospitalized for a period of 6 weeks, the physician recommended that he be discharged from the hospital with the tracheotomy tube in place. What help would the child's mother require to take care of him at home? How could you help the mother to become reassured concerning her capacity to care for her child?

5. What psychological factors may precipitate an asthmatic attack?

BIBLIOGRAPHY

Bellam, Gwendoline: Tonsillectomy without fear, Am. J. Nursing **51:** 244, 1950.

Conley, J. J.: Tracheotomy, Am. J. Nursing **52:**1078, 1952.

Cutler, Harold: Otitis media, Am. J. Nursing **53:**573, 1953.

Gibson, Frances: Laryngotracheobronchitis, Am. J. Nursing **52:** 174, 1952.

Hall, J. T., and Sadler, J. B.: Nursing care in tonsillectomy, Am. J. Nursing **47:**537, 1947.

Lewis, D. K.: Deafness, Am. J. Nursing **52:**575, 1952.

Mohr, George, Gerard, Margaret, and Ross, Helen: Summary of psychoanalytic study of asthmatic children, Psychosom. Med. Monographs **1:**81, 1939-1941.

Neffson, A.: Acute Laryngotracheobronchitis, New York, Grune & Stratton, 1949.

Smith, K. M. and Gibbs, G. E.: Aerosol therapy for infants and children, Am. J. Nursing **50:**92, 1950.

Wilson, J. L.: Dyspnea in acute respiratory disease, Am. J. Nursing **47:**15, 1947.

CHAPTER TEN

Diseases of the Circulatory System

ANATOMY AND PHYSIOLOGY

The circulatory system consists of the heart and the blood vessels. The latter include the arteries, which carry the blood away from the heart, the capillaries, which are very small and numerous and connect the terminal branches of the arteries with the veins, and the veins, which carry blood back to the heart. The capillaries are the points of exchange between the blood stream and the tissues. All other divisions of the circulatory system serve only to maintain circulation of the blood through the capillaries.

The circulating blood has two great circuits: one of these is the pulmonary; the other, the systemic circulation. The heart is divided into two parts, known as the right and the left hearts. Each acts independently of the other, although they act synchronously. The right heart receives blood which is returning from the body tissues and pumps it into the capillaries of the lungs for aeration.

The blood returns from the lungs to the left heart, which then propels it to the various parts of the body (Fig. 31).

In the normal child, blood which is returning from the body by way of the great veins (venae cavae) and fills the right side of the heart and the branches of the pulmonary artery, is venous or unoxygenated blood (dotted line in the diagrams). Its relatively low oxygen content gives it a dark purple color. Once the blood has passed through the lung capillaries and becomes fully oxygenated, it is a bright red in color. Oxygenated blood (solid lines in the diagrams) normally is found in the pulmonary veins, the left side of the heart and all the branches of the aorta and the arterial system.

The heart, the arteries and the veins are made up of involuntary muscle surrounded by a supportive layer of fibrous tissue and lined by a thin membrane composed of endothelium. In the heart, these divisions are spoken of as myocardium, pericardium and endocardium, respectively. The integrity of each is essential for the normal functioning of the heart.

The capillaries consist of the endothelial layer alone. Their walls are very thin and are permeable to certain portions of the blood but not to others.

HEART CHAMBERS

Each side of the heart is divided into 2 chambers, the auricle and the ventricle. The former receives blood from the veins and serves as a reservoir for the supply of the ventricle. The latter serves to propel the blood through the arteries, the capillaries and the veins. The endocardium is so arranged that it forms

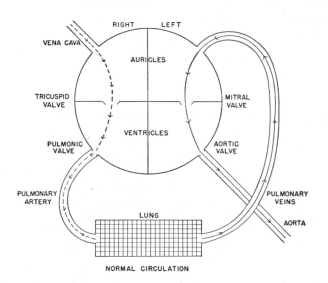

NORMAL CIRCULATION

FIG. 31. Diagram of the normal circulation of blood. Unoxygenated, or venous, blood is indicated by the dotted line from its entrance into the heart through the vena cava, thence into the right auricle, through the tricuspid valve into the right ventricle, out the pulmonic valve into the pulmonary artery and thence into the lungs, where it becomes oxygenated. The solid line indicates the course of the oxygenated blood through the pulmonary veins, the left auricle, the mitral valve, the left ventricle, the aortic valve and the aorta. The last distributes oxygenated blood to all the body tissues, where it loses oxygen in the capillary circulation, is collected by the veins and returned to the heart by way of the vena cava for recirculation. (Adapted from Cassels, D. E., and Morse, M.: Blood volume in congenital heart disease, J. Pediat. **31**:485)

2 valves in each side of the heart. One of these is between the auricle and the ventricle; the other, between the ventricle and its artery. These valves serve to prevent backward flow of blood.

ACTION OF THE HEART

The action of the heart is proportioned to the amount of work it must do. When a person is at rest, the heart contracts with a rate and a degree of force exactly sufficient to supply the tissues adequately with fresh blood. If the requirements of the tissues are increased by activity, the heart can increase its output by increasing either the rate or the strength of contraction. Usually it does both. The rate is the first to change; then the cardiac muscle responds with greater strength of contraction. Repeated demand for increased blood flow leads to strengthening of the cardiac musculature, so that it needs less increase in rate when called on for extra work. In athletes, the heart may become slightly larger than in an untrained person. This type of enlargement is known as cardiac hypertrophy and is a form of compensation or adjustment to environmental requirements. The rate of the heart beat is governed largely by the autonomic nervous system, while the force is more inherently a myocardial function. Less work is required to propel blood through the pulmonary circulation than through the systemic. As a result, the left heart is much more muscular than the right.

Diseases of the heart may be considered in relation to the effect on the heart and to the way in which they modify the heart's function.

Acute cardiac diseases may be classified as myocarditis, endocarditis or pericarditis, depending on the type of tissue chiefly affected. Often, all are involved simultaneously. Seldom does endocarditis or pericarditis occur without coexisting myocarditis.

DIAGNOSTIC PROCEDURES

Several special methods of examination are now in use which yield information about the anatomic and the physiologic state of the heart— information which in cases of congenital malformations is often essential to an exact diagnosis and to the decision to attempt surgical amelioration. These procedures are highly technical ones; only the general type of information sought can be discussed here.

Fluoroscopy. By watching the action of the heart under a fluoroscopic x-ray screen, its size, position and contours can be determined. In addition, the degree to which various portions of the outline of the heart pulsate and the amount of distention of the auricles and of the pulmonary vessels can be observed. Knowing the normal appearance of the heart, often abnormal increases in size or activity of the various chambers of the heart can be detected. Conversely, too, the lack of normal pulsation or distention also can be detected. Sometimes barium is given by mouth while the child is observed under the fluoroscope. By this method the normal indentation of the esophagus by the aorta and abnormal indentations by constricting vessels, by a right aortic arch or by a distended left auricle or ventricle can be seen. Similar information is obtainable from ordinary roentgen films of the chest, but the motion of the various portions of the heart and the great vessels cannot be observed.

Angiocardiography. In this technic the actual course of the blood through the heart and the great vessels is visualized by injecting radiopaque material into the veins and following its course through the heart by roentgenograms taken at brief intervals and in specially determined projections. Abnormal communications between various portions of the circulation may be detected in this fashion. Since the child must be held still and in proper position, usually it is necessary to use a general anesthetic.

Aortography. In this technic the radiopaque material is injected in a retrograde fashion through a needle inserted into the left brachial artery. The objects are to outline the region of the branching of the left subclavian artery from the aorta and to determine the presence of a coarctation of the aorta, an open ductus arteriosus or both.

Cardiac Catheterization. With the child anesthetized, the right brachial vein is dissected out, and a small radiopaque catheter is inserted into it and pushed up into the right auricle. By manipulation under the fluoroscope, the tip of the catheter can be directed into the right auricle, the right ventricle and the pulmonary artery. Readings of the pressure in each of these locations are made, and blood samples are obtained for chemical examination to determine the degree of oxygenation of the blood. When congenital abnormalities are present, such as an opening in the septum between the two auricles, sometimes it is possible to demonstrate these communications by probing with the tip of the catheter.

Electrocardiography. The electrocardiogram measures differences in the electric potentials of various leads taken from the heart. It often gives information about the relative activity of the 2 ventricles and about the state of health of the cardiac muscle. These inferences are drawn from an analysis of the tracings obtained. The terms "left axis deviation" or "left ventricular preponderance" indicate a relatively more vigorous activity of the left ventricle compared with the right.

MALFORMATIONS OF THE HEART (CONGENITAL HEART DISEASE)

In early embryonic life the heart consists of a straight tube which receives blood at one end and pumps it out at the other. Through a remarkable and complicated series of changes, the tube folds upon itself, forms internal septa and valves, modifies its connections with the large blood vessels which enter and leave it and transforms into the complex organ which we recognize as the fully developed heart. Nearly all the stages in this transition are completed within the first 2 to 3 months of embryonic growth. Any interference with their normal sequence of full completion results in a malformed heart.

Undoubtedly, there are many conditions of the mother which may interfere with cardiac development. Thus far, only one—rubella (German measles) during the first trimester of pregnancy—has been definitely incriminated as a cause of abnormal development.

A great variety of malformations of the heart are known. Many of these have little clinical significance, since they either do not interfere with the child's welfare or are so serious that the newborn infant is able to survive only a short time. A few types are important because they permit survival yet interfere with the child's general welfare. During the last decade the technical procedures described above have been developed. They permit accurate diagnosis of many types of congenital heart disease and surgical amelioration of some.

The classification of cardiac abnormalities is based upon their capacity to produce cyanosis. Cyanosis results from the contamination of arterial blood circulating in the systemic arteries by venous blood which enters through an abnormal channel.

ACYANOTIC CONGENITAL HEART DISEASE

A few types of malformation of the cardiovascular system are incapable of producing cyanosis because there is no abnormal communication between the pulmonary and the systemic circulations. If symptoms are present they are due to abnormalities in the course or the caliber of the vessels leaving the heart.

Coarctation of the Aorta. Coarctation is a narrowing of the aorta in a short segment just distal to the point of emergence of the left subclavian artery. The severity of symptoms depends upon the degree of constriction. When the narrowing is slight, the disorder may go unrecognized until late in childhood or

adult life, when hypertension is found in the arms and low blood pressure in the legs. Sometimes the child will fail to grow at the proper rate or will be unable to play normally, due to weakness in the legs. Severe degrees of constriction place a burden upon the heart, which is trying to pump blood through the narrow channel. Cardiac failure and death may result during early infancy.

The diagnosis is suspected from the observation of discrepant blood pressures—high in the arms and low in the legs. It can be confirmed by visualization of the aorta by roentgenogram after injection of radiopaque material (aortogram).

Treatment requires the surgical excision of the constricted segment and anastomosis of the free ends thus produced. Whenever possible, it should be performed in early childhood, since the adult cardiovascular system does not tolerate the necessary manipulations so readily.

Other Types of Acyanotic Malformation. Reduction in the caliber of the aorta may take place closer to the heart than in the usual site of coarctation.

HYPOPLASIA OF THE AORTA. This malformation is a general narrowing of the aortic arch.

SUBAORTIC STENOSIS. This is a more localized narrowing directly below the emergence of the aorta from the heart. Neither of these conditions is amenable to surgical correction.

AORTIC VALVULAR STENOSIS AND PULMONIC STENOSIS. When there is isolated narrowing of the aortic or the pulmonary valves alone, recently developed instruments and technics are available for enlarging the passageway through these valves. These conditions are known as congenital aortic valvular stenosis and pulmonic stenosis.

DOUBLE AORTIC ARCH. A double aortic arch may occur, with the two branches encircling the esóphagus, the trachea or both in such a way that swallowing or respiration is compromised. The diagnosis can be made by careful roentgen examination with opaque dye in the esophagus and the trachea. Surgical relief of symptoms may be obtained by dividing one of the encircling branches of the aorta.

POTENTIALLY CYANOTIC
CONGENITAL HEART DISEASE

In the potentially cyanotic group of malformations an abnormal communication exists between the pulmonary and the systemic circulations, but the pressure relations are such that the blood flows through this shunt from the arterial side to the venous side so that no cyanosis results. Under unusual stress, such as superimposed disease or myo-

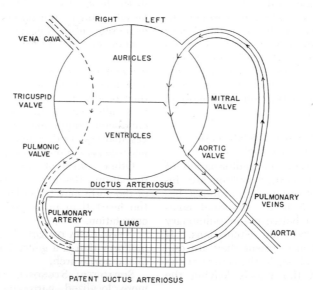

FIG. 32. Diagram of the circulation in patent ductus arteriosus. This is similar to that in Figure 31 except that oxygenated blood in the aorta can leak back through the open ductus into the pulmonary artery, thus adding to the volume of blood circulating through the lungs. Cyanosis does not develop, because the pressure relations are such that the blood in the ductus flows from the oxygenated side to the unoxygenated side, except under unusual circumstances. (Adapted from Cassels, D. E., and Morse, M: Blood volume in congenital heart disease, J. Pediat. **31**:485)

cardial failure, it is possible for the flow in the shunt to reverse its direction and produce cyanosis by admixing venous blood with arterial. When reversal of flow occurs, it is usually a terminal phenomenon; consequently, this group of disorders also is called the late cyanotic type of congenital heart disease.

Patent Ductus Arteriosus. The ductus arteriosus is a fetal connection between the pulmonary artery and the aorta. Ordinarily, this channel spontaneously constricts, closes its lumen and atrophies shortly after birth. In some infants this change fails to take place, and the fetal communication between the pulmonary and the systemic circulations persists. Symptoms result when the opening is large, because there is leakage of blood from the aorta back into the pulmonary circulation (Fig. 32). No cyanosis results, but the volume of blood which the heart must pump in order to meet the requirements of the peripheral tissues is increased. A small channel has no effect upon growth or physical activity, for the heart can hypertrophy enough to meet the slightly increased burden. When the volume of blood flowing through the ductus is large, both physical activity and growth may be hampered.

DIAGNOSIS. The diagnosis is suspected from the presence of a typical machinerylike murmur over the pulmonary artery. It is confirmed by the presence of a low diastolic blood pressure and by various roentgen maneuvers which demonstrate enlargement of the pulmonary artery and increased blood flow to the lungs or by actual visualization of the ductus itself after injection of opaque dye (angiocardiography).

SURGICAL TREATMENT. The surgical treatment consists of ligation and division of the abnormal channel. Usually it is performed after the age of 2 or 3 years. Even if symptoms are lacking, the ductus usually is closed, because its continued patency carries a risk of subacute bacterial endocarditis. In skilled hands the operative mortality is very low, and relief of symptoms can be confidently expected.

NURSING CARE. Usually the child with a patent ductus arteriosus comes into the hospital several days prior to operation for diagnostic tests and preparation. The nurse to whom he is assigned needs to establish a friendly, trusting relationship with the child to help him adapt to hospitalization and to prepare him for all the new experiences that he will have both before and after operation. Usually the child is placed in oxygen for the first 24 hours after operation. He and his parents need to see the tent and the chest Wangensteen suction apparatus which will be used postoperatively and to know why they are necessary to keep him comfortable. During the preoperative period the child is guarded carefully against infections, served a nutritious diet and encouraged to take an adequate amount of fluids.

A sedative is given, and a blood pressure reading is taken before the child goes to the operating room. After the permanent ligature or division is made, blood pressure reading discloses a rise in diastolic pressure. Blood pressure remains high for 4 to 5 days postoperatively and then stabilizes at a new level. While the child is in the operating room, the necessary equipment for postoperative care is assembled—oxygen tent, chest Wangensteen suction and a suction machine to aspirate mucus from the respiratory passages. In the first 48 hours postoperatively, the nurse must be alert for evidence of bleeding and respiratory distress. She also must keep careful watch of the suction apparatus to see that no kinking of or pressure on the tube occurs. If there is kinking or pressure on the tubing, clot formation may occur and prevent drainage. The effectiveness of the drainage apparatus also must be noted. If there is regular fluctuation of the fluid level which corresponds to the respiratory rate, it is indicative of a patent drainage system. The amount of water in the chest Wangensteen apparatus also should be noted. If the water runs to a low level, the doctor should be notified.

When chest suction is not used, vigilance to detect signs of respiratory distress is imperative. Dyspnea arises from a collection of fluid in the pleural cavity. Often, dyspnea is relieved by raising the head of the bed and turning the child onto the affected side. If dyspnea is not relieved by a change in position and the pulse and the respiration rates remain high, the nurse should notify the doctor and prepare immediately for thoracentesis.

The child should be turned every 2 hours and kept comfortable with sedatives, fluids and food as tolerated, and supportive measures should be taken to relieve his anxiety pertaining to all that he sees going on around him. Hospital personnel will view him frequently to check the oxygen tent, the suction apparatus, the dressing and the in-travenous therapy apparatus, if it is utilized. Unless the personnel's interest is interpreted to the child, he will grow anxious, wondering about the meaning of all their activities.

On the second day, when the child is given a trial period out of oxygen he will require careful observation. His pulse and respiration should be noted. Observation to detect dilatation of the alae nasi and flushing of the face should be made. Usually the child is put back into the tent for another 24 hours, after which time it is discontinued.

On the third day postoperatively the child is usually ready for quiet activity. In another few days he may be up in a wheel chair. Activity should be increased gradually and planned in accordance with the child's capacities. Usually, by the end of 10 days he can resume normal activities.

Ventricular Septal Defect. An opening in the septum between the right and the left ventricles of the heart is perhaps the most common type of congenital heart disease. Fortunately, the defect is frequently small, and no obvious interference with cardiac function results. The flow of blood from the left to the right ventricle does not produce cyanosis, but a loud harsh murmur is usually present. Accurate interpretation of this murmur is desirable to prevent unnecessary concern or unwarranted restriction of the child's activity. For most children with this defect, no treatment is required. In rare instances the placement or the size of the defect may lead to cardiac enlargement and restriction of function. At the present time surgical repair of an interventricular defect is too hazardous to be recommended.

Auricular Septal Defect. Openings in the septum between the right and the left auricle may occur. Oxygenated blood flows from the left to the right auricle through the defect and then is recirculated through the lungs (Fig. 33). A disproportion between the amount of blood circulating in the pulmonary and the systemic circulations ensues, producing enlargement of the right heart and distention of the pulmonary vessels. It has been postulated that the relatively meager flow to the rest of the body may lead to the slender delicate habitus which sometimes is observed. Susceptibility to pneumonia and rheumatic fever is increased. The diagnosis may be suspected from the presence of a loud murmur in the area of the pulmonary artery, with enlargement of the heart and roentgen evidence of congestion of the pulmonary circulation. It may be confirmed by insertion of a catheter into the right auricle and through the defect into the left auricle (cardiac catheterization). Tech-

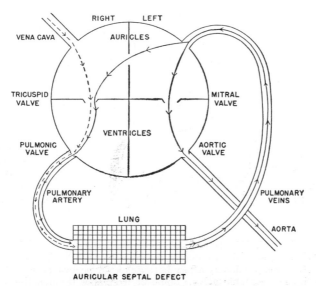

Fig. 33. Diagram of the circulation in auricular septal defect. This is similar to that of Figure 31, except that oxygenated blood returning to the left auricle can flow through the defect in the auricular septum into the right auricle, thus decreasing the volume of blood sent to the left ventricle and increasing the volume in the right side of the heart. No cyanosis develops unless the distention of the right side of the heart becomes excessive and reversal of the flow through the auricular defect takes place. (Adapted from Cassels, D. E., and Morse, M.: Blood volume in congenital heart disease, J. Pediat. **31**:485)

nics for the surgical closure of the defect are difficult and carry a high mortality at the present time.

CYANOTIC CONGENITAL HEART DISEASE

In cyanotic congenital heart disease there is a communication between the pulmonary and the systemic circulations in which the blood is flowing continually from the venous to the arterial side. The blood delivered to the periphery of the body by the aorta never is fully saturated with oxygen, and the tissues take on a bluish hue instead of the normal pink. Cyanosis may be apparent at birth and persist or it may be inapparent at birth but develop during the first year of life. In either event it tends to become more marked during the early years of life. In part this is due to an increase in the number of red cells per unit volume of blood (polycythemia), which represents an at-

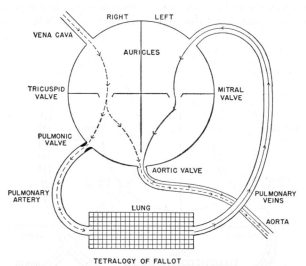

TETRALOGY OF FALLOT

FIG. 34. Diagram of the circulation in tetralogy of Fallot. Venous blood entering the right ventricle is diverted from the pulmonary artery because of the narrowed orifice at the pulmonic valve. Some of it escapes through the defect in the interventricular septum into the left ventricle and almost immediately into the abnormally placed aorta. Partly because of anatomic relations and partly because of hypertrophy of the right ventricle, the venous blood is able to flow into the aorta. A decrease in the volume of blood sent to the lungs and a continual contamination of the stream of oxygenated blood from the left ventricle result. Cyanosis is present, and an increased volume of blood is present in the greater circulation. (Adapted from Cassels, D. E., and Morse, M.: Blood volume in congenital heart disease, J. Pediat. **31**:485)

PLATE 1

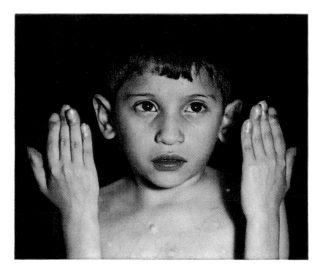

Cyanosis and clubbed fingers in a boy with tetralogy of Fallot.

tempt of the body to improve the oxygen-carrying power of the blood. When polycythemia is marked, the peripheral capillaries of the skin and the mucous membranes become distended with purple blood, the fingers and the toes may take on a clubbed shape (Plate 1), body growth is delicate and retarded, the capacity for exercise is reduced, and the child runs the hazard of complications due to spontaneous clotting of the thickened blood within his vessels. All of these symptoms are subject to considerable variation in degree in the individual child.

Tetralogy of Fallot. The most common variety of cyanotic heart disease which permits survival consists of a combination of abnormalities. Blood leaving the right ventricle toward the lungs encounters an abnormally narrow opening into the pulmonary artery (Fig. 34). In the same vicinity there is an opening in the interventricular septum which provides a ready diversion of blood into the left side of the heart and particularly into the aorta. Cyanosis arises from the contamination of the aortic contents by venous blood. The direction of flow through the shunt is determined in part by the position of the aortic opening and in part by the fact that the right ventricle has hypertrophied because of its excessive task and thus is able to overbalance the pressure of the left ventricle. Poor oxygenation of the tissues is furthered also by the fact that the rate of blood flow through the lungs is decreased. Diagnosis is made from fluoroscopic examination of the heart, which demonstrates enlargement of the chambers of the right side, decrease in size of the pulmonary artery and

decrease in blood flow through the lungs.

Usually the physical activity of the child with tetralogy of Fallot is impaired. He walks or plays for a few minutes, grows tired and gets into a squatting position which relieves his dyspnea for some unknown reason. In spite of the fact that these children have a chronic circulatory disturbance to the brain with some degree of relative anoxia, many of them are of average or above-average intelligence. Fainting spells and occasionally convulsions may occur when the degree of anoxia is increased temporarily.

The child with tetralogy of Fallot is usually irritable, overdependent and prone to emotional instability. It is understandable why he reacts in this way. From birth his parents have been concerned about his defect, his physical health and his prognosis for survival. The child with tetralogy of Fallot grows blue when he cries. Therefore, his parents prolong gratification when normally he should be learning to tolerate frustration. He refuses to do things for himself partly because he fatigues easily and partly because his mother feels that she must protect him from all experiences which are difficult or frustrating. The child with a congenital heart defect starts life under adverse circumstances, both physically and psychologically. Empathy with the child is an essential quality in his nursing care.

SURGICAL TREATMENT. The original "blue-baby operation" of Blalock and Taussig was designed to ameliorate this abnormality. In this operation a branch of the aorta is anastomosed to the pulmonary artery. In older children the subclavian artery is used. In children under 2 years of age the subclavian artery is too small to be used, and the innominate artery is selected to achieve the shunt. The Blalock and Taussig operation does not correct the original defects but adds a compensating one by connecting a systemic artery to the pulmonary artery. This increases the blood flow to the lungs, reduces cyanosis and improves the tolerance for exercise.

The Potts operation also achieves the above result. The Potts operation makes a direct connection between the aorta and the pulmonary artery. The aorta has higher pressure and forces blood into the pulmonary artery, from whence it will flow through the lungs for oxygenation.

NURSING CARE. During the preoperative period the child should have a nurse who can accept him with his individual personality patterns and needs. He will need a great deal of help in becoming familiar with the hospital, his nurse, the doctors and the routines. He will be subjected to diagnostic procedures—oxygen saturation and exercise tolerance tests, roentgen pictures and barium swallow and fluoroscopic examination. He will adapt himself more readily if time is spent letting him stir up the barium and chocolate syrup and permitting him to discover that the drink is similar to cocoa. Permitting him to examine the fluoroscopic machine while the lights are on will do much to eliminate the frightening aspects of an examination in the dark.

The child with this type of defect is undernourished, underdeveloped and susceptible to respiratory infections—especially to pneumonia. For this reason he needs protection from patients and personnel with respiratory infections. He also needs an adequate diet and fluid intake. These children usually have capricious appetites. Serving small quantities in an attractive fashion in an atmosphere of friendliness brings infinitely better results than urging.

The child's parents also will need help in the preoperative period. The doctor explains the operation, the complications that may occur and the prognosis. However, there will be many questions directed toward the nurse and many signs which indicate the parents' need for preparation, support and hope. Sometimes their overprotectiveness may be difficult to bear. However, if the nurse can visualize imaginatively what they have experienced in the months or the years before, she will understand why overprotectiveness and anxiety have become a habitual response to the problems that they have had to bear.

The parents not only will need answers to their questions but they also should be prepared for what they will see when their child returns from the operating room. They should know the length of time that the operation will take. Waiting for one's child to return from the operating room is tedious and anxiety provoking—and especially so when the parents know that the prognosis is unpredictable. Informing them of the child's condition at intervals relieves anxiety, supports them at a critical time and gives them hope.

When the child returns from the operating room, he must be placed in an oxygen tent. When intratracheal anesthesia is used, the child must be watched for signs of tracheal irritation. It is manifested by cyanosis, increased pulse rate, labored breathing or restlessness. When signs of tracheal irritation develop, steam inhalations must be provided to bring relief from dyspnea. If edema of the larynx develops, a tracheotomy may become necessary. Vital signs are taken every hour. If the Blalock-Taussig operation has been performed, blood-pressure readings must be taken from the arm opposite to the operated side. The child must be turned at frequent intervals. Sedatives are given freely to keep the child at rest. Penicillin is administered to prevent infections. Observation to detect postoperative hemiplegia is necessary. It is not a common complication but it can occur from spontaneous clotting of blood during dehydration after operation. Coramine, adrenalin and a thoracentesis tray should be in the room for emergency use. An accumulation of bloody fluid in the chest may cause listlessness, diminished breath sounds and increased pulse rate. If a thoracentesis is done, the amount of fluid withdrawn and the child's response to the treatment should be noted on the chart. The child's color should be noted and changes recorded. Fluids may be given as tolerated, followed by a soft to general diet. Mouth and skin care gives comfort. Encouraging the child to cough up mucus prevents atelectasis and is important to do at 2-hour intervals.

When the operation is successful, the child recuperates rapidly. Usually oxygen is needed for 4 or 5 days. Then the child is ready for graduated amounts of activity. Marked changes in behavior will become evident. The operation increases his vigor, and often he begins to assert himself, to become aggressive and to demand to do things for himself. These changes are striking and often frightening to the parents who repeatedly have responded with fear when the child became active.

The nurse will need to help the parents to accept their child's increased need for independence and self-assertion. With reassurance and insight they will learn to observe his increased capacities and see that soon he will be ready for many new kinds of socializing experiences. The parents will need help to change their feelings about their child before they can institute new methods of guidance. This takes time, along with advice and direction that are given understandingly. Gradually they will see and feel that their child has become more normal. The nurse can increase their powers of observation by pointing out his enjoyment of self-directed activity and his freedom from signs of untoward reactions during periods of activity.

Other Varieties of Cyanotic Heart Disease. Eisenmenger Complex. This is similar to the tetralogy of Fallot except for the absence of narrowing of the pulmonary artery. Operative procedures will not improve this type of defect at the present time.

Pulmonary Stenosis with Auricular Septal Defect. This can be improved markedly by new measures which are designed to enlarge the pulmonic opening. In general, shunting operations are not effective for this abnormality. Most of the other cyanotic types of congenital heart disease do not permit survival for more than a brief period of time.

Nursing Care. The type of nursing care required will vary considerably, depending upon the degree of functional incapacity. Infants or children with severely handicapping malformations require the type of care described later in this chapter for children with heart failure or with chronic valvular heart disease. Those in whom the malformation is mild should be encouraged to utilize their exercise capacity to the limit of tolerance. For many this will mean a normal life; for some it may require diversion of interests from competitive sports to more sedentary pursuits. Often the problem for the child lies mainly in convincing the parents to let him participate in activities commensurate with his functional capacity instead of overprotecting him and regarding him as a cardiac invalid.

FUNCTIONAL HEART CONDITIONS

FUNCTIONAL MURMUR

Murmurs heard over the heart in the absence of organic disease of the heart are known as functional or accidental murmurs. In some instances, functional murmurs are dependent on anemia. These murmurs disappear when the hemoglobin has been brought to a normal value. Accidental murmurs not related to anemia are very common in childhood. Their cause is not well understood, and they have no significance or importance. Accidental murmurs are of only moderate intensity, are

heard usually in systole and when the child is lying down. The intensity of the murmur varies with the heart rate, the murmur disappearing with a rapid rate. A child may have an accidental murmur over a period of years without related symptoms.

The only importance of the functional murmur is in relation to the diagnosis and the decision that it is functional rather than organic.

SINUS ARRHYTHMIA

That which determines the heart rate under normal conditions is the sinoauricular node. In embryologic life this is known as the sinus. Sinus arrhythmia is a change in heart rate produced by reflexes acting on the sinoauricular node. The usual reflex cause of this change in rhythm is respiration. In the presence of sinus arrhythmia, the heart rate increases with inspiration and decreases with expiration. This type of cardiac irregularity is very common in childhood, so common that it is considered a normal condition. It disappears in the presence of tachycardia from any cause.

TACHYCARDIA

Tachycardia, or rapid heart rate, may be an accompaniment of heart disease or it may occur from various causes when the heart is entirely normal. Increased heart rate occurs with fear, excitement, exercise and fever. When tachycardia is functional and fever is not present, the heart and the pulse rates become normal during sleep. They do not become normal during sleep in hyperthyroidism, rheumatic carditis or in the condition known as paroxysmal tachycardia. When a child first comes under medical or nursing care for any reason, he may have tachycardia from fear and excitement incident to the occasion. In order to obtain a satisfactory and significant pulse rate, the child must be calmed, or one must wait until he is asleep. If the heart rate is increased from any cause above 150 to the minute for a protracted period, the myocardium becomes weakened, and severe damage may result. Paroxysmal tachycardia is a condition which is relatively rare in childhood; the heart rate is increased often to 200 or more to the minute for no known reason. An attack may last a few minutes or for several days. Quinidine and Mecholyl are drugs used to prevent the attacks or stop them when they occur.

ACUTE RHEUMATIC CARDITIS

The term rheumatic carditis is used in preference to rheumatic endocarditis, which was employed formerly, for the reason that the changes in the heart never are limited to the endocardium in the acute stages of the disease. The myocardium always is affected, and often the pericardium also. Rheumatic carditis is an inflammation of · the heart which occurs as a part of rheumatic fever, not as a complication.

ETIOLOGY

The mechanism that causes rheumatic carditis also causes rheumatic fever and is discussed under the latter disease.

Fully nine tenths of all the heart disease that occurs in the first 4 decades of life is rheumatic, and in nearly three fourths of these cases the cardiac disease had its onset before 15. It is rare in the first years of life, common after 5 and has its greatest incidence of onset between 7 and 10. Its distribution between the sexes is approximately equal. The frequency of its occurrence varies with the geographic location. In surveys of hospital admissions, the proportion has varied from 0.1 to 5.5 per cent. Among college students, a mean average of 1.2 per cent has been found. The seriousness, as well as the frequency, of the disease is indicated by mortality statistics, which are more accurately known than is the morbidity. The mortality has varied from 5 to more than 9 for each 100,000 population, according to the area of the country. In the last year for which reports are available (1949), the mortality rate in the United States as a whole was 4.6 per 100,000 for children in the age range of 5 to 14. Only accidents and neoplasms were reported more frequently as the cause of death in school-age children.

PATHOLOGY

In the beginning of rheumatic carditis and during its exacerbations, rheumatic nodules (see rheumatic fever) form in the various heart structures. Subsequently, some localized endothelial proliferation takes place, and frequently small excrescences, consisting largely of fibrin (vegetations), occur on the heart valves and the chordae tendineae. The left auriculoventricular (mitral) valve is the one most often affected; the aortic valve is the next. The vegetations interfere with good closure and function of the valves, thus throwing an added load on the heart muscle in order to maintain circulation. The function of the myocardium is disturbed directly by the inflammatory changes within its structure. Thus, frequently the work demanded of the heart muscle exceeds its capacity, with the result that the heart may increase in size by dilatation. The circulatory inadequacy which results is reflected in the symptoms exhibited by the child.

SYMPTOMS

The symptoms of rheumatic carditis are proportionate quantitatively and qualitatively to the severity of the carditis. In cases of mild disease, the symptoms are in part those of a prolonged low-grade infection. The usual picture is one of irregular low-grade fever, pallor, moderate anemia and poor nutrition, with a history of preceding poor appetite, loss of weight and easy fatigue. All these symptoms are vague as far as indicating carditis is concerned. If other rheumatic manifestations are present, the significance of the symptoms may become apparent, but mild carditis easily may escape recognition when a careful physical examination is lacking. On closer observation one may find slight dyspnea on exertion and pulse and respiration rates out of proportion to the temperature. A soft systolic murmur usually is to be heard over the apex of the heart, the point where murmurs produced by lesions of the mitral valve are heard best. Often epistaxis occurs in the early stage of the disease.

When the carditis is more severe, the child is definitely ill. He prefers, or finds it necessary, to remain in bed. Usually the face is flushed, with perhaps some cyanosis. The temperature may be high in the very

acute disease or range up to 101° or 102° F. with disease of moderate severity. The temperature is always irregular. The white-blood-cell count is increased definitely and sometimes greatly. Cardiac damage is severe, and pain over the precordium is frequent. Abdominal pain also is often present. Because of the myocardial weakness and the concomitant valvular lesions, the heart dilates, and evidences of inadequate circulation appear. Failure of the heart in this manner is known as decompensation. Decompensation causes very rapid pulse and respiration rates, dyspnea, pallor and cyanosis. It also permits a back pressure of the blood in the venous system, which causes enlargement of the liver and, in more severe decompensation, edema and ascites.

When the cardiac valves are involved, the sounds produced by the heart are modified, causing murmurs. From the timing and the location of the murmur one may determine the valve affected; from the character of the murmur the condition of the valve may be estimated. The stronger the action of the heart and the greater the scarring of the valve, the louder and rougher the murmur will be. The amount of myocardial inflammation is indicated by the weakening, the spacing and the rapidity of the heart sounds, as well as by the amount of dilatation. Enlargement of the heart may be caused by stretching of weakened heart muscle, or it may be the result of hypertrophy consequent to cardiac damage by preceding attacks of carditis. An associated pericarditis may cause accumulation of fluid around the heart, simulating cardiac enlargement.

PROGNOSIS

The normal healing powers of the body tend to check the cardiac inflammation, particularly if outlying infections subside and cardiac work is kept at a minimum. Thus, children may become cured after a period of several months. Recovery from the first attack is usual. However, carditis, like other rheumatic manifestations, has a strong tendency to recur. The child may die as a result of failing circulation in the midst of one of these attacks, or, if he recovers from the illness, the summation of damage to the valves with associated scarring may lead to permanent valve deformity and dysfunction with its consequent invalidism because of inability to withstand the effects of even moderate exercise. On the other hand, from apparently severe valvular lesions in the absence of further recurrences he may recover ultimately to the extent that no dysfunction exists and even the murmurs largely disappear.

TREATMENT

The treatment of active rheumatic carditis attempts to spare the heart as much work as possible until the acute inflammatory reaction in its muscle has subsided completely. The measures which reduce cardiac work include (1) continuous and absolute bed rest, (2) the relief of pain, fever and anxiety insofar as possible and (3) appropriate treatment of cardiac failure when it is present. The success of these aspects of treatment depends in large measure upon the nurse and the other persons who care for the child. Details of nursing care are considered in a separate section at the end of this chapter. The treatment of cardiac failure also is considered in a separate section.

Measures that suppress the rheumatic inflammatory process are an important adjunct to the treatment outlined above. Salicylates or cortisone or ACTH, when used in proper dosage, will terminate fever and pain and reduce cardiac activity in most instances. What effect these measures have in limiting the ultimate degree of cardiac damage is still a matter of dispute. Their withdrawal before the end of the usual period during which spontaneous subsidence of rheumatic activity might be expected results in an immediate return of symptoms. Whether suppression of rheumatic activity does or does not limit the ultimate damage to cardiac valves and muscle, it is an important temporary expedient which lessens cardiac work by the reduction of fever and the relief of pain, anxiety and discomfort.

Both the salicylates and the hormones have undesirable side effects which must be recognized and eliminated before the disturbances which they create add to the burden of cardiac work. High dosage of salicylates may result in gastrointestinal upsets, ringing in the ears, headaches or disturbances of mental state. Stimulation of respiration can cause alkalosis through hyperventilation. Acidosis also may occur when there is excessive accumulation of salicylates in the blood. The manner in which children respond to salicylate dosage is a highly individual matter. Some can tolerate large doses without disturbance; others are easily upset by relatively small quantities.

Administration of cortisone and ACTH also is restricted by toxic manifestations. The bodily appearance may change through the rounding of facial contours (moon face), localized fat deposits, the appearance of acne or excessive hair and by weight increase with linear marks appearing in the stretched skin (striae). More serious to the child with rheumatic carditis are hypertension and the tendency to accumulate salt and water within the tissues. The latter may be counteracted by restricting the dietary intake of salt and by the periodic administration of mercurial diuretics. When mental or emotional disturbances occur during hormone therapy, they must be regarded as a serious complication which probably demands withdrawal of the drug.

During the acute stage of rheumatic carditis the maintenance of nutrition presents a serious problem. The sick child eats poorly, yet needs essential nutrients to combat his disease. Hormone therapy usually is attended by an increase in appetite which is superior to that observed when salicylates are used. Blood or plasma transfusions in small amounts are sometimes very helpful in improving nutrition.

As the acute stage subsides and the heart becomes compensated, less rigorous restriction of activity is required, but confinement to bed is continued for as long as any evidence of activity of the disease persists or for as long as compensation is incomplete. The criteria for determining persistence of activity of the disease are stated under rheumatic fever. After the child has been permitted out of bed for brief periods and has been given bathroom privi-leges, the pulse rate is a fairly good criterion as to the degree of compensation of the heart. Other tests of cardiac function may be applied, such as noting how quickly the pulse rate returns to its former level after a brief period of exercise. Restriction of bodily activity for many months has been a common custom. Such radical restriction is unnecessary, provided that all evidence of infection, including laboratory evidence, has disappeared and provided that the state of nutrition is excellent because of previous close attention to it. In most instances, unlimited activity may be allowed 6 weeks after the child has been permitted to be out of bed. When heart damage persists, the activity of the child always should be restricted within the limits of easy tolerance, as discussed subsequently.

The general measures which are discussed in Chapter 18 for the prevention of recurrences of rheumatic episodes are most important for children who have suffered from carditis.

CHRONIC VALVULAR DISEASE

Damage to the heart valves, usually produced by rheumatic carditis, leads to changes which alter the normal functioning of the valves. When the child has recovered from the active or the acute inflammation of carditis, the residual heart damage with scarring of the valves is termed chronic valvular disease. It results in changes in the remainder of the circulatory system to compensate for the valvular changes.

Two types of valvular damage may be produced. One of these consists of a puckering or a partial destruction or a binding down of the valve leaves, which results in an inability of the valve to close tightly and so allows a leakage of the blood in the circulation in the direction opposite to that in which it normally goes. This type of defect occurs most frequently at the mitral valve. At this site the condition is known as mitral insufficiency, and the backward flow of blood is spoken of as mitral regurgitation.

The other type of valve damage consists of a narrowing of the valve orifice by scar contraction or fusion of valve leaflets so that the leaflets cannot open completely. Such a lesion constitutes a stenosis and prevents easy passage of blood through the heart.

As a result of these changes, the heart must do more work. This goal is accomplished usually by increase of musculature or hypertrophy. If hypertrophy is insufficient, the heart rate also is increased.

SYMPTOMS

When compensation is adequate, chronic valvular disease produces no symptoms. Examination will reveal cardiac murmurs and an enlarged heart. Symptoms arise when for any reason compensation is inadequate. Decompensation is discussed subsequently. In the absence of cardiac insufficiency or decompensation, children with chronic valvular disease need only to avoid exertion beyond their cardiac capacity and to guard against further cardiac damage.

MANAGEMENT

It is necessary for some children with heart disease to lead a guarded and restricted life. However, it is always desirable that they lead a life as nearly normal as possible. Such children should be examined at suitable intervals to determine whether the regimen followed is adequate or unnecessarily severe. They should have such supervision as would detect at their onset any deleterious conditions. Not only the habits of life but the mental attitude toward life needs careful consideration and adjustment. The chief function of childhood is preparation for adult life, and an important part of the preparation is formal education. A lack of understanding between medical supervisor and educator may result in unnecessary neglect of the child's education.

Too often the instruction to the parent or the child is of a negative type with admonition as to what not to do, for example, "Do not run stairs and do not play hard." Instruction of this type may well produce psychological harm. What is needed is advice as to constructive use of time. The child should be told what to do rather than what not to do. Let him have his unrestricted periods. For such restriction as is necessary, definite rest periods should be prescribed.

MYOCARDITIS

Under the term myocarditis are included acute and chronic inflammations and degenerations of the heart muscle. In childhood, myocarditis is encountered most frequently as a manifestation of rheumatic fever. It occurs also with diphtheria that is severe or has been treated late and with other severe acute infections.

PECULIARITIES OF HEART MUSCLE

Disorders of the myocardium are understood more easily if the peculiarities of heart muscle are kept in mind. This tissue has the ability to contract; it holds itself in constant readiness to contract—a condition termed tonicity. It has the ability to stimulate itself to contract and thus is automatic. Its contractions follow each other in orderly sequence or rhythm. Stimulation produced or applied at any point is conducted to all parts of the myocardium and causes a contraction of the whole heart. If the heart contracts at all, it contracts completely.

SYMPTOMS

Myocarditis may cause disturbances of any or all of the stated properties of the heart. One common manifestation is weakened contractility, necessitating a more rapid heart rate. The pulse becomes noticeably weaker. On auscultation the first heart sound is faint, the two heart sounds become of almost equal intensity at the apex, and the spacing between the first and the second sounds becomes approximately equal. What is termed a gallop rhythm frequently develops. A splitting of the heart sounds results in a rhythm that sounds like a galloping horse.

The ability of the heart muscle to transmit a wave of contraction to all its parts may become impaired. Such disturbances of conduction may result in irregular pulse, and sometimes the heart chambers cease to contract synchronously. One type of conduction difficulty is known as auricular fibrillation or flutter and is characterized by very rapid and ineffective contractions of the auricles with occasional irregular ventricular contraction. In some instances, a blocking of conduction

from one part of the heart to another occurs. This also leads to lack of synchronism and may result in complete independence of contraction in the auricle and the ventricle. The latter is much slower than the normal rate, often from 30 to 40 to the minute. The ventricular rate may be determined by counting the pulse, the auricular rate, from pulse tracings made from the external jugular vein and from the electrocardiogram.

TREATMENT

The treatment in cases of myocarditis is similar to that in rheumatic carditis. In addition, there is an attempt to remove or relieve the causative factor. If cardiac failure should occur, the treatment is as described subsequently under cardiac decompensation. Some varieties of myocarditis, such as that secondary to diphtheria, have a high mortality rate associated with them. With other varieties (e.g., rheumatic) the chances for recovery often are excellent.

PERICARDITIS

The pericardium is a thin layer of serous tissue which forms a double-walled sac, the inner layer covering the heart and the outer layer lining the space in which the heart lies. The free surfaces are moist and smooth.

Pericarditis or inflammation of this membrane may be of various types and come from several causes. It is not common in infancy or early childhood. When it does occur at such an early age, it most frequently results from the extension of a pneumonic or a pleural infection. This produces commonly a suppurative type of pericarditis which causes a high mortality rate, particularly in infancy. Occasionally, pericarditis caused by tuberculosis is encountered. Though pericarditis occurs from these and other causes, by far the most frequent factor in the production of this disorder in childhood is rheumatic fever, especially after 4 or 5 years of age.

Rheumatic Pericarditis

This type is characterized early by an exudate of fibrin and cells on both free surfaces of the pericardium. With movement of the heart the two roughened surfaces rub together, producing what is heard on auscultation as a scratching sound. Subsequently, the exudate consists also of fluid, which is clear or only slightly cloudy. The quantity of fluid usually is small, though at times it may be large, producing pericarditis with effusion.

Symptoms. Rheumatic pericarditis always is accompanied by myocarditis with its associated symptoms. Local pain and tenderness usually are present. As the inflammation subsides, a strong tendency exists to form adhesions between the two pericardial layers. The adhesions may be only slight or they may be sufficiently extensive to obliterate the entire pericardial sac. The adhesions do not seem to interfere seriously with cardiac function, especially if the inflammation and the adhesive process have not extended to structures beyond the parietal pericardium. Adhesions which fix firmly to the parietal pericardium are more frequently dependent on other than rheumatic disease. Such massive adhesions interfere greatly with the heart action. Because of

the increased work, the heart is compelled to hypertrophy. If hypertrophy is insufficient, decompensation results.

Treatment. The treatment of rheumatic pericarditis is that of rheumatic carditis. Rarely is drainage of pericardial fluid necessary. Suppurative pericarditis may require surgical drainage, but usually, no matter what is done, the outlook is poor.

CARDIAC DECOMPENSATION

A damaged heart or one subjected to excessive strain is said to be compensated when it has hypertrophied and adjusted its performance sufficiently to overcome its handicap completely. If it fails to maintain an adequate circulation, it is decompensated.

Etiology

The work of maintaining a high blood pressure may exceed the heart's capacity, although this is an infrequent cause of decompensation in children except during nephritis. The most frequent cause is active rheumatic carditis with its attendant myocarditis and myocardial weakening. Chronic valvular disease may be sufficiently severe to be in itself a cause of decompensation, although, more often than not, decompensation occurs in this condition only with a recurrence of the infection.

Symptoms

When the circulation is inadequate, blood accumulates in the venous system. In the lungs, the congestion of the vessels causes symptoms resembling bronchitis. Small amounts of blood may appear in the sputum. Congestion of the systemic venous system causes digestive disturbances, enlargement of the liver and accumulation of fluid in the tissue spaces (edema) and in the serous cavities (ascites). Nausea and vomiting may be the first outstanding symptoms of decompensation. The congestion of the liver may lead to dysfunction sufficient to cause jaundice. Only rarely does the ascites become great enough to embarrass respiration or heart action.

An adequate gas exchange between the blood and the tissues is impossible in the presence of circulatory failure. Cyanosis and dyspnea result. Cyanosis is noted best in the lips and the fingertips; dyspnea may be so severe as to require the child to maintain a sitting posture.

TREATMENT

The treatment of decompensation consists of reducing to a minimum the amount of work required of the heart, administering cardiac stimulants to help the heart meet the circulatory needs and, finally, when compensation has been attained, providing favorable conditions for the heart to recover as much reserve as possible. The child should be in bed, absolutely at rest and lying flat unless dyspnea prevents it. Not only rest but also an abundance of sleep is necessary. Sedative drugs usually are strongly indicated, and no hesitancy need be shown in the use of morphine. In fact, morphine is a very important drug in this condition. The early administration of oxygen is very valuable. In cases of most severe decompensation, removal of blood from the circulation may be desirable unless anemia is present. However, removal of blood is seldom necessary when the other

measures mentioned are carried out appropriately.

Digitalis is the cardiac stimulant used. Digitalis serves to slow the heart rate by prolonging diastole, thus allowing more cardiac rest and at the same time permitting better ventricular filling. Digitalis increases cardiac tone. It increases the extent of ventricular contraction and relieves or prevents dilatation beyond the physiologic limit, making possible maximum cardiac output. Digitalis is given best in large doses for the first day or two. After that its administration should be continued in smaller amounts. A period of a day or two is required for the drug to become fully effective. The administration of the large dosage for the initial period is designated as digitalization. Precise dosage varies with the preparation of digitalis and the speed with which an effect is desired. The initial saturating dose must be computed carefully to avoid toxic symptoms when the delayed effects appear. The benefits of digitalis may be erased by such symptoms.

Great care must be exercised in the digitalization of children who have had previous treatment, in order to avoid overdigitalization. Moderate excess of digitalis causes premature heartbeats and vomiting. Other irregularities of conduction of the impulse in the heart may be observed. In more severe digitalis intoxication, heart block is likely to occur. In the event of overdosage, administration of the drug should be discontinued temporarily, then resumed at a lower dosage than previously. The administration should be discontinued when compensation is well established. A few children may require the continued administration of digitalis over a long period in order to maintain compensation.

The heart does not respond sufficiently to the preceding measures in all instances. In the presence of edema and ascites, certain other measures may be indicated. One of these is the administration of a diuretic in an attempt to cause elimination of some of the excess fluid. Theophylline is valuable for this purpose. Mercurial diuretics are in common use. A diet containing little salt and considerable carbohydrate, limited in fluid, with most of the fluid in the form of milk, has been found useful for many of these children.

After all signs of decompensation have disappeared, the child should refrain from activity until some cardiac reserve has been attained. Then activity should be permitted gradually. If the pulse rate becomes much accelerated or remains increased after exercise, the exercise has been too severe or too prolonged. It may be that the child never will have the normal degree of cardiac reserve and that his activities always must be somewhat restricted. Any noteworthy recurrence of decompensation is an indication for renewed convalescent care for weeks or months and calls for prolonged restriction of activity. It is to be remembered that in rheumatic heart disease, decompensation is brought about most frequently by active rheumatic infection. Recurrences of decompensation usually depend on recurrences or exacerbations of the infection. A primary duty to the children is to find and treat all infectious foci and to make every attempt to manage their lives in such a manner that respiratory infections are avoided.

NURSING CARE OF THE CHILD WITH HEART DISEASE

Since reduction of the load carried by the heart is of primary importance for the child with active heart disease, all nursing care is directed toward that goal. The child in severe decompensation presents a typical picture: his pulse is rapid; respirations are fast, shallow and labored; his color ranges from pallor to severe cyanosis; a hacking cough indicates mitral insufficiency and his heart is enlarged; he is alert, restless and apprehensive.

REST

Rest is the first requisite in acute cardiac decompensation. He should have rest in bed, should be moved as little as possible and should do nothing for himself which brings fatigue. The nurse's movements should be sure, smooth and unhurried. The child should be told when the nurse is going to insert the thermometer, lift him in bed, roll him to his side or perform any other act, as quick, unexpected movements startle him and increase his apprehension. Elevation of the head rest often relieves dyspnea. Support of the arms at the sides by pillows takes the weight of the arms from the shoulders. This also helps to overcome the tendency to fold the arms over the abdomen, which causes undesirable pressure, and it allows better chest expansion. Poor muscle tone and fatigue predispose the child to postural defects, and measures to support the body help to prevent poor posture.

Every possible measure should be taken to alleviate anxiety and to inspire confidence, as emotional calm is as essential as physical comfort and restriction of exercise. All nursing care should be planned carefully to provide for maximum amounts of rest. By thoughtful organization of essential nursing care the hypnotic effect of sedative drugs administered may be prolonged greatly.

ESSENTIAL NURSING CARE

This includes careful recording of the temperature and the pulse and the respiration rates. The pulse rate indicates the progress of the child and, to obtain an accurate measure, it should be observed for a full minute before the thermometer is inserted. When sleeping pulses are requested, the nurse must be sure that the child is not wakened.

A high temperature, increased perspiration and edema make care of the skin a prime requisite. The back and the buttocks need particular care and should be washed and rubbed with alcohol 3 times daily. Rubber rings or cotton "doughnuts" are useful in preventing pressure areas which develop easily, especially in edematous children. Change in position is essential for good skin care and it also helps in aeration of the lungs. When joints are painful and swollen, a cradle to raise the bedclothing from them will give added comfort.

GOOD MOUTH CARE

Good mouth care needs to be given, especially if the child is receiving limited fluids or is dyspneic and is breathing through his mouth. Lemon juice and glycerine, half and half, is a good lubricant for dry tongue, gums and lips after they have been cleaned.

RECORDING INTAKE AND OUTPUT

Recording the intake and the output of these children also requires the careful attention of the nurse. When intake is limited, a schedule should be made which will give the child a proportion of the total amount ordered at short intervals during the day and during the night when he wakes up feeling thirsty.

The nurse is responsible also for the nutrition of the child, often a serious problem, for these children have poor appetites and often their capacity is limited because of heart enlargement and decompensation. In the acute stage, a liquid diet of high caloric value usually is given. Later, as the child's physical condition and appetite improve, a high-protein, high-vitamin diet is introduced gradually.

PREVENTION OF INFECTIONS

These children are especially susceptible to infections, and association with other sick children should be supervised closely. Visitors and personnel with sore throats never should be permitted near the child with heart disease.

ADMINISTRATION OF OXYGEN

Administration of oxygen is usually the next remedial measure after rest is instituted. This is performed most satisfactorily by an oxygen tent; as it is less confining, the child can see the personnel, and a good concentration of oxygen is assured. A temperature of between 65° and 70° F. should be maintained in the tent, and the child should be protected with appropriate body covering. Explaining the purpose of the tent to the child before he is put into it will allay fears so frequently associated with confinement in a small, enclosed space.

PARACENTESIS

Paracentesis of the pericardial sac gives immediate relief to the heart if a great amount of fluid has collected because of pericarditis. Paracentesis of the abdominal cavity likewise may be indicated for relief of respiratory difficulty caused by ascites.

DRUGS

The drugs prescribed are chiefly digitalis and salicylates. Digitalis slows and strengthens the heart and so improves circulation. Before each dose of this drug is given, the pulse rate should be observed. If it has gone down markedly or has changed in quality, the doctor's approval should be secured before the drug is given. Anorexia, nausea and vomiting are the chief toxic symptoms.

The toxic manifestations of overdosage with salicylates, cortisone and ACTH have been described under acute rheumatic carditis. The nurse should be thoroughly familiar with these untoward reactions, which may demand a change in therapeutic plans.

CONVALESCENT CARE

The child convalescing from heart disease offers a real challenge to the nurse. She must keep him happy and growing but at the same time confine his activities to the limits permitted by the degree of cardiac compensation.

Attempting to carry out the order for bed rest in a negative way by constant insistence on rest is detrimental to the child's mental health. The child who has spent long periods in bed feels no need for rest and therefore has little or no interest in it. Constant use of the word merely calls attention to his handicapped body and makes him more anxious. There develop between nurse and child nagging situations which produce a negative attitude rather than a desire to co-operate. Frequent use of "don't" also tends to arouse antagonism and influences the development of personality problems as devastating as his disease. The negative direction "don't" serves only to give the child the idea of doing the forbidden thing.

Teaching the child about his disease and guiding him into quiet, interesting and absorbing activities helps him to accept the limitations which recuperation requires. Little by little through the use of artful, positive direction and teaching which helps him to understand his disease and his need for rest, the nurse gradually can build up in the child a sense of responsibility for his own actions. The acutely ill child may be told stories, shown pictures, read to, anything that requires no effort on his part. As he recuperates, he may hold the book, turn the pages, cut pictures from magazine pages and direct the placement of them in a scrapbook. Later he can color, fingerpaint, mold clay, work simple puzzles, use paper dolls, dress dolls and do schoolwork. Play periods should be of short duration. His play should eliminate emotional strain and be interspersed with periods of music and stories which have been planned to provide relaxation and rest.

A graduated program of activity with gradual increase in exercise should coincide with the rate of his physical progress. A period of a few weeks to many months is required, depending on the course of the disease and the return of cardiac efficiency.

Time out of bed should be increased gradually. When the child first is permitted to be up, a chair without wheels should be provided to prevent overactivity. A child who has been bedridden for a long period cannot be expected to maintain quiet when he is tempted with a chair that can transport him to places he has long wanted to explore. At first, he should be placed in a chair near a window with play materials that interest him and ensure quiet activity. Then, when the nurse can be in constant attendance, excursions in a wheel chair will revive his spirits and give him something more constructive to think about. Later, when his condition has improved, he can be placed in a wheel chair and given limited freedom to move about. The pulse rate should be observed before he is lifted into the chair and again when his position has been made comfortable. If his pulse does not return to normal within 5 minutes, he should be put back into bed. If his temperature rises in the evening, his sleep seems disturbed, or his behavior indicates undue fatigue, it probably means that a longer rest period is required.

A study of the child's physical and psychological needs, his home and family circumstances should be made to determine the appropriate location for convalescent care. This is one of the many services that a social service department can give to a hospital to increase its usefulness to its child patients. When the child's own home can provide individualized care, convalescent care there is to be preferred. A child thrives best in his own family when the home provides the security necessary for personal and social adjustment in addition to satisfying his physical needs for food, clothing and shelter.

During the convalescent period, whether the child is being cared for in the convalescent hospital, in his own home or in a foster one, consideration must be given to the promotion of his normal development. His environment must provide emotional security, opportunities for play, work and group life as well as continued supervision of his physical health. The continuation of his schoolwork will prevent a feeling of inadequacy when he returns to school and has to compete with his former classmates. In some cities, the board of education provides visiting teachers for children unable to attend school. There exist for handicapped children schools which meet their needs of transportation, special classes and a program planned in accordance with their individual capacities.

When school opportunities are not available or the home is found to be lacking in the essentials necessary to satisfy a child's needs, care in a convalescent hospital or a foster home may be considered advisable. The convalescent hospital provides association with other handicapped children. In many instances such an environment helps the child to adjust himself more easily to limited activity and to face his problems in

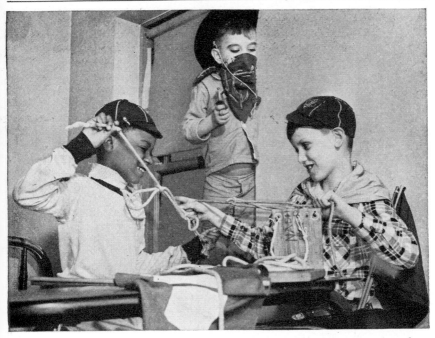

FIG. 35. The play of boys with cardiac disease is similar to the play of normal children. (La Rabida Jackson Park Sanitarium for Children with Cardiac Disease, Chicago, and The Chicago Daily Sun Times)

a more wholesome way. Schoolwork and group activities appropriate to his capacity and interests can be supplied more easily (Figs. 35 to 39). The group provides friendship and a sense of belonging and stimulates his interest in school and play activities. In a convalescent home or hospital, a child's physical condition can be supervised more adequately. When the earliest signs of respiratory infection are detected, bed rest can be resumed and thereby recurrences can be minimized.

Care in a foster home is sometimes necessary for either of two reasons: because convalescent-hospital care is unavailable or because study of a child indicates his need for the type of nurturing that is supplied by a smaller and more intimate family group. The latter is especially true of the child whose previous home background has not been sufficiently stable to give him the affection and the security that he needed for normal personality development. When plans for foster-home care are being made, participation of the child should be encouraged to prevent the experience from becoming traumatic to him. Placing an unprepared child in a strange family setting tends to increase insecurity and in some instances might signify to him rejection by those whom he

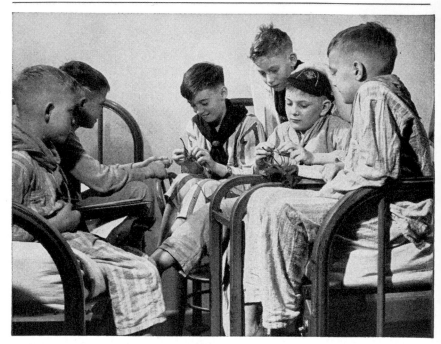

Fig. 36. Scout activities are a part of the activity program at the La Rabida Jackson Park Sanitarium. (La Rabida Sanitarium, Chicago, and The Chicago Daily Sun Times)

needs the most. Visits by foster parents prior to discharge from the hospital gives the group opportunity to become acquainted and build up the child's sense of security which facilitates adjustment into a new family situation. Continued supervision of the foster home is required to observe the child's response and adjustment to it. The child's family should be encouraged to maintain relations with him. As soon as adjustments which suit the child's needs can be made in his own home, he should be returned to that environment.

Wherever the convalescent child with cardiac disease is being cared

for, development of his personality must receive adequate emphasis. Re-establishing independence after a long period of helplessness requires thoughtful guidance. He should have supervision, but those who are entrusted with this responsibility must give it without crippling him psychologically. There are children who find it difficult to give up the privileged position that sickness brings. When this characteristic is observed in a child, it indicates his need for motivation to want to participate in normal activities. He needs to discover the rewards of getting well. He also should be given freedom to enjoy activities with other children.

Sometimes nurses unknowingly keep children dependent upon them. They do things for children that they are quite able to do for themselves. They reward dependence and provide too little freedom for them to develop relationships with their age-mates.

Those who care for children who are convalescing from heart disease need an understanding of their developmental needs, an appreciation of their capacities and limitations and the capacity to help them accept their handicaps in a realistic way. Personnel who supervise the health of these children must be convinced of their capacity to live normal, useful lives. They must provide an environment which meets their emotional, social and spiritual needs. They need continued contact with their families and preparation for home-going and growth-producing experiences. Without a wholesome environment, psychological crippling will impose a second handicap which may be infinitely more self-limiting than the physical disease.

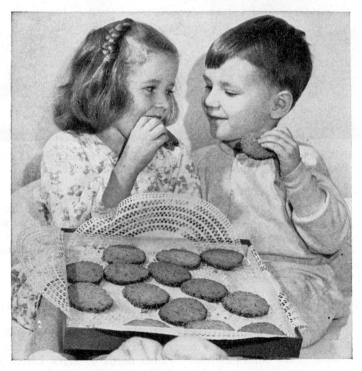

Fig. 37. Two children with cardiac disease enjoying party food and the company of each other. (La Rabida Jackson Park Sanitarium, Chicago, and The Chicago Daily Sun Times)

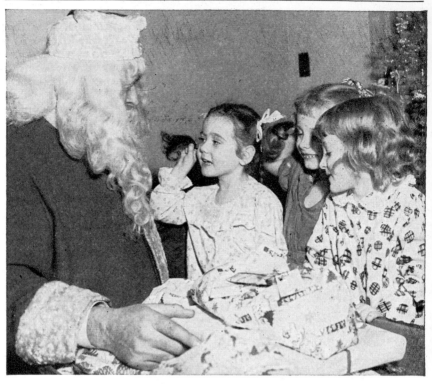

Fig. 38. Christmas festivities are important for children in hospitals. (La Rabida Jackson Park Sanitarium, Chicago, and The Chicago Daily Sun Times)

FOLLOW-UP CARE

Continued health supervision is desirable to prevent recurrences. Parents need to know the necessity for frequent clinic visits, adequate dental care and a regimen of living which provides protection from infection and adequate rest, diet, school activities and play. The school nurse and the teacher need information which will assist them in understanding the child's individual requirements. Team work between the personnel in the hospital, the family physician or the physician in the division of services for crippled children, the school nurse and the teacher is essential in the care of the child who has had cardiac disease.

SITUATIONS FOR FURTHER STUDY

1. What are the symptoms of tetralogy of Fallot?

2. What do you think a 5-year-old child with patent ductus arteriosus needs to know before going to the operating room?

3. Prepare a child with patent ductus arteriosus for operation.

Write a report of your approach, your verbal preparation, the child's response to you and all you were saying and your reactions to this experience. Include your observations of the child's response to going to the operating room, to having the anesthetic and to the experiences of the immediate postoperative period.

4. Write a description of a child who has tetralogy of Fallot. De-scribe his physical appearance, his behavior, his response to nurses, doctors and the tests that he has had in the hospital. Include your observations of his behavior after operation. In what ways is his be-havior different from that which you observed in the preoperative period? Describe his parents' response to his change in behavior? How did you help them to see that operation had

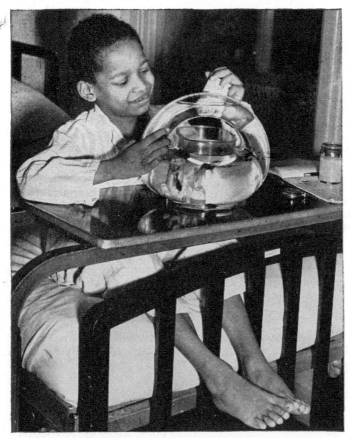

Fig. 39. Confinement to bed is more tolerable when interesting projects are available. (La Rabida Jackson Park Sanitarium, Chicago, and The Chicago Daily Sun Times)

changed his physical condition and made it possible for him to lead a more normal life?

5. What symptoms in a school-age child would lead you to suspect that the child was in the beginning stages of rheumatic fever?

6. What are the social and the emotional needs of the school-age child who is convalescing from heart disease?

7. What anxieties might a school-age child with rheumatic carditis experience? How might the nurse function in alleviating his anxiety?

8. What might be possible reasons why a school-age boy with rheumatic fever would show resistance to the order for absolute bed rest? What would you do if you noticed this kind of resistance in one of your patients?

BIBLIOGRAPHY

Blake, Florence: Development and care during the school-age period, chap. 7, p. 301, *in* The Child, His Parents and the Nurse, Philadelphia, Lippincott, 1954.

Cohen, Ethel: Medical-social problems of rheumatic children, Am. J. Pub. Health 31:819, 1941.

Dodds, Maryella: Have fun . . . get well! (pamphlet), New York, Am. Heart A., 1953.

Gross, R. E.: Surgery of Infancy and Childhood, chaps. 60-64, Philadelphia, Saunders, 1953.

Hansen, A. E.: Rheumatic fever, Am. J. Nursing 53:168, 1953.

Jetter, L. E.: Some emotional aspects of prolonged illness in children, Pub. Health Nursing 40: 257, 1948.

Josselyn, I. M.: Emotional implications of rheumatic heart disease' in children, Am. J. Orthopsychiat. 11:87, 1949.

Overholser, M. T.: The congenital cardiac program, Am. J. Nursing 53:1,478, 1953.

Pierson, D. E.: Nursing care of a child with tetralogy of Fallot, Am. J. Nursing 47:301, 1947.

Potts, W. J.: Tetralogy of Fallot, Am. J. Nursing 47:298, 1947.

Sadler, Sabra: Rheumatic Fever Nursing Care in Pictures, Philadelphia, Lippincott, 1949.

Sadler, Sabra, and Seibel, Elizabeth: The child with acute rheumatic fever and his nursing care, Am. J. Nursing 46:170, 1946.

Smith, E. M.: A nursing staff prepares for cardiac surgery, Am. J. Nursing 49:589, 1949.

Wallace, Mildred: Care of the child with tetralogy of Fallot, Am. J. Nursing 52:195, 1952.

Yasumura, Michi, and Baldwin, J. S.: Occupational therapy for the rheumatic and cardiac children, Am. J. Occup. Therapy 1:62, 1953.

Convalescent care for children (pamphlet) Chicago, Nat. Soc. Crippled Child., 1946.

Diseases of the Genito-urinary System

PHYSIOLOGY OF THE KIDNEY
ABNORMALITIES OF RENAL FUNCTION
CONGENITAL MALFORMATIONS OF
   THE KIDNEY AND THE URETER
NEPHRITIS
WILMS'S TUMOR

ABNORMALITIES OF BLADDER
   FUNCTION
INFECTIONS OF THE GENITO-URINARY
   TRACT
MALFORMATIONS OF THE LOWER
   GENITO-URINARY TRACT
SITUATIONS FOR FURTHER STUDY

PHYSIOLOGY OF THE KIDNEY

The functioning units of the kidney are the nephrons, of which approximately 2 million exist. Each nephron is composed of a glomerulus, a convoluted tubule, a collecting tubule and a blood supply (Fig. 40). A glomerulus consists of a globular network of capillaries encased in a sac. This capillary tuft is supplied by a small artery (an afferent or entering arteriole), and blood leaves the glomerulus by another (efferent) arteriole. The capillary tuft within the glomerulus acts as a filter, fluid entering the glomerular sac from the capillaries by reason of pressure of the blood in excess of the pressure in the sac. The filtrate contains a high proportion of all the plasma contents except the protein and the cellular elements. It contains waste products

as well as materials which are highly useful to the body.

The glomerular sac empties by way of a tubule which runs a very tortuous course (convoluted tubule). The first series of convolutions, lying near the glomerulus, comprises the proximal convoluted tubule. Then the tubule runs from the cortex of the kidney, where all glomeruli are located, into the medulla of the kidney and turns back (loop of Henle) to form in the cortex another series of convolutions (distal convoluted tubule). The tubule enters a collecting tubule which also collects from other nephrons. Then the collecting tubule passes through the medulla to empty into the pelvis of the kidney.

The efferent arteriole from the glomerulus supplies a capillary network which surrounds the convoluted tubule. From the convoluted tubule, materials which the body needs are resorbed into the blood of the capillary network surrounding it. Only the remaining relatively small amount of fluid containing waste products passes into the collecting tubule for excretion. After performing their functions of absorption, the capillaries of the tubule become venules to carry blood away from the kidney.

In the adult, approximately 1,500 cc. of blood pass through the nephrons each minute, an amount equal to 30 per cent of the heart output and greater than that for any other organ except the lungs. Glomerular filtrate forms at the rate of approximately 125 cc. a minute, a volume one twelfth that of the blood passing through the glomeruli. By reason of loss of this filtrate, the plasma efferent from the glomeruli is concen-

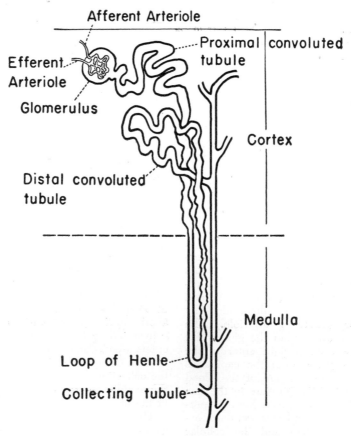

Fig. 40. Schematic representation of a nephron.

trated approximately 25 per cent, the volume of blood cells remaining the same. As the filtrate courses through the convoluted tubules, a high proportion is resorbed, and only from 1 to 2 per cent is available finally for excretion as urine. Resorption occurs in large part through osmosis resulting from the greater concentration of materials in the tubular than in the glomerular capillaries and because of a lower blood pressure in the tubular than in the glomerular capillaries. In smaller but important parts the filtrate is resorbed because of the presence of the posterior pituitary antidiuretic hormone. The resorption of sodium is subject also to the influence of the adrenal cortical hormone desoxy-corticosterone, this substance producing absorption. Through these various means, all the glucose, 99 per cent of the water and of the sodium and some of the urea of the filtrate are resorbed.

One of the important functions of the kidney is to excrete waste products, the chief of which are urea, carbonic and other organic acids and phosphates. An important one, present in smaller amount, is uric acid. These materials are excreted by the mechanisms which have been discussed. In addition, certain substances can be excreted into the urine selectively by the tubules.

Another important function of the kidney is to conserve basic substances for the body while excreting waste. To a considerable extent the base of bicarbonate can be resorbed, leaving the carbon dioxide in the filtrate. Most of the phosphate in the blood is dibasic (e.g., Na_2HPO_4). The dibasic phosphates can be converted by the tubules to the mono-basic phosphates (e.g., NaH_2PO_4), thus conserving base by excreting an acid instead of a neutral material. Also, the tubular epithelium can form ammonia from amino acids to replace base for excretion of acids, thus further conserving base for the body.

Variations in the amount of urine produced ordinarily are the result of changes in the amount of water resorbed by the tubules. Except for disturbances in which the glomeruli are diseased, the amount of glomerular filtrate produced remains fairly constant. Rather, increases in urine volume depend upon a fall in the amount of tubular reabsorption of the filtrate. Thus, excessive water ingestion dilutes the blood and causes a decrease in production of pituitary antidiuretic hormone, and the tubules allow more water to escape, or a mercurial diuretic partially poisons the resorptive activity of the tubules and more water escapes, or the presence of abnormal amounts of sugar, urea or other substances in the filtrate interferes with the resorption of water from the tubules.

The adequacy of renal function is measured by a variety of clinical tests. Determination of the level of urea or *nonprotein nitrogen* in the blood indicates the ability of the kidney to dispose of the waste products of protein metabolism. The *urea clearance test* is a more refined method of measuring this aspect of kidney function. The ability of the kidney to increase the *concentration of the urine* following a standard period of fluid restriction is another useful clinical test. The ability of the tubules to excrete an injected dye also may be tested by use of the *phenolsulfonphthalein excretion test*. During infancy these tests indicate that the kidney is immature and unable to perform such functions as efficiently as the kidney of the older child or the adult. After the age of 2 this functional difference is no longer apparent.

ABNORMALITIES OF RENAL FUNCTION

A number of terms are used to describe abnormalities of function of the urinary tract. Those that imply disturbance of kidney function are considered below. Others that relate to disorders of the lower urinary tract will be mentioned subsequently.

ANURIA

Anuria is the absence of urine. It usually results from failure of the kidney to excrete but occasionally it is due to obstruction of the lower urinary tract. It occurs rather commonly in the newborn infant for periods up to 36 hours after birth and is not significant of renal disease except in the rare circumstance of congenital absence of the kidneys. In older children it usually is associated with the onset of nephritis or severe kidney infections. Occasionally it follows mercurial poisoning, transfusion reactions, severe burns, prolonged shock or sulfonamide intoxication. In children it is generally a self-limited phenomenon which is handled best by carefully controlled administration of water and electrolytes instead of the more dramatic procedures of peritoneal lavage or the use of an artificial kidney.

OLIGURIA

Oliguria is decreased urinary flow. It is seen in dehydration and during

certain stages of the several types of nephritis. The management depends upon the underlying condition.

POLYURIA

An abnormal increase in the volume of urine may result from excessive fluid intake or administration, from poorly controlled diabetes mellitus or from diabetes insipidus.

ALBUMINURIA

Albuminuria is detected by chemical examination of the urine. It results when the glomerular membrane permits passage of the smaller protein molecules from the blood stream into the glomerular filtrate and thence the urine. In a heavy or a persistent amount, albuminuria usually indicates renal disease, such as nephritis, nephrosis or pyelonephritis. It is found transiently in newborn infants and may be found in mild degree in normal children.

Postural Albuminuria. This benign condition is discovered occasionally on routine urinalysis. Albumin appears in the urine when the child is standing or exercising but not when he is recumbent. The disturbance frequently disappears after puberty and has no known relation to renal disease. It requires no treatment, but a careful exclusion of other causes of albuminuria is demanded.

CYLINDRURIA

This term indicates the presence of abnormal numbers of casts in the urine. These are microscopic plugs which form in the kidney tubules when the rate of urine flow is slow or when albuminuria is present. They often contain cellular elements which are valuable clues to the type of renal disturbance.

HEMATURIA

Hematuria signifies the presence of red blood cells in the urine. When the concentration of cells is large the urine may appear grossly bloody or may have a brown or smoky tinge. Smaller degrees of hematuria can be discovered only by microscopic examination. Hematuria usually signifies glomerular disease in the child. Bleeding into the lower urinary tract can and does occur but is relatively infrequent among children. A number of processes may alter the glomerular membrane in such a way as to permit the passage of red blood cells. Glomerular bleeding in children is most commonly due to nephritis, trauma, infection, blood dyscrasia or sulfonamide overdosage.

AZOTEMIA

This term indicates an increase of the nonprotein nitrogen constituents in the blood above the arbitrary level of 35 mgm. per 100 ml. It indicates that the kidneys are unable to clear the blood of protein waste products at the usual speed. While most often found during renal disease, azotemia also may result when the blood flow to the kidneys is insufficient, as in cardiac failure or severe dehydration or to a minor extent when specimens are obtained after a heavy protein meal.

UREMIA

This term implies azotemia which is associated with severe impairment of renal function and usually is accompanied by symptoms which include nausea, headache, anorexia, diarrhea, fatigue, acidosis, anemia and bleeding tendencies. The management depends upon the nature of the underlying renal disease.

CONGENITAL MALFORMATIONS OF THE KIDNEY AND THE URETER

APLASIA AND HYPOPLASIA OF THE KIDNEY

Congenital absence of both kidneys is incompatible with life for more than a few hours and generally is associated with other malformations. Congenital absence of one kidney causes no disability if the remaining kidney is normal. It is frequent enough to require identification of another kidney before nephrectomy is performed. Hypoplasia of one or both kidneys results in disease which simulates chronic pyelonephritis and is considered under the section on infection.

POLYCYSTIC KIDNEY

This disorder is the result of abnormal development of the kidney tubules, many of which consist of dilated fluid-filled cysts which do not contribute to kidney function. They usually enlarge the kidney. Symptoms relate to the loss of renal function. When the malformation is severe, renal failure may occur during early infancy, but in many instances the disability is mild enough to permit the child to survive for many years, even into the third or the fourth decade. No useful treatment is known.

OTHER MALFORMATIONS

Anomalous formation of the upper urinary tract is quite common and is found in some degree in nearly 10 per cent of autopsies performed on children. Many of the malformations are of no consequence to the child but when they result in stasis of urine flow, they are prone to become chronically infected or to produce pain from obstruction. Such conditions as hydronephrosis, double kidney or ureter, dilated ureter and the disorders mentioned above can be identified only by careful urologic study. Attention usually is attracted to them by the appearance of urinary-tract infection, which is discussed in a later section. The need for and the technics of surgical correction vary with the type of anatomic and functional disorder.

NEPHRITIS

In order to present the various disease conditions which should be considered under the term "nephritis," it is desirable to have a classification of the types of disease for convenience in discussion and understanding. Unfortunately, complete general agreement does not exist as to an appropriate classification. For the purpose of this presentation, a classification which at least serves as a basis for discussing the various types has been chosen.

In some respects, nephritis of children differs much from that of adults. The child's kidneys have a power of regeneration after injury far greater than do those of the adult. The commonest type of nephritis in childhood (acute glomerular) is the least common among adults and is the most benign of all the varieties. Nephritis of the older person is likely to be complicated by degenerative changes, whereas such changes are not common in childhood. Pure nephrosis that is fully reparable seems to occur only in children. Nephrosis of adults is usually a part of chronic nephritis, which ultimately leads to irreparable and fatal kidney damage. Those

classifications dealing with adults largely or exclusively are likely to contain statements concerning nephritis which are wholly true for adults but do not apply to children.

ACUTE GLOMERULAR NEPHRITIS (ACUTE HEMORRHAGIC NEPHRITIS)

Acute glomerular nephritis is characterized by changes in the glomerular capillaries which permit the passage of blood cells and protein into the glomerular filtrate. The finding of blood in the urine is a constant feature of the disease. Associated changes in other parts of the body are commonly but not necessarily present. These include edema, hypertension, azotemia and the secondary phenomena which may result from them.

Etiology. The disease is dependent on a recently preceding streptococcic infection, usually in the upper respiratory tract and most frequently in the tonsils and the adjacent lymph nodes. It is one of the possible complications of scarlet fever, occurring in the second or the third week of this disease. It also may occur secondary to streptococcic infections of the skin (impetigo, infected eczema or scabies). It occurs at any age but is most frequent in midchildhood. The nephritis is a result of a toxic effect of streptococcic infection which affects all capillaries, including those of the glomeruli.

Symptoms. When the preceding streptococcic infection is recognized, a latent period of roughly 1 to 3 weeks ensues between its onset and the appearance of symptoms of nephritis. It is probable that many children have nephritis in such mild form that it goes unrecognized. Usually, the initial symptoms are puffiness of the face or grossly bloody urine or headache and vomiting. These symptoms may occur alone or in combination. Occasionally, the disease is announced by dyspnea due to impending heart failure. Oliguria is frequent but transient; anuria occurs rarely. Later in the disease, chronic fatigue, anemia and malnutrition may constitute the chief symptoms.

In the majority of affected children the symptoms rapidly reach their maximum intensity and trail off within a week or two, leaving the child symptomatically well but with evidence of the continuing disease from the various laboratory tests. Azotemia is seldom responsible for symptoms unless its severity is sufficient to produce uremia. The chief mechanism responsible for the symptomatology is the consequence of a general vascular disturbance which leads to edema and spasm of arterioles. Combined with hypertension, these processes lead to varying degrees of cerebral edema and myocardial insufficiency. Occasionally in children serious or even fatal complications ensue — hypertensive encephalopathy with convulsions or coma, or congestive heart failure.

Diagnosis. Usually, the history and the symptoms alone strongly suggest the diagnosis. Examination of the urine should disclose red blood cells, albumin and casts. If the casts contain red blood cells, there is no doubt about the diagnosis. Hypertension and azotemia may or may not be present.

Prognosis. Recovery from acute glomerulonephritis is to be expected in nearly all children. Even among those in whom the disease is severe enough to require hospitalization,

about 85 per cent recover completely. Mild illnesses last as little as 2 to 3 weeks; in the more obstinate cases evidence of continuing renal disease may last from 12 to 18 months before recovery takes place. In exceptional instances the disease is progressive and takes on the characteristics of chronic nephritis. A small number of children succumb to the early effects of hypertensive encephalopathy or heart failure.

Treatment. INFECTION. Although antibiotic therapy is of no avail in the treatment of the nephritis itself, complete eradication of the beta hemolytic streptococcus infection which preceded should be assured through the use of penicillin.

BED REST. During the acute stage and for as long as appreciable amounts of blood appear in the urine, the child should be kept at bed rest. If the disease is prolonged and enters a subacute stage in which there are minimal findings in the urine, the child may be allowed complete activity but should be protected from further infection and from chilling, which seems to reactivate the nephritic process.

DIET. Contrary to previous belief, the diet need not be restricted in respect to protein but should contain a full complement of all nutrients as soon as the appetite returns. In the presence of edema, salt intake usually is restricted. Except during evidence of cardiac failure no fluid restrictions need be imposed.

CARDIAC FAILURE. The management of cardiac failure is essentially the same as described in the preceding chapter. Morphine, oxygen and digitalis may be required. Diuretics are contraindicated in the presence of nephritis.

HYPERTENSION. The control of hypertension is a very important aspect of treatment. Magnesium sulfate may be given for this purpose by mouth, intramuscularly or intravenously, depending upon the severity of the cerebral symptoms. Prevention of convulsions is highly desirable, so that oral administration of a 50 per cent solution in doses of 1 or 2 ounces usually is given as soon as appreciable elevation of the blood pressure is detected. The drug has surprisingly little cathartic action during the course of nephritis. The rectal route may be substituted for the oral if vomiting is present or if the child refuses to take the medication. At higher levels of blood pressure, magnesium sulfate is given intramuscularly in a 25 per cent solution at a dosage of about 0.2 ml. per Kg. of body weight. If symptoms are severe or other forms of administration have been ineffective, the drug may be given slowly intravenously in a 2 per cent solution at a dosage of 10 ml. per Kg. Overdosage with magnesium sulfate may produce respiratory depression, which can be counteracted by intravenous administration of a soluble calcium solution which should be readily available whenever intramuscular or intravenous treatment is being employed.

Nursing Care. The child should be dressed warmly enough to prevent chilling. While rest in bed is required, play activities should be provided to keep the child happily occupied. The blood pressure should be observed at intervals during the day and the night during the early stage of the disease. Any elevation

should be reported immediately. When an elevation in blood pressure is noted, increased observation is indicated to detect signs of cerebral symptoms. When the child's blood pressure is high and he begins to show cerebral symptoms, cribsides or a crib bed should be provided for his protection. Equipment to give magnesium sulfate intravenously and intramuscularly should be in readiness in the child's room.

NEPHROSIS
(LIPID NEPHROSIS, NEPHROTIC SYNDROME)

Nephrosis is a disease which is peculiar to young children. It is characterized by generalized edema associated with a heavy loss of albumin in the urine, by a fall in the level of the blood proteins, chiefly involving the albumin fraction, and by a rise in the level of blood lipids including cholesterol. Hypertension, azotemia and hematuria are not usually present in the early stages of the disease.

Symptoms. EDEMA. The disease usually appears insidiously without any antecedent infection, beginning as the slow, asymptomatic accumulation of edema, which is noticed first about the eyes. As the swelling advances, it may involve the legs, the arms and the back to varying degrees. Accumulation of fluid in the peritoneal cavity and the scrotum is frequent (Fig. 41). Shifting of the edematous areas is common, depending to some extent upon the position of the child during sleep or during waking activity. With moderate stretching of the skin over the subcutaneous fluid, there is pronounced pallor which is out of proportion to the degree of anemia; with severe degrees of edema, striae may appear from overstretching—striae which simulate those seen on the abdomen of the pregnant woman.

MALNUTRITION. In spite of their appearance, which is often grotesque, nephrotic children usually maintain a surprising cheerfulness and evenness of disposition. Excessive fluid accumulations impede their activity and appetite and may embarrass respirations by limiting the excursion of the diaphragm. As the disease continues, inapparent malnutrition takes place, which is revealed clearly only when diuresis and loss of subcutaneous edema occur.

ANEMIA of moderate degree usually appears during the course of the illness.

POOR RESISTANCE TO INFECTION. This is characteristic. Before modern chemotherapy, death occurred in a considerable proportion of children with nephrosis because of the ravages of septicemia, peritonitis and meningitis. Formerly, streptococci and pneumococci were usually responsible for these severe infections; more recently, there has been an increasing prevalence of other organisms.

NEPHROTIC CRISIS. A nephrotic crisis simulates peritonitis by producing abdominal pain, fever and sometimes an erysipeloid skin eruption. These events may occur without demonstrable infection. They usually subside within a few days and may be followed by a spontaneous diuresis.

When the course of nephrosis is complicated by one of the contagious diseases such as measles or chickenpox, spontaneous diuresis

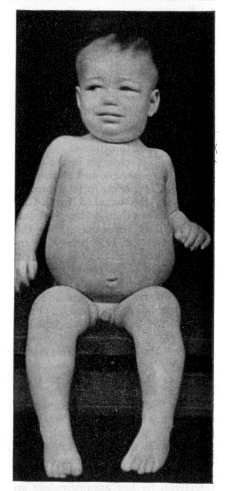

FIG. 41. Edema of nephrosis.

and loss of edema may result. Although the remission is ordinarily temporary, occasionally it is permanent.

Laboratory Findings. URINE. In the urine the constant findings are those of heavy albuminuria with casts and white blood cells. Red cells may appear transiently, in small amounts persistently, or in larger numbers when the disease is changing its characteristics toward those of chronic nephritis. The child usually retains the ability to concentrate the urine. The urea clearance test of kidney function is commonly normal, sometimes supernormal. Lipid granules are almost always present in the urine and aid in diagnosis of the disease.

BLOOD. The changes in the blood involve the proteins and the lipids. There is a reduction in total protein level from the usual 6 to 8 Gm. per cent to less than 4 Gm. per cent. Most of this reduction is in the albumin fraction, which may be reduced to less than 1 Gm. per cent. The levels of blood lipids, including cholesterol, are usually at least double the normal values and frequently produce a cloudy appearance of the blood plasma when it separates.

Course and Prognosis. The course of nephrosis invariably is prolonged unless death occurs from an early complication. Few children endure a course that is less than 18 months. During this period there may be fluctuations in the severity of symptoms, even to the extent of complete remission. If the child can be carried safely through the threatening infections, he has approximately an even chance between surviving with a complete cure or having his disease change its characteristics and assume the features of chronic nephritis with its invariably fatal outcome.

Etiology. Among those who deal with sick children, there is little disagreement that nephrosis constitutes an entity which is quite distinct from other varieties of renal disease. Yet there is no uniformity of opinion about its etiology and there are many points of disagreement about the mechanism of its abnormal physiology. Unlike acute glomerular nephritis, there is no relation to streptococcal infection, healing is delayed and uncertain, and renal function is usually good at the onset. Peculiarities of protein and lipid metabolism and of the distribution of electrolytes remain unexplained. The peculiar effect of acute infection in producing a remission also requires an explanation. At the present time the disease continues to be a lively topic of speculation and investigation.

Treatment. The general plan of management of the child with nephrosis varies according to the convictions of individual physicians. Some feel that it is essential to try to modify the course of the disease by active methods to induce diuresis and support blood protein levels. Others believe that such measures have but little long-term effect upon the illness. They believe that it is better to bank on the spontaneous healing which will occur in many children, in the meanwhile supporting the child's nutrition, combatting infection and providing relief from excessive fluid accumulations by periodic abdominal paracentesis.

DIET. As in every other chronic disease, the diet should be complete. The dietary components which have received greatest attention are protein, salt and water. A generous protein allowance is desirable. To the customary need for protein must be added that which results from constant loss in the urine. Very high protein diets are not taken well and are utilized no better than those of more moderate content. A suitable allowance is from 3 to 3.5 Gm. for each Kg. Limitation of salt intake by making no salt additions to the diet is appropriate, but extreme or prolonged limitation of salt is dangerous. There is no advantage in water restriction.

INFECTIONS. Appropriate attention must be given to existing focal infections, and the child's regimen should be so regulated as to reduce his chances of acquiring respiratory disease. Prompt recognition of major infections is imperative, for antibiotic treatment must be started promptly.

ACTIVITY. Insofar as possible it is wise to permit the child freedom of activity in order to maintain his and his parents' morale during the long course of the disease. Bed rest and confinement to a hospital should be avoided whenever possible.

PLASMA PROTEINS. Attempts to support the level of plasma proteins by transfusion, plasma infusions or the injection of salt-free albumin have not met with impressive success. Most of the injected protein appears promptly in the urine and has no lasting effect upon the course of the illness.

DIURESIS. A great variety of measures have been used to produce diuresis. Many of them are occasionally or temporarily effective. The list includes plasma and albumin injections, mercurial diuretics, calcium and potassium salts, salts which alter the acid-base balance of the blood, transmission of measles and other infectious diseases to the patient and more recently cortisone and ACTH.

Nursing Care. This is the most important part of the management of a child with nephrosis. The illness is chronic, and effective treatment measures are few. In these circumstances, the day-to-day care becomes highly important. During the stage when edema is present, the appetite is poor. Serving small quantities of special-diet foods initially and permitting the child to help himself to additional amounts frequently stimulates his appetite. Catering to a capricious appetite is necessary to encourage the child to eat the food that is necessary for his maintenance and final recovery. The use of attractive dishes and colored straws often appeals to the child who has little or no inclination to eat.

During periods of marked edema, care of the skin is especially important. When the external male genitalia are extremely edematous, special local care becomes necessary. The genitalia should be bathed several times daily and dusted with a soothing powder. The scrotum should be supported by a cotton pad held in place by a T-binder lightly applied. Cotton to separate the skin surfaces will prevent intertrigo from developing. When the child is lying on his side, pressure on the edematous organs can be eliminated by placing a pillow between his knees. When edema of the eyelids is marked, circulation of lacrimal secretion over the eyes is impaired. Warm normal saline irrigations can be used to keep the eyes free from exudate. By maintaining head elevation during parts of the day, eyelid edema usually subsides sufficiently to give the child a greater degree of comfort.

The child with nephrosis should be weighed 2 or 3 times weekly to note changes in the degree of edema. Accurate records should be kept of intake and output. Every effort must be made to avoid respiratory infections.

When ascites is present to a marked degree, abdominal paracentesis is required to relieve the pressure symptoms. If the child is prepared in such a way that he is helped to understand that the discomfort of the procedure will be less than the discomfort from the collection of fluid in his abdominal cavity, he usually will co-operate and assist by maintaining quiet during the procedure.

Puncturing the bladder during the paracentesis can be avoided if the child is placed on a bedpan and encouraged to void just prior to the treatment.

Sterile equipment required for an abdominal paracentesis consists of hypodermic syringe, hypodermic and aspiration needles, procaine (Novocain), scalpel, cannula, trocar, rubber tubing, needleholder, suture needles, sutures, forceps, gloves, towels, graduated receptacle, cotton balls, gauze squares and an abdominal dressing.

Unsterile equipment consists of a preparation tray, test tubes, a pail for the collection of fluid, a scultetus or abdominal binder and safety pins.

The child should be placed close to the edge of the examining table. Two nurses are required to assist in this procedure. One nurse prepares the area, collects samples of ascitic fluid for culture and checks the child's pulse, respirations and color during the procedure. The second nurse is responsible for maintaining the child's position. When the child's co-operation has been se-

cured, no restraint is necessary. Satisfactory position usually can be maintained if the nurse stands behind the child, supports his back with her body and clasps his hands which are held at his side. By suggesting that the child close his eyes or turn his head away from the tray of equipment, fear may be lessened.

After the doctor has anesthetized the area with procaine and has made a small incision through the skin, he inserts the cannula and the trocar until fluid begins to flow from the peritoneal cavity. Then the doctor attaches the rubber tubing to the cannula, regulates the flow to prevent sudden withdrawal of fluid and directs the flow into the graduated receptacle. Sudden and rapid withdrawal of fluid reduces intra-abdominal pressure, causes the blood to distend the deep abdominal veins and reduces the normal supply of blood in the heart. If too much fluid is withdrawn, symptoms of shock develop. When sufficient fluid has been withdrawn to reduce pressure symptoms, the cannula is removed, sutures are taken, and the area is cleansed with alcohol and covered with a dressing. After a scultetus or an abdominal binder has been applied snugly, the child is returned to his bed. After the treatment, the amount of drainage from the wound and the child's condition should be observed and charted.

For most and sometimes all of the long period of illness these children have no prostration or discomfort. Play activities suitable for their age and interest must be provided. When the degree of edema lessens and the child is permitted to be out of bed, activities in a playroom will be enjoyed greatly and will contribute toward making his hospital stay constructive.

Before the child is discharged from the hospital, parental guidance will be necessary to ensure adequate continued care. The mother will require help to understand the child's diet, the measures necessary to prevent upper respiratory infections and the need for continued medical supervision.

CHRONIC NEPHRITIS
(CHRONIC GLOMERULAR NEPHRITIS)

Chronic nephritis is a terminal illness which is the result of progressive destruction of nephrons, leading to severe loss of renal function. Although the clinical manifestations are fairly uniform, the avenues by which individual children enter are diverse.

Etiology. There is no uniformity of opinion about the etiology of chronic nephritis, and it is probable that the term encompasses the end result of several different disease entities. Some children are discovered to have well-advanced chronic nephritis without having suffered any recognizable renal disease previously. Others first pass through a period of nephrosis which gradually changes over to chronic nephritis. A few suffer from chronic or recurrent bacterial infection of the kidney. Rarely does the child pass directly from a classic episode of acute glomerular nephritis into the progressive form of the disease.

Symptoms. When there has been no recognized renal disease previously, the symptoms are insidious, and the onset is gradual. Fatigue, anemia, headache and mild degrees of edema of the face or the feet are the most common early symptoms. Often the disease is discovered accidentally during a routine urine examination or during a physical examination which reveals the presence of mild hypertension. In the early stages symptoms are frequently mild or intermittent, and the child is able to pursue normal activities. The terminal symptoms are those of uremia or hypertension. Activity may be hampered by severe headache, nausea, fatigue or acidosis. In the final days of his illness the child usually passes into coma due to hypertension or uremia.

Diagnosis. The diagnosis of chronic nephritis depends upon the interpretation of laboratory tests. The earliest abnormalities are found in the urine, where albumin and casts are regularly present, together with varying degrees of hematuria. The urea-clearance, phenolsulfonphthalein and urine-concentration tests indicate marked loss of renal function. In the later stages of the disease, blood-chemical determinations show retention of nitrogen products (uremia), acidosis and the accumulation of phosphates and creatinine above their usual levels. The blood pressure, particularly the diastolic pressure, usually is elevated.

Course and Prognosis. Recovery from fully developed chronic nephritis is not to be expected. The course may last only a few weeks after discovery of the disease or may permit survival over a period of many years. In very unusual instances children have been known to reach a point of permanent stabilization of the disease.

Treatment. No treatment is known which will stem the progress of chronic nephritis toward a fatal termination. When the diagnosis has been established with certainty, the most charitable attitude is to permit the child to follow normal activities within the limits of his physical comfort. This regimen allows him the maximum enjoyment of his remaining months or years and supports his morale by tendering false assurance of favorable progress.

General hygienic measures are important. The diet should be designed to maintain optimal nutrition. Salt restriction should be imposed if there is edema. Prevention and prompt treatment of all infectious illnesses should be provided. During the periods of hypertensive or uremic symptoms, hospitalization usually is required to provide comfort through such measures as sedation, transfusion, relief of heart failure and correction of acidosis.

WILMS'S TUMOR

Wilms's tumor is one of the most frequent types of neoplasm seen among children. It is an adenosarcoma arising from fetal rests in the kidney, i.e., from abnormal bits of tissue which are left behind during early embryonic life and have the capacity to begin unrestrained cancerous growth after the child is born. For this reason, Wilms's tumor is seen mainly in the first year of life and almost exclusively during the first five years. It appears as a mass in the kidney region which is discovered accidentally by the parent or the examining physician. Usually the mass has reached considerable size by the time it is discovered. Since the tumor has a strong predilection to extend locally through the kidney capsule or the renal vein and to disseminate to other parts of the body by the blood stream, prompt recognition is imperative. The diagnosis usually can be confirmed by intravenous pyelography, which shows displacement and distortion of the pelvis of the kidney.

Treatment consists of prompt surgical removal of the tumor, followed or preceded by x-ray treatment to the area about it. Unfortunately, many Wilms's tumors already have metastasized, usually to the lungs, by the time the original tumor is discovered and treated. Irradiation of the pulmonary metastases is temporarily effective but seldom permanently curative. Even with prompt recognition and removal of the tumor, the prognosis is doubtful. Less than 25 per cent of such children survive for 3 years.

ABNORMALITIES OF BLADDER FUNCTION

DESCRIPTIVE TERMS

Several terms are employed to describe abnormalities of the manner of passing urine from the bladder.

Pollakiuria refers to an increase in the frequency of urination. It may accompany polyuria when the total volume of urine is increased or may be associated with dysuria when frequent painful discharge of small amounts of urine results. In some instances there is neither increased volume nor pain, and the frequent passage of urine appears to be related to nervous tension instead.

Dysuria signifies painful urination. It is found most often with infections of the lower urinary tract, which are discussed in a later section. Mechanical irritants such as foreign bodies in the bladder or the vagina, burns about the external genitalia or pinworm infestations are responsible at times for painful urination.

Incontinence implies lack of voluntary control over the discharge of urine from the bladder. It is a normal feature of the young infant who has not yet acquired voluntary control. It may accompany severe mental retardation; it is seen during severe prostrating illnesses and is a feature of a number of neurologic disorders which impair the operation of the lower spinal cord or the peripheral nerves that serve the bladder. The latter conditions include spina bifida, transverse myelitis, spinal cord injury and occasionally poliomyelitis.

Enuresis is distinguished from incontinence because it is involuntary micturition occurring in an individual, who, by reason of age, intelligence and lack of neurologic disability, might be expected to have control over his bladder function.

Neurologic Bladder

The complexities of the nervous control over bladder function are not completely understood. Co-ordinated activity of the intrinsic musculature of the bladder is regulated in part by involuntary centers in the lower spinal cord through the autonomic nervous system and in part by higher voluntary centers in the brain. Normally, the sphincter muscle at the outlet of the bladder is kept tightly closed by involuntary signals from the spinal cord. As the bladder fills with urine, its distention beyond a certain point calls forth contraction waves in the muscula-

ture which eventually are felt by the higher centers in the brain. Through a voluntary act, the sphincter tone then is relaxed and the bladder contracts unopposed, discharging its content of urine. Then the sphincter closes and comes back under the automatic control of the spinal cord, while the bladder refills with urine.

During sudden acute afflictions of the spinal cord such as myelitis, poliomyelitis or injury, the normal mechanism is disturbed by the loss of sensory awareness of bladder distention and by the impairment of voluntary control over the relaxation of the sphincter. The bladder distends progressively until the volume and the pressure of urine are sufficient to broach the sphincter without the mediation of voluntary relaxation. Overflow incontinence with dribbling results. The cardinal principle in the management of acute retention of this sort is prevention of infection within the stagnant pool of urine. Chemotherapy and antibiotics usually are prescribed to prevent this occurrence, and catheterization of the bladder is avoided whenever possible. When the cord injury is a temporary one, the return of normal function can be expected within a period of 1 to 4 weeks.

When the interference with nervous control is permanent, due to congenital abnormality or the persistence of an acquired disorder of the spinal cord, the clinical manifestations vary somewhat. If the spasticity of the sphincter predominates, retention persists, but usually the overflow dribbling is replaced by periodic partial emptying of the bladder, which is not under voluntary control. Under these circumstances the chronic obstruction to urine flow results in abnormally high pressures in the bladder and hence in ureters and kidney pelves which may enlarge the kidneys slowly and destroy their functioning tissue gradually.

Management of this type of chronic neurologic bladder usually requires some form of relief from chronic obstruction. This may be afforded by indwelling catheters or by artificial openings into the bladder (cystotomy). Sometimes the neurologic disturbance produces a lax sphincter which is unable to hold back urine. Under these circumstances the bladder is small and spastic and contains little or no urine. In both varieties of chronic disorder the hazard of chronic or recurring infection of the urinary tract is so great as to be almost unavoidable. Periodic or continuous administration of antibiotics or chemotherapy may eliminate infection temporarily or reduce its severity. Although many of these patients live for years in spite of the effects of chronic infection and back pressure upon the kidneys, their prospects of reaching adult life are limited.

ENURESIS

The term enuresis is applied to instances of involuntary micturition among persons who might be expected to have urinary control because of age, training, mentality and absence of physical defects which cause incontinence. Enuresis may be nocturnal, diurnal or both.

Etiology. Involuntary micturition is normal in infancy. Many children acquire day control by the age of 2½ to 3½ and night control by 3½ to

4½. Control may be acquired earlier or later, depending upon the child's neuromuscular development and upon the guidance he is receiving. Mentally deficient children acquire control slowly or not at all. Certain organic lesions of the spinal cord, such as transverse myelitis or congenital malformations, lead to permanent incontinence. These conditions can be distinguished from enuresis readily.

In some children, enuresis may be only a continuance of the uninhibited infantile pattern of micturition. In other children, control is gained for a time and then lost. Enuresis is commonly a result of environmental factors and conflict in interpersonal relationships.

Various secondary or exciting causes have been stated. Among these may be enumerated the following: polyuria from excessive water drinking, concentrated highly acid urine, inflammation of the bladder with or without a calculus and numerous conditions acting reflexly, such as phimosis, preputial adhesions, narrowed meatus, pinworms, constipation and adenoids. It is doubtful if these or any other physical condition acting reflexly can cause enuresis alone. It is possible that some of them at times may be factors. It is desirable to remedy all, whether enuresis is present or not. The correction of these defects usually has no effect on established enuresis. Furthermore, the majority of children with enuresis have no such defects.

Symptoms. Enuresis does not affect the health, although at times poor health and enuresis are associated. Good habits are more difficult to acquire in the presence of poor health. Enuresis may persist up to 8 or 10 years of age. Seldom does it continue beyond puberty. With frequent voiding, a reduced bladder capacity may result and become a factor in the continuance of the habit. The longer enuresis has been established, the more difficult it is to control.

Treatment. The varieties of treatment which have been advocated are numerous. It is possible that all can be classified under the term "psychotherapy." Each clinician develops his own methods, which are adapted to his manner of practice and are successful for him. His own assurance of the effectiveness of the method employed would seem to be a large factor in its success.

A study of the child and the interpersonal relationships he has experienced within his family is necessary before any guidance of the child or his parents can begin. Obtaining a history of the training regimen that the child has experienced is important in understanding the parental attitudes to which the child has been subjected. It is the child who requires treatment. Enuresis is only a symptom of underlying conflict. In many instances, treatment in a child-guidance center is indicated and necessary.

When the services of a therapist are not available, every effort to correct the environmental factors which have produced enuresis should be made. There is no formula that will cure enuresis. The child in his family setting must be studied and treated in a way that meets his emotional requirements. The parents will need help in changing their attitudes toward the child and his symptoms. The child also needs help to change his attitudes toward his symptoms. However, this cannot be accomplished directly. It can come only through a good interpersonal relationship with his doctor —a relationship which helps him to feel that he is being guided by someone who is genuinely interested in the way he feels about himself and his intimate relationships with those within his family.

Obtaining the child's interest in acquiring increased control of his bodily functions eventually must be aroused and maintained. He needs help to feel that he can develop increased control and that the responsibility for control is his. At the same time he should be helped to feel that both the doctor and his parents are interested in and desirous of helping him to accept the responsibility entailed in developing the controls that are appropriate for his age. Scolding and punishment accomplish nothing; they merely increase his conflicts and tension and make the symptom more pronounced. Neither fear nor humiliation should be associated with the treatment. Humiliation tells the child he is "bad." He is not bad or inferior; he is merely the victim of interpersonal relationships that have failed to meet his emotional needs. He needs help, not condemnation.

Drugs have been used with limited success in helping the child to overcome enuresis. Occasionally, atropine and its derivatives may reduce bladder irritability and improve sphincter tone. However, reliance upon drug therapy is avoiding the main issue, which in nearly every instance is one of psychological orientation.

INFECTIONS OF THE GENITO-URINARY TRACT

PYURIA

A number of terms are employed to designate the presence of infection within the urinary apparatus. Pyelonephritis implies that the inflammation is primarily in the kidney parenchyma; pyelitis indicates the pelvis of the kidney; ureteritis, the ureter; cystitis, the bladder. The more indefinite term "pyuria" is preferable, for infection within the tract usually is not confined to a single location, nor is it possible always to localize the major site exactly.

Etiology. Pyuria is more common in infants than in older children and more common in girls than in boys. Colon bacilli are the infecting organisms in from 75 to 80 per cent of the cases; streptococci and staphylococci, in most of the remainder. The infecting bacteria may reach the urinary tract by way of the blood or from below by ascent from the exterior. Some controversy exists as to which of these routes is the more common. A widely held view is that staphylococci and streptococci reach the urinary tract by way of the blood, with the primary infection in the kidney, and that infections with the colon bacillus are chiefly of the ascending type. The wearing of diapers and the relatively short urethra of girl infants as compared with that of boys seem to be sufficient to account for the greater frequency of the disease in girl babies.

Obstruction in the urinary tract plays a highly important role in urinary infection. Once infection has occurred, obstruction aggravates the condition and is an important factor in making the infection severe and chronic. Most often, in childhood the obstruction is produced by some congenital malformation, seldom by stone. A relationship exists between urinary infection and infections of the upper respiratory tract and gastro-intestinal disturbances, particularly diarrhea.

Symptoms. The symptoms of pyuria are extremely varied. In the infant and the young child they are not localizing. In the older child they may simulate those of appendicitis, meningitis, pneumonia or other febrile illnesses. Fever is almost always present with acute attacks and frequently is marked by rapid fluctuations, with chills or convulsions during the rising portion of the fever curve. Leukocytosis is generally present.

With chronic pyuria or pyuria which persists beyond the initial attack, the systemic manifestations of fever, chills and general malaise are usually milder or completely lacking, in spite of heavy infection of the urine.

Unlike older children, the newborn infant is affected with equal frequency in the two sexes. It is assumed that such infections are the result of blood-borne bacteria. In the older infant or child, pyuria in the male is much less common than in the female, and its occurrence almost invariably means the presence of some anatomic or functional malformation of the urinary tract.

Diagnosis. The clue to diagnosis lies in the discovery of pus upon microscopic examination of the urine. Pus must be present in abnormal amount, and there must be assurance that it did not come from preputial or vaginal secretions. When there is doubt, a clean or a catheterized specimen of urine is required. The latter procedure has the advantage of permitting accurate culture of the urine in order to identify the bacterium responsible and to test its sensitivity to various chemotherapeutic and antibiotic agents.

Prognosis. The prognosis of uncomplicated pyuria is good. In many cases in which no obstruction or urinary retention exists, the pyuria and the bacilluria will cease spontaneously or with little treatment, when associated parenteral infection or gastro-intestinal disturbance has subsided. The cases of most troublesome and persistent infection are those in which obstruction exists. Obstruction alone leads ultimately to kidney failure. When infection is present in addition, kidney failure is hastened.

Treatment. Control of pyuria requires the elimination of the infecting organisms from the urinary tract. Sulfonamides are highly satisfactory in the treatment of most acute attacks; sulfadiazine and gantrisin have the greatest popularity. Because these substances are concentrated by the kidney, an effective level in the urine can be obtained with moderate doses. In some instances the infecting organism is not readily susceptible to these substances or has acquired resistance to them. Then rational treatment must be guided by isolating the infecting bacteria and testing its sensitivity to the many antibiotic agents that are now available. In long-standing or recurrent pyuria, bacteria of the proteus and the pseudomonas families may be encountered. These organisms not infrequently defy the most carefully planned antibiotic attack.

With the possible exception of the initial attack of simple pyuria in girls, all cases should be studied carefully for the presence of abnormalities of the anatomy or the physiology of the urinary tract so that, whenever feasible, situations that produce stasis of urine can be corrected in the hope of forestalling future episodes of pyuria. Such studies usually begin with an x-ray visualization of the upper urinary tract by intravenous pyelography. An opaque dye such as Diodrast or Neoiopax is injected into the blood stream of the child after a period of partial dehydration and roentgenograms of the abdomen are taken at intervals thereafter. Usually the outline of the kidneys and the ureters can be discovered by this method, and some indication of the excretory power of each kidney can be obtained. The lower portion of the urinary tract may be visualized by a cystogram. This procedure involves the injection of an opaque dye into the bladder through a catheter in the urethra. Then x-ray films are taken which demonstrate the size and the shape of the bladder and sometimes reveal the ureters if their orifices are abnormally patulous. A satisfactory understanding of the abnormality sometimes requires the additional information provided by cystoscopy with retrograde pyelography. Direct visualization of the bladder and the urethra is possible; urine may be collected from the two kidneys independently for study, and better x-ray visualization of the ureters and the kidney pelves can be made when catheters

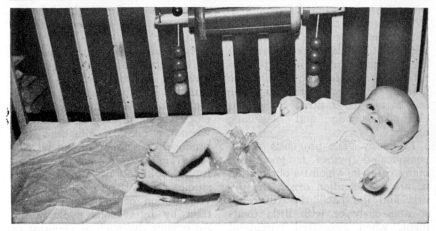

FIG. 42. Illustrating the use of a plastic specimen diaper.

are passed up into the upper portions of the tract. Unfortunately, the procedure of cystoscopy is painful and upsetting to small children and usually cannot be done without a general anesthetic.

Nursing Care. Specimens of urine will be desired from infants and children with pyelitis. Several methods of collecting specimens from infants are used. For a young infant the Tomac plastic urine specimen diaper* (Fig. 42) is a simple, comfortable method of obtaining a sample of urine. When the head of the bed is elevated, a specimen can be collected without restraining the infant. A test tube or wide-mouthed bottle can be attached by means of adhesive plaster to the male genitalia (Fig. 43). A bird-seed receptacle can be used similarly for girls (Figs. 44 and 45). For girls, other devices, such as wedging a small basin between the thighs or

* Obtainable from American Hospital Supply Corporation, Evanston, Ill.

allowing the child to be in a slightly cupped square of plastic material, also may be used.

In some institutions specimen binders are used to keep the test tube or the receptacle over the genitalia (Fig. 46). For a quiet, young infant, no restraints are necessary; for older and active infants, ankle and wrist restraints are required. The binder with the attached test tube is pinned securely around the lower abdomen. Then the test tube is placed over the penis, and the binder tapes are brought across the perineum and pinned to the side of the waist band (Fig. 47). The binder used for collecting specimens from female infants is applied in a similar manner. The receptacle is placed above the anus and over the genitalia and held in position by pinning the center tab snugly to the back of the waist band. Elevating the head of the crib facilitates the collection of specimens. Care must be taken to prevent contamination

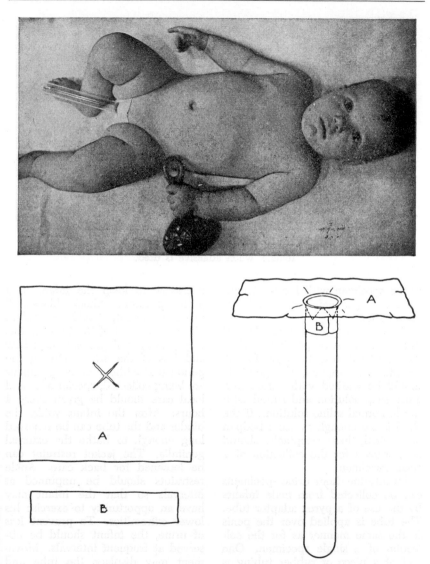

Fig. 43. (Top) Apparatus applied for the collection of urine, single specimen, male, when adhesive is used. (Bottom) Equipment for the collection of urine, single specimen, male. (A) Adhesive for the purpose of attaching the tube to the child. (B) An adhesive strip for attaching the tube to the larger piece of adhesive.

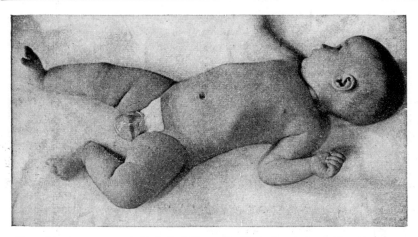

FIG. 44. Apparatus applied for the collection of urine, single specimen, female, when adhesive is used.

of the specimen with feces. A contaminated specimen is unsuitable for examination.

Often clean specimens are desired from children with pyelitis. Before the sterilized test tube or female receptacle is applied, the genitalia should be washed with cotton and green-soap solution and rinsed with sterile normal saline solution. If the child is old enough to use a bedpan or a urinal, these receptacles should be sterilized for the collection of a clean specimen.

Twenty-four hour urine specimens can be collected from male infants by the use of a pyrex adaptor tube. The tube is applied over the penis in the same manner as for the collection of a single specimen. One end of a piece of rubber tubing is attached to the open end of the adaptor tube; the other end is taped just inside the bottle, which is hung at the foot of the infant's crib. Jacket and ankle restraints are necessary to keep the infant in a prone position. Shock blocks, 6 inches in height, should be used to elevate the head of the bed. In this way gravity will prevent back flow and loss of the urine. During the period that 24-hour urine specimens are being collected, special back and local care should be given every 4 hours. After the infant voids, the binder and the tube can be removed long enough to bathe the external genitalia. The jacket restraint can be loosened for back care. Ankle restraints should be unpinned at intervals so that the infant may have an opportunity to exercise his lower extremities. To prevent loss of urine, the infant should be observed at frequent intervals. Movement may displace the tube and make readjustment necessary.

If a sterile specimen is required for culture, catheterization is required. The following sterile equipment is necessary for the procedure:

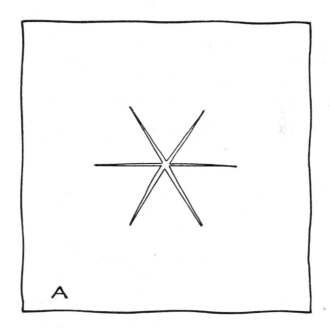

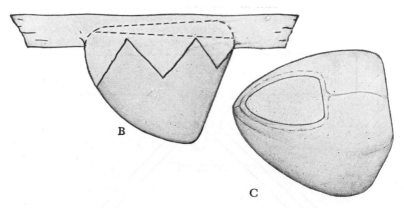

Fig. 45. (A) Showing the method of cutting a square of adhesive. (B) The method of attaching the receptacle to the adhesive. (C) Glass receptacle.

2 catheters (size 8 or 10 Fr.), gloves, towels, kidney basin, 1 glass with 2 drams of tr. Zephiran, basins of green-soap and normal saline solution, 3 applicators, cotton balls and culture tubes standing in a round basin.

If the sterile specimen is desired from an older child who understands the procedure sufficiently to co-operate, the catheterization pro-

cedure is the same as for an adult. Co-operation of the child is essential, as relaxation is necessary if a catheterized specimen is to be obtained. Explaining the procedure to the child, showing her the equipment and asking her to help by breathing deeply through her mouth usually brings co-operation and produces the relaxation necessary to introduce the catheter into the

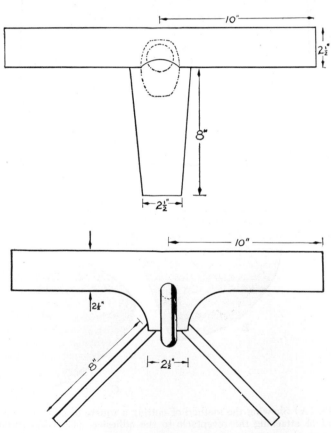

FIG. 46. (*Top*) T-binder with bird-seed cup for collection of urine from female infant. (*Bottom*) T-binder with test tube attached for collection of urine from male infant.

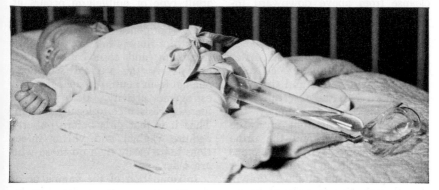

Fig. 47. Collecting single specimen of urine from male infant when binder is used. Receptacle for female also is shown.

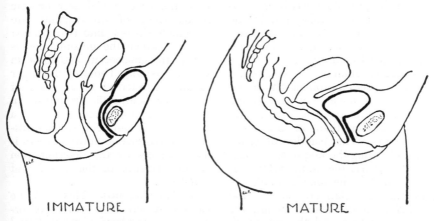

IMMATURE   MATURE

Fig. 48. Showing the relative position of the bladder and the direction of the course of the urethra (heavy lines) in the infant and the mature female.

bladder. When a specimen is required from a young child who cannot be prepared, two nurses are necessary to carry out the procedure safely. One nurse will be required to help the child lie quietly. A second nurse will carry out the procedure after she has scrubbed her hands and put on the sterile gloves. The bowl holding the standing test tubes should be placed on the sterile towel which previously had been placed in front of the perineum. One hand is used to hold the labia separated. The other hand is used to cleanse and to apply the tr. Zephiran to the meatus and the surrounding area. In cleansing the external genitalia, a cotton ball should be used only once. It should cleanse from above downward toward the anus and then be discarded. The cotton balls must be handled carefully. The gloved hands must remain uncontaminated. After the tip of the catheter has been lubricated with saline and the wide end placed into the test tube, the catheter is passed through the meatus into the urethra until the bladder is reached and the urine begins to flow. When specimens have been collected, the catheter can be pinched off and withdrawn. If catheterization is ordered to relieve distention, the catheter is not withdrawn until urine ceases to flow. When the procedure has been completed, the test tube should be covered with sterile gauze squares, placed in a specimen bottle and sent to the laboratory.

Catheterization of the young child often produces a problem for the inexperienced nurse. In the young infant, the bladder is higher and more anterior than in the adult (Fig. 48). The bladder descends rapidly during the first 3 years, then slowly. It has the adult position at 20 years. In the female adult, the urethra is relatively short and straight. In the female infant, the urethra hooks round the symphysis in a "C" shape. When the meatus is located, the catheter should be introduced and directed downward instead of in the direction necessary to reach the bladder of an adult patient.

Vulvovaginitis

In girls before puberty, the mucosa of the vagina and the vulva is covered with a relatively thin layer of epithelium as compared with that of the adult. The change to the adult type of epithelium occurs at puberty through increase in estrogenic hormones which stimulate growth of the epithelium, producing thickening and cornification. Also, at puberty the vaginal secretions change from neutral to acid through estrogenic activity. Both changes increase resistance to local infection. Thus it is that girls before puberty acquire vaginal and vulvar infections more easily than do those who are older.

Inflammation of the vagina or of the vagina and the vulva is relatively frequent in childhood and especially is this true among girls from the lower social or economic strata. Cases of vulvovaginitis are commonly divided into two groups: those in which the inflammation is due to the gonococcus and those in which it is not. Those of the latter group are referred to as cases of simple or nonspecific vaginitis. In both types, the child presents a more or less purulent vaginal discharge. Distinction between them is made wholly by the determination of the presence or the absence of gonococci.

Simple Vaginitis. This may be caused by any of a variety of organisms—organisms normally found in the lower intestinal tract are usually responsible. Streptococci which are simultaneously infecting the respiratory tract are occasionally isolated. Frequently, simple vaginitis is due primarily to lack of cleanliness with resultant secondary implantation of bacteria. Less often, it is due to masturbation or to insertion of objects into the vagina. Simple vaginitis is not communicable and responds readily to treatment. In some instances, a daily tub bath with local cleansing is sufficient. In other instances, a short period of treatment with simple douches produces prompt recovery. Almost any cleansing douche is satisfactory. It may be a solution of sodium chloride, boric acid or sodium bicarbonate. Sulfonamide therapy is effective and in some instances may be preferable to treatment by douches. Penicillin is effective if hemolytic streptococci are present.

Gonococcic Vaginitis. This would be rare in childhood were it not a contagious disease for girls. If the infection is newly acquired and acute, there is complaint referable to the local inflammation, especially pain on micturition because of urethritis and vulvitis. There also may be a certain amount of constitutional disturbance with fever. In some cases, proctitis also is present. After a time all symptoms disappear, and there remains only continued vaginal discharge. Periods of visible discharge may alternate with periods of latency during which no discharge is seen, although the infection is still present, as shown by culture or smear.

When untreated, gonorrhea in girls resembles the same disease in women in its chronicity and its latent periods. It is dissimilar in that secondary pelvic inflammatory disease and involvement of the glands of Skene and Bartholin and of the glandular structures of the endocervix are very rare in childhood. Although an adult may be a source of contagion to a child, the infection is not contagious in the same sense among adults.

In its chronic form, gonorrheal vaginitis in childhood seldom has any ill effect on the health nor has

it usually any local symptoms other than discharge.

Intramuscular injection of penicillin in doses of 300,000 units per day or more is regularly effective in the treatment of gonorrheal vaginitis. Cure may be effected in as brief a period as 3 or 4 days. During the early stages of treatment, isolation technic must be observed to prevent the spread of infection to other female children in the environment.

INFECTIONS OF THE PENIS AND THE URETHRA IN THE MALE

Meatal Ulcer. Circumcized infants not infrequently develop small ulcerations of the meatus of the urethra from the irritant and macerating effect of wet diapers. The small ulcer which usually forms just inside the meatus tends to crust over and sometimes will partially block the opening. Often it is washed off during the act of voiding, and a small drop of blood may be noted in the diaper or at the tip of the penis. Occasionally, voiding is painful. Treatment consists of thorough drying of the tip of the penis by leaving it exposed as much of the day as possible until the ulcer has a chance to heal. In rare instances a persistent ulceration will result in scarring and constriction of the terminal urethra, which requires dilatation.

Balanoposthitis. Uncircumcized males in whom cleansing of the glans and the prepuce of the penis is neglected may develop nonspecific infection of the mucous membrane of these structures. The infection yields promptly to adequate cleansing and warm applications. When edema is severe and the prepuce cannot be retracted to permit cleansing, a dorsal slit operation may be required to permit adequate drainage.

Urethritis and Prostatitis. Occasionally, balanoposthitis may extend upward into the urethra. Gonorrheal urethritis also is known to occur in older boys and runs the same clinical course as in the adult male. Treatment is by intramuscular injection of penicillin.

A nonspecific variety of prostatitis may be seen in adolescent boys. The symptoms are those of dysuria and hematuria without fever. The disorder may be related to excessive masturbation either as a cause or as an incitant. Expectant treatment is usually sufficient, for the disease runs a brief, self-limited course of a few days.

MALFORMATIONS OF THE LOWER GENITO-URINARY TRACT

Exstrophy of the Bladder

All the various malformations of the bladder are rare, and only one of them, exstrophy of the bladder, will be discussed. This condition is caused by failure of union between the two sides of the lower abdomen, a failure which produces a fissure in the mid-line from the umbilicus to the genitalia. The defect includes the abdominal wall, the anterior wall of the bladder, the symphysis pubis and the urethra. The posterior and the lateral surfaces of the bladder are exposed, and the ureteral outlets are visible. The condition is more common in boys than in girls. In boys, usually a groove is present in the anterior surface of the penis; in girls the clitoris is divided, and the labia may be separated. Other congenital malformations may be associated.

Treatment consists of operative removal of the bladder, the ureters first having been transplanted to the colon. A suitable age for the operation is 6 months.

MALFORMATIONS OF THE MALE GENITALIA

Undescended Testicle (Cryptorchidism). Early in fetal life the testicles develop within the abdomen near and below the kidneys. In most instances, they descend into the scrotum during the last 2 months. In some instances, they are still in the inguinal canal at the time of birth and occasionally within the abdomen. Those undescended at birth usually descend during the first few weeks after birth, but may descend at any time up to the period of adolescence. When nondescent is bilateral, the testes nearly always descend before puberty. When it is unilateral, approximately half descend at puberty or soon afterward. Undescended testicle is to be found in only about 0.3 per cent of men by the time full maturity is reached.

At puberty, the testes normally increase in size and develop spermatogenic and increased androgenic activity. An undescended testis develops at puberty in the same manner for a short time, but eventually the sperm-forming cells degenerate, with sterility as a result if both testes are affected. Although slight decrease in androgenic activity may occur, the body and the secondary sexual characteristics develop normally. The temperature at which the testis is maintained seems to be the controlling factor in its spermatogenic activity, scrotal temperature being lower than that of the body. A testicle in the inguinal canal is more subject to injury than when in the scrotum—both external injury and that from torsion and strangulation. An undescended testis produces a psychological handicap.

TREATMENT is required only in those instances in which descent does not occur at puberty, except for the unusual instances in which degeneration occurs before puberty. Many physicians wait until puberty before instituting treatment. Others treat at from 10 to 11 years old, a period preceding puberty development, in order to avoid the possibility of prepuberal degeneration. Normal puberty development results from a hormone produced by the anterior pituitary gland. An active principle similar in action to the pituitary hormone can be obtained from human pregnancy urine. This material, known as chorionic gonadotropic hormone, may be responsible for descent of the testis before birth. It is the hormone used in the treatment of undescended testis. The hormone is given in doses of from 200 to 500 units 2 or 3 times a week, the total not exceeding 6,000 units, and over a period not exceeding 6 weeks. Treatment in excess of these amounts is likely to produce precocious puberty. In some instances, the treatment is repeated after an interval of several months. Hormone treatment causes descent in possibly half the cases and possibly only in those instances in which the testes would have descended subsequently without treatment.

Those who fail to respond to hormone treatment require operation to bring the testis into the scrotum.

Surgical treatment should be given as soon as the hormone treatment has been stopped and while the testis and its cord are still increased in size as a result of the treatment. Operation is not uniformly successful in producing a good result.

Hydrocele. In the male infant, the testis descends from the abdominal cavity into the scrotum, carrying with it the parietal peritoneum and thus forming a tube from the abdomen to the scrotum. Normally the upper end of the tube closes, the lower end remaining as a testicular covering (tunica vaginalis). A hydrocele exists when this sac is filled with fluid. If a small communication with the peritoneal cavity exists, the hydrocele is reducible. Hydrocele may be limited to the testicular region or to the spermatic cord or it may include both these regions, depending on what portion of the peritoneal process has become obliterated. This type of hydrocele is congenital. It usually disappears spontaneously in the course of a few weeks or months. If not, simple aspiration is usually all that is required. In a few instances, surgical removal of the sac may be indicated. Acquired hydrocele may result from inflammation of or trauma to the tunica vaginalis and is very uncommon in childhood.

Epispadias. Epispadias is a malformation in which the urethra opens at any point along the top or the dorsal surface of the penis or even at its base. In the more pronounced of the malformations, the usual procedure is to transplant the ureters into the colon at any early age.

Hypospadias. Hypospadias is a malformation in which the urethra opens on the undersurface of the penis proximal to the normal place of opening. The defect is remediable by plastic surgery, which usually is done at early school age but may be deferred until after puberty, when the parts have reached their mature stage.

Preputial Adhesions. Adhesions of the prepuce to the glans are very common and should be broken up at an early age. After this procedure, a small amount of antiseptic ointment should be applied, particularly if bleeding has occurred, and the prepuce should be retracted daily for cleansing and to prevent reformation of the adhesions.

Phimosis signifies a narrowed outlet through the foreskin of the penis. It is to be distinguished from the term "redundant" prepuce, which is applied to an unusually long foreskin irrespective of narrowing and also from the term "adherent" prepuce, in which condition adhesions exist between the foreskin and the glans. Phimosis rarely is sufficiently severe to obstruct the outflow of urine and is not a cause of symptoms, either local or general. Phimosis is undesirable chiefly because it does not permit suitable cleanliness. In some instances the content of the preputial sac is invaded by bacteria to the extent of causing a local infection (balanitis). Phimosis may be corrected either by circumcision or by stretching. Preputial adhesions usually are present. When stretching is the procedure employed, the subsequent management is similar to that for preputial adhesions. Care must be taken not to permit paraphimosis, which is a condition in which the tight ring of foreskin formerly in front of the glans is left posterior to the glans, resulting in severe edema of the distal parts and requiring prompt attention and possibly surgical relief.

CIRCUMCISION consists of surgical removal of that part of the foreskin which lies in front of the glans. The preferable time for circumcision is on the sixth or the seventh day after birth. When done at this time, healing is well under way by the time the mother is discharged from obstetric care. At a later age the procedure becomes a bigger task and may require the use of a local or a general anesthetic.

After the procedure is completed, the cut edges are covered with gauze impregnated with petrolatum. The postoperative treatment consists in keeping the wound clean.

The necessity for circumcision is seldom one of medical urgency. Since it may create considerable emotional disturbance in the young child, the operation should be undertaken in early infancy if the parents wish it done. When the child is left uncircumcized and the parents change their minds at a later date, it is preferable to wait until the boy himself can have some part in the decision and has an understanding of its implications.

MALFORMATIONS OF THE FEMALE GENITALIA

Malformations of the female genitalia are relatively rare. Few of them occur with sufficient frequency to merit discussion here. Rarely is the hymen imperforate. It should be opened at any age that it is discovered in order to prevent accumulation of secretions in the vagina. Adhesions about the clitoris usually are not a cause of disturbance and they are easily broken up in infancy. Hermaphrodism is a condition in which the gonads of each sex are present, a condition extremely rare. Somewhat more common is pseudohermaphrodism, in which determination of sex by inspection is difficult and in which the gonads of only one sex are present. It occurs in both sexes. Determination of the true sex may require laparotomy. Only after the sex has been determined definitely should plastic operations be performed. Pseudohermaphrodism in the female is simulated with overactivity of the adrenal cortex.

SITUATIONS FOR FURTHER STUDY

1. How does nephritis in children differ from that in adults?

2. How can nephritis be prevented in childhood?

3. What are the complications of nephritis? What are the complications of nephrosis?

4. What preparation would a 4-year-old girl require for an intravenous pyelogram?

5. An 8-year-old child has been brought to the children's clinic because of enuresis. Observe the doctor's interview, talk with the parents and the child and consider the following points: How did the mother describe the child's problem? Did she talk about it in the child's presence? Has he always had enuresis? If not, when did it begin? What was the family situation when enuresis began? How did the mother attempt to help the child establish control? When did she begin to institute training? What problems developed at that time? What was the mother's reaction to the child's enuresis? How has she attempted to help the child overcome it? What was the child's reaction to his problem? Did he feel ashamed, guilty, or did he seem anxious to be helped to overcome it? What type of parent-child relationship existed? Were any physical abnormalities found on examination? How did the child respond to the examination? What guidance did the doctor suggest? Do you feel that the mother received sufficient insight to utilize the doctor's recommendations? What further help will the parents and the child require?

BIBLIOGRAPHY

Campbell, Meredith: Clinical Pediatric Urology, Philadelphia, Saunders, 1951.

Gerard, M. W.: Enuresis: a study in etiology, Am. J. Orthopsychiat. 9: 48, 1939.

Heyman, Walter: Renal disorders in infants and children, Am. J. Nursing 48:436, 1948.

Wright, Lucille, and Prince, C. L.: Hypospadias: nursing care in surgical repair, Am. J. Nursing 46: 686, 1946.

Diseases of the Nervous System

◇◇◇

SPINA BIFIDA
HYDROCEPHALUS
MENTAL DEFICIENCY
MOTOR DISABILITIES OF CEREBRAL
   ORIGIN
SEIZURES
BRAIN TUMOR

INFECTIONS
HEREDITARY DEGENERATIVE DIS-
   ORDERS OF THE NERVOUS AND THE
   MUSCULAR SYSTEMS
MISCELLANEOUS NEUROLOGIC
   DISTURBANCES
SITUATIONS FOR FURTHER STUDY

The nervous system consists of an intricate complex of nerve centers and pathways (the brain and the spinal cord) which is confined within a protective bony shell (the skull and the vertebral column) and sends out branches (the peripheral nerves) to all parts of the body. Through the anterior motor nerves, the brain and the spinal cord control the activity of muscles and organs; through the posterior sensory nerves they receive sensations from them and also from the skin and the organs of special sense. Intellect, mind, memory, feeling and personality all are related intimately to the function of the brain.

Structural or functional disturbances of the central nervous system occur in bewildering numbers. Their complexities can be understood only with the aid of an extensive knowledge of the anatomy and the physiology of the nervous system. In a brief text of this sort it will be possible to mention only a few of the representative types. For more detailed consideration the reader is referred to the texts suggested in the bibliography.

SPINA BIFIDA

Spina bifida is a malformation of the spine in which the posterior portion of the bony canal containing the spinal cord is completely or partially lacking because of failure of the vertebral laminae to develop or to fuse. Some degree of this defect is relatively common, especially in the lumbar region. When it exists without associated changes in the cord or the meninges, it is known as spina bifida occulta and, being symptomless, it is not discovered unless sought.

A more serious condition is a protrusion of the cord and its membranes (myelomeningocele) or the cord membranes alone (meningocele) through the defect to form an external cystic tumor, which is present at birth. The tumor is rounded, fluctuating, more or less compressible, and contains cerebrospinal fluid. It is commonly about the size of half of a small orange and most frequently is located in the lumbar or the sacral region. The wall of a meningocele is made up of spinal membranes and skin. In a myelomeningocele (Fig. 49), a portion of the cord is spread out and embedded in the cyst wall. Commonly, the condition is associated with increased pressure of the cerebrospinal fluid, so that the tumor tends to increase in size, the wall becoming thinner. With continued enlargement the tumor may rupture spontaneously or more commonly it is the seat of ulcerations, often perforating, consequent on the poor blood supply. Rupture or ulcerative perforation usually leads to meningitis. Spina bifida with meningocele causes no symptoms. If the cord is included in the cyst wall, urinary and fecal incontinence and paralysis of the legs are likely to result.

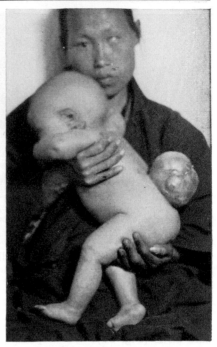

FIG. 49. Meningomyelocele.

TREATMENT

The treatment of simple meningocele is surgical removal of the sac with plastic reinforcement of the tissues over the fissure. Operation usually is not advisable for meningomyelocele when paralyses are present, except for the purpose of avoiding infections or at times for cosmetic effect.

PROGNOSIS

The only instances of favorable result from operation are those of simple meningocele in which hydrocephalus is not present or does not develop after operation. Hydrocephalus is a common accompaniment of spina bifida with tumor, in some instances developing spontaneously and in others as soon as the sac is removed. Hydrocephalus occurs or increases with such frequency after operation that the operative results are most discouraging. However, hydrocephalus associated with spina bifida is more amenable to treatment than that from other causes.

NURSING CARE

When the covering over the tumor is very thin, the surface must be kept clean and protected from pressure. In the period preceding operation, nursing measures to prevent or to clear infection must be

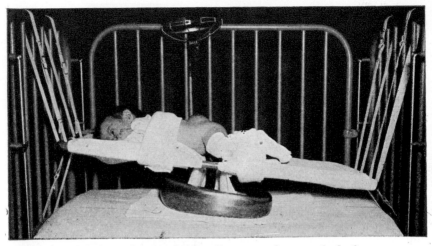

FIG. 50. A baby with spina bifida, illustrating also a method of care on a frame.

carried out. Placement on an infant Bradford frame facilitates care, exposes the tumor and prevents pressure on it (Fig. 50). To keep the infant in position over the frame opening, ankle and chest restraint is necessary. Diapers folded as cravats can be placed around the chest and also around one ankle, under the frame and over the other ankle. To prevent deformity, a small pillow made of abdominal pads should be placed under the lower portion of the legs to keep the toes and the feet from pressing into the hard surface of the frame.

When the spinal cord is included in the tumor wall, urine and feces are excreted constantly. Therefore, care to prevent excoriations around the perineum becomes necessary. Folded diapers under the abdomen and under the legs, over the edge and into a receptacle beneath the frame opening protect the frame covers and permit easy change to keep the infant dry. Cleansing the perineum and the groins with oiled cotton each time the diapers are changed will keep the skin in good condition.

When an infant is kept in this position for long periods of time, attention to the skin of the face and the knees becomes imperative if excoriation is to be prevented. If paralysis of the lower extremities is present, abrasion of the knees does not occur frequently, but if the infant's motor development is normal, frequent knee movement may cause skin irritation. Stockings prevent skin irritation in many instances. Good care of the knees and the skin of the face with applications of zinc-oxide ointment to the tip of the nose, the chin and the cheeks will prevent abrasions.

Various methods to prevent or to clear infection of the tumor mass may be used. Cleanliness with exposure to light may be all that is necessary. Alcohol, antibiotic or petrolatum gauze dressings may be desired. If used, they should be changed frequently enough to keep them sterile and the area free of exudate.

During the preoperative period the infant should be held for feedings. It gives him needed position change and affection and facilitates feeding and bubbling. The infant should be handled gently, for the tumor area is sensitive. The tumor should be covered with a sterile towel and the infant held in such a way that pressure on the area can be eliminated. Observation as to his weight and his behavior before and after feedings will serve as a guide to his need for food. Optimum nutritional state is necessary before surgical intervention, and more frequent feedings may be necessary to satisfy his needs.

The sac may be excised, or the meninges may be folded in to preserve the absorbing surface of the sac before the skin is closed over them. In either type of operation the principles of postoperative care remain the same. In the period immediately after operation, symptoms of shock should be watched for, and appropriate treatment given if they occur. The dressing must be kept clean and free from feces, and the prone position must be maintained by the same method as is used in the preoperative period. No covering directly over the infant should be be used, as it will become soiled.

If the infant's temperature is subnormal, a light should be placed over the infant, and the bed should be covered with blankets, encasing the child in a heated unit. When the infant's temperature is subnormal and unstable, care in an incubator may be indicated. A Bradford frame may be simulated by pinning firm material across the frame of the bassinet inside the incubator. Temperature of the incubator should be regulated according to the individual needs of the infant.

Nursing measures used preoperatively should be continued, with the exception of the position used to feed the infant. Until sutures are removed, the baby should be fed on his frame, which is now hung so that his head is from 3 to 5 inches lower than his body. The chest restraint can be loosened, and the infant may be turned slightly to make feeding less difficult for him. The same method should be used to bathe the undersurface of his body.

During the postoperative period, observation as to whether or not the head circumference is increasing guides the physician and the nurse in the type of advice that the parents will need upon the baby's discharge from the hospital. Many times, operation is performed in the neonatal period. Therefore, the mother will require help in understanding the total needs of her child. The infant has been born with an anomaly: the development of wholesome attitudes toward it can be influenced by the nurse.

HYDROCEPHALUS

Hydrocephalus (Fig. 51) is a condition in which the amount of cerebrospinal fluid is increased greatly above normal, resulting in increased size of the head and characteristic pressure changes in the brain.

In the older child whose skull sutures have united, lesions which would cause hydrocephalus if they

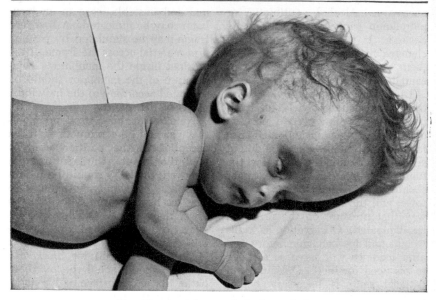

Fig. 51. An infant with hydrocephalus.

occurred in infancy result fatally before gross changes in the brain occur. Increased intracranial pressure in the older child is not referred to commonly as hydrocephalus.

ETIOLOGY

Cerebrospinal fluid is secreted by a network of veins (choroid plexus) situated in each of the lateral ventricles. From the ventricles it passes downward and posteriorly by way of the foramina of Monro, the aqueduct of Sylvius, the fourth ventricle and the foramina of Luschka and Magendie. At the base of the brain the fluid passes into the subarachnoid space which almost completely surrounds the brain and the spinal cord. From this space it is reabsorbed into the large venous sinuses on top of the brain. Normally, a balance exists between secretion and absorption.

Noncommunicating Hydrocephalus. If all or any large part of the subarachnoid absorbing space is shut off by any cause so that fluid from the ventricles does not circulate, the rate of absorption cannot keep pace with the rate of secretion, and noncommunicating hydrocephalus results. The obstruction may be in the path between the ventricles and the base of the brain from occlusion of the aqueduct of Sylvius.

Communicating Hydrocephalus. In some instances, obstruction is caused by adhesions between the meninges about the base of the brain. The adhesions may be from some unknown prenatal cause, they may be secondary to intracranial hemorrhage from birth injury or they may occur as a result of recognized meningitis after birth. The adhesions may obstruct the foramina at the base of the brain completely, so that no absorption can take place, or they may surround the foramina without obstructing them so that fluid can enter the spinal subarachnoid space freely, but not the cerebral space. The latter event gives rise to what is termed communicating hydrocephalus. By this is meant that communication exists between the ventricles and the spinal space and that fluid can be obtained freely by spinal puncture. Even though hydrocephalus may be communicating, it is still obstructive.

In cases of spina bifida, the medulla and part of the cerebellum may be pulled into the foramen magnum because of attachment of the cord at the site of the spine defect and growth in length of the spine. The tissues pulled into the foramen thereby are changed characteristically in shape and position (Arnold-Chiari deformity). It is the obstruction of flow over the cortex that causes the hydrocephalus so common in those with spina bifida.

SYMPTOMS

The progressive accumulation of unabsorbed fluid distends the ventricles and causes the head to enlarge and the brain cortex to become thin. With continued enlargement of the head the skull sutures separate. The infant becomes increasingly helpless, first because of inability to support the large head, later because of damage to the brain and because of malnutrition which always accompanies severe degrees of hydrocephalus. During the late stage, pressure sores are frequent unless most carefully avoided by changes of position and protecting pads. Death finally occurs from either progressive malnutrition or intercurrent infection.

DIAGNOSIS

The head may be larger than normal at birth, but more often no change is noticed until several weeks after birth. The finding that the head is larger than normal is strongly suggestive of hydrocephalus. Question as to diagnosis arises only in the early stages when the head size is not greatly in excess of normal. The diagnosis can be made certain by encephalogram (skull roentgenogram taken after the spinal fluid in the ventricles has been replaced with air), which shows the dilated ventricles. Increase in head size of an inch or more a month is also good evidence of hydrocephalus.

Occasionally, hydrocephalus is caused by meningovascular syphilis. This variety is not obstructive in a mechanical sense and never becomes extreme. Because of its failure to progress beyond a moderate degree and because of the characteristic cerebrospinal fluid changes, syphilitic hydrocephalus seldom would be confused with the usual obstructive types.

TREATMENT

In a few instances, hydrocephalus undergoes spontaneous arrest, a balance between secretion and absorption having been reached by some means. When the hydrocephalus is of moderate degree, it is well to defer radical surgical treatment until the rate of head growth can be determined. Operation may be unnecessary.

Since the cause of hydrocephalus is entirely mechanical, not much is to be expected of any kind of treatment except mechanical. Surgical treatment offers the only hope of cure and occasionally is effective. However, the operative mortality is high, and unfortunately the results are frequently disappointing or only temporarily successful. Procedures which are used include (1) removal or destruction of the choroid plexus to decrease the production of spinal fluid, (2) shunting operations which attempt to lead off the accumulated fluid through artificial openings in the ventricular system or through catheters to absorbing areas such as the tissues of the neck, the mastoid antrum, the peritoneal cavity or the ureter and (3) removal of a portion of the occipital bone and the vertebral lamina in the presence of the Arnold-Chiari deformity to provide decompression and improve the circulation of spinal fluid.

NURSING CARE

Preoperatively, the chief nursing problems are concerned with the maintenance of nutrition and the prevention of pressure sores on the head. Babies with hydrocephalus often have increasing nutritional failure as the hydrocephalus progresses. Important are feeding schedules which avoid vomiting and at the same time permit an adequate intake of food.

As the head increases in size the baby becomes more helpless. He cannot hold up his head to assume a sitting position and ultimately cannot move the head much while lying in bed. The head must be moved for him, and this must be done often enough to prevent pressure sores. Special care of the scalp and the use of a lamb's-wool pillow are measures suggested. Unless the head is enormous and heavy, holding the infant for feedings will relieve pressure for short periods.

After operation, the temperature and the pulse and the respiratory rates should be observed every half hour during the first 24 hours so that symptoms of shock may be detected and treated early. During the first day, pronounced rise in temperature may be noted. When the rise in temperature is marked, alcohol sponges (35 per cent alcohol) may help to control it. Clothing should be minimal, and bed covering should be removed. Fluids are given continuously by the intravenous route until fluid and nutritional needs can be satisfied orally. Nursing measures should be directed toward keeping the solution running in at the prescribed rate of flow and keeping the extremity used for injection adequately immobilized. A suction set should be in readiness, for mucous secretions may cause respiratory difficulties. Convulsions after operation may occur and should be watched for.

The infant should lie on the unoperated side to prevent pressure from within being exerted on the bone flap. Because positions are limited, every precaution should be taken to prevent pressure sores from developing. The ear may become the site of a pressure ulcer, and before the head bandage is applied cotton should be placed behind and over the ear. After approximately 1 week the infant may be held for feedings, but the position on the unoperated side should be continued until healing of the wound site is complete.

Spinal punctures to remove some cerebrospinal fluid to lessen pressure symptoms may be necessary at periods after operation. The nurse's functions in this procedure are described subsequently.

Operation may be unsuccessful, and, if so, the problem of caring for the child with hydrocephalus in the home or in an institution will require consideration.

MENTAL DEFICIENCY

ETIOLOGY

The failure of a child to develop normal intellectual capacity nearly always is due to structural defects within the brain. These defects may be the result of gross malformations of brain structure. However, more often, they depend upon the loss of brain cells through injury, anoxia or infection or upon the congenital absence of such cells. Since the cells of the brain are susceptible to a wide variety of noxious influences, mental deficiency is seen as an accompaniment of or sequel to a similarly large number of disorders. It will be possible to cite some representative examples only.

Heredity is clearly responsible for some instances of mental deficiency, for its occurrence may be traced through other members of the family in some instances.

Maternal Infection. Maternal infection during pregnancy (rubella) may be responsible for maldevelopment of the brain.

Prenatal Infection. Prenatal infection with syphilis is sometimes responsible for brain damage.

Birth Trauma. Birth trauma with the associated anoxia and hemorrhage is regarded as a frequent cause and may result in additional motor disorders.

Anoxia after birth may occur during severe atelectasis or anemia.

Toxic Effects. The "toxic effects" of bilirubin or other substances produced during the course of erythroblastosis fetalis may damage brain and result in the condition known as kernicterus.

Infection of the Central Nervous System. Beyond the newborn period infection of the central nervous system is the most common precursor of mental deficiency. Meningitis and the several varieties of encephalitis are the most frequent causes of acquired mental deficiency.

Degenerative Diseases and Thyroid Deficiency. Mental deficiency is a part of the degenerative diseases such as Schilder's or Tay-Sachs disease and accompanies some metabolic diseases such as thyroid deficiency. A spurious type of mental retardation is seen among children with severe emotional disturbances.

SYMPTOMS

The cardinal symptom of mental deficiency is failure to reach the normal developmental milestones at the appropriate age. The appearance of symptoms depends in large measure upon the severity of the defect. A few types, such as mongolism and microcephaly, are identifiable at birth, due to the presence of characteristic physical defects. However, usually the disorder is not suspected during the early months of life unless the defect is quite severe. The first inkling of abnormality comes with delay in grasping, sitting, standing and walking. Slowness to talk and difficulty in self-feeding and toilet training appear later. The infant's behavior may be very placid, so that he is regarded as a "good" baby, or he may present the opposite extreme of restlessness, hyperactivity, irritability and sleep disturbances. Drooling of saliva is common. Convulsions, feeding difficulties and spasticity of muscles are sometimes the first indications of defective development.

When the defect is of lesser severity the child may pass through infancy and the preschool years without showing obvious symptoms. This difficulty may become apparent only when he attempts to cope with the abstract concepts of his school work.

DIAGNOSIS

As indicated above, only the more severe grades of mental deficiency can be diagnosed with confidence in infancy. Caution is necessary in the interpretation of delay in motor performance, for there is a wide variation from the average among intellectually normal children. It is important to be sure that delay in motor achievement is not due to associated physical disability, to the effects of chronic illness or to severe malnutrition. Poor hearing or vision may complicate the diagnosis by hampering the development of normal skills in an otherwise competent child.

Beyond the period of infancy, standardized mental tests permit an estimate of the severity of the intellectual defect. The intelligence quotient or "I.Q." is computed by dividing the child's mental age as measured by the test by his chronologic age and multiplying by 100.

Mental deficiency is classified on the basis of such tests into the following general types:

Idiot .... 0 to 24 I.Q.
Imbecile .... 25 to 49 I.Q.
Moron .... 50 to 74 I.Q.
Borderline .... 75 to 90 I.Q.

The interpretation of intelligence tests is not a simple matter, as was stated in Chapter 3. Whenever the results are doubtful, repeated testing in 6 to 12 months is desirable as a confirmation. The test always must be regarded as a minimum measure of the child's intelligence, since any interfering factors tend to depress his achievement.

PROGNOSIS

Except in the severe degrees of mental deficiency or those associated with disturbances of motor control, the prognosis for life is about the same as that for normal children. The outlook for the child's adjustment in society will depend in large measure upon the degree of his deficiency. Idiots and imbeciles require permanent care and supervision. Morons are generally able to make a living; those of borderline intelligence ordinarily get along quite well in jobs suited to their capacities.

MANAGEMENT

With the exception of mental retardation which is due to thyroid deficiency there is no useful treatment which will alter the underlying defect. Some improvement can be expected from adequate control of convulsions when these are present and from the removal of unwarranted pressures applied to the child by parents or teachers who have an unrealistic concept of his ability.

Lacking any effective treatment, the objectives of management are to arrange an environment for the child in which he can utilize his limited powers to the best advantage. For seriously retarded children there is little to be done except to arrange for custodial care. Moderately retarded children generally benefit from placement in institutions which are equipped to give patient training and to exploit their manual skills. Most such children are happier if removed from the competition of intellectually normal children. Those of lesser defect will require special schooling with emphasis upon the development of manual skills in order to pursue trades to which they are suited.

Discussion of the problem with parents is often a difficult and delicate procedure. Whenever there is reasonable doubt about the diagnosis of mental retardation, the parents must be spared the anguish which the diagnosis creates. When there is no doubt about the diagnosis the parents must be told in order that reasonable plans can be made for the child. Such plans will have to vary somewhat, depending upon the parents' reaction to the child's handicap and upon the facilities that are available in the area in which they live.

Nursing Care

Mentally deficient children are in the hospital usually either for more accurate diagnosis of their mental condition or for some coincidental illness. It is to be expected that the hospital stay will be brief, and the chief nursing problems are concerned with current nursing care. Usually they are not in the hospital long enough to have effective teaching in new habit formation, although often such teaching is much needed and should be given when the period of hospitalization is prolonged.

The problems of nursing care vary with the age of the child, the degree of mental deficiency and the behavior patterns of the child. Thus a wide range of situations is possible.

The chief problem with the infant usually is in the feeding. Often these infants take food poorly and tend to refuse any food that is not fluid. If possible, they should be taught to take new foods and to have the varied diet customary for the age. The physical and emotional care is the same as for the normal infant. Even though he does not respond overtly to all forms of stimulation, he feels and requires emotional warmth equally as much as the normal child.

It is the young child who is likely to cause the greatest difficulty. Many are happy, quiet and contented. They are well behaved and, although more or less irresponsible, do not get into trouble. Others are noisy, irritable and destructive and need constant, consistent supervision to redirect them and to prevent self-injury. Closely confining restraints are undesirable, but in some instances a closely fitted canvas top to the crib or some similar device becomes necessary in order to restrict activity and particularly to avoid self-injury from falling out of bed. Some of these children cannot feed themselves yet and must be fed.

Although the older child may present behavior problems, usually these are not serious. They are chiefly from irresponsibility. Patience, understanding of his capacities and consistency in management will prevent problems from becoming fixed. Constructive play activities during the hospital stay will help to focus his attention on acceptable behavior.

Mentally deficient children are late in learning to talk. Some are so deficient that they never talk, although when they are older they develop various ways of making their wants known. For the younger group the various needs must be anticipated.

MONGOLISM

One group of mentally defective children usually can be recognized at birth by virtue of the associated physical defects which they present. The facial characteristics simulate those of persons of Oriental races, hence the name (Fig. 52). The face is round, with close-set eyes

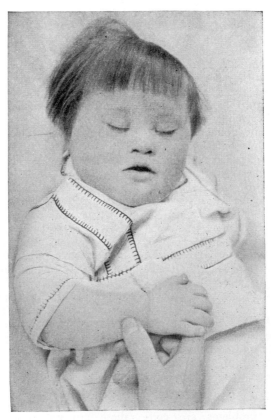

FIG. 52. Mongolism, showing the characteristic facies and short curved little finger.

which slant upward at their lateral extremities. Epicanthus is usually present. The head is small in circumference and grows at an abnormally slow rate. It is flattened in the anteroposterior diameter. Posteriorly, the infant has a flat occiput with broad and pudgy neck. Anteriorly, the nose is flat, and the cavities of the nasopharynx and the mouth are shallow in the anteroposterior diameter. The tongue is often large and protruded constantly. There may be marbling of the irides of the eyes. The muscles are lax, and the joints are loose, so that hyperextension is possible with the assumption of bizarre postures without apparent discomfort to the child. The hands are usually broad, with short and incurved fifth fingers and abnormalities of the creases of the palm. The great toe of the foot often is separated from the other toes by a wider space than normal through which runs a deep skin crease. Other abnormalities may include congenital malformations of the heart and umbilical hernia.

Mongolism (also called mongolian idiocy or mongolian imbecility) occurs with greatest frequency in the children of women who are approaching the end of their childbearing period. The mongolian child is very often the product of the last pregnancy possible for the individual woman. In a minority of the cases, the mongolian child occurs first in the sequence of pregnancies of a young woman. Under these circumstances the subsequent children are almost always normal. Rarely, mongolian children may appear in the middle of a succession of pregnancies or twice in the same family. The cause is unknown, but

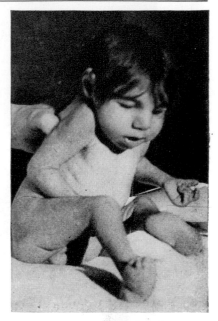

Fig. 53. Microcephalic idiocy.

it is presumed to be due to a widespread defect in the early development of the embryo.

Mongolian children develop slowly, generally have placid dispositions and can be expected to perform menial tasks only. They seldom reach a development level greater than 7 years. They are unusually prone to infections that carry an increased risk for them. In spite of modern antibiotic therapy their prognosis for life is less than that of the normal child.

MICROCEPHALY

An uncommon variety of mental deficiency which can be recognized at birth is microcephaly (Fig. 53). The newborn microcephalic infant has a skull that is obviously smaller

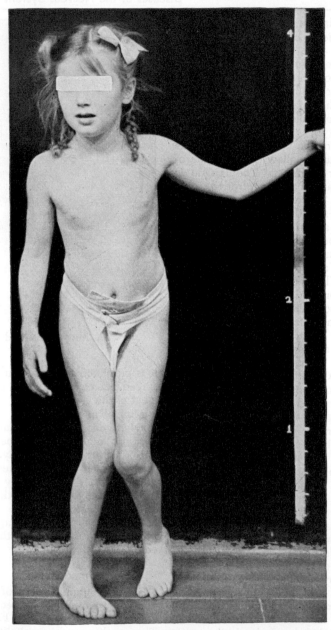

FIG. 54. Girl with spastic paralysis, showing spasticity of the
legs, with abductor spasm.

in volume than it should be and measures less in circumference than does the chest. The skull usually is flattened in the frontal region and sometimes comes to a point on top. The primary defect is in the brain itself, which has failed to develop properly. The skull size is merely a reflection of the abnormal size of the brain beneath. Such infants are retarded severely and seldom learn to talk. Sometimes their motor development is within reasonably normal limits.

MOTOR DISABILITIES OF CEREBRAL ORIGIN (CEREBRAL PALSIES)

"Cerebral palsy" is commonly but unwisely used as a comprehensive diagnostic term for children who have difficulty with voluntary muscle control. It erroneously implies that such children suffer from a specific disease entity which has some uniformity of etiology, symptomatology, prognosis or therapy. Such is not the case. On the one hand, the use of an all-inclusive label may unnecessarily stigmatize the child who has a mild disability and a good prognosis; on the other hand, it may encourage the parents of a hopelessly disabled child to pursue the chimera of recovery because of the knowledge that others with the same diagnosis have improved under treatment or have made a good adjustment in society.

ETIOLOGY

In a few children with motor disability the etiologic mechanism is clear and not subject to debate. In such children the symptoms begin after a specific postnatal illness. The most common cause is encephalitis, either primary or as a complication of one of the contagious diseases. Other precursors of motor disability are brain damage due to lead poisoning or to severe febrile illness, such as pneumonia, complications of meningitis, head injury, and kernicterus, the cerebral complication of erythroblastosis fetalis.

However, more numerous than these are the instances of motor defect in which natal or prenatal disturbances are thought to be at fault. There is considerable disagreement concerning the relative importance of abnormal brain development during fetal life and the potentially damaging mechanisms of birth—narcosis, anoxia, trauma and hemorrhage. The presumptive mechanism may be apparent in certain children, but it is necessary to admit that in a great many the relative importance of the prenatal and natal factors cannot be designated.

CLINICAL MANIFESTATIONS

Spasticity. The most frequent manifestation of motor disability is spasticity (Fig. 54). In this condition the voluntary muscles lose their normal fluidity and respond with difficulty to either the voluntary efforts of the child or the passive efforts of the examiner to alter their position. Abnormally strong tonus of certain muscle groups keeps the extremities and other portions of the body in characteristic attitudes which are altered jerkily by voluntary efforts. Spasticity is most often apparent in the lower extremities, where it tends to point the toes and cross the legs. In the arms it usually produces some clenching of the fist, flexion of the forearm and adduction of the upper arm against the chest wall. In severely affected children there may be an involvement of the muscles of the trunk which keep the back arched and the head extended.

All degrees of severity of the symptom are observed. Severe generalized spasticity results in a rigid, physically helpless child. Very mild degrees may not be apparent to casual observation and can be detected only by a careful neurologic examination. In some instances spasticity may be limited to one side of the body or to one extremity. The eye muscles may participate with the production of a convergent squint. In severely affected infants and children, swallowing may be difficult or impossible, due to the involvement of muscles of the face, the tongue, the jaw and the pharynx.

Weakness. Localized and diffuse weakness of muscles often is mixed in with the more obvious symptoms of spasticity. In some children the signs of brain damage are exclusively those of general or local weakness without associated spasticity.

Involuntary Movements. Several varieties of involuntary movement may be seen, usually in conjunction with other manifestations of brain damage.

CHOREA consists of quick, brief movements of a localized portion of the body, most commonly an arm or the face.

ATHETOSIS is a slow, prolonged, writhing movement of the extremities.

CHOREO-ATHETOSIS. Frequently, athetosis is combined with chorea and the resulting motions are designated as choreo-athetosis.

TREMOR. A persistent vibration of an extremity is called a tremor.

Associated Disturbances. Children with motor disability frequently have the additional problems of convulsions or mental retardation or behavior disturbances. These aspects are probably a concomitant of the brain damage which has produced the motor disturbance. They are of varying importance to individual children and have no necessary relationship to the severity of the motor disturbance. A child with severe choreo-athetosis may have normal or even superior intelligence; one with mild spasticity may be severely retarded. Their management must be considered in relation to the child's total problem.

DIAGNOSIS

Motor disability of cerebral origin may be recognized shortly after birth when the symptoms are severe. The early appearance of afebrile convulsions, feeding difficulties or spasticity in the first few months of life may raise the suspicion of brain damage which is confirmed by the subsequent failure of the child to follow the normal pattern of motor development. Except for the milder and the localized varieties of motor disability, all manifestations, such as spasticity, weakness and involuntary movement, interfere with the achievement of sitting, walking, talking, feeding and other co-ordinated muscle activities. Often it is the failure in such performance that first attracts attention to the possibility of brain damage. While the presence of motor disability is an adequate explanation for developmental failure, it does not necessarily imply that the more complex functions of the brain are damaged. It is imperative to evaluate the intellectual capacity of the child separately in order to guide his management. This is often a very difficult task, because the motor disability may hamper his ability to communicate and vitiates many of the performances required by the standard intelligence tests.

TREATMENT AND NURSING CARE

No form of therapy can be expected to restore the cerebral defect. Appropriate management must be based upon a realistic appraisal of the individual child's assets and ultimate potentialities. If convulsions are present they should be controlled by the measures discussed in the next section.

In the period of infancy, the child with cerebral palsy may show difficulty in sucking, swallowing and learning to eat solid foods. A hyperactive reflex often initiates the gag reflex, with resultant vomiting. Often his whole body tightens up, and when feedings are not given slowly enough, vomiting and aspiration may result. Gradually he will need to be taught to eat solid foods. At first, swallowing them will produce difficulties, but patience and calmness when they are refused, spit out or vomited eventually will help him to learn to eat them.

Respiratory difficulties and body spasticity in early life are not uncommon. The changes in respiration may be due to mucus or to the cerebral lesion. Often, the infant lies with his back arched, and spasticity may make movement difficult. Frequent change of position lessens his irritability and discomfort.

In the management of the child with cerebral palsy, one of the first objectives is the prevention of contractures. If contractures develop or seem to be imminent, the baby should be provided with corrective splints. For most babies these may be worn only at night. A back support or corset may be needed to enable the baby to sit. Leg splints usually are used in the daytime if the Achilles group of muscles go into spasm whenever the baby is placed on his feet.

During this early period in the child's life, the parents will require help in understanding the particular needs of their child with cerebral palsy. If they can be helped to accept the child, in the period of infancy, to gain security in their ability to satisfy his needs and to see the effects of oversolicitude on his emotional development, an important contribution to the child's mental health will be made. It will influence attitude development, a point which will have profound effect on the child's attitude toward himself and upon later feelings concerning his handicap.

Many times parents hesitate to hospitalize their child for the correction or the prevention of further deformity. Economic factors may influence their feeling, and when this is the case, the help of a community agency such as State Services to Crippled Children should be enlisted. However, many times fears exist because of a lack of knowledge as to procedure, period of hopitalization, outcome or adjustment of the child outside the home.

The nurse who understands the parents of handicapped children, can help them gradually to feel a need to secure medical care for their child. She also can allay fears that prevent them from utilizing community resources that function to provide the handicapped child with opportunities equal to those of the normal child. Often the nurse will need to initiate the co-operation of community agencies when she observes the child's need for continued medical care.

Several periods of hospitalization may be required. Often those periods are long ones, and opportunities for psychological growth, as well as good physical nursing care, must be provided. A child recuperates quickly from surgical operation. If a Sprengel operation to sever the nerves leading to the spastic extremities has been performed, the child will be in a cast that covers the lower half of his body. If he has not matured to a stage of bowel and bladder control, care on a Bradford frame will be indicated. If an operation has been performed to lengthen the Achilles tendon, casts from below the knee over the foot will be applied. If this operation has been performed, more play opportunities can be provided, for the child can be placed in a chair where he can enter into group activities. Other surgical procedures are employed to overcome the adductor spasm that produces the "scissors" gait so frequently seen in the child with cerebral palsy.

The child's mental capacities should be known. It is not the intelligence quotient but a knowledge of his potentialities that will assist the adult in planning an environment that will ensure optimum individual growth. A true picture of his mental ability is an intricate task, because the cerebral defect interferes with both verbal and motor expression. However, a test given by an experienced psychologist tells far more than casual observation.

Emotionally, the child with cerebral palsy seems to be unstable; there are reasons why this is so. Some of the instability may be due to inherent factors, but much of it results from the kind of guidance he has had during the formative years of his life. It is much more difficult for the child with cerebral palsy than for the normal child to get his basic human needs satisfied. He has a drive to explore, to master himself and his environment, but his physical limitations often prevent him from having the normal experiences of childhood. It takes imagination and ingenuity to help him find ways to learn. Unless his mother faces his handicaps and finds ways for him to have play experiences, intense frustration and insecurity from lack of mastery and self-fulfillment will result. Often the need for recognition is unsatisfied because of his unattractive appearance, which may be grotesque. Many parents, siblings and playmates find him difficult to accept. He becomes the object of ridicule and jests by his playmates and schoolmates and he is incapable of doing the things that other children can do. They see his body and its abnormal functioning instead of his person. As a result he is deprived of a vital ingredient for emotional growth—the responsiveness of others. Frequently, he is unable to express himself creatively, which is another basic need for personality integration. Often he has speech difficulties and is limited in his ability to communicate verbally with others. He also may have eye defects which produce reading difficulties and prevent him from having vicarious experiences through the media of movies, television or books. Learning to write presents problems because of muscular in-co-ordination. Sometimes his need for affection is completely unsatisfied because his parents and others are unable to accept him as he is. Many times he is overprotected rather than guided in a way that meets his individual changing needs.

Assisting the child to a stage of greater independence is a slow process but a very possible one in most instances. Opportunities to learn must be presented. He must be helped to do those things that he is capable of doing, yet too much must not be expected of him. The child with cerebral palsy can learn to feed himself. Feeding him is a skill; teaching him to do it himself is an art. It requires patience, faith in his ability, an understanding of his limitations and ingenuity in finding suitable equipment and methods of teaching that make the process of eating an easier and more enjoyable experience. The child also can learn to do many other things. Observation of skilled nursery school teachers as they teach children with cerebral palsy to do things for themselves, to express their inner creativeness and learn to communicate with others will provide unlimited educational opportunities for the inexperienced mother or nurse.

Teaching the child to relax and take frequent rest periods is important because he fatigues easily. Soft music in a room with few stimuli, with a person who talks quietly in a reassuring manner and helps him to feel that she is trying to help, produces the desired effect. Excitement of all types immediately before bedtime and technics that produce resistance should be eliminated. Discipline must be redirective and given with understanding. Irritation and impatience create tension that makes self-control almost impossible. The child needs to feel that his mother, nurse or teacher is truly interested in *him*. Although his speech is difficult to understand, it will increase his self-esteem and sense of security if the adults in his environment learn to understand his attempts to communicate verbally with them. Responsiveness on the part of the adults lessens tension and brings increased relaxation, emotional comfort and the capacity to use all his powers.

Many of the child's needs can become satisfied in play. His interests should be encouraged from the time they first are manifested. The child needs encouragement to feel that his interests are important. If the nurse uses ingenuity in finding play materials, and if the child is helped to use them constructively, he will acquire belief in his powers. With help he may excel to such a degree that his need for recognition becomes satisfied. Self-expression also can become possible through careful selection of materials and guidance in their use.

Play experiences should assist him to recreational productivity and provide opportunities for socialization. Play within a group is necessary. It will satisfy his need for friends and for normal social play experiences. It will help him to identify himself with a group outside his home, a need that must be fulfilled in the school-age period if wholesome emotional development is to occur.

The nurse's attitude toward the child with cerebral palsy will influence the group's acceptance of him. In the beginning, the nurse may have to direct the activity in a way that provides opportunity for him to participate in it. If she prevents him from meeting defeat, the group eventually will plan ways to utilize his abilities.

Educational opportunities should be provided in accordance with the child's abilities. The advantages of schools especially adapted to deal with his physical handicaps and to provide physiotherapy and muscle re-education are indicated. The child who is mildly incapacitated may be expected to attend a regular school but may require guidance in the selection of an occupation which is commensurate with his potentialities. Education is essential for the normally intelligent child. Through it he can develop his interests and eventually find ways of losing himself in an all-absorbing life task. With education and wisely directed guidance he can learn to excel in some realm. Succeeding is a necessary factor in eliminating feelings of inferiority that underlie attitudes of self-pity, the most injurious of all emotional feelings.

During childhood, growth-producing experiences which provide opportunities for satisfaction in the growing-up process must be provided. It is possible for the child with cerebral palsy to have normal personality development if environmental influences are conducive to it. Whether or not maladjustment occurs depends upon the number and the severity of the problems that

he must face. The child is severely limited only insofar as he has accompanying personality limitations. If opportunities for growth are denied him, he will suffer untold misery from feelings of inadequacy and incompetency, which will bring disturbances in his relationships with other people.

Guidance that helps the child face reality must begin in infancy and grow in proportion to the child's capacity to utilize it in finding constructive modes of adjustment. Denying his handicap impedes his progress toward self-understanding. When the adult recognizes the child's problem with him, he can approach it with the feeling that he has help and support to overcome it. He must recognize his problem and deal with it if he is to understand and learn to cope with it in a constructive manner.

The period of adolescence is a volcanic experience for a normal child, but for the child with cerebral palsy, surmounting the development tasks of the period is infinitely more difficult. Establishing heterosexuality, emancipating himself from his family and selecting and preparing for a career pose problems of great magnitude. In adolescence the social aspects of his handicap take on new proportions. If he has not been helped to accept the reality of his handicap prior to adolescence, he may show signs of acute emotional distress. He should be encouraged in social activities with both sexes to establish heterosexuality, to give him opportunities to emancipate himself from his parents and to prevent introversion.

The nurse's responsibility extends to those in the school and the community. She can explain the cause of the child's disability to the teacher, increase her insight into his psychological and physical needs and interpret his prognosis for future adjustment. She also can influence the attitudes of lay people toward the crippled child. The nurse who recognizes that the crippled child's needs are like those of the normal child will utilize her insight to help others accept him and find ways to meet his educational needs and accept his problem.

SEIZURES
(CONVULSIVE DISORDERS)

The term seizures is used to encompass a number of varieties of episodic disturbance of brain function. Most seizures are accompanied by loss of consciousness; many of them, by abnormal muscle tone. In children the most common variety of seizure is a convulsion, but other varieties of spells, attacks, fits and abnormal states also are seen. These phenomena of diverse and uncertain etiology are grouped together because of the conviction that they all represent periods of disorganization of the normal physiologic state of the brain.

Seizures create two general types of medical problems—the management of an acute convulsion and the study and the control of recurring attacks.

SINGLE CONVULSIONS

Symptoms. Convulsions usually are sudden in onset, though in some instances their imminence may be suspected by the general behavior of the child. In a typical case, the entire body becomes stiff, and consciousness is lost. More or less skin pallor is present. The eyes tend to be fixed in some one position, perhaps rolled up or crossed. As a part of the general tonic state, the head is held backward, the back is more or less arched, the arms are flexed, and the hands are clenched. Immediately after the general stiffening of the body, twitching or clonic movements occur. These may be generalized in the beginning or may start in some part and extend to all parts of the body. The clonic movements consist chiefly of quick, jerking to-and-fro movements of the extremities and similar spasmodic movements of the muscles of the face. The spasm includes the muscles of respiration, so that breathing is irregular and ineffectual, and cyanosis results. Inability to swallow saliva may produce frothing at the mouth and rattling in the throat. The pulse becomes weak and often irregular. Convulsions may be very brief or may last a half hour or more. Usually after a few minutes the convulsive movements become weaker and finally cease. The body relaxes, and consciousness returns. If the convulsion was severe, the child may remain somewhat stuporous, and at times certain parts appear to be paralyzed temporarily.

A convulsion may not be repeated or it may recur in a few minutes or hours. In some cases, convulsions may recur frequently over a period of several days. All are not so severe as the preceding description indicates. They may be lacking in several of the described features and may be of very short duration. In some instances, convulsions may involve only part of the body; in other instances of repeated convulsions, one part may be affected during one convulsion and other parts during other convulsions. Partial involvement of the body in this manner is not necessarily evidence of a localized intracranial lesion.

Etiology and Prognosis. A convulsion is a symptom of an underlying disorder and not itself a disease. The prognosis both for life and for the patient's mental and neurologic future depends upon the setting in which the convulsion occurs. Often the significance of an acute convulsion can be determined only in the light of future developments.

FEBRILE CONVULSIONS. Some infants and young children have convulsions at the onset of infectious diseases when the temperature is beginning to rise. These are commonly but somewhat inexactly called febrile convulsions. The phenomenon is somewhat analogous to the chill that takes place in adults under similar circumstances of disease but it depends upon the susceptibility of the individual patient to convulse. The infection itself may be a trivial one; a rapidly rising or excessively high fever triggers the convulsion without necessarily implying that the disease is a serious one. Children who have such a tendency ordinarily lose it as they grow older, so that febrile convulsions generally are not observed in children beyond the age of 4 or 5. Such convulsions are alarming but rarely fatal. When they are occasional, brief and limited to the period of early childhood and feverish illnesses, they probably have no adverse effect upon the child's ultimate development.

INFECTION OF THE CENTRAL NERVOUS SYSTEM. In the presence of fever, an acute convulsion some-

times announces the presence of infection of the central nervous system. Meningitis, encephalitis, tetanus, rabies, cerebral sinus thrombosis and brain abscess are examples. The prognosis will depend upon the particular variety of infection and the adequacy of treatment that can be marshaled to combat it.

INCREASED INTRACRANIAL PRESSURE. Acute convulsions may be seen associated with an increased intracranial pressure from causes other than infection—intracranial bleeding, brain tumor, uremia, lead encephalopathy. Here the immediate prognosis for life and the later prognosis for complete recovery of function are relatively poor.

TOXIC AND METABOLIC DISORDERS. Many toxic and metabolic disorders can be listed as causes of acute convulsions. Kernicterus in association with erythroblastosis of the newborn, rachitic or parathyroid tetany, insulin reactions, asphyxia and inhalation anesthesia, alkalosis, hypertension and prolonged treatment with ACTH are some of the disturbances which may have convulsions associated. Prognosis depends upon the ability to recognize the precipitating disorder and to bring it under control.

NO ASSOCIATED DISTURBANCE. Many acute convulsions have no associated disturbance. Some of them represent the first in a series of recurring episodes which are considered in a following section.

Treatment. Most acute convulsions are the unexpected harbinger of an illness. The majority are brief and self-limited and subside spontaneously, no matter what is done. When they are brought to medical attention, immediate sedation usually is indicated to ensure their termination. Many drugs have been used in the past, but the safest and easiest to administer is sodium phenobarbital by subcutaneous injection. Doses from ½ to 3 grains may be used, depending upon the size of the infant or the child. If the fever is high, the use of a tepid bath or a sponging to reduce the temperature gradually is rational.

If simple measures fail to terminate the convulsion within a period of ½ to 1 hour, rectal anesthesia with avertin may be employed. Search for associated disease requiring independent treatment always is indicated, whether the convulsion ceases spontaneously or not.

Nursing Care. Protection of the child from injury is one of the first considerations during a convulsion. Regardless of age, a crib bed is essential. If the convulsions are severe the cribsides should be padded. Inspection of the child's toys to remove those that might produce injury during a seizure should be made. To prevent suffocation, soft pillows should not be allowed. A padded tongue depressor should be in readiness to place between the teeth to prevent biting of the tongue. If convulsions produce increased secretion from the pharynx, a suction set should be kept in readiness. In some instances, oxygen may be necessary for extreme respiratory difficulty produced by muscular in-co-ordination.

Placement of the child where continued observations may be made is important for the protection of the child and for recording behavior that is helpful in making a diagnosis. Prior to the convulsion there may be an aura. The older child may tell the nurse of the experience. He may complain of tingling sensations, of seeing light, of hearing sounds or of dizziness, or he merely may utter a shrill cry. The young child is not able to express his sensory experience in words but instead may show changes in his behavior. He may become more irritable and restless or more destructive or he may become apathetic and listless. Whenever changes in behavior occur, keener observation should follow.

There is nothing that a nurse can do to stop a convulsion; her duty lies in observing and recording it in all its detail and in protecting the child from injury. In describing the movements, the term "twitching" should be used when the movements are clonic or jerking and "contraction" when the child holds himself in a tonic or a contracted and stiffened state. Observations as to the following should be made: behavior state preceding onset; length of the seizure in minutes; the site where the twitching or the contraction began and the parts of the body involved; eye movements and pupillary changes; types of movement; degree of perspiration; incontinence before, during or after the seizure; pulse and respiration rates; posture of the body; color; secretions from the mouth; the first and the last areas to relax; behavior at the end of the convulsion. If the child is old enough to talk, the state of consciousness can be observed. Degree of memory for recent events, type of speech and amount of co-ordination are observations that are needed to detect the extent of cerebral dysfunction produced by the seizure. After the convulsion the child should be placed in bed if he is not already there. Usually he will sleep for long periods, the time depending on the severity of the seizure.

After one convulsion the child should be protected against recurrence by continuing administration of sedatives until the danger of recurrence seems to be past.

RECURRENT SEIZURES

Persons who have recurring seizures of one sort or another often are said to be victims of epilepsy. To the average lay person this ancient appellation connotes a disease that is hereditary, incurable, socially disgraceful and a precursor of mental deterioration. While it is true that some unfortunate sufferers are so fated, it is manifestly unjust and undesirable to stigmatize the much larger number who have infrequent seizures or are able to control their seizures completely. These individuals may have normal or even superior intelligence and may lead useful and productive lives. Epilepsy does not denote a specific disease entity. It is much preferable to avoid the use of the term entirely and to speak of individual varieties of recurrent seizure patterns.

Nearly three fourths of those who eventually suffer from recurrent seizures do so in childhood; a significant number begin to have seizures before the age of 5. Untreated seizures tend to become more frequent and more severe. However, if a therapeutic regimen can be discovered which will keep the child free of attacks over a long period of time, it is often possible to withdraw the drugs gradually without return of symptoms.

Varieties of Recurrent Seizure. Recurrent seizures may be manifested in a great variety of ways. Because the basic mechanism of a seizure still is understood imperfectly, there is some difference of opinion about the implications of the different types.

GENERALIZED CONVULSIONS, MAJOR CONVULSIONS OR GRAND MAL. The symptoms of a generalized convulsion have been described in the preceding section. Such seizures also are called major convulsions or grand mal attacks. There is always loss of consciousness and postural muscle tone, followed by tonic or clonic movements of the extremities. Older children and adults who have generalized convulsions often describe a constellation of warning symptoms known as an aura. Peculiar feelings, sights, sounds, tastes, smells or involuntary muscle contractions may occur a few seconds before consciousness is lost and may lead the victim to utter a warning cry or noise before he falls. Headache and deep sleep not infrequently follow a generalized convulsion.

AKINETIC SEIZURE. An akinetic seizure is similar to a generalized convulsion except that there is no clonic jerking or tonic contraction of the extremities. The child loses consciousness and postural tone and falls limply.

LIGHTNING MAJOR CONVULSION. In young children less than 2 years old, a variant type of seizure called a lightning major convulsion sometimes is seen. It consists of a very rapid forward ducking of the head with simultaneous pulling of the arms and the legs onto the abdomen. The duration is often so brief that the significance of the movement may not be recognized. Such convulsions may occur in bursts, are usually difficult to control and often portend mental retardation.

FOCAL CONVULSIONS. In focal convulsions consciousness may be retained and postural tone preserved while involuntary convulsive movements of an extremity progress from its tip toward its connection with the body (jacksonian fit). Episodic sensory disturbances may replace the muscle movements in this type of seizure, so that it appears as a temporary disturbance of sight, smell, hearing or taste or as pallor, flushing, hypertension, abdominal pain, changes in heart rate and other manifestations. Differentiation of the last group from other varieties of bodily disorder may be very difficult.

MINOR CONVULSIONS OR PETIT MAL. Minor convulsions or petit mal attacks consist of very brief absences or loss of consciousness without loss of postural tone or abnormal muscle movements. The victim momentarily stops whatever he is doing for a few seconds and then resumes where he left off. He is frequently unaware of the fact that he has had a brief seizure.

PSYCHOMOTOR ATTACKS OR EPILEPTIC EQUIVALENTS. Various abnormalities of behavior of recurrent and often bizarre type are regarded as psychomotor attacks or epileptic equivalents. The child has no memory of the peculiarity of behavior. Psychomotor attacks usually occur in children who are having other types of seizure in addition.

Recurrent seizures of more than one variety may occur in the same child. For instance, akinetic seizures may precede the appearance of generalized convulsions. A high percentage of children with uncontrolled petit mal attacks eventually will develop generalized convulsions in addition to or instead of the initial form of seizure.

Diagnostic Considerations. Children who have recurrent seizures often require special study either (1) to ascertain that the episodes are really seizures or (2) to attempt to discover an anatomic or physiologic reason for them. When the child suffers from characteristic generalized convulsions there is seldom any doubt about their nature, but recognition of minor attacks and psychomotor attacks may be more difficult. Supporting evidence can be obtained by the use of the electroencephalograph, a machine which records the cyclic changes in the electric potentials of the brain. The procedure is somewhat analogous to the electrocardiogram applied to the study of heart disease. Most individuals with seizures display abnormal patterns of "brain waves" not only during the seizures but between attacks. In some instances the shape of the waves may be altered by having the child hyperventilate his lungs—a technic which occasionally precipitates an actual seizure. Electro-encephalograms are complex curves which require considerable experience for proper interpretation. Although it is usually true that an individual with seizures has an abnormal pattern, this is not invariably so. Conversely, some persons who never manifest seizures may have abnormal tracings. Electro-encephalograms also may be used to localize areas of abnormal brain discharges in some instances where operative correction is contemplated.

Diagnostic procedures are indicated in many children whose recurrent seizures are suspected of having an anatomic or physiologic basis. In addition to electro-encephalography, which may confirm the presence of seizures and occasionally localize their site of origin, x-ray visualization of the skull is usually desirable. Various abnormalities of shape, proportions and calcification of the cranial bones may give clues to an underlying disorder. A view of the gross structure of the brain itself may be obtained by removing the spinal fluid and replacing it with air (encephalography). The roentgenograms taken subsequently outline the cavities within the ventricular system and around the surface of the brain and often disclose structural abnormalities.

When there is suspicion of previous infection of the nervous system, various types of specific diagnostic tests may be indicated to exclude virus encephalitis, tuberculosis, syphilis or toxoplasmosis. Abnormalities of carbohydrate metabolism leading to periods of hypoglycemia or of calcium metabolism leading to tetany require special biochemical study. Rickets and lead poisoning produce changes in the x-ray appearance of the ends of the long bones, which may afford etiologic clues.

Treatment. A small number of children with recurrent seizures will be found to have a remediable underlying condition, the correction of which will terminate the seizures. But in most instances the seizures are of unknown causation or are associated with some disturbance which cannot be modified. The main problems in therapy consist of the discovery of a drug regimen that will abolish the seizures or reduce them to a minimum and the guidance of parents and child to an acceptance of a realistic way of life.

Phenobarbital is the most widely used drug for the prevention of recurrent seizures. It is almost devoid of toxic effects and has a large factor of safety which permits liberal dosage even in small children. Its disadvantage is that it is not very effective against petit mal attacks or psychomotor seizures. In large dosage it may cause drowsiness or unsteadiness. For the control of generalized convulsions it may be given in doses of 1 to 3 grains per day, depending upon the size of the child and the frequency of convulsions. The total dose usually is divided into 2 or 3 portions. A level of drug is sought which will prevent attacks without producing drowsiness or unsteadiness. When there is a tendency for the child to have an attack at a certain period of the day, accurate timing of his medicine is necessary to forestall seizures. Attacks that occur during or upon waking from sleep pose a difficult problem that may be solved by administering enteric coated capsules the effect of which is delayed. If a successful regimen can be found, it should be continued until the child has had at least 2 years free from seizures. Slow withdrawal of medication then may be attempted.

When phenobarbital is unsuccessful in controlling generalized convulsions or produces too much drowsiness for the school-age child, other drugs may be used instead of or in combination with it. Dilantin is most commonly used as an adjuvant to or substitute for phenobarbital. The dosage is from 1 to 5 grains per day, depending upon the age of the child. Toxic effects are observed more frequently than when phenobarbital alone is used. These include ataxia, rash and hypertrophy of the gums. A closely related drug is Mesantoin, which has the additional hazard of depressing the blood-forming elements in the bone marrow, a toxic effect which must be sought by periodic leukocyte and differential blood counts in order to terminate the use of the drug at the first sign of difficulty.

Generally, minor convulsions are controlled effectively by Tridione. The dosage ranges from 5 to 20 grains a day. Its ability to terminate petit mal is often dramatic. Disadvantages lie in the side effects which it may produce—rashes, drowsiness, a peculiar sensation of glare and infrequently depression of the blood-forming organs. Paradione is a closely related compound which may be used in its place.

For focal and psychomotor seizures Dilantin is usually the drug of choice. Phenurone is sometimes useful but is a much more toxic substance.

In children who suffer from both petit mal and major convulsions, a therapeutic problem arises in that Dilantin generally tends to aggravate minor convulsions while suppressing the major attacks, while Tridione may stimulate major seizures while controlling minor attacks.

Bromides and ketogenic diets are mainly of historical interest in the control of seizures. In unusual in-stances the former may be required for the control of major convulsions. The latter will work in the control of petit mal attacks but are very difficult to maintain.

Nursing Care. The nurse has a number of obligations toward the child who is hospitalized for treatment or investigation of recurrent convulsions. She contributes important information by accurate observation of the child and recording the number and the variety of his seizures. She can help to regulate his daily life in such a manner as to avoid unnecessary excitement and provide him with as much healthy diversion as his condition will permit. She must be cognizant of the possible toxic effects of the drugs that he is taking and observe him for such adverse symptoms. In addition she may have to help him through diagnostic procedures such as a lumbar puncture or an encephalogram.

Encephalograms are used as a part of the diagnostic regimen in an attempt to find an anatomic cause for the seizures. Cerebrospinal fluid is replaced by air through a spinal puncture needle in order to obtain contrast roentgenograms of the brain. One method for this procedure is to withdraw 10 cc. of fluid and replace with 5 cc. of air, after which 10 cc. of fluid is replaced with 10 cc. of air, and this process is repeated until no more fluid is obtained. Approximately 100 cc. of air may be injected in this manner. Normally, the air will fill the ventricles and spread over the cortex. A roentgenogram shows the outline of the ventricles and of the cortical convolutions. Distortions and changes from the normal outlines indicate the location and often the nature of the lesion.

Preparing the child psychologically for this procedure is necessary. A preliminary hypodermic of a sedative and an Avertin anesthesia preceded by a cleansing enema usually are ordered. Both procedures should be explained to him, and he should understand the effect that will be produced by the Avertin. In some instances, children are made ill by this procedure. Headache may be a complaint, and some degree of prostration or shock may appear. Older children react to the aftermath of an encephalogram much better if they have been forewarned of the discomfort that they may experience. Before the anesthesia is given, the blood pressure should be determined. Avertin reduces blood pressure, and the significance of the readings after the procedure is based on the readings prior to anesthesia.

Sterile equipment for an encephalogram consists of spinal-puncture needles, gloves, 20-cc. syringe, medicine glass, spinal manometer and 3-way stopcock, glass graduate, lumbar puncture drape sheet, cotton balls and a gauze dressing to cover the site of puncture.

Two nurses are required for the treatment. The child must be held on the treatment table in a sitting position to allow the injected air to rise and replace the cerebrospinal fluid. Position can be maintained more easily if a stool covered with a pillow is placed over his lap and his body is bent forward to rest on it. A second nurse assists the doctor, collects samples of spinal fluid, records the amount withdrawn and the amount of air injected and watches for change in the child's pulse and respiration rates.

After the injection of air, the child should be wrapped in a blanket and transported in an upright position to the x-ray department for skull films. A tray containing hypodermic equipment and stimulants should be taken with the child, as emergency stimulants may be indicated by a change in color, pulse and respiration rates and blood-pressure reading. Pulse and respiration rates, temperature and blood pressure should be observed frequently until stabilized. Symptoms of shock and increased intracranial pressure should be watched for.

In many institutions, fluids are given parenterally on return from the x-ray examination to replace fluids lost by withholding nourishment and by perspiration during the procedure. Oral intake of fluid is usually low in the first 24 hours after this diagnostic procedure. Administering oxygen 100 per cent by mask for 2 minutes at hourly intervals for the first 6 to 8 hours aids in the absorption of the injected air, decreases headache and prevents nausea. Helping the child to see the benefits of remaining flat in bed prevents discomfort from headache.

In the presence of brain tumor, a ventriculography is done instead of encephalography. Cerebrospinal fluid is replaced by air through a needle passed into the lateral ventricles through trephine openings in the skull. Ventricular needles, rubber tubing and a 3-way stopcock replace the lumbar puncture needles for this procedure. Maintaining an upright position is not necessary for this procedure.

Postoperative care is the same as for encephalography. However, occasionally it is necessary to remove from the ventricles air that is producing symptoms of increased intracranial pressure. For this reason, a sterile ventricular set should be kept in the child's room for 48 hours after the procedure.

The "whole" child, not merely his seizures, must be studied and treated. The child's personality is influenced by his response to problems and situations created by his disease. The convulsion itself does not lead easily or early to personality disintegration. Nor do convulsions always occur in persons with a particular personality type. It is chiefly the significance of the convulsion to the child in his little world that affects his personality development.

Often the child with recurrent seizures is described as being emotionally unstable, egocentric, tempestuous in emotional response, selfish and moody. If these traits are existent in the personality make-up of a child, they indicate a need for delving beneath the surface to discover the genesis of his eruptive behavior. Eliminating the pressure points that cause his undesirable behavior will do much toward decreasing the number of attacks and helping him to become better adjusted. This does not mean that his attacks are psychogenic in origin but it does mean that unwise guidance tends to cause emotional feelings that can precipitate an attack. Such behavior traits as the above are not peculiar to the child with seizures; they are seen as frequently in normal children who come from environments that are inadequate for their needs.

The nurse interested in the well-being of the child must extend that interest into the home and into his community. Unless convulsions are severe and uncontrolled, school experience with normal children should not be denied him. Teachers who have learned how to handle a child in a convulsion and have understanding of his home background and insight into his needs exert a profound influence on the child's peers and often through them on those in their homes. They help the community to accept him, a point which increases his security and belief in himself and gives him a feeling of "belongingness." Feeling for himself is influenced by the attitudes of his family and the reactions of his group toward him.

At home and in school, relationship experiences that produce anxiety, fear and problems too great for the child to solve must be eliminated to bring him peace of mind. The more problems there are for which he cannot find satisfying solutions, the less probable is the therapeutic value of any drug.

Assisting the child, his parents and his community in accepting him as he is constitutes one of the greatest responsibilities that society can have. The child must do his own adjusting, but society can assist him in making a comfortable and constructive adjustment to his handicap.

The National Epilepsy League in Chicago does a great deal to help the parents of children with seizures. They provide pamphlet material and direct parents to sources of help in their communities. Personnel in branches of the organization counsels parents and works with nurses and teachers in the schools.

BRAIN TUMOR

Brain tumor is a result of abnormal growth of cells already present in the brain or of malignant cells transported to the brain from their origin elsewhere in the body. Most brain tumors are of the first group.

ETIOLOGY

Brain tumors are approximately one sixth as frequent in children as in adults; nevertheless, they are relatively frequent among the tumors of the body. Most of the brain tumors of children occur in the posterior fossa of the skull cavity, whereas most of the tumors of adults occur above the tentorium. Fully three fourths of the tumors of childhood are composed of glial cells (glioma). These cells are of various types which differ in their invasive ability. The most common type is slow growing and not invasive. The type of glial cell is known as astrocyte, and the tumor is an astrocytoma. These tumors usually are in the cerebellum.

SYMPTOMS

Most of the symptoms are caused by increase in intracranial pressure. Tumors of the posterior fossa are almost certain to cause hydrocephalus from obstruction of the outflow of cerebrospinal fluid from the basal foramina. Increased intracranial pressure is likely to cause headache and vomiting. Among the nerve changes resulting, one easy to detect is swelling of the head of the optic nerve, as observed by ophthalmoscopic examination ("choked disk"). After a period of persistent swelling, the optic nerve atrophies, causing permanent blindness. In young children, the skull sutures are not united. Therefore, the sutures may separate as a result of the increased pressure and thus somewhat delay some of the more severe pressure effects. Increased intracranial pressure is likely to cause slowing of the pulse and may cause increase in blood pressure. Fretfulness, irritability and changes in disposition are common results, followed later by mental dullness and drowsiness. Older children may complain of dizziness.

Symptoms from local destructive effects of the tumor vary greatly and may be lacking. Cerebellar tumors often cause nystagmus and disturbances in gait and ability to stand. Localizing symptoms are produced more often by tumors above the tentorium. Convulsions are common with cerebral and rare with cerebellar tumors.

DIAGNOSIS

Tumors of the brain have an insidious beginning, and often early diagnosis is impossible. The course is progressive, and soon or late symptoms suggesting the condition appear. The course of some of the slow-growing tumors at times may be as long as several years before serious symptoms appear. In other instances of tumor, perhaps only a few weeks elapse. The coexistence of headache, vomiting and choked disks is highly suggestive of brain tumor, but these 3 conditions appear together late in the disease. A ventriculogram or an encephalogram is helpful in making the diagnosis and locating the tumor. In some instances, electro-encephalogram also is helpful. Evidence of increased intracranial pressure may be obtained by direct measurement of the cerebrospinal fluid pressure and in many instances by x-ray examination of the skull. The skull may show separation of the sutures in the younger children and atrophy of bone in the same pattern as the brain convolutions in the older children. Symptoms identical with those of brain tumor may be produced by brain abscess, encephalitis and certain degenerative diseases of the brain. Examination of the cerebrospinal fluid is often helpful in making a differential diagnosis.

Treatment

The treatment of brain tumor is surgical removal when this procedure is feasible. An invasive tumor cannot be removed completely and it is certain to recur after operation. Some of the tumors of children are enucleated easily and removed completely. With such tumors the prognosis is good if the child survives the operative procedure.

Nursing Care

When a child comes under observation because of possible brain tumor, the nurse should observe symptoms that may be helpful in localizing the lesion. The child of school or adolescent age will talk of his symptoms; the younger child cannot. But if the nurse is observant, she will note behavior that results from partial blindness, visual hallucinations, headache and intracranial pressure. Pulse and respiration rates, temperature and blood pressure should be observed at short intervals, and changes should be reported promptly. Observations as to the following should be made: mental state, drowsiness, sleepiness, irritability, pupillary changes (fixation or dilatation), vomiting with or without nausea, quality of speech, yawning, hiccoughing, sphincter control and details of convulsions.

When the diagnosis of brain tumor has been made, nursing measures to prepare the child for operation are indicated. Good nutrition influences the postoperative course, and frequent nourishing feedings should be given in the days prior to operation. Vomiting usually is unaccompanied by nausea, and in many instances the child is hungry and can be refed. Optimism and encouragement are necessary in the preoperative period, and every effort should be made to prepare the child psychologically, to understand him as an individual and to gain his confidence so that he may be relieved of emotional tension in the period when physical discomfort makes co-operation difficult. A preoperative enema may be contraindicated because it may increase intracranial pressure. Preoperative drugs may include atropine, but morphine seldom is given because of its depressant action on the central nervous system.

A crib bed should be provided for all children with brain tumor in both the preoperative and the postoperative periods. When the child returns from the operating room he should be placed in bed off the operative site, on his side, with his head level. The nasopharynx must be kept free of secretions and vomitus. The suction catheter should of firm rubber and should be held closed to prevent injury to the mucous membrane as it is passed through the nose into the throat and then opened to produce suction.

Knowledge of the anesthetic used will guide the nurse in understanding the significance of the recorded temperature, blood pressure and pulse and respiration rates. Observations of these phenomena should be made every 15 minutes until the child's condition justifies longer intervals. If the operative procedure has been extensive, symptoms of surgical shock may be striking. In applying external heat, warm blankets are preferable to hot-water bags, as these children burn easily because of their sensory and motor disturbances. Raising the foot of the bed is considered inadvisable, due to the possibility of increasing intracranial pressure and bleeding. Emergency stimulants, oxygen inhalations, intravenous fluids and small blood transfusions may be indicated, and apparatus to give these supportive measures should be in readiness. Measures to raise blood pressure rapidly to normal levels are not desirable because rapid change predisposes to intracranial bleeding.

When operation has been preceded by a ventriculogram, a sterile ventricular tap setup to remove cerebrospinal fluid which may contain blood and produce both increased pressure and rise in temperature must be included in the equipment always available at the child's bedside. A ventricular tap setup includes ventricular needles, spinal manometer and 3-way stopcock, 20-cc. syringe, rubber catheter (cut off to 3 in. in length, including the wide end), gauze squares, Kelly clamp, lumbar-puncture drape, towels, medicine glass, emesis basin, gloves and materials for a collodion and gauze roll-dressing. Test tubes and a bacterial culture medium

should be available to collect samples of cerebrospinal fluid for culture and to determine progress of the bleeding by noting changes in its color from time to time.

If the dressing becomes moistened with blood or cerebrospinal fluid, the doctor may wish to be notified so that the dressing can be changed. Escape of spinal fluid is often advantageous, since it reduces the intracranial pressure. If the child is young or restless, elbow restraints must be applied to prevent him from disturbing his dressing. Before wrist and ankle restraints are applied to children who are dangerously restless, every method possible should be used to allay their fears and anxieties, for they not only make them uncomfortable, but they also increase intracranial pressure.

Hyperthermia may be due to trauma, disturbance of the heat-regulating center or to intracranial edema. Control of hyperthermia requires constant vigilance and intensive nursing care. The child's temperature should be taken hourly. When it begins to rise above 101° F., he should be undressed and covered with a sheet. Room temperature should be regulated as changes in temperature occur. When the temperature rises to 101.4°, the sheet over the child should be replaced by a diaper to cover the pubic area. Icebags under the axilla, near the groins and around the trunk often will assist in reducing the temperature. However, if the temperature reaches 101.6° F., tepid-water sponge baths are indicated. The bed should be protected by a bath blanket or bath towels if the child is small, and water at 85° F. should be used initially and then reduced to 75° F. When sponging, only the parts of the body that are warm should be included. The parts that are cold to touch should be covered with a light blanket until warm, when sponging of these parts may be included. When the temperature registers 102.5° F., rectal ice-water enemas may be desirable. The size of the catheter and the amount of water introduced will be dependent upon the age of the child. The water should run in slowly. Then the tube should be clamped off and after 10 minutes reopened for siphonage and to introduce more water. After this process has been repeated 3 or 4 times, the tube should be removed gently and the temperature taken in 30 minutes. If the temperature continues to rise to a level of 103° F., warm-alcohol sponge baths may be given every half hour. For a markedly elevated temperature (104° F. or over), small retention enemas with aspirin will produce diaphoresis and temperature reduction. In all the above procedure, it is not expected that the temperature will be reduced to normal; keeping it within a reasonably low range only is desired. Lumbar punctures to remove blood and fluid may be necessary to reduce temperature.

The child's temperature must be taken at half-hour intervals during the period of hyperthermia to prevent it from dropping too rapidly. If it drops as much as 1 degree below the level of the starting point, the temperature-reducing procedures should be discontinued. If it drops to a subnormal level, the child should be dressed and covered with blankets. However, care must be taken to prevent overheating him to such a degree that his temperature again rises to above 100° F.

Trauma during surgery may produce edema of the face and the eyelids. If the edema is great, circulation of lachrimal secretion over the eye may be impaired and the eye may become dry and subsequently infected. Drops of sterile sweet oil prevent corneal dryness, gentle warm-saline irrigations keep them free of exudate, and elbow restraints keep the child's hands away from his irritated eyes. Swelling of the eyelids can be controlled partially by the application of cold compresses. Care in application should be used to prevent dampening the head dressing.

The extent of the external facial and scalp edema may be indicative of the amount of intracranial edema that exists. When marked external edema develops, with accompanying drowsiness and pupillary change, the nurse should be increasingly watchful for additional signs of intracranial pressure requiring prompt treatment.

When nausea subsides, fluids can be given by mouth. To prevent aspiration, only small sips of water should be given until the swallowing reflex is known to be functioning. A rubber-tipped or a cellophane drinking tube should be used, and when nourishing fluids can be tolerated, amounts should be increased gradually. Too rapid ingestion of fluids is to be guarded against, because vomiting, which increases intracranial pressure, may be induced. Until the child's fluid and food requirements are satisfied orally, infusions are continued.

If the swallowing reflex is absent, gavage feedings may be given. Usually, the catheter is introduced and left in place for a 24-hour period. By withdrawing it an inch or two for saline cleansing of the catheter and the nostril, irritation from the tube can be prevented. When tube feedings are given, distention should be watched for.

As the child's condition improves, solid foods can be introduced. Often encouragement is necessary to help the child eat increasingly larger amounts of foods of high calorie and vitamin content.

Unless meticulous mouth care is given frequently, discomfort results. Use of a tongue depressor to keep the mouth open when cleansing the teeth, the gums and the tongue makes the procedure a safer one.

To prevent pressure sores of the head and the body and hypostatic pneumonia, the child's position should be changed hourly. Pressure sores of the head and the ears develop easily, and cotton "doughnuts" to lie on prevent them from occurring. Until the use of suction is unnecessary, the child should be kept off his back to prevent aspiration. After that period, he can be placed in any position that eliminates pressure over the operative site. His back should be washed and massaged thoroughly every 4 hours. A good preparation for use is a combination of zinc-oxide ointment and castor oil. When changing his position, his head should be supported, and turning should be done slowly and carefully. Quick movements produce vertigo and increase in blood pressure.

In cases in which there is paralysis or spasticity of the extremities, support of the parts with pillows, rolls or other means is necessary.

Need for measures to prevent foot drop and pressure sores of the ankles, the heels and the knees often exists; when indicated, these measures must be employed.

There is no nursing more intensive or detailed than that required for a child who has had a craniotomy. Intelligent observation resulting in appropriate nursing and a determination to continue supportive nursing, regardless of the seeming outcome, are part of the skill and the spirit which are required to nurse these children. Although to the observer he may appear to be unconscious, conversation that might have a deleterious effect on the child never must occur.

The child's parents need much consideration. If they have been prepared previous to operation, the sight of their child with his bandaged edematous head and the emergency procedures so often required will not be so frightening to them. They must be helped, too, to handle their emotions in the presence of their child.

His convalescent care should include guidance that assists him to a greater stage of independence and should provide him with opportunities for more normal living. As function of the body returns, it should be noted, and graduated opportunities to use it should be provided. During the acute stage of his illness he has been waited on, and his needs have been anticipated constantly; now in convalescence he needs to learn gradually to do things and play by himself and with others and to share his nurse with others. If in this period the parents observe his increasing abilities, they will continue to foster independence at home. Return visits during the ensuing years are necessary to check progress after removal of brain tumors.

INFECTIONS

MENINGITIS

Inflammations of the meninges are classified according to the bacterial exciting cause. The differential diagnosis is made chiefly by identifying the causative organism in cerebrospinal fluid obtained by lumbar puncture.

Tuberculous Meningitis. ETIOLOGY. Tuberculous meningitis is caused by the tubercle bacillus *(Mycobacterium tuberculosis)*, which gains access to the meninges from a focus elsewhere in the body. The disease may occur in association with a generalized miliary tuberculous infection, in which case the symptoms of miliary tuberculosis are likely to be masked by those of meningitis. It often occurs also when symptoms and signs of tuberculosis elsewhere are not manifest and when a careful examination reveals perhaps nothing more than a hilus gland infection. Thus, tuberculous meningitis may appear in a child who previously had had apparently excellent health and nutrition. Tuberculous meningitis may occur at any age, but it is encountered with the greatest frequency under 5 years of age.

SYMPTOMS. The onset is gradual and insidious in most instances and is manifest by some variety of change in behavior. These changes vary with the person and probably are brought about chiefly by increased intracranial pressure caused by an increased amount of cerebrospinal fluid. The child is likely to become cross and irritable. The play habits and reactions to associates change. Drowsiness and mental dullness are common. Because of the increased intracranial pressure, vomiting, anorexia and constipation are frequent, especially in infants, and headache becomes a complaint of older children. The temperature

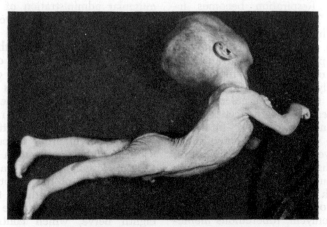

FIG. 55. Opisthotonus position in a baby with meningitis.

during this period is elevated only slightly. These symptoms of the early stage do not give very definite indication of the cause of the difficulty but after perhaps a week, sometimes longer, the symptoms become more severe and point more definitely to their intracranial origin. Drowsiness and headache increase. Hyperesthesia appears, and the child prefers to remain undisturbed. Intolerance of noises and bright lights frequently develops. In some cases, the child screams now and then, the so-called hydrocephalic cry. The reflexes are increased, the pupils are of normal size or small, the neck is stiff, the head is held back, and very often the extremities also are held rigidly (Fig. 55). Convulsions sometimes occur. This period of more severe illness has been called the irritative stage. Gradually, the illness goes through a transition into what is known as the paralytic stage. The stupor becomes more marked and continuous and eventually becomes so deep that the child cannot be aroused. Respiration becomes irregular. The pupils are large and fixed. The reflexes diminish until they no longer can be elicited. Various paralyses, often transitory, may be noted. Muscle movements are chiefly automatic and not purposeful. General muscular relaxation increases. Death occurs either quietly in deep coma or in a few instances with terminal convulsions. At the very end, the temperature, which has been relatively low throughout the illness, rises rapidly to a high point.

PROGNOSIS. Before the discovery of streptomycin, tuberculous menin-gitis was almost invariably fatal. At the present time it is impossible to say how effective streptomycin and the adjuvant drugs used with it will be in the cure of tuberculous meningitis, for widely divergent results are reported from different countries and from different clinics within the United States. Treatment is more likely to be successful with older children than with infants. The best results are reported when treatment can be initiated very early in the course of the disease. Infants under 1 year old and older children who are already in coma at the time of diagnosis recover in less than 25 per cent of the cases. Under the most favorable circumstances, recovery without residual effect may be expected in more than half of the patients treated.

TREATMENT AND NURSING CARE. Because of the serious danger to life and to mentality, antituberculous drugs must be used in maximum quantities over long periods of time. Therapeutic regimens differ in detail, but most include daily intramuscular administration of streptomycin or dihydrostreptomycin combined with oral isoniazid or one of its derivatives and a third adjuvant such as promizole or para-aminosalicylic acid. Long duration of treatment usually means at least 4 to 6 months and sometimes a year or two. Some treatment regimens include intrathecal injections of streptomycin in order to carry the drug in high concentration directly to the lesions in the meninges. Whenever one of the streptomycins is used for such lengths of time the very real risk of damage to the eighth nerve, which controls the functions of hearing and equilibration, must be recognized and accepted as necessary.

Treatment may be handicapped by the formation of meningeal adhesions which prevent the free circulation of spinal fluid and in consequence produce hydrocephalus. Various surgical measures and intraspinal injection of enzyme preparations such as streptodornase, streptokinase, papain and other materials have been used with indifferent success in counteracting this complication.

During the prolonged treatment, nursing measures to care for the skin and prevent pressure sores are necessary during the early stages of the disease. Also, nutrition must be maintained by careful feeding, sometimes requiring gavage technic. If the child recovers with residual neurologic difficulties, the same sort of rehabilitative measures as those outlined for the child with motor disabilities must be used. Deafness may be a permanent handicap. Loss of equilibrium is usually a temporary disability for which the child learns to compensate.

Meningococcic Meningitis (Epidemic Meninigitis, Cerebrospinal Fever, Spotted Fever). ETIOLOGY. Meningococcic meningitis is caused by the diplococcus, *Neisseria intracellularis* or *meningococcus.* This organism gains entrance to the body by way of the nose and the throat and during the early stage of the disease may be cultured from this locality and from the blood. Therefore, the disease is naturally transmissible. Great variation is shown at times in the ease and the frequency of transmission. Most of the time meningococcic meningitis exists as an occasional sporadic disease but at other times it becomes widely epidemic. In approximately three fourths of all cases, this disease occurs in children under 10 years of age and in nearly half of them, in children under 5.

SYMPTOMS. As with other infectious diseases, this one has its abortive, mild, severe and malignant forms. The symptoms of only the common form will be described.

After a short incubation period, usually less than a week, prodromal symptoms lasting a day or two may appear. More commonly the onset is sudden, with vomiting, prostration, headache, pain in the neck, the back and the legs and frequently convulsions. Although present, fever seldom is high. The head is bent backward, and the neck and the back are held rigidly. A position of marked opisthotonos may be assumed. The child prefers to be undisturbed, and movement causes much discomfort. Delirium is common. Stupor and coma appear in the more severe illnesses but are not so common in those of ordinary severity. Fretfulness and irritability may alternate with periods of drowsiness or stupor. Herpes may appear about the mouth.

An eruption of purpuric spots varying from pinhead size to large ecchymotic blotches is characteristic of the meningococcus bacteremia that generally accompanies the meningitis. In a few instances the rash is very extensive and is associated with signs of shock which progress rapidly to a fatal termination, presumably due to adrenal failure (Waterhouse-Friderichsen syndrome).

DIAGNOSIS. The diagnosis is made by examination of the cerebrospinal fluid. One or several of the symptoms and the signs enumerated constitute the indication for spinal puncture. This is particularly true of neck rigidity and other signs pointing to irritation of the nervous system. In an infant, the fontanel is full or bulging.

Lumbar puncture reveals increased quantity and pressure of cerebrospinal fluid. At the onset of the illness, the fluid may be fairly clear, although showing a definite increase in cells. However, very quickly the fluid is cloudy from the large number of pus cells present. These statements are true also of other varieties of purulent meningitis. The difference between the fluid of meningococcic meningitis and that of other purulent forms is solely in the variety of organism present as the cause.

In most cases of purulent meningitis, the causative organism is easily demonstrable in a stained smear prepared from the cerebrospinal fluid. In the few instances in which the organism cannot be found readily, the chances are great that the illness is caused by the meningococcus. The meningococcus is a gram-negative diplococcus and is found chiefly within the pus cells. The causative organism of no other common variety of meningitis has these characteristics. Usually the meningococci can be grown and identified by cultural methods when they are too scarce to be found easily by direct examination.

PROGNOSIS. Before the use of specific serum the mortality rate was approximately 70 per cent. With serum treatment the rate was reduced to 30 per cent or less. With sulfonamide therapy the death rate is approximately 10 per cent. The mortality rate varies with the age of the child and with the promptness with which therapy is instituted. When appropriate treatment is given on the first or the second day of the disease, the death rate is low. The mortality rate is much higher in the first year than in the second, and higher in the second year than later. With prompt and effective treatment, complications are uncommon. On the other hand, some of the complications are serious. They include mental deterioration, various paralyses and, in infants, hydrocephalus.

TREATMENT. Until the advent of the sulfonamide drugs, the treatment consisted of the use of specific serum developed by immunizing the horse with cultures of the meningococcus. Serum now has been supplanted almost completely by the sulfonamide drugs. Oral administration is satisfactory, although a more prompt effect is obtained by giving a soluble preparation intravenously for the first dose. Sulfadiazine is the preparation usually preferred. It is given in full dosage, which varies in relation to body weight according to the age of the child.

Penicillin also is highly effective and may be used for those who are sensitive to sulfadiazine.

Symptomatic treatment consists chiefly of good nursing care. Spinal puncture may be required occasionally in convalescence for the relief of pressure, should pressure symptoms develop.

Influenza Bacillus Meningitis. Except during times when epidemic meningococcus meningitis is present, influenza bacillus meningitis is the most common form of purulent infection of the meninges in children.

ETIOLOGY. The disease is caused by the *Hemophilus influenzae,* a gram-negative rod which differs markedly in size and shape under various circumstances of cultivation. The same organism causes respiratory infections among children and in particular is responsible for a severe variety of croup.

SYMPTOMS. The early symptoms are similar to those of meningococcus meningitis except that the purpuric rash is absent. In infants the onset is likely to be more insidious, with unexplained fever, vomiting, lassitude or peculiar cry or behavior as the presenting complaints. In older children the disturbance advances rapidly toward stupor or coma with the usual evidences of meningitis.

PROGNOSIS. Before the discovery of antibiotics, the fatality rate from influenza meningitis was nearly 100 per cent. Prompt diagnosis and treatment now permits survival of 80 to 90 per cent of the victims. Delayed or inadequate treatment carries an increasing hazard of neurologic sequelae, even if life is spared. Despite optimal treatment, some of the infants afflicted fail to make a complete recovery.

TREATMENT. Since 1940 a number of substances have been discovered which are capable of curing children with influenza meningitis. Antibacterial rabbit serum, sulfadiazine, streptomycin, chlortetracycline, oxytetracycline, tetracycline and chloramphenicol are included in the list. Because of the propensity of the influenza bacillus to acquire resistance to many of these agents before treatment can be completed, it is now considered prudent to use at least two of the substances simultaneously. Serum is expensive and difficult to obtain. Streptomycin is toxic to the eighth cranial nerve and does not enter the spinal fluid rapidly. Consequently, the preferred method of treatment at the present time is full dosage of sulfadiazine and one of the tetracycline antibiotics in addition. At the beginning of treatment these substances usually have to be given by parenteral routes—intramuscularly or intravenously—because of vomiting or coma. Once improvement begins, they may be given orally. Treatment must be continued until repeated spinal fluid cultures have been shown to be free of influenza bacilli.

Other Types of Meningitis. Any one of several varieties of bacteria may cause a purulent type of meningitis similar to meningococcic meningitis. The more common varieties of organism are the pneumococcus, the streptococcus, the staphylococcus and the organisms which normally inhabit the intestinal tract. Without specific treatment the outcome is uniformly fatal. The bacteria usually enter the meninges by way of the blood stream, except when there is direct extension from an infected mastoid or cranial sinus cavity. The onset is usually sudden, and the symptoms include vomiting, convulsions and stiffness of the neck with eventual stupor and coma.

PNEUMOCOCCIC MENINGITIS. This disorder is seen most frequently in small infants as a complication of pneumonia, otitis media or mastoiditis. Unless it is treated promptly it is rapidly fatal. The symptoms are similar to those of other types of meningitis. Rapid recognition of the disease is usually possible, for the pneumococci are found in large numbers in the spinal fluid and are identified easily by microscopic examination. Treatment consists of heavy dosage with penicillin and sulfadiazine administered by a parenteral route at first and continued until the patient has had sterile spinal fluid for at least a week, since this variety of meningitis is prone to recur if treatment is stopped too soon. The results of treatment depend upon the speed of recognition of the disease. When full treatment is begun within the first few hours of symptoms, recovery may occur in as many as 75 per cent of the children affected.

STREPTOCOCCUS MENINGITIS. During hemolytic streptococcus infections the meninges are invaded in rare instances. The symptoms and the management of this variety of meningitis are almost identical with those of pneumococcus meningitis.

STAPHYLOCOCCUS MENINGITIS. This organism may gain entrance to the spinal fluid from trauma to the skull, from erosion of the sac of a myelomeningocele or in the course of a blood-stream infection with the staphylococcus. The symptoms and the diagnosis of staphylococcus meningitis are similar to those described previously. Treatment is complicated by the fact that the staphylococci present in the environment are not uniformly sensitive to any one antibiotic. It is essential to test each strain, as it is isolated from the patient, for its sensitivity to all the available antibiotics. This procedure takes a day or two to complete in the laboratory. Hence, it is desirable to treat with more than one antibiotic from the start until the best agent can be identified accurately. In general, the newer the antibiotic, the less likely is the staphylococcus to be resistant to it. Penicillin is effective against approximately half of the strains of staphylococcus at the present writing and should be used in conjunction with another substance, such as erythromycin.

INTESTINAL ORGANISMS. In small infants, in chronically debilitated children and in those who have wound infections following neurosurgical procedures, meningitis may occur due to a wide variety of organisms which ordinarily are found in the intestinal tract—colon bacilli, proteus, pseudomonas, salmonella, Streptococcus faecalis, for example. The meningitis so produced tends to be a relatively low-grade chronic process. Treatment depends upon identification of the organism (or organisms, for sometimes mixed infections are found) and laboratory determination of the most appropriate antibiotic, as in the case of staphylococcus meningitis. The difficulty of suspecting and recognizing meningitis in the newborn infant has been discussed in Chapter 7.

Nursing Care of Meningitis. Children with meningitis have all degrees of prostration and illness according to the stage of the disease. In the early stage of purulent meningitis before improvement from therapy has begun, one may have to deal with convulsions, delirium, stupor, cyanosis and urinary retention.

The convulsions of meningitis are managed as previously discussed in this chapter. Cyanosis requires administration of oxygen. When stupor is present, special attention is required for management of the food and fluid intake. Depending on the general condition of the child, the food may be given by gavage or, if vomiting is severe, it may be administered parenterally.

Records should be kept suitable for prompt detection of urinary retention, which may require catheterization. Fecal retention also should be watched for, although it does not have the major importance that urinary retention does.

The child with meningitis may be restless or, if disease is fulminating, his movements are limited, and unless he is moved he lies on one side, his back arched in the position of opisthotonos. Good skin care and frequent turning will lessen the incidence of complicating upper respiratory infection and pressure sores about the ears and over the hips. Tepid-water sponge baths may be necessary to control high temperature and to make the child more comfortable. If fever is present and orally administered fluids are not tolerated, special mouth care is indicated. If the meningitis is tuberculous or of other types that are severe, suction apparatus and stimulants should be on hand for emergency use.

Lumbar punctures are done for diagnostic purposes and to determine the progress of the disease, to give medication intrathecally and to relieve pressure symptoms if they develop. The sterile equipment required consists of lumbar-puncture needles, drape sheet, spinal manometer and 3-way stopcock, hypodermic syringe, needles and procaine, cotton balls, dressing, gloves, medicine glass and medication as desired by the attending physician. Test tubes for spinal-fluid samples should be available. After the procedure the equipment contaminated with spinal fluid should be washed in soap and water, soaked in an antiseptic solution and boiled. When antimeningococcus serum is given, adrenalin should be on hand in the event of anaphylactic shock.

The technic for spinal puncture in the child differs in no essential way from that in the adult. However, the adult usually can be persuaded to lie quietly, while more often than not this is impossible with children. It is desirable that as much co-operation as possible be obtained from the child, and the situation should be discussed with him to that end if he is old enough to understand and if his consciousness is not clouded by his infection. Even with co-operation, holding usually is desirable to avoid the trauma which might be produced by unexpected and involuntary movement. The manner of holding the child is important; in fact, the success of the puncture depends about as much on the holding as on the skill of the operator. The child usually is in a recumbent position on the right side, the thighs and the legs flexed and the back arched in a curve with the convexity posteriorly. Restraint in a good position is accomplished most effectively when the holder places his right arm about the thighs and his left arm about the neck, bringing the hands together in a locked position at the front of the child (Fig. 56). The struggle can be minimized still further, if necessary, by leaning forward, thus placing some weight on the body of the

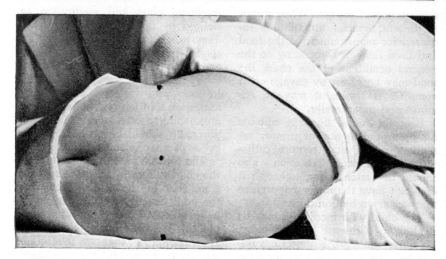

Fig. 56. Illustrating spinal puncture. This shows a method of holding the child and the puncture site.

child. For obtaining cerebrospinal fluid the puncture usually is made between the third and the fourth or between the fourth and the fifth lumbar vertebrae. The appropriate site of puncture may be located by drawing a line across the back at the level of the crests of the ilium. The vertebral space nearest this line is chosen.

At times, as when the spinal canal is blocked, it becomes desirable to make the puncture at the top of the spine. This procedure is designated "cisternal puncture." The space containing the cerebrospinal fluid (the cistern) is entered by inserting the needle immediately below the edge of the skull, with the needle pointing toward a line between the two ear canals.

Sometimes spinal or perhaps cisternal puncture is done for diagnostic purposes when the child is not sick, as in the case of latent syphilis, for example. If such children are permitted to remain ambulatory, often headache and perhaps vomiting occur. Reactions of this type are avoided by keeping the child recumbent for a period of from 8 to 12 hours.

During convalescence, return of function of the extremities should be observed and when it occurs it should be recorded. During this period, too, behavior that might indicate complicating brain abnormality, deafness or symptoms in the infant of developing hydrocephalus should be noted.

ENCEPHALITIS

Encephalitis is a diffuse inflammation of the brain. In some instances the spinal cord is affected also, and the disease is then called encephalomyelitis. There are many inconsistencies in the current use of these terms, for at some times they are applied to diseases that have well-recognized bacterial or viral etiology; at other times they describe conditions in which a known or a presumed toxin is at fault; in still other instances the term is not used in spite of the fact that the disease has all the typical features of encephalitis. From this confusion of terms it is possible to separate out one group of disorders which is due to specific virus infection of the brain and is transmitted in epidemic form by mosquitoes or mites, a second group which represents a complication of some of the contagious diseases and of vaccination procedures, and a third group which results from the influence of known and unknown soluble toxins upon the brain tissue. In a separate listing, the encephalitides which masquerade under some other name will be enumerated.

Virus Encephalitis Transmitted by Insects and Mites. Epidemiology. Since 1930 a number of specific viruses have been shown to cause epidemics of encephalitis in the United States and other parts of the world. Viruses isolated from specific geographic areas can be separated from one another in the laboratory, although the diseases they produce are clinically very similar. Each has acquired the name of the general area and circumstances under which it was first discovered—St. Louis, western (U. S.) equine, eastern (U. S.) equine, Japanese B, Russian spring-summer. The term "equine" indicates that this form of encephalitis exists primarily in horses rather than in man. Now it is known that each of these forms is transmitted from animal to man by a particular variety of mosquito or mite. In some instances the epidemics are restricted to certain times of the year (usually summer) because of the life cycle of the insect required for the spread of the infection.

Symptoms. The onset of the disease is generally abrupt, with fever, vomiting, stiff neck, convulsions, delirium and coma present in varying degree. In some instances there may be a preceding period of illness that simulates influenza. In many respects the symptoms imitate meningitis, and the distinction must be made from examination of the spinal fluid, which contains relatively few cells, usually lymphocytes instead of polymorphonuclear leukocytes, and is sterile on bacterial culture. The fatality rate and the incidence of enduring neurologic disturbances is higher among infants than in older children or adults. Exact figures depend upon the variety of agent responsible for the encephalitis.

Diagnosis. Usually this is made from the clinical picture and the examination of the spinal fluid. At a later stage in the illness, specific virus antibodies appear in the blood which can be used for laboratory confirmation of the type of illness.

Treatment. No specific treatment is known. General good nursing care, control of convulsions and support of nutrition are indicated until the disease subsides spontaneously.

Encephalitis Following Contagious Disease or Prophylactic Injections. During the course of some of the contagious diseases, symptoms of irritation of the brain may appear at a time when convalescence otherwise might be expected. Such symptoms may be mild—delirium, headache, stiff neck, increase in fever—

or more serious events such as convulsions, coma, or paralysis of the eye muscles, the extremities or the bladder. Measles is the contagious disease which is complicated most often by encephalitis. Fortunately, complete recovery takes place in more than 80 per cent of the children thus affected. Occasionally, a similar complication is seen following chickenpox, rubella, smallpox and the process of vaccination against smallpox. During the course of pertussis an unusually severe form of encephalitis may result in infants which leads to prolonged convulsions, stupor or generalized rigidity and usually results in severe mental retardation.

After prophylactic injections against rabies there is a significant incidence of paralysis, usually involving the lower extremities and the bladder. Symptoms commonly begin about 3 weeks after the injections are given and often start with peculiar sensations in the feet, later progressing to paralysis of the legs. Between 10 and 20 per cent of such individuals succumb. The survivors usually make a fairly complete recovery. This unfortunate complication must be recognized in considering whether or not to give rabies prophylaxis to a child who has been bitten by an animal.

In a very few instances severe encephalitis has been described following prophylactic injections against pertussis. The number of such cases is so small that the complication can be disregarded as a significant risk in conducting programs of pertussis vaccination.

Toxic Encephalitis. During the course of acute infectious diseases such as pneumonia, small infants at times may exhibit bizarre and dramatic symptoms of cerebral irritation. These take the form of extreme irritability, diffuse muscular twitching, generalized convulsions or nystagmoid movements of the eyes. The manifestations presumably are due to some toxin produced during the course of the illness. At times recovery is completed as the original infection is brought under control; at other times there may be permanent damage of the brain, with residual mental deficiency. Lead poisoning produces a toxic encephalitis that is characterized by generalized convulsions which are very difficult to control. Treatment is sometimes effective, but too often recovery is followed by persisting neurologic difficulties and mental deficiency.

Tetanus and chorea might be classified as forms of toxic encephalitis.

Other Varieties of Encephalitis. Among the diseases which are really forms of encephalitis but are not so designated are rabies, poliomyelitis and lymphocytic choriomeningitis, a disease which is rare. Mumps often is complicated by encephalitic symptoms; infectious mononucleosis and herpes sometimes are followed by signs of cerebral inflammation.

Encephalitis lethargica (von Economo's encephalitis) is a disorder of considerable historical interest. It appeared in epidemic form during World War I, producing acute symptoms somewhat like those described above for the specific virus encephalitides. In addition, it adopted a chronic form which appeared over a space of years and resulted in a wide variety of peculiar disabilities, of which parkinsonism is one and oculogyric crises is another.

In recent years the acute stage of this disease seldom is recognized, but some of the more chronic manifestations are still apparent. No specific virus infection has been demonstrated as a cause, although such an etiology has been suspected for a long time. Many instances of mental retardation and peculiarities of behavior are ascribed to chronic encephalitis. The retrospective diagnosis of this condition is often difficult and tenuous.

HEREDITARY DEGENERATIVE DISORDERS OF THE NERVOUS AND THE MUSCULAR SYSTEMS

A large number of disorders are recognized among children as hereditarily transmitted processes which, during infancy or childhood, lead to progressive loss of muscular or neurologic function. Fortunately, these disturbances are relatively rare. Unfortunately, their accurate identification is difficult and even may require study by a specialist in child neurology. The nurse cannot be expected to remember the exotic names and complex pathologic processes with which these disorders are endowed, nor can they be treated with any completeness in a brief text. A few representative types of disorder will be described briefly. More detailed information must be sought through the use of standard pediatric or neurology texts. Most of these degenerative disorders lead inexorably to death or important permanent handicap. Only a few can be alleviated by any useful form of treatment. Some terminate life during early infancy; others appear during early or even late childhood and produce disability which is carried into a fairly long adult lifetime.

AMAUROTIC FAMILIAL IDIOCY (TAY-SACHS)

This disorder affects infants, frequently of Jewish families, and leads to arrested and then regressing mental development around the age of 6 months. Characteristic changes are visible in the fundus of the eye. The degenerative changes progress so rapidly that life seldom is spared for more than a year after the diagnosis is made. In amaurotic familial idiocy, lipid degeneration is confined mainly to the central nervous system.

Niemann-Pick Disease. This is closely related but attended by additional widespread deposition of lipid substances in organs such as the spleen, the liver, the lungs and the lymph nodes.

Gaucher's Disease. This is an allied but less frequently fatal disease in which the nervous system usually is spared, and a long and fairly normal life is possible.

GARGOYLISM (HUNTER'S SYNDROME, LIPOCHONDRODYSTROPHY)

In this hereditary disorder there are widespread changes in the body due to abnormal lipid deposits in the brain, the spleen, the liver, the bone marrow and the cornea of the eyes. It is recognized easily by the gradual appearance of facial features and body characteristics which are almost identical in all affected children. The appearance is much like that of the Duchess in the popular illustrations of *Alice in Wonderland*. Mental retardation is usually definite but moderate, and the disease often permits the child to survive for a number of years.

OTHER FORMS OF CEREBRAL
DEGENERATIVE DISEASE

Schilder's Disease. Among infants a rapidly fatal disturbance known as Schilder's disease is seen occasionally. Generally it is marked by frequent and severe convulsions, loss of vision or hearing and retardation which progresses within a few months to coma and complete helplessness. No treatment is known.

Wilson's Disease. Among older children the degenerations include Wilson's disease, which combines cirrhosis of the liver with progressively increasing tremor and muscular rigidity.

Dystonia Musculorum Deformans

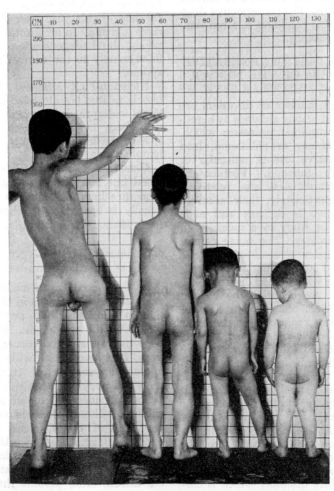

FIG. 57. Pseudohypertrophic muscular dystrophy in four brothers.

(Torsion Spasm). This peculiar twisting spasm of muscles usually begins in one leg and progresses to the point where the child is bedfast.

Friedreich's Ataxia. In this disease there is unsteadiness of gait and tremor of the extremities, which advances very slowly, and, during childhood at least, may not interfere seriously with activities.

These are only a few of many bizarre and fortunately rare disorders that are encountered.

AMYOTONIA CONGENITA

Two forms of this disorder are recognized; both may be observed

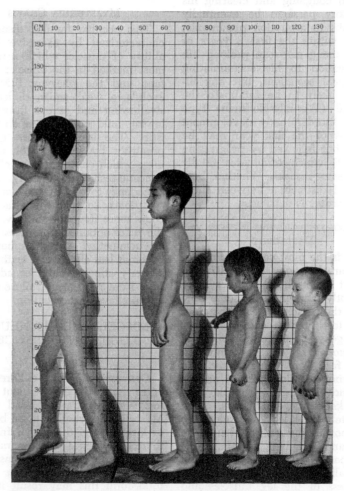

FIG. 58. Pseudohypertrophic muscular dystrophy in four brothers.

in the same family. The outstanding feature is generalized weakness of muscles without loss of intelligence. In the congenital form (Oppenheim), weakness is present from birth and prevents the child from learning to hold up his head, to sit or to make any forceful voluntary movements. Because of his difficulty in coughing and clearing his respiratory passages he eventually succumbs to aspiration pneumonia, usually within the first 2 years of life. Nursing care can prolong life by attention to his accumulating pharyngeal secretions, but any illness is likely to be fatal. In the acquired (Werdnig-Hoffman) type of the disorder, early development for most of the first year may be normal but followed by progressing weakness which terminates fatally for the same reasons. Whether there is a real distinction between these two disorders is debated.

Pseudohypertrophic Muscular Dystrophy

This is the most common form of muscular dystrophy (Figs. 57 and 58). It affects boys 8 times more frequently than girls. At some time during the preschool years the child begins to show weakness in his legs which generally is accompanied by enlargement of the calf muscles, which feel firm and rubbery. To arise from a sitting posture on the floor such children learn that they must kneel on all fours, then straighten their legs and gain the erect posture by putting hands on knees and "climbing up the legs." This performance is typical and practically diagnostic of the disease. Weakness of the leg muscles and later of the arm and the shoulder

muscles progresses gradually, and the victim usually succumbs by early adult life to some intercurrent disease. Periods of bed rest are to be avoided whenever possible, for muscle strength tends to deteriorate more rapidly unless activity is maintained. At present no useful treatment has been discovered.

Myasthenia Gravis

This peculiar familial disorder is characterized by excessive fatiguability of muscle, which usually is most marked in the muscles of the face and the pharynx. Drooping eyelids, a weak smile, difficulty in swallowing and severe fatigue following mild exercise are characteristic. The symptoms are relieved promptly by injection of neostigmine which constitutes the chief diagnostic test. Unfortunately, there is a tendency toward progression of the symptoms, so that the attacks become more frequent and severe and the relief obtained from neostigmine or octamethyl pyrophosphoramide becomes less effective. Death in the severely affected child or adult results from respiratory failure during an unrelieved exacerbation.

MISCELLANEOUS NEUROLOGIC DISTURBANCES

Trauma

Concussion. Few children traverse the early years without suffering some variety of head injury. Most of these result only in bruising or laceration of the scalp. In a few there is evidence of temporary disturbance of cerebral functions which is referred to as concussion. In its mild form this may result in temporary dizziness, headache, vomiting or brief loss of consciousness. Sometimes there may be disturbances of vision or of motion of the eyes. Children usually recover rapidly from simple concussion and within a period of a day or two are restored to normal. The important point in management of concussion is to make sure during the early hours after the injury that no intracranial bleeding has resulted from the trauma.

The first 2 to 6 hours after injury is the critical period in which careful observation is required. During this time impending coma must be watched for. The parent or the nurse should test the child's state of consciousness by arousing him periodically. In the hospital, accurate observation of pulse, respirations and blood pressure is desirable. Drastic change in these measurements or inability to arouse the child demand prompt investigation. If signs of bleeding are confirmed, neurosurgical exploration usually is indicated. Even though it be attended by a period of unconsciousness, only a very small fraction of children who suffer head injury will have bleeding, but this small fraction presents a dire emergency.

Skull Fracture. The management of skull fracture is primarily a neurosurgical problem. In many instances there is a linear crack in the skull which causes no displacement of the bones and is not associated with bleeding. Management in such instances is the same as for concussion. More serious disturbances result when the break in the bones occasions tearing of blood vessels or distortion of the brain by compression. Some form of operative relief usually is indicated in such instances. Recognition of depression of a skull fracture depends upon roentgen examination or upon the presence of localizing neurologic findings which indicate abnormal pressure upon specific areas of the brain. With severe injuries the problem of managing shock and intracranial pressure is often of primary importance.

SUBDURAL HEMATOMA

Etiology. The brain is covered by a delicate filmy membrane which encloses the surrounding layer of cerebrospinal fluid. This membrane is known as the pia-arachnoid. Bleeding into the space which it encloses is called subarachnoid hemorrhage, and the blood usually is found circulating freely in the spinal fluid. Between the arachnoid and the tough membrane (dura mater) which lines the inner surface of the skull, there is a potential space (subdural space) which is normally empty because the arachnoid is in close apposition to the dura. Under certain conditions such as trauma or some form of hemorrhagic disorder, bleeding from small vessels may occur into the subdural space. The extent of the bleeding is limited by the pressures required to push away the brain in order to make room for the clot. Once formed, the clot usually liquefies. Its high protein-content tends to draw more fluid into the space within the membrane which surrounds the clot. Thus, a slowly enlarging space-occupying mass exists within the rigid confines of the skull and creates an increase in the intracranial pressure. Subdural hematoma in older children is almost always the result of trauma. In infants it often is found in the absence of any obvious trauma other than the more or less normal events of birth and early infancy. It is more likely to be found in poorly nourished infants or those with bleeding tendencies. However, this is not exclusively the case, for it also is seen in otherwise healthy infants.

Symptoms. The bleeding usually takes place rather slowly, so that the symptoms appear insidiously. Abnormal enlargement of the head, slow developmental progress, irritability, convulsions, vomiting and poor weight gain may be present. In many of the infants, hemorrhages are seen in the eye-grounds and some degree of swelling of the optic nerve head betrays the presence of an increase in intracranial pressure. Occasionally, the bleeding takes place rapidly, and the child passes into a state of shock, coma or uncontrolled convulsions.

Diagnosis. Diagnosis is suspected from the enlargement of the head and from the symptomatology. The finding of hemorrhages in the eye-grounds of an infant is almost certain to mean the presence of a subdural hematoma. Confirmation of the clinical suspicion is obtained by inserting a needle through the dura of the skull and withdrawing yellow, chocolate or bloody fluid from the liquefied clot. In infants with open suture lines, such taps are performed easily between the margins of two separated cranial bones. In older children, exploratory burr holes must be made by the neurosurgeon.

Treatment and Nursing Care. Subdural hematoma is primarily a neurosurgical problem. In older children a craniotomy has to be done, and the clot and its surrounding

membrane must be removed. In infants often the same procedure is indicated, but in some instances repeated aspirations through the dura will effect a cure without the need for a craniotomy. Postoperative nursing care is similar to that which is employed after brain-tumor operations. It should be emphasized that early recognition and prompt treatment of this disorder are necessary to permit normal growth of the brain during infancy. Where the diagnosis is overlooked and treatment is delayed too long, permanent damage to the brain and irreversible mental deficiency result.

INFECTIOUS POLYNEURITIS

Infectious polyneuritis is a disorder characterized by generalized, often extensive weakness and pain in various muscle groups. It is ordinarily a self-limited disease which progresses for a period of 2 to 4 weeks and then abates. During this interval there may be considerable atrophy of the involved muscles. The chief importance of this disorder is its confusion with poliomyelitis. Distinction between the two diseases is made from the presence of sensory changes in infectious polyneuritis and from the appearance of the spinal fluid, which usually contains a marked increase in protein but little or no increase in cells. Nursing care of polyneuritis is similar to that for poliomyelitis.

TIC (HABIT SPASM)

A habit spasm or tic is a simple or complex muscular movement which is repeated over and over in the same manner. Tics differ from choreal movements in that the latter are without order or purpose and never are repeated twice in the same order of progression. Tics most frequently involve the face, but often also the neck, the shoulders or some other part of the body. They may take the form of blinking of the eyes, a facial grimace, shrugging of the shoulders or other movements, or a combination of some of these. Tics begin as voluntary movements and are repeated until they become habitual and involuntary. Even in the habitual and involuntary stage, the movements can be repeated voluntarily on request. The movements may have had their origin in imitation of another or they may have started as the result of some local irritation or discomfort; they continue long after the exciting cause has disappeared. A tic may leave one part of the body and appear in another. As in chorea, the movements are increased by excitement and cease during sleep. Drugs and disciplinary measures are ineffectual in the treatment of tics. The parents should be urged to ignore the symptom as much as possible and to expend their efforts toward relieving general factors in the child's life which may be contributing to his feelings of insecurity or unhappiness. If changes in environmental circumstances do not bring cessation of the tic, it probably indicates the need for psychiatric therapy. It is particularly important to differentiate the movements from those of rheumatic chorea, since the treatment of the latter disorder is quite different.

SPASMUS NUTANS (NODDING SPASM)

This queer affliction is confined to infants and runs a self-limited course of a few months. Its cause is unknown, and it is seen with decreasing frequency in recent years. The manifestations consist of a peculiar shaking of the head from side to side or up and down, together with nystagmoid movements of the eyes and a tendency to cock the head on one side when looking at objects. No treatment is known or necessary.

SITUATIONS FOR FURTHER STUDY

1. If an infant was born at home with spina bifida and you were in attendance, how could you help the mother to meet the disappointment of giving birth to an infant with a congenital anomaly? What information could you give her concerning the infant's prognosis? After receiving the doctor's orders as to specific care of the spina bifida tumor mass, what guidance would be required to ensure adequate care before hospitalization for operation?

2. During hospitalization, after a child's mental capacity was established as inferior, if the parents were unable to accept the diagnosis, what problems could you anticipate would result for the child? How would the failure of the parents to accept the fact of his limitations affect the relationship between the child and his siblings?

3. Study a child with seizures. How has he accepted his handicap? How could you help him to adjust to it? Does he seem to be emotionally stable or unstable? What were his adjustment problems in the hospital? Does he say anything that might indicate the attitude of his peers toward him? Does he talk of his convulsions? What does he say? Or does he try to hide the fact that he

has them when he is with a group of children? Does he in any way indicate his relationship to his parents, brothers and sisters? What reaction do you have to the parents' attitude toward this child? Are there ways in which you could help them to accept the child's handicap and develop his individual capacities? Visit the child's school and talk to his teacher to determine his progress in school and the teacher's attitude toward him. If the child shows problems of adjustment, what community resources are available for his help? How would you interpret the function of the agency to the child? How would you interpret it to his parents to help them understand the need of seeking its aid?

4. Write to the National Epilepsy League, Room 715, 130 N. Wells, Chicago 6, Ill., and obtain literature concerning the needs of the child with seizures. Use it in observing and working with the child you are studying.

5. Write to the National Society for Crippled Children, Inc., 11 S. LaSalle Street, Chicago 3, Ill., for pamphlet material pertaining to the mental hygiene needs of the child with cerebral palsy. Use the literature in studying a nursery or a public school for crippled children.

6. Visit a nursery school for children with cerebral palsy and write a report which answers the following questions: In what ways were the children like normal children? Describe ways in which the teachers helped the children to be more independent, to express themselves creatively and to communicate verbally with them and with other children? How had they adapted equipment to meet the needs of the

children? What was the teacher's philosophy in working with the children? What emotional attitudes did the teacher have which helped the children to succeed in gaining increased self-mastery?

7. Study a child of school age with spastic paralysis. What limitations are imposed because of his handicap? What is he capable of doing? Compare his capacities with those of a normal child of the same age. In what ways could you teach him to become more independent? Does the child seem to be normal mentally? If intelligence tests have been given, study the results to increase your insight into his potentialities. What characteristics does he have that would make intelligence testing difficult? What are your observations when the hospital schoolteacher is with him? What help could she give you in understanding him and in gaining insight into ways in which you could be of greater help to him? How has he accepted his handicap? Does his crippling condition affect the parent-child relationship? What is his reaction to other children and what is their reaction to him? How could you help him in increasing association with other children? How could you direct the play activities of the group so that his powers could be utilized in group play? What are his interests? Can he express them? What play materials could you present that he could use to express himself in such a way that some of his basic needs might be satisfied? How does he respond to attention and recognition? How does he seek them? If you were supervising this child's care in the home, what would be your objectives and how

would you approach the problem of attaining them? What are the community resources available for his care?

8. What early symptoms might be indicative of the presence of a brain tumor in a preschool child?

BIBLIOGRAPHY

Abel, Marjorie: Feeding the child with cerebral palsy, Am. J. Nursing **50**:558, 1950.

Bridge, E. M.: Epilepsy and Convulsive Disorders in Children, New York, McGraw-Hill, 1949.

Carlson, E. R.: Born That Way, New York, Day, 1941.

Carter, J. D.: Children's expressed attitudes toward their epilepsy, Nerv. Child **6**:11, 1947.

Cruickshank, W. M.: The mental hygiene approach to the handicapped child, Am. J. Occup. Therapy **1**:215, 1947.

Ford, F. R.: Diseases of the Nervous System in Infancy, Childhood and Adolescence, ed. 3, Springfield, Ill., Thomas, 1952.

Glick, Selma, and Donnell, Catherine: Nonmedical problems of the child with cerebral palsy, Nursing Outlook **1**:101, 1953.

Gratke, Juliette: Help them help themselves (pamphlet), Texas Soc. for Crippled Children, 3703 Worth St., Dallas, Texas, 1947.

Grulee, C. G., and Eley, R. C.: The Child in Health and Disease, ed. 2, Baltimore, Williams & Wilkins, 1952.

Holt, L. E., Jr., and McIntosh, R.: Pediatrics, ed. 12, p. 1019, New York, Appleton, 1953.

Ingraham, F. D.: Spina Bifida and Cranium Bifidum, Cambridge, Mass., Harvard, 1943.

Jones, M. H.: The cerebral palsy child, Am. J. Nursing **46**:465, 1946.

Kerr, Marion: Nursing responsibilities in cerebral palsy, Am. J. Nursing **46**:469, 1946.

Lewis, R. S., Straus, A. A., and Lehtinen, L. E.: The Other Child, New York, Grune, 1951.

Nelson, W. E.: Textbook of Pediatrics, ed. 5, p. 1291, Philadelphia, Saunders, 1950.

Perlstein, M. A., and Barnett, H. E.: Nature and recognition of cerebral palsy in infancy, J.A.M.A. **148**:1389, 1952.

Roseman, Ephraim, and Taylor, Anne: Progress in the treatment of epilepsy, Am. J. Nursing **52**:437, 1952.

Ryan, Elizabeth K.: Nursing care of the patient with spina bifida, Am. J. Nursing **51**:28, 1951.

Shriner, Mildred: Foundations for walking (pamphlet), National Society for Crippled Children and Adults, Inc., 11 S. LaSalle St., Chicago, Ill.

Stewart, Mary: The child with cerebral palsy and the nurse, Am. J. Nursing **52**:1228, 1952.

Westlund, Norman, and Polumbo, Adelaide: Parental rejection of crippled children, Am. J. Orthopsychiat. **16**:271, 1946.

Diseases of the Skin

◇◇◇

CONGENITAL AND HEREDITARY DISORDERS OF THE SKIN

Disorders of the skin that have a congenital or hereditary basis are numerous and diverse in characteristics. In Chapter 7 some of the more common aberrations seen in the newborn infant are described, and the significance to the child is indicated. Individual variations in the pigmentation, the texture, the reactivity to stimuli and the degree of oiliness of the skin are so great as to defy comprehensive description. The more serious congenital disturbances are too rare to warrant inclusion in a short text, and the reader should consult one of the treatises on dermatology for a full description and illustrations.

INFECTIONS OF THE SKIN

BACTERIAL INFECTION

Impetigo Contagiosa. Impetigo contagiosa is a skin disease caused by an infection that invades the superficial layers of the skin. The infection tends to spread from one area to another on the affected person. It is transferred easily to other persons by direct or indirect contact. Both streptococci and staphylococci are causative agents. The individual lesion varies in size from 3 mm. to 3 cm. or more. It appears first as a vesicle located superficially in the skin, with a loose and often wrinkled, rather than a tense and distended, top. Soon purulent material can be seen through the skin covering. The skin immediately surrounding the lesions shows no change from the normal. The pustule ruptures easily, and the exudate over the lesion tends to dry and form a crust. The crust eventually falls off, leaving an area slightly reddened. Soon all trace of the presence of the lesion disappears. The individual lesion runs its course in a week or two, but the disease has no uniform duration. Because of continued auto-inoculation, it may persist for many weeks.

The number of lesions on the body varies greatly, the total number depending on the amount of reinoculation from earlier lesions. Exposed parts (hands and face) are chiefly affected, but the lesions may be in any location, especially in babies. No symptoms of consequence are associated with the disease, and rarely are complications or sequelae encountered. In a few cases of severe impetigo, acute hemorrhagic nephritis has occurred as a complication. When the infection occurs in the newborn, the lesions usually are large blisters, and often the condition is designated as pemphigus neonatorum.

The treatment consists of removal of the crusts and the tops of bullous lesions and the application of some germicide. The crusts may be removed by washing gently with warm boric-acid solution. Perhaps the germicide most extensively used is an ointment containing 3 per cent ammoniated mercury. The ointment should be applied at least twice daily to those areas where it cannot be protected by dressings from being rubbed off. Often other types of germicide are preferred, such as a 3 per cent aqueous solution of gentian violet or silver nitrate in concentrations up to 5 per cent. These solutions are painted on and not used as wet dressings. Antibiotic ointments are usually quite effective. Preparations containing bacitracin, polymyxin, chlortetracycline, erythromycin and neomycin are employed commonly. Ointments containing sulfonamides and penicillin are generally less effective and are more likely to result in sensitization of the child. When local therapy is not effective within a few days, it may be necessary to give an appropriate antibiotic systemically. If the im-

petigo is superimposed upon scabies or pediculosis, the underlying condition also should be treated.

Furunculosis is a condition in which multiple small abscesses or boils are present in the skin. While a furuncle may occur at any age, multiple lesions, constituting furunculosis, occur chiefly in infants and especially in infants who are malnourished. The furuncles are caused by pyogenic bacteria, chiefly staphylococci, which gain entrance to the skin by way of the hair follicles. They are most common about the head but may occur in any location and may be generalized.

Symptoms of furunculosis in a baby are few or lacking. Little or no fever is present in most instances. No doubt, furunculosis produces some constitutional effects, but such effects are vague and usually undetectable.

In the management of the skin disease, meticulous cleanliness is important. The hair should be shaved around any lesions on the scalp, and that area should be cleansed with green-soap solution several times daily. Incision is indicated only after the furuncle has pointed. In some instances, it may be desirable to hasten maturation of the lesions by the use of hot compresses. Draining furuncles should be covered in order to avoid spread of the infection. The dressing should be changed frequently enough to keep the drainage from the surrounding area. Elbow restraints may be necessary to prevent the infant from removing the dressing and transplanting the infection to other areas of the skin. Application of an antibiotic ointment may assist in destroying the infecting organisms as they emerge in the contents of the boil. Systemic treatment is often desirable. The selection of the antibiotic to be used can be made best by isolation of the infecting organism from the pus expressed from within the furuncle and determination of the sensitivities of the particular agent recovered. Staphylococci in particular have become resistant to many of the commonly used antibiotics.

FUNGUS INFECTIONS (RINGWORM OR TINEA)

Superficial fungus infections of the skin commonly are called ringworm and technically are known as tinea. The varieties of tinea are designated by the part of the body or the shape of the resulting lesion. Thus, ringworm of the scalp is tinea tonsurans or capitis; of the body, tinea circinata; of the nails, tinea unguium or onychomycosis; of the inguinal region, tinea cruris; of the feet, tinea pedis or dermatophytosis or athlete's foot. A number of fungi, some of which are obtained from young domestic animals, may be involved. Accurate identification of the fungus requires special laboratory facilities but is sometimes essential to direct adequate treatment.

Ringworm of the Scalp. This infection may have its start at the site of a single hair, but the lesion increases in extent up to an inch or two in diameter. The patches are roughly circular. The base of the hair is invaded by the spores of the fungus. The hair becomes brittle and breaks off close to the skin, leaving the area apparently bald. The skin of the area is scaly and shows no other evidence of inflammation except that secondary infec-tion may occur with the formation of pustules in the hair follicles. Mycelia of the fungus are found in the scales.

The treatment is unsatisfactory in that response to it is slow. The lesions should be washed thoroughly every day, and local application should be made. The application may be tincture of iodine, a sulfur ointment or some other fungicide, according to preference. Complete removal of the hair of the area hastens recovery. The hair may be removed with forceps or by x-ray irradiation. The latter must be used with caution in order to avoid permanent baldness. In pustular ringworm, the hairs pull easily, and removal by forceps is a satisfactory method of treatment.

If the ringworm has been acquired from animal pets or farm animals, as is common in rural areas, the lesion is more likely to be inflammatory and pustular. In such cases there is an elevated, intensely red, pus-exuding inflammation with much crusting. The application of strong fungicides, iodine or sulfur preparations to this variety of scalp ringworm is contraindicated. Application of bland wet dressings, such as potassium permanganate or boric acid, is preferable. Unlike the less inflammatory form of the disease, this type tends to be self-limited. Too vigorous treatment is more likely to result in sensitivity reactions, scarring and permanent baldness.

Ringworm of the Body. This differs unimportantly from ringworm of the scalp, except that hair is not affected so obviously. The lesion occurs also on the face. In any location the lesion extends by enlargement at the edges: the newer part is pinkish and slightly elevated; the older part at the center is paler or pigmented and moderately scaly. Thus the lesion may be suggestive of a ring. Itching may be present, but little inflammation is apparent except where the origin was animal, and then there may be much inflammation. The responsible fungus is found in the scales. A customary treatment consists of the application of Whitfield's ointment, which relieves the itching promptly. However, the cure of the lesion requires a long period of applications of some fungicidal substance, such as tincture of iodine or an ointment containing undecylinic acid (Desenex).

Ringworm of the Feet. This infection is located most often between the toes. The moisture of these regions prevents the usual scale formation; instead, the macerated superficial epithelium tends to desquamate, leaving a raw surface with fissures and often with vesicles. The itching is likely to be intense. Like all ringworm, the disease is contagious. It is acquired in gymnasiums, at swimming pools and other similar places where people go barefooted. For the purpose of avoiding this infection, it is desirable to wear foot covering when walking where others walk barefooted. Also, it is important to keep infected persons away from places where people are likely to walk barefooted.

Treatment for the ordinary type, such as occurs between the toes or on the soles of the feet, consists of application of an ointment such as Desenex. Other and often more vigorous methods of treatment are advocated by various physicians. The more vigorous methods are much more likely to cause treatment dermatitis. In addition to treatment of the skin, the foot coverings previously worn should be sterilized or discarded. Thin, ventilated shoes help to avoid the sweating that aggravates the condition.

VIRUS INFECTIONS

Warts. Warts or verrucae are overgrowths of the superficial layers of the skin which are thought to be due to infection with a rather indolent virus. They may occur on any portion of the body and are usually of no great importance except for the cosmetic appearance. When they are present on the feet or at points of pressure they may become tender and uncomfortable.

Most warts eventually will disappear spontaneously but they frequently endure for many months or years. On occasion, suggestion or the application of superstitious remedies* seems to be effective in causing their disappearance. When they are painful they generally are destroyed by chemicals or an electrocautery or by x-ray treatment. Unfortunately, they tend to recur after treatment and may leave scars. Unless the indications for removal are important, it is best to leave warts alone.

Herpes Simplex. The common fever blisters or cold sores are due to infection of the outermost layers of the skin with a specific virus. Small, thin-walled blisters usually appear first but rupture very quickly. The common site is in the skin about the

---

* Tom Sawyer had an infallible incantation which would work if the victim swung a dead cat about his head three times in a graveyard at midnight on a moonless night.

mouth and the nose, but occasionally herpetic lesions may occur elsewhere. In rare instances they may be generalized over the whole body. Herpes infection often remains dormant in individuals during health and then flares up when acute illness, fatigue, menstruation or some other event temporarily depresses the general resistance. When normal vigor returns the lesions clear, but the virus infection probably persists in inapparent form. Treatment consists in the application of soothing ointments.

Herpes Zoster. This disorder, commonly known as shingles, consists of a group of itching or painful blisters that are confined to the distribution of one of the sensory nerves emanating from the posterior root ganglia of the spinal cord. It is recognized by its sharp limitation to one side of the body within a skin area corresponding to a dermatome. It is now thought that herpes zoster is caused by the same virus as chickenpox and that it often represents a second attack of chickenpox in a person who had his first attack years ago. The disease is not very common in children.

INFESTATIONS AND BITES

Pediculosis. Three varieties of lice are found inhabiting the hair or the clothing of children.

PEDICULOSIS CAPITAS. The most common form is pediculosis capitis, in which the lice dwell in the hair of the scalp and lay their eggs or nits on the shafts of the hairs. The lice themselves are often difficult to see, but the nits are small, fixed, ovoid, white bodies which can be seen with the naked eye. Scalp lice cause itching which eventually may lead to infection of the scalp by pyogenic bacteria at sites of trauma from constant scratching.

PEDICULOSIS CORPORIS. Body lice (pediculosis corporis) actually live in the clothes but irritate by their excursions onto the skin surfaces for the purpose of biting and feeding.

PEDICULOSIS PUBIS. Pubic or crab lice (pediculosis pubis) dwell in the pubic hair of older people but may invade the eyelashes or the eyebrows of younger children. The nits are seen easily; the lice themselves are found less commonly.

Modern treatment of louse infestation is relatively simple and quite effective. Clothes can be laundered or dusted with 5 per cent DDT in talc, which kills both lice and nits. Various preparations for use in the hair are available. Topocide contains DDT and benzylbenzoate as its main constituents; Kwell and Eurax contain other types of synthetic pesticide. Usually, 2 applications about 12 hours apart are sufficient to eradicate the lice and the nits.

Scabies is a contagious skin disease caused by *Acarus scabiei (Sarcoptes scabiei)* or itch mite. The human disease is caused exclusively by the female acarus, which burrows into the skin for the purpose of depositing eggs. The parts of the body involved are chiefly those in which the skin is thin and moist. In the older person, one may expect to find the lesions most abundant between the fingers, on the underside of the wrists, in the axillae and about the genitalia. In the infant, they may be almost anywhere. The most characteristic lesion in infants is the infected burrow on the palm, present as a small pustule with the black wavy line of the burrow on the surface. The primary lesions are the burrows produced by the travels of the acarus. These usually are less than one half inch in length. With a hand lens they are seen as dark or black lines, the color being produced by fecal deposits of the parasite. Typical burrows may be difficult to find because of secondary inflammation. Scabies causes severe itching. The reaction of the parasite, together with infection produced by scratching, causes inflammatory changes which may take the form of papules, vesicles or pustules.

The treatment of scabies is similar to that for pediculosis as noted above. Occasionally, the modern agents are not available, and the old-fashioned sulfur ointment (5 per cent) may be used. It is important to discover all of the infested members in a family so that they may be treated simultaneously in order to kill all the mites within the household and prevent return of the disturbance.

Ticks (and mites) are small arthropods which have biting and sucking parts and attach themselves to man or animals for the purpose of sucking the blood. After satiating themselves they let go and drop off. In the process of feeding they may transmit virus or rickettsial infection to a child or may cause paralysis or fever by the injection of toxic substances. These latter events depend upon the presence of poisons or infections within the particular tick which is biting. In the United States, most ticks are harmless, and the bite is inconsequential except for the local discomfort. Some of the diseases which may be transmitted by ticks or mites are Rocky Moun-

tain spotted fever, St. Louis encephalitis, typhus fever and rickettsialpox. The rather uncommon circumstance of tick paralysis clears up rapidly when the tick is discovered and removed.

Bites and Stings. Children playing outdoors are often the victims of bites and stings from a number of types of insect. In general, these produce only pain or itching at the site of assault. Occasionally, a sting by a bee or wasp produces a dramatic sudden swelling that is due presumably to hypersensitiveness to the injected material. In rare instances, fatal stings have been observed due to this mechanism. In certain geographic regions mosquitoes may be responsible for the transmission of diseases such as malaria, encephalitis or yellow fever. Fleas, chiggers and bedbugs are common nuisances which ordinarily do not result in disease transmission.

DISORDERS DUE TO PHYSICAL AND CHEMICAL AGENTS

REACTION TO BODY EXCRETIONS

Miliaria (miliaria rubra, "prickly heat") is the result of inflammation about the sweat glands in association with sweating from any cause, whether summer heat, excessive clothing or febrile illness. It is more common in babies than in those older. It is manifest by a bright-red papular rash. Some of the lesions may be topped by a small vesicle; others may become pustular. The rash tends to be most prominent about the neck and the body folds.

Treatment includes management of the hygiene to avoid sweating. Frequent bathing without soap is useful. Some simple dusting powder should be applied to the affected areas. The occasional use of calamine lotion is helpful, especially if itching is present.

Intertrigo is an inflammation of the skin which occurs in body folds where moisture accumulates and two moist surfaces remain in contact. It is more common in the obese and in infants. The infant's skin reacts more easily to irritation than does the skin of the older person. In infants, intertrigo may occur in the axilla, between the upper parts of the thighs, in the folds of the groin and the neck and in any other location where two skin surfaces come together. The affected skin is red and sometimes more or less raw from the loss of the outermost layer of skin. Intertrigo may be both prevented and treated by keeping the skin dry and clean in the body folds. Exposure of the affected areas to permit complete evaporation of moisture is desirable whenever possible. Clothing should be light and porous, and any material such as plastic or rubber diaper coverings which holds in moisture must be avoided until the lesions heal. In some cases the intertrigo becomes infected secondarily by skin bacteria or fungi. Application of mild antiseptics, antibiotics or fungicides may be necessary.

Diaper Rashes. In infancy, irritation or excoriation of the skin beneath the diapers is a common annoyance. In addition to the irritant effect of moisture from sweat and urine, there may be the burning erythema produced by organic acids in the stool or by ammonia which results from bacterial decomposition of the urine.

Diarrheal stools contain large amounts of organic acids which may result in a chemical burn of the skin if allowed to remain in contact with it for any appreciable length of time. The lesions produced have a characteristic distribution which conforms to the area of soiling by the stool. Dermatitis from this cause clears up when the diarrhea is brought under control. Prompt cleansing of the skin, preferably with a bland oil, helps to prevent this form of diaper rash. Mechanical protection against the next stool may be given by smearing a layer of protective ointment over the affected area. A number of proprietary preparations are available for this purpose.

Diaper irritation from urine generally is due to the formation of ammonia by bacterial action on the urea normally present as a constituent of urine. The bacillus responsible is a common inhabitant of the intestinal tract, particularly of the artificially fed infant. Since it readily contaminates the perineum and the buttocks of the infant it has easy access to urine in the wet diaper unless this is replaced rapidly by a dry one. The distribution of ammonia dermatitis corresponds to the spread of urine—mainly over the buttocks in an infant who habitually sleeps on his back, mainly over the anterior abdominal wall in an infant who sleeps face down.

ULCERATION OF THE URINARY MEATUS. This is a common disorder of circumcised male infants which probably depends upon the same general mechanism. It may occur even in the absence of any associated diaper rash. A small ulcer is produced just at or just within the opening of the urinary meatus at the tip of the penis. A small crust forms over this ulcer, which is washed away easily by the stream of urine, producing pain and the appearance of a small drop of blood on the diaper. If the crust remains firmly attached, the urinary stream may be diverted to one side, or occasionally the opening will be blocked temporarily.

Treatment of ammonia dermatitis consists in thorough drying of the affected parts by persistent exposure to the air and by application of bland oils and protective ointments. Prevention may be achieved by measures designed to interfere with the growth of the bacteria which produce ammonia. Diapers may be given a final rinse in boric acid, 1:5,000 mercuric chloride solution or one of the proprietary antiseptics prepared for this purpose. Whichever substance is used, the diaper should be hung up wet so that the antiseptic can remain in the diaper in good concentration.

Seborrheic Dermatitis. In the common form of this disorder, surface lipids, scales, serum and dirt accumulate into yellowish crusts on the scalp in infants which, if neglected, may become thick, irritated or secondarily infected. Periodic removal of the crusts and the scales with a soap and water shampoo or the application of a bland oil is sufficient for mild accumulations. Ointments containing salicylic acid or sulfur are useful in removing heavy scales. The tendency toward seborrheic dermatitis of the scalp usually decreases when the infant reaches a year of age. Occasionally, other parts of the body are affected.

EXOGENOUS IRRITANTS

A very large number of substances are capable of stimulating a sensitivity reaction after repeated contact with the skin. Infants and young children are generally more likely to acquire such sensitization because of their relatively thin skins. In its mild form this contact dermatitis or allergic dermatitis appears as an area of redness with mild itching. In a more severe form it may result in swelling or even blistering. The main problem in treatment is to discover the offending substance and prevent further contact with it. Bleaches and detergent soaps used in laundering clothing or diapers are perhaps the most common sources of trouble today. Occasionally, such items as rubber pants or sheeting, plastic substances, cosmetics, adhesive gum, nail polish, iodine, or dyes from clothing are found to be responsible. Poison ivy or poison oak causes a form of contact dermatitis which results when the individual becomes sensitized to the oil present in the leaves of these plants.

BURNS

General Considerations. Burns are relatively frequent in childhood and when of more than slight extent are serious. The effects are general and not limited to the burned area.

SHOCK. The first serious effect is that of shock, the symptoms of which appear soon after the accident. The usual symptoms of shock include rapid pulse rate, subnormal temperature, pallor, prostration and low blood pressure. If the child survives the shock, the symptoms disappear to a large extent within 12 hours.

TOXIC STATE. The second serious effect is a toxic state which develops within from 1 to 2 days. It is characterized clinically by prostration, fever and a rapid pulse rate. Cyanosis, vomiting and edema may occur. The urine decreases in volume, sometimes to complete suppression. These symptoms may become progressively worse and lead to coma and death. In other cases, they may continue for days or weeks. No general agreement exists as to the cause of the toxic symptoms. They may be due in part to delayed effects of the initial shock, which disturb the function of such vital organs as the kidney and the liver, in part to severe electrolyte imbalance or in part to the absorption of toxic substances from the destroyed tissue or from bacteria invading the burned area.

From 65 to 75 per cent of the deaths from burns occur in the first 48 hours. If as much as 20 per cent of the body surface is burned, shock is almost certain to develop unless active measures are taken to prevent it. When a third to a half of the total skin surface is involved, the chances for recovery are slim.

CONVALESCENCE. Children who are burned extensively and yet survive the early dangers of shock and toxicity face a long period of convalescence and complicated care. Attempts must be made to prevent secondary infection of the wound, to provide protection for the delicate epithelium which grows in to replace dead tissue and to prevent the formation of contracting scars and keloids during the healing stage.

When the tissue destruction is deep and the gap too wide to be bridged by natural healing, skin grafts must be made to cover the defect. Many of these procedures require prolonged and arduous immobilization. Both the effects of the original burning and those of protracted convalescence interfere with nutrition by hampering the regeneration of serum proteins and red blood cells. Prolonged inactivity and discomfort are likely to interfere with the child's appetite and make it difficult for him to take in the necessary nutriments to speed his recovery. In addition to physical rehabilitation there is much to be done in maintaining his morale and helping him to accept whatever residual handicap and disfigurement he may have to bear. At all stages the management of severe burns is a complicated and difficult procedure.

Management of Shock and Toxicity. In severe burns the first consideration must be given to the prevention of shock (or the treatment, if shock has appeared already) and of the toxic state that may ensue. In some instances, local treatment of the burn will be deferred until these dangers are over. Where it is necessary to carry out a débridement early, adequate anesthesia or sedation is essential not only for humanitarian reasons but also to minimize pain which may otherwise aggravate shock.

In shock the blood volume becomes reduced, due to the passage of its fluid element, the plasma, through the walls of the blood vessels and into the tissues. The circulating blood then becomes reduced in amount, and as a consequence the circulation becomes sluggish. The normal function of vital organs may be impaired by anoxia and by slow interchange of nutriments and waste products with the blood stream. The loss of plasma in the blood results in an increased concentration of the red blood cells. This affords a simple means of measuring the severity of the shock and the effectiveness of its treatment. Either the red blood-cell count or the hematocrit of the blood may be used as a rough guide. The main element of treatment is to attempt to restore blood volume by the intravenous injection of plasma in amounts large enough to counteract the losses through the capillary walls. In addition, the patient may require oxygen to combat anoxia and sedation to relieve pain. Adequate but not excessive external heat should be applied to maintain body temperature without causing dilatation of peripheral vessels.

Once the blood volume has been supported adequately, it may be necessary to provide additional parenteral fluids such as salt solution, glucose or sodium lactate in order to maintain an adequate fluid intake, promote urine formation and counteract acidosis.

Nursing Care. THE INITIAL STAGE. During the early care of a burned patient the nurse's activities must be concentrated upon close observation of the vital signs, such as body temperature, pulse, respirations, blood pressure and the state of the peripheral circulation, in order that she may inform the doctor of changes in the child's condition. In addition, she must do what she can to make her patient comfortable and to give him encouragement and support.

PHYSICAL HYGIENE. First-degree burns produce only simple erythema and require nothing more than local application of an ointment or an oily dressing to relieve pain. Unless they are extensive there is often no need for hospitalization or elaborate treatment. Burns of greater intensity and extent require careful attention.

Difference of opinion exists concerning cleansing and preparation of the burned area for the first dressing. Some advocate thorough surgical cleansing, while others maintain that no need for washing exists and that washing should be restricted to the unburned areas. Some advocate the opening of blisters and débridement (removal of contaminated, macerated or lacerated tissue); others maintain that débridement is unnecessary and that the blebs protect the underlying tissue. Simplicity in treatment is advantageous and should be practiced to the extent compatible with the welfare of the child.

The methods of further management are multiple; the one chosen will depend on the preferences of the physician in charge. The goal in any case is the avoidance of infection and the promotion of healing. Some prefer ointment dressing exclusively (boric acid or antibiotic ointment or gentian violet jelly), regardless of the location of the burn. It is generally agreed that this type of dressing is greatly to be preferred for burns of the face, the hands, the joints, the genitalia and the perineum. When used for other parts of the body, it is common custom to retain the ointment in place by a snug-fitting bandage and leave the dressing undisturbed for a period of from 5 to 10 days before changing, except that the bandage is re-

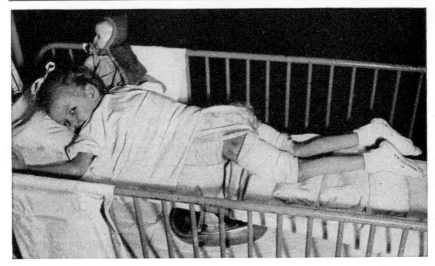

FIG. 59. Illustrating the care of a burned child on a Bradford frame. Waterproof material is used to protect from contamination the burned areas on the thighs. To collect urine specimens from an incontinent child, waterproof material should be used to construct the trough leading into the bedpan.

tightened to snugness from time to time.

Other methods of managing burns include wet dressings, exposure to air and the formation of eschars by early spraying of the burned area with gentian violet, tannic acid, silver nitrate or other substances which coagulate the proteins and form a protective crust. Since skin grafting will not be successful unless a clean, uninfected granulating base can be obtained, it is desirable to try to prevent infection of the burn whenever possible. If this fails, careful bacteriologic study of the invading bacteria and their sensitivities to various antibiotic agents is indicated so that appropriate local or general treatment can be given. Similar scrupulous care is necessary after the grafts have been placed.

Selection of the exact method of treatment must be varied to suit individual needs. Nursing care also must vary. The plan of nursing care will be influenced by the type of treatment instituted, by the location and the extent of the burned areas and by the age and the needs of the particular child. The use of a Bradford frame in extensive trunk-and-extremity burns is highly desirable (Fig. 59). Contractures can be prevented by maintaining good posture; urine specimens can be collected when the child is incontinent; and wound contamination from feces and urine can be lessened or prevented. If the head of the Bradford frame is hung higher than the foot, gravity will produce a downward flow of urine. By using 2 pieces of waterproof material, each 6 x 18 in., to form a trough leading into a bedpan placed beneath the opening of the frame, urine can be collected more easily. One piece of the material should be placed under the buttocks and over the edge of the frame, while the other should be secured over the pubes and brought down over the perineum and into the bedpan. To determine kidney function, accurate measurement of urine must be recorded.

Pressure areas can be prevented by turning these children at 3-hour intervals and giving them skin care. When 2 beds with Bradford frames are available for a burned child, discomfort from moving can be reduced. Instead of lifting him on to a stretcher while his frame is being recovered, he can be turned and lifted directly onto a clean frame. Skin around the burned area can be kept free from irritating exudate and in good condition by frequent cleansing, massaging and application of petrolatum. When the lower extremities are burned, pressure on the heels can be prevented by supporting the thighs on small pillows to elevate the heels from the frame or the bed.

Measures to prevent foot drop are required. When the child is lying on his abdomen, a pillow placed beneath his thighs will keep his feet in good position.

Every precaution must be taken to prevent infection, which retards healing and growth of the grafts. Gown-and-mask technic should be used to prevent cross-infection, and the hands should be washed thoroughly before any care is given. Sterilized linen placed over the Bradford frame or the bed and over the dressings is an added preventive

measure. When the child is young, and the burned area is irritating, arm restraints may be required to keep him from infecting the area with his hands. However, many times, snug coverings which keep the wound inaccessible can be applied. If the child is not too ill, suitable play materials will interest him and divert his attention from the skin irritation. When dressings are changed without anesthesia, a face mask should be put on the child to prevent self-contamination.

When the buttocks and the genitalia are burned, care to lessen dressing contamination and to promote healing is indicated. If enemas are necessary, waterproof materials must be used to prevent dressing contamination. After bowel evacuation, the perineum should be cleansed with cotton balls and oil, and in some instances careful irrigation of the area with warm normal saline solution will help to cleanse the fecal material completely from the burned area. When the penis and the scrotum are burned, frequent cleansing and application of dressings saturated with 1 per cent Mercurochrome reduce the incidence of infection. When the child is on his abdomen, a diaper sling under the frame opening will support the edematous organs and maintain the position of the dressing.

Maintaining a desired position is necessary to prevent contractures and to keep a grafted area at rest. When the neck is burned anteriorly, a roll under the shoulders will hyperextend it and prevent disfiguring contractures. Sandbags or specially applied restraints may be indicated for immobilization. Constant supervision is essential to readjust appliances which prevent crippling complications that require traction or plastic surgery to correct.

NUTRITION. Frequent feeding of foods high in calories, protein and iron is imperative to lessen the degree of hypoproteinemia and anemia. During the early stages of the illness, loss of nitrogen is great. It is lost when it passes from the surrounding areas into the burned tissue, when it is excreted from the body by way of the urinary tract, and when exudate is formed. Frequently, poor appetite is encountered, and when protein intake is insufficient hypoproteinemia develops rapidly. In some instances amigen, a casein digest, is given orally. Through use of this material larger amounts of protein may be given than when unhydrolyzed protein alone is used. Often, vitamins B and C are given to accelerate healing and to stimulate appetite. Iron therapy is used when anemia begins to develop. Grafts do not grow well when the red blood-cell count and the hemoglobin are low.

Encouraging ingestion of fluids aids the body in eliminating toxins, maintains body-fluid requirements and prevents kidney damage when sulfonamide therapy is used to prevent or control infection. During the first few days, thirst from dehydration may be increased, and care must be taken not to give fluids too rapidly, for nausea and vomiting are produced easily. After this period, encouragement is usually necessary to keep the intake at desired levels. Accurate intake records must be kept. When intake is compared with output, the onset of kidney impairment may be detected.

EMOTIONAL SUPPORT. Long periods of immobilization, isolation from family and playmates and painful and frightening experiences involve mental attitudes that must be understood if the burned child is to be nursed intelligently and completely. The accident itself is a harrowing experience for the child. If it resulted from doing things that his parents had cautioned him not to do, the trauma to his psyche may be nearly as great as the trauma to his body. The child needs reassurance and understanding to build up his tolerance to all the experiences that are to come. A burned child requires frequent trips to the operating room for dressing changes and for grafting; the type of preparation that he receives may influence the course of his illness. If he anticipates the trips with horror and apprehension, the anxiety produced will affect his personality, his appetite and his total well-being. Evidences of regressive behavior and problems of nursing will become increasingly more evident. The nurse should discover the child's fears and discomfort. She must help him to face them and to use whatever resources he has to meet them.

The child needs help in handling dreaded experiences. Children react differently to painful experiences. Some seem outwardly to accept them, yet on closer observation one sees signs of anxiety. To react to pain with shrieks is more trying to the nurse in attendance, yet it may be that child's way of reacting to pain, and it may give him far greater release than if he were to remain silent. If a nurse whom the child enjoys accompanies him to the operating room and remains to make his waiting time pleasurable, trips there can be made pleasant. When operating-room nurses and attendants greet the child in a friendly fashion and talk to him of interesting things, anticipation at seeing friends there may supplant his former dread. When the ordeal is over, showing recognition of improvement in the way he met the situation increases his courage and helps him to continue handling his disagreeable experiences constructively.

Unless arms and hands are burned, equipment for independent play should be provided. A folded sheet brought under the Bradford frame and pinned to the sides of the crib will form a hammock that will provide support for the child's arms and space for his toys. The use of the hammock will prevent position changes which result when a child retrieves his fallen playthings from beneath the frame.

The child will enjoy being read to and played with, and his need for companionship should be met. Placing his bed so that he may look out of the door or the window or into a ward of convalescent children will stimulate his individual activities and increase his desire to get well enough to join the group. In the convalescent period he will need the companionship of children and an environment that gives him increasingly more opportunities to prepare him for life at home.

Through conversation or observation of the parent-child relationship, feelings of guilt often will be detected in the parents. If the accident resulted from lack of supervision during play or because the parents failed to teach their child or failed to remove dangerous objects from his environment, parental remorse undoubtedly will be felt. Parental feelings of guilt may be expressed verbally but more often they are expressed unconsciously as they attempt to compensate by oversolicitude. If the feelings of guilt are strong and if they adversely influence their attitudes toward the child, help of a therapist may be necessary to lessen or overcome them.

Assisting in a program of burn prevention is the responsibility of the hospital and the public-health nurse. The mortality rate due to preventable accidents that produce burns is tremendously high. Little children are social beings. They enjoy the kitchen because they are with their mothers and because there is much there to interest them. For this reason kitchens must be made safe. Preschool children should be taught caution in the use of matches and in observing bonfires. Fires are fascinating to children, and negative admonition will not stifle their interest in them. Instead, positive direction should be given to teach children *how* to light a match and *when* they may do it and to teach them *how* to watch a fire safely. Adults must be taught to keep inflammable materials out of children's reach and to supervise all bonfires in their neighborhood. If these measures could be instituted, the incidence of burns would be reduced markedly.

ECZEMA

Eczema is a dermatitis caused by internal or external irritants and having distinctive characteristics which make it differ from the dermatitis of bacterial inflammation. It tends to run a chronic course with periods of remission and exacerbation. Eczema occurs at all ages but it is considerably more frequent in infancy than at any time later. In the majority of cases, the eczema appears before 6 months of age, though seldom in the first month.

MANIFESTATIONS

Eczema of infancy differs from that occurring later in its greater severity and in the distribution and the general nature of the lesions. The common type of infantile eczema occurs most often in fat or well-nourished babies. The lesions are most severe on the face but they may appear also on the scalp, the forearms, the legs and the trunk. In the early stages and in exacerbations, the superficial epithelium is lost, and the skin surface is raw and oozing. The exudate tends to dry, forming crusts. The skin is not thickened.

A less common type, more frequent in malnourished babies, is characterized by a reddened, thickened, scaly skin. The lesions of this type may appear anywhere on the body. This latter type is the most common in older children, except that it is more likely to be limited in the body folds, especially at the elbows and the knees.

Infantile eczema is accompanied by considerable itching or burning, and as a consequence the baby, if permitted, will rub or scratch much of the time, thus aggravating the condition markedly. Remissions and exacerbations of the eczema occur at irregular intervals. The eczema usually is much worse in winter and better in summer, often disappearing entirely in the warm months only to recur in the fall. In the majority of instances, the skin heals between 1 and 2 years of age, and the eczema does not recur.

ETIOLOGY

The cause of infantile eczema cannot be stated with the definiteness and the accuracy that one desires. That allergy is a large factor in many instances is an acceptable belief, but any claim that it is the cause in all cases is not supportable by the evidence at hand. Approximately three fourths of the older babies with eczema have positive reactions to various proteins when applied to the skin by customary testing methods. Babies in the first half year, especially those under 4 months, seldom present good evidence of skin sensitivity to test proteins, even though the eczema may be caused by these proteins. The food proteins to which infants most commonly are found sensitive are egg white; various cereals, especially wheat; cow's milk; fruit, especially apple and orange; and potato.

Even though a considerable proportion of babies with eczema have positive skin reactions to test proteins, only about one third or fewer of them will obtain relief from their eczema when removal of the supposedly offending protein from the diet is the only therapeutic measure employed. Factors other than allergy seem to play an important role. The skin of the infant is more sensitive and delicate than that of the child and reacts to milder stimuli. A large factor in the increased sensitivity of the infant is the large water content of the body, in which the skin shares. The extracellular or the interstitial water of the body of the infant is fully twice that of the adult, and the skin normally contains as much water as that of an edematous adult. Thus it is that many infants can have eczema without aHergy and that treatment other than removal of the responsible allergen is necessary. Thus, also, is explained why eczema is aggravated by the trauma of rubbing and scratching, by local infections which are acquired so easily in the affected areas of skin and by sudden marked changes in temperature such as those to which the baby is exposed when taken outdoors in winter.

Dietary Factors Other Than Allergens

There are those who believe that eczema is caused or aggravated by dietary factors apparently unrelated to allergy, such as an excess of fat, an excess of sugar or an excess of total food. It is difficult to state the exact degree of truth in such a belief. In general, it may be stated that the eczema of well-nourished babies decreases when the babies lose weight, and that weight loss may result when the diet is restricted sufficiently in any of the ways stated. In ordinary circumstances this should not be considered a good method of management. Any success it may have probably is dependent on loss of water from the body and therefore from the skin. Interstitial water never exists alone but always has in solution definite quantities of certain salts, chiefly sodium chloride. Therefore, any type of diet that tends to increase salt retention also would increase the water content of the skin and aggravate the eczema. The converse likewise would be true.

Babies with eczema have been found to have a low unsaturated fatty acid content of the blood, and the feeding of fats high in unsaturated fatty acid content has been suggested in treatment. Such therapy has not met with much clinical success. However, a diet relatively high in fat and low in carbohydrate (ketogenic type) has a dehydrating effect and could be beneficial in eczema.

Nursing Care of Infantile Eczema

Ideally, the infant with eczema should be restrained as little as is absolutely necessary to prevent scratching and infection. It has been observed that these infants cry less than other babies. When they are frustrated, angry and unhappy they scratch instead of crying. If a nurse is in constant attendance, she can follow his cues and give him affection or food or help him find a satisfying activity according to his specific need at the moment. The baby with eczema improves physically and psychologically when he has a continuous warm relationship with a nurse who recognizes his need to express his feelings overtly and to use his powers in independent, learning activities.

Restraint. When constant attendance is not possible, it is necessary to employ some means that will prevent scratching or rubbing. Elbow cuffs that prevent flexion at the elbows are of assistance, but usually the arms must be held with additional restraint to prevent rubbing of the face with the upper arms. Restraints must be applied securely and in a kind fashion. They must be adjusted securely because his discomfort and desire for activity drive

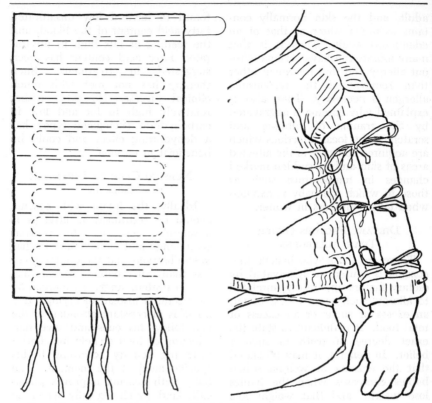

Fig. 60. Elbow cuff restraint. (*Left*) Elbow cuff for use in treatment of eczema. (*Right*) Elbow cuff applied.

him to find methods of freeing himself. A few minutes without restraint may undo the nursing of the past weeks and produce open lesions that become infected easily. They must be applied in a kind fashion to minimize feelings of anger at being restrained.

A good type of elbow cuff is one splinted with tongue blades (Fig. 60). It is more comfortable for young infants to have the tongue blades cut to about 4 inches in length. In order to retain the cuff securely, the shirt sleeves should be folded over the lower end of the cuff and pinned to it. Ankle restraints are necessary if eczema is present in the legs. When the weather is warm or when the infant tends to perspire profusely, it is advisable to eliminate the use of the shirt. To keep the cuff restraints in position, a 4-inch strip of old linen can be brought across the shoulders and down the arms and then pinned back over the cuff.

Protection by Pliofilm. When an infant tends to rub his face on his shoulders, a bib of Pliofilm prevents

FIG. 61. A method of restraint and the use of a face mask to keep dressings or ointment in place are illustrated with the use of a doll.

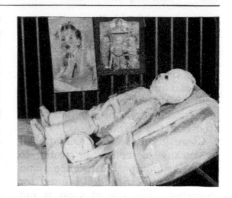

excoriations. Such a bib may be made of an 8-inch square of Pliofilm with tabs of adhesive and tape at the corners for pinning it into position. In some institutions, Pliofilm covers over the head of the mattress have been used with excellent results. When the Pliofilm bib and mattress covers are used, the infant can be turned from side to side and on his abdomen without danger of increasing the severity of the lesions. Changes in position are important in the prevention of respiratory infections, a complication to which the infant with eczema is very susceptible. Elevating the head of the bed aids in the prevention of otitis media.

Local Applications. The selection of appropriate dermatologic remedies and their meticulous application are useful in all cases of eczema and, in addition to other general measures discussed, are sufficient in many instances to bring about recovery without recourse to radical dietary changes. If the skin is moderately infected when the baby comes under care, an antiseptic ointment, such as 3 per cent ammoniated mercury ointment, may be used until the infection has disappeared. Oint-

ments containing antibiotics may be required. In instances of more severe infection, wet packs of normal salt solution serve better than an ointment. If the skin is not infected or if the infection has been treated effectively, a protective or soothing ointment is indicated. Such an ointment may be 2 per cent ichthyol or Lassar's paste. If satisfactory improvement is not obtained with the soothing ointment, a stimulating ointment, such as 6 per cent tar ointment or carbonis detergens cream, is indicated, but only after the protective ointment has failed. When tar ointment is used, exposure to the sun should be avoided because the ointment contains a photosensitizing fraction that produces skin irritation as a result of exposure to sunshine.

Ointments should be applied thickly, and reapplications should be made whenever necessary. Applying the ointment with long strokes has been found to produce a more soothing effect.

In order to ensure satisfactory retention of ointments or wet dressings applied to the face, it may be necessary to use a mask (Fig. 61). A mask is prepared by cutting holes in a piece of old linen or cotton stocking, the holes corresponding in shape and location to the eyes, the nose and the mouth. The mask should be large enough to go around the head and should be held in position with attached tapes. Binding and friction must be avoided when adjusting the mask.

Cleansing the Skin. Oil applied by means of cotton or water to which sodium bicarbonate and starch have been added is used for cleansing. The use of soap is not advisable. When ointments are being used, it is customary to cleanse the skin once daily or less frequently. Cleansing should be done gently without rubbing. If itching is intense and restraint is being used, only one extremity at a time can be released for cleansing.

Sometimes a colloidal bath is desired. In preparation, an infant-sized tub is filled with water at 95° F., and one quarter cup each of soluble starch and sodium bicarbonate is mixed in thoroughly. Floating toys should be at hand to divert the infant's attention and prevent scratching during the procedure. A diaper should be placed in the bottom of the tub to prevent the baby from slipping, and a firm hold is necessary to prevent the child from feeling insecure in the tub. During the time the infant is in the tub (15 to 20 minutes), the washcloth should be used to pour water over the infant's head and body. Rubbing the skin may produce a paroxysm of itching.

Diet. Usually it is not possible at the first examination to determine whether or not infantile eczema is on an allergic basis. Whether or not special dietary measures are insti-

tuted at the beginning of treatment, they may be employed if response to local treatment is not definite and prompt. More than half the babies with eczema will respond to local treatment without dietary change. If the eczema is dependent on allergy to foods, the offending foods should be omitted from the diet, while at the same time the diet should be kept "complete."

One good method of management is to use what is known as an elimination diet. This is accomplished by starting with a simple basic diet which is hypo-allergic to the extent that improvement in the eczema is permitted and then adding one food at a time to determine the infant's reaction to each food. In such a scheme, new foods should be introduced in small amounts. The diet and the skin changes should be charted in full in order to determine the foods to which the baby is sensitive.

The chief article of the basic diet should be some form of milk or milk substitute. Prolonged or high heating of protein alters its character in such a way that it is less allergenic, often sufficiently less that babies who are sensitive to the raw protein can take the cooked protein without disturbance. It is the alteration produced by heat that gives to evaporated and dried milk a considerable degree of usefulness in the management of babies with allergic eczema. Babies sensitive to cow's milk often are able to take goat's milk. Synthetic "milks" are commercially available. Some of these are prepared from soybeans. One is prepared from hydrolized casein. Regardless of which of these various foods may be chosen, the formula must be supplemented by vitamins C and D and perhaps other essentials, depending on the food chosen. In the dietary management of babies with eczema, foods are to be avoided on the basis of actual demonstration by feeding, not on the basis of skin tests.

Psychological Aspects. Eczema is rarely dependent completely upon sensitivity to foods but often is aggravated by either internal or external environmental irritants. Feathers, wool, kapok and certain dusts may irritate the child. The common factors among these materials should be eliminated. Stuffed toys may contain allergenic factors. Emotional factors also may play a part in producing eczema. Many investigators who have studied children with eczema have found emotional disturbances in the mother-child relationship. Dunbar concluded that a climate of "smother love" was the characteristic emotional climate to which the child with eczema was subjected. She felt that many of these children experienced conflict between their desire for affection and their fear lest they be hurt if they sought it. Other investigators found these children overprotected and recipients of domineering love. Some believed that a frustrated need for love was one of the dynamic factors operating to produce the condition.

A baby with eczema should be held for feedings the same as one does in the case of a normal child. Such holding gives him a change in position and the affection that he needs for normal emotional growth. Time of feeding should be gauged by his need for food. Awakening a baby with eczema brings frustration and an increased need to scratch. Often excellent results are obtained by giving the baby increased opportunity to suck. It reduces tension and brings relaxation. A pacifier has been found to be effective in bringing the baby increased comfort. However, other sources of pleasure also must be provided. He needs both stimulation from a satisfying, nonsmothering type of relationship with a parent figure and sufficient opportunity to meet his need for sucking.

In preventing scratching, the nurse must not lose sight of the fact that her patient is a human being who needs the same satisfactions and opportunities for learning as does the normal infant. He needs freedom for self-directed play and opportunities to develop his independence. Restraints should be removed each time the infant is fed, and his arms and legs should be exercised. If he is old enough to be interested in self-feeding, his interest in learning should be encouraged. As soon as the skin lesions show sufficient improvement, the outer restraints should be removed and the infant allowed to move about and play freely under close supervision. Toys suited to his individual needs should be introduced. Diversion prevents scratching and gives the infant needed experience with play materials. When the cuff restraints are first removed, the hands may be covered for short periods with rubber gloves, the fingers of which have been tied off. The glove cuffs may be pinned to the shirt. Thus, relatively free activity becomes possible without danger of injury. Fingernails and toenails should be kept cut short at all times. Then if he resorts to scratching when unrestricted, he will not damage himself so severely.

When nursing a child with eczema the nurse also should direct her interest to the needs of the mother. The nurse not only needs to reflect upon her feelings toward the eczematous child but also she should consider her response to his mother. Either the nurse can increase the mother's feelings of inadequacy, guilt and resentment or she can understand the mother's need to overprotect or reject overtly. If she understands the mother she can increase her feelings of competence, lessen her guilt and resentment and help her to develop more positive feelings toward her child. Before the mother assumes complete charge of her infant she will need detailed instructions and demonstrations concerning his care and assurance that she is capable of providing it. The young mother often fears lest she is incapable of caring for her child. She may see his condition as evidence of her failure. She may hesitate to restrain and to restrict his diet because it frustrates her deep need to overprotect. Many mothers fear that their infants are afflicted with a chronic disease that may produce scars and prevent normal development. An understanding nurse can allay these fears. She also can help these mothers find ways to restrict scratching that are less punishing.

Nervous mannerisms are seen frequently in children with eczema. The long periods of restriction with constant frustrations tend to produce emotional instability, insecurity, aggression, extroversion, restlessness and an unusual drive to dominate.

Parental anxiety often is reflected in their behavior. When frustrated in play, these children not uncommonly revert to scratching, even though their skin shows little or no irritation. Some studies have indicated superior mental ability in these children. If this is true, it is not to be wondered at that they are eager to investigate their environment when once freed from the restraints that have limited and angered them. To prevent these nervous mannerisms, it is necessary that the nurse understand the problems of the mother and help her to feel the need to give her child more opportunities to develop his independence in play and in learning to do things for himself.

MISCELLANEOUS SKIN DISORDERS

ACNE VULGARIS

A disturbance of the pilosebaceous apparatus appears in late childhood or adolescence in a high percentage of children. Under the influence of the sexual hormones of the maturing person an activation of the sebaceous glands occurs which results in an increased production of oily sebum. At the same time there is a tendency for the orifices of the glands to become blocked by dark inspissated material (blackheads or comedones), around which may develop an inflammatory reaction, often with pustule formation. Acne vulgaris is usually prominent about the forehead, the face and the neck. It also may be present on the shoulders and the back and occasionally on the chest. Its extent is quite variable. Some children have little or none during the whole course of their adolescence and early adult lives. Others are affected severely, with permanent scarring of the skin as a consequence of the repeated formation of pustules. Administration of cortisone or ACTH often produces a similar eruption even in young children, but there is seldom any associated infection.

Treatment of mild acne consists of frequent bathing of the skin to remove oil and bacteria and to encourage drying. For the latter purpose various washes that cause mild peeling are useful. Exposure to ultraviolet light is also beneficial, either from the sun or from a lamp. The diet is of some importance in the aggravation of lesions, and the natural tendency of the adolescent to gorge himself with carbohydrate foods must be discouraged if the inflammatory reaction is to be controlled adequately. Expression of the contents of comedones and pustules usually is done by the physician. In severe cases, judicious use of x-ray treatment may be required.

ALOPECIA

Alopecia or loss of hair may be observed in children of various ages. Usually the cause is unknown, and the condition is temporary. Patches of the scalp hair come out spontaneously, leaving a bald area. In some instances congenital defects of the skin lie beneath such bald areas. In others the baldness is the result of the child's pulling his hair out by the roots, in which case the possibility that he is swallowing it and producing a hair ball (trichobezoar) in the stomach must be considered. Tinea of the scalp also must be excluded as a cause of such bald areas. In rare instances, all of the scalp hair comes out following one of the infectious diseases.

PITYRIASIS ROSEA

This is an asymptomatic, faint, generalized eruption of unknown cause, the only importance of which is the possibility of its confusion with other eruptions. It usually begins with a single small oval slightly scaly patch on the trunk, which is followed a week or so later by a number of similar lesions all over the trunk. There is no fever or other evidence of disease. The patches may last as long as 2 months and then disappear.

URTICARIA

Urticaria or hives may occur in children of almost any age. In its classic form it is a manifestation of sensitivity to some substance taken in the food or as medicine or injected by an insect. The individual spots are pleomorphic bright-red wheals which often have a small raised white center and itch intensely. They may be few in number or generalized over the whole body. In extensive cases there may be fever. In some instances urticaria can be traced to a specific substance, and attacks may recur each time the sensitized child has contact with such a food or medication. In other instances, isolated attacks of urticaria occur for which no cause can be discovered and they never recur. Such subjects may not show any other evidence of allergic manifestations. Treatment usually consists of topical application of lotions to relieve itching. Adrenalin, antihistaminics or cortisone may be used in severe afflictions.

DRUG ERUPTIONS

Many of the medicines commonly used in the treatment of disease in children are capable of producing skin eruptions if the child becomes sensitive to them. Various forms of eruption may occur. For example, atropine produces a generalized flush somewhat like scarlet fever; sulfathiazole may produce an eruption like measles; penicillin may be responsible for urticaria. In general, once a drug eruption has appeared in a given child, the same lesions are likely to recur if the substance is given again. Of course, treatment depends upon the accurate recognition of the offending substance and its scrupulous avoidance in the future.

SITUATIONS FOR FURTHER STUDY

1. Outline the instructions you would give a mother if she were going to treat her child with scabies at home.

2. How do you imagine a baby with eczema views hospitalization and his treatment?

3. How do you react to the care of a baby with eczema?

4. How do you suppose a mother of a baby with eczema feels about his condition and the responsibilities his care entails?

5. Before an infant with eczema is discharged from the hospital, what help would his mother require? If you were to go into the home where an infant with eczema was being cared for, what observations would you make? If the infant were 11 months old and required elbow restraints only, what play equipment would you suggest for his use?

6. After removing restraints from an infant 16 months old who is convalescing from eczema, observe his activity with appropriate play materials. How long does he remain interested in one toy? What does he do with it? What type of toy interests him the most? Does he scratch during the supervised playtime? If he does scratch, what behavior preceded it? After reapplying restraints, how does he react? Does he accept his restraints more easily after a period of satisfying play or does he resent having his play discontinued?

7. Study mortality rates of burns. At what age period is the rate highest? What are some of the causes of burns in the periods of infancy, childhood and adolescence? When making home visits, how could you help a mother learn to keep her infant's environment safe? What would you teach a mother that would prevent accidents from burns?

BIBLIOGRAPHY

Andrews, G. C.: Diseases of the Skin, ed. 3, Philadelphia, Saunders, 1946.

Armistead, N. B.: Preventing deformities following severe burns, Am. J. Nursing 50:162, 1950.

Becker, S. W., and Obermayer, M. E.: Modern Dermatology and Syphilology, Philadelphia, Lippincott, 1941.

Bozian, M. W.: Nursing care of patients having dermatologic conditions, Am. J. Nursing 52:873, 1952.

Deutsch, F., and Nadell, R.: Psychosomatic aspects of dermatology with special consideration of allergic phenomena, Nerv. Child 5: 339, 1946.

Dunbar, H. F.: Mind and Body: Psychosomatic Medicine, p. 190, New York, Random, 1947.

Herschfield, J. W.: The treatment of thermal burns, Am. J. Nursing **46:** 156, 1946.

Lofthouse, E. M.: Infantile eczema, Am. J. Nursing **49:**500, 1949.

MacKee, G. M., and Cipollaro, A. C.: Skin Diseases in Children, New York, Hoeber, 1946.

Miller, M. L.: A psychological study of a case of eczema and a case of neurodermatitis, Psychosom. Med. **4:**82, 1942.

Ormsby, O. S., and Montgomery, H.: Diseases of the Skin, Philadelphia, Lea, 1948

Stone, H. M.: Psychological factors in infantile eczema, Am. J. Nursing **53:**449, 1953.

Wallinger, Elsie: Burns and their nursing care, Am. J. Nursing **42:** 1000, 1942.

Woodhead, Barbara: The psychological aspects of allergic skin reactions in childhood, Arch. Dis. Childhood **21:**98, 1946.

Diseases of the Eye

CONGENITAL AND NEONATAL
   ABNORMALITIES
INFLAMMATORY DISORDERS

THE VISUALLY HANDICAPPED CHILD
SITUATIONS FOR FURTHER STUDY

CONGENITAL AND NEONATAL ABNORMALITIES

CATARACT

Cataract is a condition in which part or all of the lens of the eye is opaque. The affected part of the lens appears white. Any cataract that is present at birth or appears early in life is included in the congenital group. In some instances, cataract is familial; in others, it is nutritional in origin; in still others it is traumatic, perhaps from birth injury in some cases. The occurrence of rubella in the mother during the first trimester of pregnancy is known to cause congenital cataract in a high proportion of babies. Partial cataract may be anterior, central or posterior in the lens. The only symptoms of cataract are those pertaining to interference with vision. The only treatment is surgical. Needling of the lens causes it to be absorbed, leaving the path of vision clear but also leaving the eye without power of accommodation.

Cataracts affecting the entire lens require operation. Whether or not operation is indicated in partial cata-

ract depends on the amount of useful vision present. Most partial cataracts do not progress, but a careful watch must be kept to detect those that do increase, in order that appropriate surgical treatment may be given when indicated.

Nursing Care. There are differences of opinion as to the amount of restraint that is necessary for the child postoperatively. Some surgeons feel that attempts at restriction result in more tension and attempted movement than does complete freedom. They suture adequately and eliminate the need for body restraint, recommending only the use of elbow restraints to prevent the child from removing the dressings. Other surgeons feel that immobilization is essential. They recommend the use of jacket and elbow restraints to prevent the infant from disturbing his dressings and to keep him from sitting up or turning onto his abdomen. Often sandbags are used on each side of his head to immobilize it completely.

The infant must be fed on his bed until orders that permit him to be moved into a sitting position are given. Fluids should be given in small amounts until tolerance for larger quantities is noted. Every measure should be taken to prevent vomiting, which may result in aspiration and increased intraocular pressure.

Care should be taken to prevent startling the infant when he is approached. Talking pleasantly to him before the cribside is lowered lessens the danger of frightening him with an abrupt approach to his bedside. The infant who requires immobilization will miss the comfort he formerly felt when he was held for feedings, play, affection and parental enjoyment. Substitute satisfactions must be provided during the period when immobilization is necessary. Stroking the infant's head, talking to him in gentle, soothing tones and carrying out all measures that ensure physical comfort will lessen his need for sedatives, which are required when he is restless, tearful and irritable.

Squint (Strabismus)

Squint is a condition in which the eyes cannot be used at the same time for looking at an object; such a person is said to be cross-eyed. Normally, the lines of vision (visual axes) of the eyes are parallel when the object is at a distance of 20 feet or more. When looking at a nearer object, the visual axes converge to meet the object. In squint, the visual axis of only one eye goes to the object. The other eye is the squinting eye.

Many varieties of squint exist. Squint from prenatal causes may become apparent at any time from birth to the sixth year. Develop-

ment of squint after this time usually is caused by disease. Sometimes the muscles that move the eye outward or those that move the eye inward are overactive or underactive, and the resulting condition may be referred to as paralytic squint. When squint is caused by underaction of the muscles of one eye, the affected eye does not have as full ocular movements as the fellow eye. In nonparalytic squint the squinting eye moves with the eye used for vision, but always with a visual axis not corresponding to that of the seeing eye, a condition known as concomitant squint. Concomitant squint may be either monocular or alternating. In monocular squint, one eye is used constantly for vision and the other eye is turned either inward (convergent squint) or outward (divergent squint). In alternating squint, either eye is used for vision and the other eye becomes the squinting eye.

Concomitant squint usually is due to errors of refraction. When the eyes change fixation from a distant to a near object, the pupils contract, the lenses change power for an exact focus, and the eyes converge. The error of refraction may be such that the focus (accommodation) is not accurate at the same time that both eyes are able to fix accurately on the object. The child must choose between accurate fixation with poor vision and accurate accommodation with double vision. The choice resulting in squint may be made at any time in early infancy.

When both eyes cannot be brought to bear on an object, double vision (diplopia) results, and the images in the eyes differ. The person with squint quickly learns to disregard the image in the squinting eye. As a result, vision in the squinting eye may be reduced markedly. Usually the false image of the squinting eye is suppressed by the time the child comes under care.

Because of danger to vision, as well as for cosmetic effect, treatment for squint should be undertaken as soon as the condition is observed. Usually, the earlier the treatment is undertaken, the better the results, and, conversely, the later the treatments, the slower the progress and the less satisfactory the final status. The objectives of treatment are to improve the vision of the poorly functioning eye, to produce or restore single vision when both eyes are focusing together and to correct the deformity.

In early infancy the better eye should be occluded by a patch or a cover until the baby is old enough to wear glasses, which may be at the age of from 12 to 14 months. With use of the poorer eye the vision should improve and often it can be brought to normal. Correction of the refractive error helps to restore single vision and is fully effective in many instances. For some children, correction of the deformity by operation may be necessary, but operation is not indicated until maximum improvement by glasses and training has been attained, usually not before 3 or 4 years of age. Correction of the deformity early, particularly before the child goes to school, is important for psychologic reasons. Otherwise, the child is taunted, becomes embarrassed and is likely to develop personality changes with an inferiority or a defense complex. After operation, if this has been necessary, further treatment must

be given in the use of the eyes together.

Spurious Squint. During the early months of life, infants are not expected to maintain parallel vision at all times. Brief periods of convergent or divergent squint usually have little significance. Frequently, too, parents and relatives may be misled by an optical illusion which causes them to believe that the young infant with a broad nose and epicanthal fold is suffering from convergent squint, when actually he is using parallel vision. The explanation lies in the fact that during lateral gaze, the eye that is turning toward the nose appears to go too far inward because the epicanthal fold obscures more of the white sclera than the observer thinks that it should. The superficial conclusion of squint is drawn easily. A simple test will permit a distinction between real and spurious squint. If a bright point of light is directed into the infant's eyes, the reflections from the two corneas should be seen in the same relative position with respect to the center of the pupil in each eye. If the eyes are not parallel there will be an obvious difference between them.

Nursing Care. When operation is necessary to correct strabismus it is advisable to hospitalize the child a few days before it is performed. The child needs to become adjusted to the hospital and to the nurses who will attend him postoperatively. Some surgeons have ceased to use eye dressings postoperatively to prevent psychic trauma. They feel that it must be terrifying to receive a general anesthetic and awaken blinded by eye dressings. Other surgeons feel that eye dressings are essential postoperatively. In these instances the child needs to become accustomed to the feeling of elbow restraints and to dressings that completely occlude his vision *before* he is anesthetized. His nurse also must anticipate the fears that he may experience after operation (of awakening in the dark and of permanent loss of vision, for instance) and give him preparation to meet them. When nausea has ceased, a regular diet can be introduced. Children with eye dressings enjoy having their food described as they are being fed. They also enjoy the feeling of independence that comes when their restraints are removed and they are permitted to feed themselves the finger foods provided on their trays.

In most instances longer visiting periods are necessary for the child who has had an operation on his eyes. This is especially true when eye dressings have been applied. Temporary loss of vision produces panic in many children. The child's mother can allay his fears more effectively than the nurse because the latter has had too short a time to establish a relationship that brings the security and the satisfactions that he needs.

During the period when dressings cover both eyes, the child can be entertained by music and stories. Radios, which are a great source of pleasure and entertainment, should be provided when eye dressings make play activities impossible.

Fortunately, the period of blindness is short, but unless nurses safeguard the child from frightening experiences during the period of hospitalization by permitting his mother to be with him, a feeling of insecurity may develop. Insecurity may last beyond the time when successful correction of the deformity has been achieved.

When exercises are recommended postoperatively, the nurse should assist the mother in understanding their importance. If the child is attending school at the time of operation, it is advisable to notify the school nurse so that she may follow the child's care and ensure continuation of the orthoptic training.

RETROLENTAL FIBROPLASIA

Retrolental fibroplasia is an important cause of blindness which is seen almost exclusively in prematurely born infants; it is really a neonatally acquired disease rather than a congenital malformation. It is discussed briefly in Chapter 7.

INFLAMMATORY DISORDERS

CONJUNCTIVITIS

Inflammations of the conjunctiva result from a great many causes. Some of the disturbances are characteristic of the newborn period (gonococcal conjunctivitis, inclusion blenorrhea, chemical conjunctivitis, obstruction of the nasolacrimal duct); they have been considered in Chapter 7. Others are the result of vitamin deficiency and will be described in Chapter 26. Bacterial, virus and allergic factors account for the more common varieties of conjunctival inflammation.

Bacterial Conjunctivitis. Bacteria that are responsible for upper respiratory tract infections (streptococci, pneumococci, influenza bacilli and staphylococci) rather commonly invade the conjunctival sac to produce symptoms of itching, photophobia, redness of the eyeball and the lids and purulent secretion and crusting of the lids. Often the loose tissues about the eyes become swollen out of all proportion to the importance of the infection. Treatment with an appropriate antibiotic salve or drops is usually effective within a day or two. Important complications are rare, although ulceration of the cornea may take place during pneumococcal infections. The influenza bacillus sometimes produces a low-grade inflammation without much purulent exudate, which is readily transmissible among school children and is known commonly as "pink eye." Chronic staphylococcus infections may be associated with the formation of styes on the lids which respond slowly to local treatment and tend to recur.

Viruses are the cause of inclusion blenorrhea, trachoma and the primary conjunctivitis of measles.

INCLUSION BLENORRHEA. This disease is more common in the newborn period than at other times. In the newborn the infection is acquired from the vagina of the mother. The disease becomes manifest in from 7 to 12 days after birth. The acute stage has a duration of from 2 to 3 weeks and is followed by a chronic stage lasting from 6 weeks to 6 months. It is a harmless disease in that no serious complications or sequelae develop. The diagnosis is made by finding inclusion bodies in epithelial cells scraped from the conjunctiva and stained. Local antiseptics have no effect. Sulfonamide in standard dosage for 10 days is effective in control.

TRACHOMA is a result of a virus infection which is endemic in some parts of this country. The inflammation of the conjunctiva and the cornea is low-grade and chronic, often lasting over many years. Inclusion bodies are found in conjunctival scrapings. In the early stages of the disease the conjunctivitis is catarrhal or only moderately purulent. As the inflammation becomes chronic, follicles of hypertrophied conjunctival epithelium appear, and blood vessels invade the cornea. In the course of time, these lesions are associated with scarring in the conjunctiva and clouding of the cornea; such damage is permanent. Formerly, no treatment used was wholly satisfactory. At present, sulfonamide seems to be curative in that the virus is destroyed and the disease process is arrested. Existing scarring is likely to remain. Approximately half the standard dosage of sulfonamide is given for about 3 weeks.

Allergic Conjunctivitis. This inflammation occurs as a result of conjunctival sensitivity to any one of a number of materials. The most common variety is that associated with hay fever. At times the conjunctiva alone is affected, producing a lesion known as vernal conjunctivitis. Allergic conjunctivitis of these types is seasonal and recurrent. It is associated with itching and lacrimation. The treatment consists of avoiding the offending antigens, if possible, and of local application of epinephrine or ephedrine as needed. In general, allergic conjunctivitis causes a diffuse reaction throughout the conjunctiva. It may be caused by drugs used for general or local treatment.

Foreign Bodies. Foreign bodies that enter the conjunctival sac usually produce a rapid inflammatory reaction with excessive lacrimation and pain when the object impinges upon the cornea. Sometimes the tearing is sufficient to float the object out of the eye. Sometimes it can be located by inspection of the eye and can be removed easily. At other times the detection and the removal of a foreign body is a difficult procedure which requires the special skill of an ophthalmologist. A persistent unilateral conjunctivitis of sudden onset always should arouse the suspicion of the presence of a foreign body.

KERATITIS

Keratitis or inflammation of the cornea may be superficial or deep (interstitial). Almost all of the organisms that cause conjunctivitis may on occasion cause a keratitis which is much more painful and serious than conjunctival inflammation. Superficial keratitis is associated with severe pain, marked redness and frequently reduced vision. In healing, a scar that permanently impairs vision may remain in the cornea.

Phlyctenular Keratoconjunctivitis. Presumably this inflammation is the result of allergy, but the more intense reaction is localized in one or more phlyctenules or small papules

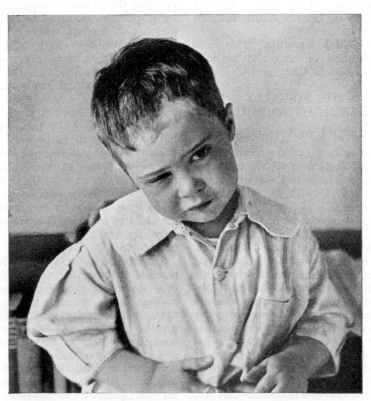

FIG. 62. Photophobia of phlyctenular keratoconjunctivitis, a condition occasionally found in association with sensitivity to tuberculin.

which are the characteristic lesion of the disease and occur on the conjunctiva or the cornea or both. Phlyctenular keratoconjunctivitis occurs chiefly in those who have had a tuberculous infection and usually show a marked skin sensitivity to tuberculin. The initiating factor has not been determined with certainty. Eventually, the papule disappears by ulceration and subsequent healing. On healing, a corneal lesion may produce a small area of opacity, a more or less permanent scar. During the acute stage, the chief symptoms are intense photophobia and lacrimation (Fig. 62). Present methods of treatment are unsatisfactory.

Interstitial Keratitis. This late complication of congenital syphilis is described in Chapter 18.

THE VISUALLY HANDICAPPED CHILD

RECOGNITION OF VISUAL DEFECTS

The analysis and the correction of visual defects is a highly technical specialty which can be performed only by those with special training. When there is obvious deformity or abnormal movement of the eyes the child usually is brought quickly under the care of such a specialist. But in many instances the visual defect is a subtle one which is discovered only through the astute observations of parents, nurses, doctors or schoolteachers. In some instances early discovery and proper management are essential to preserve bilateral vision; in other instances it is necessary to prevent problems of social and educational adjustment. Most of the visual defects that are

not grossly apparent depend upon errors of refraction in one or both eyes. A few are due to abnormal development or disease of the retina and its vascular or nervous supply.

Visual defects in infants may easily go unnoticed for several weeks or months. Early suspicions may be aroused after the infant has reached the age of 2 months if he fails to observe objects or to follow them with his eyes or to blink when they are brought close to his eyes. During the second half of the first year the child's failure to locate distant objects and his propensity for bringing things very close to his face for inspection may lead to the suspicion that he has severe myopia. In the school-age child, failure to learn, headaches, head-tilting or behavior disorders may be the first indication of a visual handicap.

As indicated above, a child who has a severe refractive error may begin to squint. More importantly, he may begin to favor his better eye and slowly lose the vision in the other eye because of disuse. Unless the poor vision in the defective eye is discovered early and efforts are made to correct it or to encourage the child to use the eye some of the time, its vision may be lost irretrievably.

Unfortunately, it is not always possible to assume that the child's eyes are under proper care merely because he is wearing glasses. In some instances the original fitting may be unskillful. In other circumstances the parents may have assumed that one examination and correction was all that ever would be needed and have failed to return for the periodic examinations requested. In some instances the child's refractive error keeps changing over a period of years, and the initial pair of glasses becomes obsolete.

PSYCHOLOGIC CONSIDERATIONS

Minor or correctable visual defects seldom create important problems of adjustment. Glasses have become so common among school children that the average child soon accepts the fact that he must wear them and makes an easy adjustment. When the visual handicap is moderately severe it may be necessary to place the child in a sight-saving class where special equipment and technics are available. Vocational guidance and training often are required to fit him for a realistic job or profession that recognizes his limitations. Both the parents and the child may need professional help in reaching an acceptance of the restriction of vocational and social opportunity which his handicap imposes upon him.

The parents of infants who are discovered to have serious visual defects or total blindness nearly always require help in adjusting to the handicap suffered by the child. In some instances they react with an unnecessary restriction of the child's activities which prevents normal physical development. In addition, such parents require assistance in providing the child with proper stimulations and opportunities to develop independence and technics of self-help. Later on, special teaching is required so that the child can learn Braille and develop vocational skills that will make him self-supporting in later life. These ac-

tivities usually are provided in special schools run by the local or the state government.

SITUATIONS FOR
FURTHER STUDY

1. Is the in-co-ordination of eye movements observed in the 6-month-old infant normal?

2. At what age should a mother seek medical attention for her infant with strabismus?

3. What care is necessary after operation to correct strabismus?

4. How could you help a 3-year-old child to accept eyedrops without untoward emotional response?

5. If a 5-year-old child who had had a repair of strabismus had his restraints but not his dressing removed, what diversion could you suggest that required no sight?

6. How do you imagine a 3-year-old child feels when he awakens from an anesthetic in a strange place, with strange people, with painful eyes and restraints and blinded from the application of dressings over both eyes?

7. What is orthoptic training? How does it aid in the correction of strabismus?

8. Write to the American Foundation for the Blind, 15 West 16th Street, New York 11, N. Y., and obtain pamphlets pertaining to the psychological needs of the blind child. Prepare a paper describing the care that a blind child requires during the preschool period of personality growth.

BIBLIOGRAPHY

Elonen, A. S., Norris, Miriam, and Craine, M. V.: The preschool blind child project of the University of Chicago Medical Clinics (pamphlet), Am. Found. for the Blind, 15 W. 16th St., New York 11, N. Y., 1952.

Lancaster, W. B.: Crossed eyes in children, Am. J. Nursing 50:535, 1950.

The preschool child who is blind

(Children's Bureau Folder No. 39), Washington, D. C., Govt. Print. Off., 1953.

Weaver, H. E.: The nurse and sight conservation, Am. J. Nursing 51: 553, 1951.

Weiss, M. O.: Psychological aspects of nursing care for eye patients, Am. J. Nursing 50:218, 1950.

Diseases of the Glands of Internal Secretion

◇◇◇

GENERAL DISCUSSION
NORMAL SEXUAL DEVELOPMENT
PRECOCIOUS SEXUAL DEVELOPMENT
HYPOTHYROIDISM

HYPERTHYROIDISM
DIABETES MELLITUS
DIABETES INSIPIDUS
SITUATIONS FOR FURTHER STUDY

GENERAL DISCUSSION

The glands of internal secretion or the endocrine glands are the thyroid, the parathyroid, the adrenal and the pituitary glands, the ovary, the testis, the islands of Langerhans of the pancreas, and sometimes included in this list are the pineal gland and the thymus. The function of the pineal gland is not known definitely. Persons who show calcification of the pineal body by roentgenogram without referable symptoms indicating a lack of need for this body are encountered occasionally. The thymus is a lymphoid organ and probably has no endocrine function.

The endocrine glands secrete hormones that are absorbed into the blood. These hormones are "chemical messengers" which have their effect on other organs of the body. Hormones of several glands may act together and enhance the effects of the others. Again, they may act antagonistically, maintaining a balance of activity.

The pituitary hormones activate or inhibit secretion in so many other endocrine glands that sometimes the pituitary is spoken of as the master gland. The pituitary gland or the hypophysis has two parts, an anterior and a posterior lobe, each with separate functions. When injected, posterior lobe preparations cause increased blood pressure, increased intestinal tonicity and peristalsis, increased respiratory rate and powerful contraction of the uterus, and they have an antidiuretic effect in diabetes insipidus. The most important hormones of the anterior lobe are those that promote growth and those that increase the function of the generative, the adrenal and the thyroid glands. Many other effects have been recorded.

Several of the hormones of the anterior lobe of the pituitary have been isolated in relatively pure form.

Of these, the adrenocorticotrophic hormone (ACTH) which stimulates the cortex of the adrenal glands is the most widely used in treatment of children. The gonadotrophic hormones, which stimulate the generative organs and the thyrotropic hormone, which increases the activity of the thyroid gland, are also available for therapeutic use. A growth hormone has been isolated, but its effect appears to be confined to experimental animals.

The effect of hormones in some instances depends on the ability of the receptor organ to respond. Abnormally increased secretion of the growth-promoting hormone of the anterior lobe of the pituitary gland results in exaggerated symmetric growth of the body (gigantism) if the epiphyses have not yet fused; as a consequence, the bones have capacity for growth in length. After fusion of the epiphyses, the increased secretion results in acromegaly, a condition of distorted growth in which various parts of the body increase in size without increase in body length.

Carbohydrate metabolism is controlled by the pancreas and the pituitary, the adrenal and the thyroid glands. The internal secretion of the pancreas, insulin, regulates the storage of glucose as glycogen. One of the pituitary hormones is antagonistic to insulin. Hyperpituitarism produces hyperglycemia and glycosuria. Hypopituitarism has the opposite effect. Adrenalin causes increase in blood sugar by calling out the glycogen stores from the liver and has other effects on sugar metabolism. The thyroid hormone causes increased combustion of sugar.

Anterior pituitary hormone stimulates the thyroid gland to increased secretion. Hyperthyroidism may be produced in this manner. Conversely, through lack of stimulation of the thyroid, decreased pituitary secretion lowers the basal metabolic rate and may produce hypothyroidism.

Growth and maturation of the body are dependent on proper functioning of the pituitary, the thyroid, the adrenal and the gonad or the sex glands. The pituitary is concerned directly with growth and also indirectly through stimulation of the gonads and the thyroid. The general maintenance of growth of body organs, especially of epiphyseal and periosteal bone growth, is the chief function of the growth-promoting hormone of the pituitary. The thyroid also directly affects growth because of its effect on metabolism.

The parathyroid glands control the level of blood calcium, using bone as the reservoir of calcium. Hypoparathyroidism produces tetany from low blood calcium. In addition to producing high blood levels and high rate of excretion of calcium, hyperparathyroidism causes disappearance of bone mineral, with resulting osteoporosis.

The adrenal glands have a medulla and a cortex. The medulla produces adrenalin or epinephrine, a material which increases blood pressure, increases the conversion of glycogen to glucose, stimulates the thyroid and inhibits the internal secretion of the pancreas. The cortex of the adrenal produces hormones essential for the metabolism of sodium, water and carbohydrate. Deficiency causes Addison's disease. An excess causes precocious puberty with masculinizing changes, regardless of sex. In Addison's disease, the major effect of cortical deficiency is on the kidney, which loses its ability to excrete certain materials, such as potassium, and to stop excreting sodium and chloride when these should be retained.

NORMAL SEXUAL DEVELOPMENT

The physical changes characteristic of puberty (see Chap. 3) are dependent on the presence of gonadal or sex hormones that are formed as a result of stimulation of the gonads by the gonadotropic hormones of the pituitary gland. The amount of secretion of gonadotropic hormones by the pituitary is negligible in early childhood but increases in late childhood to give the impetus to puberty development. These pituitary hormones maintain gonadal activity for many years.

The sex characteristics, particularly the secondary characteristics, are determined by the type of hormone formed in the greatest quantity and by the relative proportions of the two types of sex hormones. The sex hormones, both male and female, are similar chemically. Each person elaborates both types of hormones. The male sex hormones are called androgens and the female hormones, estrogens. Androgens give the body the male configuration and cause the normal hypertrophy of the male sex organs. Estrogens give the body the female configuration and cause normal hypertrophy of all female sex organs. Both types of gonadal hormones stimulate fusion of the epiphyses through repression of the pituitary growth hormone,

bringing growth in length to a stop. The process of epiphyseal fusion is slow, so that growth proceeds for a considerable time after puberty. The gonadal hormones have a powerful influence on psychic attitudes and general health.

The endocrine sex mechanisms in boys are relatively simple in comparison with the complicated cyclic changes which take place with menstruation in girls. The gonadotropic hormones of the pituitary not only stimulate the production of estrogen by the ovary but also stimulate the maturation of ova. As soon as the ovum begins to ripen, the follicle in which it is developing secretes further amounts of estrogen. This increased amount of estrogen causes increased growth of the inner lining of the uterus (endometrium) and increase in its vascularity. After the ovum has matured fully and has been extruded, the follicle site becomes filled with cells to form what is known as a corpus luteum. This is formed under the stimulus of a luteinizing hormone from the pituitary. The corpus luteum has a hormone of its own. The effect of this hormone on the uterus is to cause still further increase in the thickness, the vascularity and the gland development in the endometrium. The endometrial changes are in preparation for reception of the fertilized ovum. When the ovum is not fertilized it is not implanted in the uterus, and the corpus luteum immediately atrophies, and its hormone progesterone disappears. With the sudden decrease of progesterone, the outer portions of the hypertrophied endometrium slough off, producing menstrual flow.

In case a fertilized ovum becomes implanted, the corpus luteum persists and continues to form its hormone progesterone. Progesterone then suppresses estral rhythm, stimulates formation of the placenta and, together with estrin from the ovary, stimulates increased development of the gland and the duct tissue of the breast. A placental hormone also aids breast development. Progesterone inhibits the hormone of the pituitary, prolactin, which stimulates milk production. After the birth of the baby, progesterone disappears, and prolactin increases.

Even in the period of childhood, menstrual disorders which require hormone therapy may develop. A knowledge of the endocrine relationships is desirable in the management of these disorders. In a few instances, the use of some of these endocrine products and analgesics may be indicated for functional dysmenorrhea or excessive menstrual flow.

PRECOCIOUS SEXUAL DEVELOPMENT

CONSTITUTIONAL OR IDIOPATHIC PRECOCITY

Sexual development is regarded as being precocious when secondary sex characteristics appear before the age of 8 in girls and before the age of 10 in boys. Such an acceleration is about 4 times as common among girls as it is among boys. In both sexes the most common variety of sexual precocity is called constitutional or idiopathic precocity, signifying that there are no obvious associated abnormalities which might be presumed to set off the maturing effects of the pituitary gland prematurely.

In some instances there appears to be a hereditary predisposition within the child's family. The effects of this variety of sexual precocity may be upsetting to the family and to the child because of his abnormally mature appearance. No serious consequences result otherwise, and the child's age-mates eventually catch up to his development. The ultimate height of such boys and girls tends to be below the average, for, although a marked growth spurt usually occurs when sexual development first appears, the process also leads to early epiphyseal closure in the long bones of the skeleton, which in turn limits the duration of growth to an abnormally brief period.

INTRACRANIAL LESIONS

Intracranial lesions such as a preceding encephalitis or an unrecognized brain tumor may stimulate the precocious appearance of puberty. Usually there are other evidences of neurologic disturbance when this is the exciting cause.

TUMORS OF THE ADRENAL CORTEX

Certain tumors of the adrenal cortex in both boys and girls may elaborate an excess of androgen, in which case male secondary sex characteristics develop, including abnormal hypertrophy of the clitoris.

TUMORS OF THE GONADS

Rarely, tumors of the gonads may be responsible for precocious pubertal development. Interstitial cell tumors of the testis usually can be recognized by palpation, since they produce enlargement of one testis. Granulosa-cell tumors of the ovary are likewise discoverable by palpa-

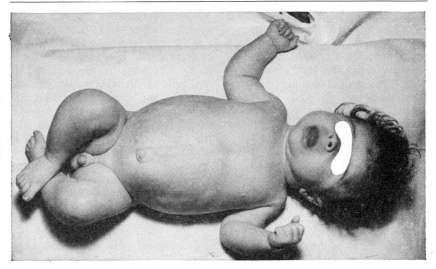

Fig. 63. A baby with cretinism.

tion. In such circumstances the tumor must be removed.

HYPOTHYROIDISM

CRETINISM

Cretinism is the condition produced by complete absence of thyroid secretion from birth. Cretinism occurs only sporadically in this country but is found endemically in goitrous regions of other countries. Sporadic cretinism is associated with congenital absence of the thyroid gland. The mother of the cretin is presumably normal. Cretins develop normally up to the time of birth because of the availability of the mother's thyroid secretion. The effects of lack of thyroid make their appearance gradually. The characteristic physical features do not appear for a period of from 3 to 5 months, although certain chemical changes in the blood characteristic of hypothyroidism could be de-

tected earlier if examination were made.

Once the condition of cretinism has developed fully it is distinctive and unmistakable, although the inexperienced often confuse it with mongolism. These children are conspicuously backward mentally and have characteristic physical abnormalities. The facial features are heavy and almost pathognomonic, although an adequate word picture of them is scarcely possible (Fig. 63). They lack the slant eyes and the epicanthic folds of the mongol. The tongue protrudes from the mouth; the voice or the cry is hoarse. Two cardinal symptoms of cretinism are absence of sweating and obstinate constipation. The skin is dry, and often the hair is coarse. Generally, growth in length is greatly retarded, the retardation showing itself chiefly in the short extremities. Because of slow bone development, the fontanel remains open far beyond the normal closing time. Roentgen examination of the bones discloses that the ossification centers appropriate for the chronologic age have failed to appear. Tooth eruption is delayed. The poor muscle tone leads to protrusion of the abdomen, and often there is an umbilical hernia.

In addition to the clinical appearance and behavior of the child, various laboratory tests may assist in confirming the suspicion that thyroid function is depressed. Radioactive iodine given by mouth fails to reach a normal concentration in the thyroid gland, as determined by the Geiger counter. Chemical examination of the blood shows an abnormally low level of iodine which is bound to protein (essentially a direct measurement of the quantity of thyroid globulin being manufactured). Blood lipids may be abnormally high. More cumbersome but useful are tests of basal metabolism and creatine excretion in the urine, both of which give low values in hypothyroidism.

Prognosis. The prognosis in cretinism depends on how early and how effectively treatment is given. If an adequate amount of thyroid is given very early, the physical growth will proceed in a normal manner, and the mental development will tend to be relatively normal. It is seldom that mental development is fully satisfactory, even with the best of treatment.

Treatment. The treatment consists of the administration of dried thyroid gland by mouth. The amount of thyroid should be the maximum that can be taken without symptoms of overdosage. A cretin infant will require from 0.5 to 1.5 grains daily. The original dose should be smaller and then the amount should be increased to tolerance. The diet should be complete and should include ample vitamin D. Without vitamin D, rickets is very likely to develop because of the very rapid rate at which the bone will grow when thyroid is first given. The symptoms of overdosage of thyroid are the same as those of hyperthyroidism, notably, vomiting, diarrhea, irritability, fever, rapid pulse and weight loss.

ACQUIRED HYPOTHYROIDISM

Occasionally, hypothyroidism of lesser degree than that of cretinism is encountered in childhood. All degrees of hypothyroidism exist, from the obvious to that detected only with special tests. When the condition is of at least moderate degree, both physical and mental growth is slowed (Fig. 64). The basal metabolic rate is decreased. The "bone age" is less than the chronologic age. Puberty is delayed. The child tends to be lethargic, the skin cool and dry and of a poor color. The cholesterol content of the blood is increased, and the phosphatase content is decreased. The creatine output in the urine is below normal.

Treatment. The treatment of these children consists of giving an appropriate dose of thyroid. The amount should be that which corrects the symptoms and less than that which produces nervousness or other evidence of hyperthyroidism. The child with hypothyroidism has good tolerance to thyroid medication. When thyroid is given in case of an erroneous diagnosis of hypothyroidism, as often happens in obesity, the toler-

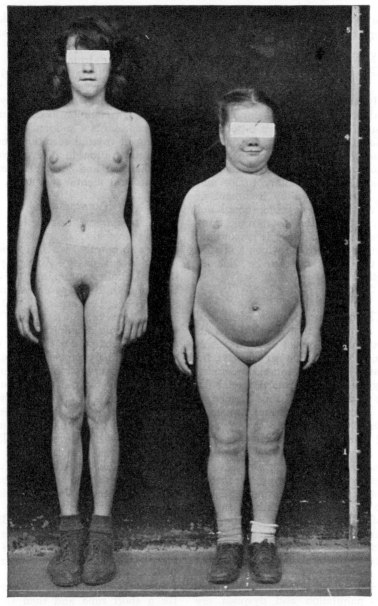

FIG. 64. Normal 12-year-old girl (*left*) contrasted with 13-year-old girl with hypothyroidism.

ance is poor, and nervousness develops quickly.

HYPERTHYROIDISM (TOXIC GOITER, EXOPHTHALMIC GOITER)

Hyperthyroidism as it occurs in childhood is more frequent in girls than in boys and has its onset most often near the time of puberty. The cause of increased thyroid secretion is not known. Toxic goiter has been observed with pituitary tumor and has been relieved by treatment of the tumor. It is possible, though not proved, that the thyrotropic hormone of the pituitary is responsible in other instances in which no lesion of the pituitary can be demonstrated.

SYMPTOMS

The onset usually is gradual. All the symptoms that develop are attributable to excess thyroid secretion. These include nervousness, increased pulse rate, muscle weakness, easy fatigue, increased metabolic rate and sweating. Fine tremor of the extended fingers and tongue is present. Despite increased appetite and food intake, many have weight loss because of increased metabolic rate. The rate of growth is increased, and the bone age ultimately advances above the chronologic age. The thyroid gland increases in size (goiter), and the eyeballs become prominent (exophthalmos). The urinary excretion is increased, and blood cholesterol is decreased from the normal. In the more severe intoxications, vomiting, diarrhea, cardiac palpitation and dyspnea are likely to be present.

The course of the disease varies, but the illness does not become dangerously severe so often in adolescents as in adults. In some instances it may become progressively and rapidly worse from the onset and cause death if no relief is given. More often, it progresses slowly with remissions. The so-called thyroid crisis is not common in children. A crisis represents a sudden large outpouring of thyroid secretion, resulting in prostration, high fever, vomiting, diarrhea and greatly increased nervous and mental symptoms.

TREATMENT

All symptoms, except the protruding eyeballs, decrease or disappear promptly when iodine is given. A customary iodine preparation is Lugol's solution, and the dose is from 5 to 10 drops daily. In the adult it may be expected that the symptoms will return despite continued iodine administration; consequently, iodine treatment is used as a preliminary procedure preparatory to the operation of removing much of the thyroid gland. In the child, continued use of iodine is more likely to be of lasting benefit, particularly when this treatment is combined with bed rest and sedative medication as indicated. In the child, continued medical treatment is well worth a trial and is successful in some instances. Hyperthyroidism in adolescence tends to be self-limited; it "burns itself out." If relapse should occur, resort to surgery can be had before the illness becomes severe. In these circumstances it is the preference of some surgeons to stop the iodine treatment for a short time and then start it again in preparation for the operation. The purpose of this procedure is to obtain relief from symptoms before operation and thus more certainly avoid a crisis.

The nonsurgical treatment of juvenile hyperthyroidism has been facilitated since the introduction of antithyroid drugs such as propylthiouracil and methylthiouracil. These substances given in doses of from 150 to 300 mgm. per day gradually will slow down the activity of the thyroid gland and in the course of 2 to 3 months may result in a decrease in basal metabolic rate and a subsidence of symptoms. If a maintenance dose can be found, then the child may carry on fairly normal activity. In some instances the drug can be withdrawn gradually after several months of treatment, without a return of symptoms. In some instances treatment is complicated by the appearance of rashes, fever or leukopenia due to the drug.

DIABETES MELLITUS

Diabetes mellitus is a condition in which part or all of the ability to utilize sugars has been lost because of deficiency of insulin, an internal secretion of the pancreas.

ETIOLOGY

The disease is less common among children than among adults and apparently more common among children in some parts of the country than in others. The primary cause of the disease remains obscure. Heredity apparently is a predisposing factor in many instances, but this factor is not obvious in many others. Occasionally, diabetes has its onset after an acute infection, but a causal relationship is not certain.

PATHOGENESIS

In diabetic children, digestion and absorption of food are unimpaired. Normally, absorbed sugar is stored as glycogen or converted into fat, and small amounts are being burned constantly to supply energy. In diabetes mellitus the ability to store, convert and burn the absorbed sugar is impaired or lost, and the sugar accumulates in the blood. When the amount in the blood increases above the renal threshold, sugar is excreted in the urine.

SYMPTOMS

The onset of diabetes is usually abrupt, since its preliminary stages may present no symptoms. Sugar may be discovered in the urine incident to a routine examination. As the disease appears, loss of weight and increased urination, thirst and hunger usually are present. The excess sugar requires water for its excretion and this accounts for the thirst and the polyuria. Since much of the food is not utilized the child loses weight, and increasing muscular weakness may be noted. When the disease has progressed rapidly from the onset, sometimes these early symptoms are of brief duration and pass unnoticed, the first observed evidence being a state of coma due to the development of severe acidosis.

Acidosis. The capacity of the body to burn fats is limited. When carbohydrate is not available for energy production, fat is mobilized for energy in amounts greater than can be burned completely. Much of the fat is oxidized incompletely, with the resultant accumulation of ketone bodies (acetone, diacetic acid and oxybutyric acid). When neutralized, these substances are only slightly toxic and are excreted readily in the urine. Their chief harmfulness arises because two of these substances are acids and require neutralization. The base is removed from the body, giving rise to acidosis, which easily becomes serious and is the usual cause of death of those with diabetes.

COURSE

When untreated or inadequately treated, the diabetic child continues to lose the ability to utilize sugar, and increasing amounts of insulin are required. The rate of downward progress is not constant for various children or even for the same child. Such factors as overexercise, infection, nervous exhaustion and excessive carbohydrate ingestion accelerate it. Soon or late, acidosis and coma supervene, and the child succumbs unless adequate emergency treatment is instituted promptly. Untreated diabetes in the young runs a relatively more rapid and more uniformly fatal course than in older patients. When the management is intelligent and consistent the diabetic child is as healthy as the normal child. Because of the thought and the care given to the diet, most diabetic children who are under good control are in a better physical state than the average nondiabetic children.

DIAGNOSIS

The symptoms that have been enumerated are strongly suggestive of the presence of diabetes but do not prove it beyond question. The finding of sugar in the urine is important but not conclusive evidence, since a few children have a low renal threshold for sugar (renal glycosuria) with entirely normal metabolism and blood sugar. The repeated finding of glycosuria, together with increased sugar in the blood, may be considered as conclusive. In such instances, in the uncommon mild case, the prediabetic phase of the disease or when one wishes to confirm or to exclude the existence of diabetes definitely, a sugar-tolerance test may be made.

Sugar-Tolerance Test. A sugar-tolerance test is useful only for diagnosis and not for the determination of the amount of sugar that may be permitted a diabetic child. The test is made before breakfast after a night of fast. Dextrose is given in solution by mouth in the amount of 1.75 Gm. for each Kgm. of body weight, or sometimes a standard dose is given regardless of age. The blood and the urine are examined before and at hourly intervals after the dextrose has been ingested. The normal child will not excrete sugar or have high blood-sugar values in these circumstances, while the diabetic child will. Normally, the blood contains some sugar at all times, the amount varying from 70 to 160 mgm. for each 100 cc., depending on the relation to meals. At slightly above this higher level sugar appears in the urine of the normal person. Sometimes a diabetic child has a renal threshold higher than normal.

PHILOSOPHY OF MANAGEMENT

Today there are two distinct ways of approaching the details of the management of a diabetic child. The traditional (strict diet or aglycosuric) method implies that the diabetic child must be controlled closely and meticulously if he is to have the best chance for a long life and freedom from the late complications of his disease. This school uses calculated, weighed diets, permits no departures from them without exact substitution of equivalent food and regulates the insulin dosage so closely that no sugar is excreted in the urine at any time. Advocates of the more recent (free diet, glycosuric) method do not believe that such exact regulation is necessary and that excretion of glucose in the urine is not by itself harmful. They feel that the child should be given freedom to follow a diet of his own choosing, provided that he avoids excesses and that his insulin need be regulated only with a view to keeping him from excreting ketone bodies. This latter school doubts that late complications are any more frequent with this type of management and feels that the child is much better off with the freedom and the lack of regimentation which their system provides. Actually, the general principles of the management of diabetes are the same in each instance, the main difference lying in the exactness with which physiologic correction is sought. Since the two approaches are quite different, each will be described.

STRICT DIET MANAGEMENT

The food requirements of the child are calculated carefully, a diet is prescribed, weighed and measured precisely, and its exact components taken at the same time each day. Insulin doses are arranged so that no sugar will be lost in the urine. Periodic adjustments of diet are made for growth and activity changes, and insulin doses are modified accordingly.

Food Requirements. The food requirements of a diabetic child are the same as those of a nondiabetic child of the same age. These are discussed elsewhere. Since the child has decreased ability to utilize carbohydrate, the concept became established that a large share of the energy requirement should be derived from fat and only a small portion from carbohydrate. However, it now is known that for diets of equal energy value the insulin requirement after stabilization of control remains the same regardless of the relative proportions of fat and carbohydrate. The older concept has been modified almost everywhere, and the general tendency is to have the relative amounts of these food components approximately the same as those found in the diet of the nondiabetic child. These more popular diets allow the child to feel less different from others and thus have a beneficial psychological value.

It is important that the foods selected to fill the specifications of protein, carbohydrate and fat be of such a nature that the mineral and vitamin needs also are supplied. According to one good method of management, the meals should be apportioned so that they are equal, each representing one third of the day's allowance. The food must be weighed carefully and all of it ingested. No other food of any nature is permitted. However, water is allowed.

Use of Insulin. In the case of some diabetic persons, adults more often than children, the nutritional requirements may be satisfied with a closely regulated amount of food which can be handled by the body without the use of insulin. The majority of diabetic children require more food than their unaided tolerance would permit. Insulin should be given in such quantities that sugar is not excreted in the urine, and blood sugar remains at an approximately normal level. When the child is receiving sufficient food and appropriate amounts of insulin he is in the same metabolic status as a nondiabetic child.

Insulin is prepared from the pancreas of animals. It is supplied in vials in solutions of various strengths designated as U20, U40, U80 and U100. These contain 20, 40, 80 and 100 units, respectively, to each cc. It is valueless by mouth and must be given hypodermically, intramuscularly or intravenously. Syringes graduated in cubic centimeters are entirely satisfactory for insulin administration, but special insulin syringes are available and are commonly used. They are graduated in terms of U20 insulin on one side and U40 on the other or in terms of U40 and U80. It should be remembered that if a certain volume of U40 insulin is required, twice this volume of U20 will be necessary to supply the same number of units, while only half the volume of U80 will be required. The dosage must be measured accurately, and to this end the syringe and the needle should be free from leaks.

DOSAGE. The dosage of insulin required varies for each child. The less the insulin supplied by the child himself, the more severe the diabetes and the more the insulin required by injection. The dosage is established by intelligently managed, trial-and-error procedure. It is important that the insulin be given as prescribed at the proper interval before a meal. The food allotment for the day is divided equally into 3 meals given the same number of hours apart, but the insulin dosage is not so divided. The child with severe diabetes usually requires 4 doses of insulin daily. A satisfactory distribution of the insulin has been found to be 35 per cent 30 minutes before breakfast, 22 per cent 30 minutes before the noon meal, 28 per cent 30 minutes before supper, and 15 per cent once during the night. When the child has mild diabetes, 3 and sometimes 2 daily doses will be satisfactory.

The initial doses of insulin frequently are based on the amount of excess sugar in the blood, and the subsequent doses on the amount of sugar lost in the urine. For this reason, it is desirable to collect the urine in 4 separate portions: (1) from breakfast to dinner, (2) from dinner to supper, (3) from supper to bedtime or the time of the night dose of insulin and (4) from previous collection until breakfast. By means of this division the adequacy of each dose of insulin is indicated. When diabetes is brought under control in this manner, it is customary to find that the child recovers some of his lost sugar tolerance, and as a consequence the insulin dosage must be lowered. Usually a stability in the insulin dosage is attained in the course of from 3 to 6 weeks, and the daily dosage becomes relatively constant. Certain uncontrollable factors, such as the amount of exercise and the occurrence of infection, may cause moderate variation from day to day. For this reason, constant checking and alertness are necessary. The insulin requirements will change also with the increased food necessary as the child grows. Blood-sugar determinations should be made at intervals, as it is possible for the blood sugar to be maintained at a level above normal and no sugar to appear in the urine.

INSULIN SHOCK. Occasions will arise when it will be evident that insulin is present in the body in excess of the immediate need. Such a condition may occur because of increased tolerance for food and a lessened need for injected insulin, because of error in calculation and administration of either the insulin or the diet, because some of the prescribed food is not eaten, is vomited or is utilized poorly because of diarrhea, or delay in eating or unusual exertion. In any of these circumstances more sugar is stored than should be, and too little is left for circulation and use. The sugar in the blood falls below normal limits, and insulin shock results. A definite group of symptoms is associated with this event. Any or all of the following may be observed: nervousness, irritability and possibly other personality changes such as silliness; a general drowsiness or lassitude; unusual hunger; either pallor or flushing, accompanied by dilation of the pupils and sweating; decreased response, perhaps leading to unconsciousness; local jerking or generalized convulsions. In mild insulin shock, only the first 3 or 4 symptoms may appear. The symptoms usually develop within a relatively short time and disappear within a few minutes after the child receives some sugar-containing food. For a mild attack, 1 ounce of orange juice and for a more severe attack, 2 ounces of orange juice should be given. If the attack persists for 15 minutes, the dose of orange juice should be repeated. If the child is unconscious or refuses to co-operate, the orange juice or the isotonic-sugar solution may be dropped into the mouth with a medicine dropper. Dextrose solution may be given intravenously. It is necessary to distinguish between insulin shock with coma and diabetic acidosis with coma. During insulin shock the urine is sugar-free, and the blood sugar is low. In diabetic acidosis, sugar is present in the urine, and the blood sugar is high.

Varieties of Insulin. The type of insulin referred to in the preceding discussion is designated as ordinary or regular insulin. Other varieties have been produced and some are in common use. Insulin has been prepared in combination with zinc in a crystalline form known as zinc-insulin crystals. It is dispensed in solution in the same unitages as ordinary insulin. A solution of zinc-insulin crystals has the same action as ordinary insulin and presents no advantage over ordinary insulin except that it is less likely to cause reaction at the injection site. Ordinary insulin, like the solution of zinc-insulin crystals, has an effect of relatively brief duration, several injections being necessary every 24 hours to keep diabetes in control. In the endeavor to produce an insulin product which would be absorbed more slowly and so have a more lasting effect, it was found that when insulin was combined with a very simple protein the desired effect was obtained. However, the resultant products are unstable and have poor keeping qualities. When they are combined with zinc, more stable products result.

PROTAMINE ZINC INSULIN. This has commercial distribution and is commonly used. The outstanding characteristic of protamine zinc insulin is its slow, continuous absorption. By its use, mild diabetes in some instances can be kept under control by a single injection daily. When the disease is sufficiently severe to require more than 1 dose of insulin daily, it is customary to give only 1 dose of protamine zinc insulin and to supplement this dose with other injections of ordinary insulin. By this means fewer total doses are required.

The advantage of fewer injections through the use of protamine zinc insulin may be outweighed by the dangers encountered in its use. Shock resulting from overdosage of ordinary insulin is recognized easily and responds readily to sugar by mouth, whereas shock from protamine zinc insulin tends to develop insidiously, become very severe and respond slowly to treatment, dextrose frequently being required by the intravenous route. The severity of the reaction and the slowness of response to treatment cause great alarm to attendants. When shock has occurred in the home, away from technical and laboratory facilities, it has resulted fatally in some instances.

GLOBIN ZINC INSULIN. This form is a more recent commercial product which is absorbed more slowly than regular insulin but more quickly than protamine zinc insulin. By its use it is possible to eliminate 1 or 2 doses of regular insulin. The night dose of regular insulin can be elim-

inated by giving about 43 per cent of the day's requirement as globin zinc insulin 1 hour before the evening meal and saving half of the milk from this meal to give from 3 to 4 hours later. This change can be made without altering the level of control.

NPH INSULIN. This is approximately a combination of two parts of regular insulin and one part protamine zinc insulin. It acts a little more slowly than globin zinc insulin, but its late effects do not persist as long as those of protamine zinc insulin.

FREE DIET MANAGEMENT

With this type of management, excretion of sugar in the urine is permitted, and the precise controls over diet and insulin are relaxed. This does not mean that supervision is abolished. Until the child and his parents learn the general principles of diabetic physiology and the vagaries of the individual child's disease, frequent consultations about diet, insulin adjustment and general hygiene are needed. Regular examination of the urine for the presence of sugar and acetone is required also.

The mother and the child are instructed in the requisites of a good diet. Although an exact intake is not prescribed, regularity and consistency are urged in order that insulin adjustment may be regulated easily. Periodically, the child's food intake is analyzed by the physician or the dietician in order to be sure that he is meeting his requirements for calories, proteins, minerals and vitamins. If he is lacking in any dietary respect, acceptable modifications of the diet are suggested. Excessive carbohydrate intake and between-meal feedings are discouraged but not forbidden.

Since exact control of glycosuria is not a goal, the administration of insulin usually can be reduced to a single injection of globin or NPH insulin once a day or a combination of protamine and regular insulin given simultaneously in 1 or 2 syringes. The urine is tested 3 or 4 times a day for both sugar and acetone. If there is intermittent glycosuria without acetone in the urine, the regulation is considered adequate. If glycosuria is continual but without acetone, periodic quantitative estimation of the amount of sugar being excreted per day is desiderable. If more than 30 Gm. are being lost in the average 24-hour period, the glycosuria is considered excessive and insulin is increased in an attempt to decrease the spillage. When acetone appears in the urine it is regarded as a danger sign which requires consultation with the physician in order to adjust the diet or the insulin or to arrange for an examination to discover an unrecognized infection. If the urine remains consistently free of sugar, usually insulin is reduced in order to avoid the appearance of insulin reactions.

The proponents of the free diet type of management of diabetes recognize the danger that parents and children will become too lax and casual in the regulation of the disease. However, they feel that in the long run most families can achieve a satisfactory regulation while avoiding the social disadvantages and the emotional rebellion which the stricter type of regimen sometimes induces.

MANAGEMENT OF SPECIAL CIRCUMSTANCES

Initial Effect of Treatment. When a diabetic child first comes under adequate care, the insulin requirement is always higher than it becomes subsequently. With the return of blood sugar to normal levels the child's ability to produce insulin increases. The insulin requirement eventually becomes stabilized, the time required depending on the closeness of control and on the state of nutrition. A longer period is required for the undernourished than for the well-nourished child.

Exercise has a striking effect in reducing the insulin requirement. Increase in muscular activity requires compensation either by increasing the food intake or by decreasing the dosage of insulin. Failure to make this compensation is the most frequent cause of insulin shock. For spasmodic increase in activity it is better to try to maintain a relatively constant dosage of insulin and give additional food at mealtime. For more prolonged periods of activity it is necessary to decrease the insulin dosage. A boy spending the summer at a camp with its active life requires much less insulin than when he returns to the sedentary life of school in the fall.

Emotional Disturbances. The effect of emotional disturbance may be as severe as that of infection and in the same direction in that the insulin requirement is increased. The insulin dosage is much easier to regulate for the emotionally stable child.

Acute Infections. During acute infections, the ability of the body to use sugar properly is lessened. As soon as the signs of any infection appear it is advantageous to increase the insulin dosage moderately in an attempt to prevent glycosuria. If glycosuria occurs, the insulin should be increased still more, and if symptoms of shock develop, the dose should be decreased. The diet should be made up of easily digested soft or liquid foods. With the more severe infections, fat should be reduced or eliminated. As convalescence takes place, the regular regimen is re-established.

Surgical Operations. Diabetic children withstand operative procedures well if proper care is given them. Details of management vary with the circumstances of operation. Insulin must be given before and during the postoperative period. Crystalline insulin usually is employed because of its short period of activity. If food cannot be tolerated, calories must be supplied by intravenous infusion of glucose. Many children can be restored to their usual regimen on the day after operation.

Acidosis. The mechanism by which acidosis develops already has been described. As long as the ketone bodies are formed in only moderate amounts and the body is able to excrete them without excessive drain on its supplies of base, acidosis does not develop. The condition then is known as ketosis. This is not a desirable or a healthful state of affairs, but the immediate danger is slight. With increased formation of ketone bodies the base of the body is depleted and acidosis develops. As it becomes severe enough to become clinically manifest, the following symptoms and signs may be noted: the respiration becomes

deep, rapid and without pause (air-hunger breathing) and remains thus until the child is in extremis, when it may become slow and shallow; the cheeks are flushed, the skin and the mouth are dry; nausea and vomiting are frequently present; thirst usually is extreme; the pulse is rapid and thready; the temperature is either normal or elevated; the white cells of the blood may be increased markedly; severe abdominal pain may be present.

As the acidosis increases in severity, the child becomes stuporous and then comatose. Death is the usual sequel to untreated diabetic coma. These various signs and symptoms usually do not appear suddenly but increase in severity rather insidiously during several days as a result of some infection or dietary mismanagement. If the urine is tested daily, as it should be, sugar and increasing amount of diacetic acid will be found, giving warning and making it possible to prevent or to relieve the acidosis promptly.

If the urine contains much diacetic acid and sugar but symptoms of acidosis have not developed, the child should be confined to bed, kept comfortably warm and given abundant fluids. The diet should consist of liquids; most of the fat-containing foods should be excluded. The dextrose equivalence of the previously prescribed diet or of a diet slightly lower in energy value should be maintained. The insulin dosage should be increased sufficiently to make the urine sugar-free. Usually this also will cause the disappearance of diacetic acid. The amount of insulin needed cannot be foretold. When the sugar excretion has lessened demonstrably, the extra insulin administration should be discontinued and the child put on the regimen described under treatment of diabetes.

If symptoms of acidosis are present, the treatment is similar to that just described but it must be more vigorous. The sugar content of the fluids ingested should be recorded, and every 2 to 4 hours the child should receive one unit of insulin for each gram of sugar ingested in the preceding period. If the child is vomiting excessively, it may be necessary to give intravenously 5 per cent dextrose in normal salt solution, to which insulin has been added, one unit for each gram of sugar. Two hundred and fifty cc. an hour can be given with benefit. In addition, extra insulin will be needed to consume the excess of sugar already present in the body. The amount needed will depend on the amount of sugar in the blood and the severity and the duration of the symptoms. Frequently, from 15 to 40 units, depending on the size of the child, will be required as soon as the diagnosis of acidosis is established. Supplementary doses of insulin should be given every hour or two. The total amount required in mid-childhood in the first 24 hours of treatment is usually from 75 to 125 units. The urine should be tested before each insulin injection, and the supplementary injections of insulin should be continued until the urine sugar is reduced markedly in amount. Concurrently, the diacetic acid should have decreased greatly or disappeared. When this has been accomplished the acidosis has been corrected. The respiration will have resumed its normal character. The administra-

tion of sugar-containing fluids and insulin should be continued until the urine is free from diacetic acid. When such large amounts of sugar are being given, it is desirable to administer thiamine in addition.

If at any time during the treatment of acidosis the urine should become entirely free from sugar, it is advisable to give an extra glass of fruit juice by mouth or from 50 to 100 cc. of 10 per cent dextrose solution intravenously. Unless the urine is examined at short intervals, it may become sugar-free, and the child may develop insulin shock. Symptoms of insulin shock might be interpreted as evidence of acidosis and lead to the administration of more insulin. Such a mistake could easily be fatal.

When acidosis is extreme, it is often useful to supplement the treatment as outlined with the intravenous administration of alkali or potential alkali. This phase of the treatment of acidosis is discussed in Chapter 19. During the period of recovery from severe acidosis it is desirable to administer solutions containing potassium, which is lost in large amounts during the acute stage of metabolic disturbance. Parenteral potassium is administered. cautiously and only after renal flow has been established. When the child is able to take oral fluids, liquids such as tea, fruit juice and milk will provide significant amounts of potassium. After the acidosis has disappeared, as evidenced by the disappearance of diacetic acid from the urine, the subsequent treatment is directed toward the re-establishment of the child on a regimen of suitable diet and insulin dosage, as already described. It is desirable to use a liquid diet for a day or two after recovery from acidosis, the fat content being kept lower than would be necessary later. Usually it is safe to give the child his calculated diet requirement within 2 or 3 days.

Nursing Care

The child who comes into the hospital for diagnosis or because he is acidotic or showing symptoms of insulin reaction will need careful observation and emotionally supporting nursing care. The symptoms that accompany the onset of diabetes, acidosis or insulin reaction are threatening. The child cannot help feeling less stable physically. He responds with changes in behavior and signs that indicate that he also is threatened psychologically. His parents and the hospital personnel are concerned about his symptoms. He responds to their concern with increased anxiety. As the nurse assists with the treatments previously discussed for the care of the child in acidosis or with symptoms of insulin reaction, she needs to be as sensitive to the child's psychological needs as she is to his need for immediate medical therapy. The child who comes into the hospital for diagnosis needs to know the purpose of each test to which he is being subjected. If he is too young or too ill to understand, he must be supported adequately, because his response to initial physical care will color his feelings about all subsequent care that he will require. If the child is well supported initially, the possibilities of developing wholesome attitudes toward his disease and its treatment will be greater.

Observation of the child's personality characteristics is essential in detecting signs that indicate a change in his physical status. The nurse must be able to distinguish between emotional upset and temporary personality change caused by low blood-sugar. If insulin shock is suspected, the child should be put to bed. If no sign of improvement is detected in 10 minutes, the physician should be notified. He may order dextrose water, orange juice or part of the milk from the next meal. Close observation should continue until the child is behaving normally.

The child with diabetes needs a routine that includes periods of rest and relaxation. In many instances he will require help in learning to relax, for often restlessness and anxiety are associated with the disease. An anxious child cannot relax. Carbohydrate metabolism can be altered by emotional disturbances. Therefore, it is obvious that the nurse should concentrate her efforts in alleviating his anxiety. Most children with diabetes have concerns about their physical status, their prognosis and the reasons why they have to have insulin and a dietary regimen that is different from that of other children. Some children feel guilty about their hostility and view their illness as punishment for misbehavior or evil thoughts and wishes. Discovering the child's concept of his disease, its treatment and the meaning that it has for him personally should precede teaching. Unless unrealistic notions are corrected, the child will derive little therapeutic value from the instruction.

The child's parents also will require guidance. Their attitudes toward the child, his disease and its treatment will become reflected in the child's feelings about himself. They will determine the kind of adjustment that he will make to his disease and the requirements of his care. Overprotection and oversolicitude increase the child's excitability. They arise from guilt and tension within the adult; they increase the child's anxiety and place undue emphasis upon the handicapping features of his disease.

When there are several children with diabetes in the ward, it is desirable to group them together for meals and for insulin administration. Instead of having their insulin at their bedside, they can have it in the treatment room. Insulin should be given first to those children who already are well adjusted to their medical regimen. This gives the child with recently diagnosed diabetes an opportunity to observe children who have adapted themselves to insulin administration.

When insulin is administered, the same care as when giving any hypodermic medication should be taken but with the following additions: the syringe should be dry before measuring the insulin; there must be no bubbles in the insulin; a cotton pledget should be held firmly over the site of injection for a few seconds to prevent leakage of insulin; and the site of injection should be selected with care. Injections may be given in the upper or the outer part of the arms and the thighs. Repeated injections in one area cause "insulin pads." To prevent them from developing, the legs and the arms should be used in rotation, and the injections should be given in rows.

Teaching the young child to cleanse the area and to choose one of the various sites of injection of insulin will stimulate his co-operation and divert his attention from the discomfort of the procedure. As he indicates his capacity, the child should be encouraged to give his own insulin. If the child is given a feeling of accomplishment with each success, he will become increasingly interested in the mechanics of the treatment. His interest and the use of his own power in giving the insulin will help him to master his fear of the procedure. Some 5-year-old children are capable of injecting the prepared insulin. With supervision, the average child between the eighth and the tenth years can be taught to measure the required dose in the syringe. Because insulin will be a daily requirement, it is imperative that the child learn to accept it in a matter-of-fact way. The manner in which the insulin is given during early years will greatly influence his feelings toward it in later years.

Specimens of urine should be collected methodically. When fractional specimens are desired, sufficient bottles plainly labeled with the date and the times at which collection began and ended (e.g., 7 to 11 A.M.) should be at hand. Gradually, the child with diabetes can learn to prepare and take the specimen to the laboratory, test it and report the results to the physician or to his mother if he is being cared for in his home.

Because the occurrence of glycosuria is such an important factor in the plan of treatment, collection of specimens may become an irksome routine for the older child and for the adult who must assume the responsibility for the preschool child.

If diabetes has developed after bladder control has been attained, little difficulty will be encountered. However, if it has not, care must be taken to prevent the personality distortions that result from coercive toilet training. The nurse or the mother must guard against over-anxiety when she is collecting specimens. It produces anxiety and tension and prevents the child from acquiring the inner controls that he desires and needs. Accomplishments should bring a satisfying response from the adults, and accidents should be accepted with patience and understanding. During preschool years the responsibility for specimens must rest with the adult. However, later it is a responsibility that the child is capable of assuming.

Infections and injuries should be prevented in such a way that the child does not come to feel that he is being overprotected because of his disease. Early symptoms of infection should be noted so that change in treatment may be begun before sugar tolerance has become greatly affected.

Although the diet is prescribed by the doctor and prepared by the dietitian, it is the nurse who helps the child accept his food happily. The child who is placed on a restricted dietary regimen must be helped to face the fact that his food in some ways differs from that served to other children or adults. Segregating him from the group because of food differences protects him from temptations that he eventually must learn to meet. It also will tend to make him feel different, which is an unwholesome attitude for him to acquire. If he is served at the table with other children, opportunities for teaching will present themselves. Little by little, the nurse can give him understanding of his particular dietary needs.

When planning menus for the child with diabetes, his food likes and dislikes should be taken into consideration. Forcing and urging a child to eat large quantities of disliked foods creates attitudes that are difficult to overcome. Personality problems may occur which are more difficult to treat than the diabetes. As the child matures, opportunities to assist in the planning and the preparation of his food should be provided.

When a child's appetite is unsatisfied the temptation to eat forbidden foods is increased, and he easily falls victim to it. The power of resistance to temptation is a matter of slow growth. A child with diabetes often is faced with a temptation that he has not learned to resist. The temptation may be greater at some times. When the blood sugar is low, the child becomes extremely hungry and is driven to satisfy his needs.

When a child gives in to temptation in the hospital or at home, he needs understanding and support. Many children give in to temptation because they have not lived long enough to develop controls from within. Scolding, labeling them as thieves or un-co-operative beings and punishing them provoke feelings of hostility, rebellion and resistance. Instead, they need help in building up their tolerance for frustration. Facing his desire for forbidden foods with him is a helpful means of supporting the child in his fight to resist temptations. When his problem is faced with him by an understanding adult he gets the strength that he needs for growth. The adult's faith in the child must be maintained consistently. When it is, the child will acquire a sense of responsibility for his own care.

Preparation for the child's home-going is imperative. In the hospital the parents' attitudes toward the child and his problems should be observed as a basis for guidance. The home should be studied so that environmental problems which might complicate his treatment or influence his adjustment to it may be eliminated. Parents of children with diabetes should receive repeated reassurance that the prognosis is favorable when adequate care is given. Many times the nurse will need to give the parents the confidence that they require in caring for the child. Until parental anxiety is relieved they will not be able to cope with their problems. Nor will they be able to accept the child as he is and provide him with the kind of support that makes it possible for him to make a constructive adjustment to the realities that he must meet.

Confidence can be developed through learning experiences that bring competence. The parents can be taught to calculate diets and to prepare and administer insulin. They also can be taught to recognize the early symptoms of acidosis and insulin shock and to carry out the emergency treatments for them, should they occur. Parents cannot know too much about their child's disease, for it is through knowledge and wholesome attitudes that self-assurance is gained. The child also needs to know about his disease and

the values of treatment in supplying his body with what he needs for health. Self-responsibility is the outgrowth of self-acceptance and knowledge. Self-understanding is the child's birthright. Denying him this privilege robs him of his right to competence!

For many mothers the administration of insulin will be the most difficult feature of the child's care. So much depends upon the mother's attitude, and it is here that the nurse can make a contribution to the mental hygiene of the family. Understanding supervision of the mother is essential. Her fear needs acceptance. Permitting her to voice her feelings will give the nurse clues concerning the meaning of the procedure to the mother. She may see the treatment as punishment. If she does, she may be inhibited in acquiring competence. If she feels that it is a punishing act, the nurse can help her to see its therapeutic value—that it is in reality an act of giving what is necessary to keep him in a state of health.

As the child with diabetes approaches maturity he will need help in reappraising and accepting himself. He should have additional support to surmount the developmental tasks of the period. Frequently feelings of despondency, of introspection and of inferiority are discovered in adolescent diabetics. They need help in acquiring a mental attitude that will enable them to face life in a reasonably contented way. There is no cure for diabetes. This fact the adolescent must face, accept and handle. Everyone has a handicap of one kind or another. The wholesome solution is to face it with the feeling that it is a surmountable problem that need not hinder the individual's capacities for self-realization and productivity.

It has been estimated that approximately 50 per cent of cases of coma occur between the ages of 10 and 15. Prepubescent physical growth accounts for some, but psychological change seems to have a greater bearing on the occurrence of complications. During preadolescence and early adolescence, self-discipline becomes more difficult. There is a strong urge for recognition, to be like others and for self-expression and independence. Parental devaluation and doubt of parental control increases, and the adolescent tends to rely on his own judgment, which too often has not become strengthened through sufficient experience. All routine to the adolescent is irksome, and the routine that diabetes requires adds duties which are viewed as "boring," "bothersome" and sometimes even "useless." He exceeds his dietary regimen, not always because of physical needs but because of psychological needs produced by growth. The adolescent is driven to express his independence, to be like others and to rebel against authority. One excess in diet produces no immediate catastrophe, but an accumulative effect is produced without his realization.

Many of the problems of adolescence could be prevented if opportunities for self-direction were given gradually as the child showed the capacity to handle them. To survive, the child with diabetes must learn self-control and must achieve the capacity to take responsibility for

himself. This growth can come only with experience that provides opportunities to develop his inner resources. Autocracy provokes rebellion and provides no freedom to acquire the capacity for self-direction. The preadolescent and the adolescent need guidance that is different from what was appropriate during the school-age period. They have grown; they want a new status and opportunities to become increasingly more independent. The teen-ager with diabetes has the same needs as the normal youngster and has equally as much capacity for acquiring self-direction. Democratic guidance will give him the support that he requires to achieve responsibility for his own behavior.

DIABETES INSIPIDUS

Diabetes insipidus is a condition in which the water excretion by the kidneys is abnormally large, with the result that the intake also must be large in compensation. The kidneys are normal but do not function normally because of lack of the controlling posterior pituitary hormone. This lack causes a lowered threshold for water. Because of the large quantity of water excreted, the urine has a very low specific gravity (1.002).

Diabetes insipidus may be caused by various conditions that disturb pituitary function. Thus, it may occur in cases of brain tumor located in or near the pituitary gland, particularly in the neighboring hypothalamic region. It may occur as a result of encephalitis or other inflammation of the hypothalamic region. In some instances it has resulted from traumatic injury to the brain. In many instances no lesion can be demonstrated, and the disease is on an idiopathic basis.

SYMPTOMS

The symptoms of the idiopathic disease may consist only of drinking and excreting large amounts of water. The nutrition may suffer because the drinking of so much water is likely to interfere with the taking of sufficient food.

TREATMENT

The treatment consists of regular daily administration of posterior pituitary hormone and of attention to the underlying brain lesion, when such exists. Such conditions as brain tumor are more dangerous to life than diabetes insipidus. Certain of the brain lesions are not amenable to treatment.

When the disease is idiopathic, administration of posterior pituitary hormone is the only treatment needed. Pituitrin may be given hypodermically in a dosage of from 0.5 to 1 cc. once or several times a day as needed. Posterior lobe material may be given intranasally, either in solution or as a powder of prepared dried gland. Insufflation of a prepared powder is usually the procedure of choice because of ease of administration and lower cost. The powder may be used as snuff or it may be given by means of a powder blower. It should not be given in such quantity at one time as to cause sneezing, and the nose should not be blown for 2 hours. The dose for the adult is approximately 40 mg. 3 or 4 times a day; the dose for the child is proportionate to size and age.

SITUATIONS FOR FURTHER STUDY

1. If diabetes were discovered while a 5-year-old child was hospitalized for treatment of appendicitis and you had the responsibility of giving his first injection of insulin, how would you proceed?

2. If a child 4 years old with diabetes were eating at the table with a group of normal children, what would you do if he reached for a cookie from the nondiabetic children's supply? If a diabetic child 8 years old were seen taking cake from the food truck, what should be done?

3. Study a teen-ager with diabetes. At what age did the diabetes develop? What is his attitude toward the disease? Is he well-informed about his needs as a diabetic? Does he accept insulin in a matter-of-fact way? Can he prepare and give it to himself independently? How well developed socially is he? Does he enjoy being with a group or does he prefer solitude? Does he show feelings of inferiority? Is he irritable or emotionally unstable? What type of situations produce excitability? Does he accept his diet pleasantly or does he make suggestions that should be used in planning his diet? What characteristics of adolescence does he manifest? How does his developmental status influence his attitude toward his diabetic regimen? What is his relationship with his parents? Have they encouraged independence and self-reliance or have they tended to overprotect or neglect his need for

growth? How have their attitudes toward him and his disease influenced his behavior? How could you increase their insight into the developmental needs of a teen-ager?

BIBLIOGRAPHY

Blake, F. G.: Development and care during the preadolescent period 10 to 12 years), p. 360, and Development and guidance during adolescence, p. 381, *in* The Child, His Parents and the Nurse, Philadelphia, Lippincott, 1954.

Brown, G. D.: The development of diabetic children with special reference to mental and personality comparisons, Child Develop. **9:** 175, 1938.

Bruch, H., and Hewelett, E.: Psychologic aspects of the medical management of diabetes in childhood, Psychosom. Med. **9:**205, 1947.

Fischer, A. E.: The emotional factors in the treatment of diabetic children, Proceedings of the Am. Diabetes Assn. **7:**217, 1947.

————: Factors responsible for emotional disturbances in diabetic children, Nerv. Child **7:**78, 1948.

Robinson, Pauline: A child with diabetes, Am. J. Nursing **51:**690, 1951.

Wilkinson, Margaret: Diabetes mellitus in adolescence, Am. J. Nursing **50:**126, 1950.

Diseases of the Blood

◇◇

PHYSIOLOGIC CONSIDERATIONS
ANEMIA
LEUKEMIA
MALIGNANT LYMPHOMA
INFECTIOUS MONONUCLEOSIS

INFECTIOUS LYMPHOCYTOSIS
PURPURA
HEMOPHILIA
SITUATIONS FOR FURTHER STUDY

PHYSIOLOGIC CONSIDERATIONS

Blood consists of a fluid portion known as plasma and of formed components or cells. The plasma comprises slightly more than 50 per cent of the volume of the blood. Among the many functions of the plasma are the carrying of food materials to all parts of the body and the carrying away of waste products for excretion.

The plasma is concerned with blood clotting. A blood clot is formed by conversion of fibrinogen of the plasma to fibrin, which forms the coagulum. Fibrin is formed under the stimulus of thrombin. Thrombin is formed from the prothrombin of the blood through the action of thromboplastin derived from damaged blood platelets and from injured tissues. The calcium of the blood also is necessary for clot formation. That part of the plasma which remains after the fibrin is separated is serum.

The formed components of the blood consist of red cells (erythro-cytes), white cells (leukocytes) and platelets (thrombocytes).

In fetal life and earliest infancy the red cells are formed in the liver, the spleen, the bone marrow and other lymphatic structures; after birth they are formed in the bone marrow. The mature red cell has no nucleus, but a nucleus is present in an early stage of its formation. In fetal life, nucleated red cells are common in the blood, and some may be found in the early days after birth, particularly in prematurely born babies.

After the earliest period of life, the finding of nucleated red cells means an abnormally rapid formation of red cells to supply a demand, as in the case of some of the anemias of infancy. A lesser degree of immaturity of red cells is shown by persistence in the cell of material known as reticulum, which is identified easily in a specially stained preparation of blood. Normally, red cells are being destroyed constantly and being replaced by new ones. As evidence of normal speed of generation and replacement, approximately 1 per cent of the red cells of the blood is reticulated (reticulocytes). An increase above this proportion indicates rapid cell generation, and, similarly, the converse is true. In the anemias, a knowledge of the proportion of reticulocytes is important for diagnosis and prognosis.

The chief function of the red cells is to carry hemglobin, and the chief purpose of hemoglobin is to take oxygen to the tissues and remove carbon dioxide for excretion by way of the lungs. Hemoglobin is formed by the reticuloendothelial cells of the bone marrow. In the normal disappearance of red cells from the blood, the cells are removed by the reticuloendothelial tissues, especially those of the spleen. The hemoglobin of the cells is broken down. The iron of the hemoglobin is split off and is largely reused. The pigment is changed to bile pigment and is excreted.

The white cells of the blood consist of granular leukocytes or granulocytes, lymphocytes and monocytes (large mononuclear leukocytes). The mature lymphocytes and monocytes have no important subdivisions. Granular or polymorphonuclear leukocytes are of 3 varieties: neutrophils, eosinophils and basophils. The granular leukocytes are formed in the bone marrow, the lymphocytes develop in the spleen, the lymph nodes and other lymphatic tissue, and the large mononuclear leukocytes have their origin in the reticuloendothelial lining of the blood sinuses of the spleen, the bone marrow, the liver and the lymph nodes.

In the course of development of granulocytes, the type of cell imme-diately preceding the mature cells is known as a myelocyte. Myelocytes differ from mature cells in their appearance and staining characteristics when a stained preparation is examined microscopically. The presence of myelocytes in the blood indicates an unusually rapid formation of granulocytes. The abundance of myelocytes characterizes the disease myelocytic leukemia.

The mature lymphocyte is small in comparison with the larger and more deeply staining immature form. The immature forms are found abundantly in lymphatic leukemia.

The white blood cells seem to have no physiologic function in health other than to serve as a part of the defense mechanism of the body against infections. They are actively motile and penetrate tissues, especially at the site of infection. An increase in the number of neutrophils in the blood is often evidence that an infection is present and is stimulating the increase. After these leukocytes have migrated to the site of infection, they ingest and destroy many, though not all, varieties of bacteria. The so-called pyogenic infections stimulate an increase in the polymorphonuclear leukocytes. Other types of infection cause an increase in the lymphocytes of the blood. The eosinophils are increased especially in parasitic infestations.

The blood platelets or thrombocytes are formed in the bone marrow. The chief function of the platelets concerns blood coagulation. Platelets adhere to injured surfaces. In a wound, they quickly become damaged. Damaging of platelets releases thromboplastin, which initiates clot formation. When platelets are decreased greatly in the blood, spontaneous bleeding or purpura results. While platelets are important in the prevention of spontaneous bleeding, they are of less importance than the injured tissues in stopping hemorrhage from a wound. Injured tissues are a more important source of thromboplastin in these circumstances. Another important function of platelets is associated with their tendency to agglutinate. Thrombi in blood vessels sometimes consist mainly of agglutinated platelets. Agglutination in the terminal vessels of a wound assists in stopping bleeding.

lion, where it remains permanently. The amount of hemoglobin at birth varies, with an average value of 17 Gm. for each 100 cc. of blood. The amount decreases for a period of from 10 to 12 weeks to 10 to 12 Gm., with subsequent increase of the lower values to approximately 12 Gm., where it tends to remain during infancy. The value rises through childhood. The rise is more rapid early in childhood and less rapid later. Adult values are reached at about 16 years of age. These values are from 14 to 16 Gm. for boys and as much as 2 Gm. less for girls. Average values vary geo-

NORMAL BLOOD VALUES AT DIFFERENT AGES

	BIRTH	12 WKS.	6 MOS.	2 YRS.	12 YRS.
Red cells (millions/cu.mm.)	4.5-5.5	3.5-4.5	4.0-4.5	4.3-4.7	4.5-5.0
Hemoglobin (grams/100 cc.)	15.5-18.5	10-12	11-13	12-13.5	13.5-15
White cells (average/cu.mm.)	20,000	12,000	12,000	10,000	8,000
Platelets (average/cu.mm.)	350,000	300,000	300,000	300,000	300,000

The number of red cells at birth varies from 4.5 to 5.5 million for each cubic millimeter of blood. The number decreases rapidly in the first 7 to 10 days, the resultant hemoglobin breakdown often causing the so-called physiologic jaundice. Subsequently, the decrease is slower. The lowest number (3.5 to 4.5 million) is reached at from 6 to 12 weeks. Then the number gradually increases and at 6 months averages between 4 and 5 million. Subsequently, the number increases to a mean value of approximately 5 mil-

graphically, the variation being dependent chiefly on the iron content of the soil and its vegetation.

The total number of white cells (exclusive of platelets) may be 20,000 or more for each cubic millimeter of blood on the day of birth. The number decreases rapidly to a total of from 10,000 to 15,000 by 2 weeks. Thereafter the decrease is slow. The number is between 9,000 and 14,000 at 1 year, between 8,000 and 13,000 at 2 years and between 7,000 and 12,000 thereafter in childhood. The large mononuclear cells, the eosinophils and the basophils maintain a small but fairly constant proportion of the total white cells throughout infancy and childhood, ranging from 1 to 4 or 5 per cent. The chief variations with age are in the relative proportions of lymphocytes and polymorphonuclear leukocytes and in the numbers of immature white cells. The proportion of immature cells may be as high as 20 per cent in the early days of life, but very few, if any, are to be found after 6 months of age. The polymorphonuclear leukocytes predominate at birth but decrease to equal the lymphocytes between 1 and 2 weeks of age. Thereafter the lymphocytes predominate until late in the second year, when the two are again equal. Subsequently, the polymorphonuclear leukocytes permanently outnumber the lymphocytes during health.

The number of platelets varies, but the variations with age are not remarkable. The number tends to be slightly higher in the first year than later. A normal value after the first year is between 200,000 and 350,000 for each cubic millimeter.

ANEMIA

GENERAL DISCUSSION

Anemia literally means without blood. Sometimes the term is used in this sense in relation to organs of the body, such as anemia of the brain, a condition in which the supply of blood to the brain is greatly reduced. More commonly the word "anemia" is used to designate a condition in which the concentration of red blood cells or of hemoglobin or of both in the circulating blood is reduced below

normal. Usually, in childhood anemia the level of hemoglobin is the more important figure to consider.

Classification. Normally, red cells and hemoglobin are formed at the same rate at which they are destroyed. Anemia occurs whenever formation is decreased or destruction is increased. In the growing child the rate of formation also must keep pace with the demands of a body which is increasing in size. Except for the circumstance in which blood is lost from the body by hemorrhage, these two mechanisms are the sole fundamental causes of anemia. However, in many conditions there is a combination of the two mechanisms (or even of three mechanisms if we include blood loss) taking place, and a strict classification of anemias on this basis is not made easily. In the table which follows, the principal mechanisms of anemia are outlined with examples of specific disorders in which these mechanisms operate as the main cause of the resulting anemia.

PRINCIPLE MECHANISMS PRODUCING
ANEMIA IN CHILDHOOD

Blood loss (hemorrhage)
    Acute (trauma, operation, purpura, hemophilia)
    Chronic (ulcerative colitis)
Inadequate rate of blood formation (hypoplasia)
    Poor hemoglobin synthesis (prematurity, iron deficiency)
    Delayed red cell maturation (megaloblastic anemia, scurvy)
    Combination of above factors
    Infection (chronic respiratory, nephritis, rheumatic fever)
    Drugs (tridione, folic acid antagonists, nitrogen mustard)
    Poisons (lead, benzol)

Bone marrow invasion (leukemia, tumors)
Other (idiopathic anemia, hypersplenism, radiation injury)
Increased blood destruction (hemolysis)
Antibody reactions (erythroblastosis, transfusion reaction)
Hereditary trait (congenital hemolytic jaundice, sickle-cell anemia, Mediterranean anemia)
Drugs (sulfanilamide, acetanilid)
Poisons (naphthalene, fava bean)
Infections (malaria, septicemia)
Other (acquired hemolytic anemia, Lederer's anemia)

Symptoms. The symptoms of anemia are similar regardless of the cause. Lassitude, listlessness and fatigability are the early manifestations. As the severity increases, pallor, weakness, tachycardia and palpitation may occur. It is surprising how well a child with chronic anemia can get along. Compensations for the low level of hemoglobin often permit fairly normal activity when the concentration is reduced to a third of the normal value. However, persistence of such levels results in mental sluggishness, irritability and cardiac enlargement. Fatal anemia is a consequence of the inability of the heart to perform its normal work.

General Treatment and Nursing Care. The management of anemia will depend upon the severity and upon the presumptive cause in the individual case. Transfusion is the obvious and most widely applicable method of correction. It is imperative and often lifesaving when acute blood loss or severe chronic anemia has progressed to the point of interfering with cardiac function. It also may be useful in supplying missing blood elements other than red blood cells and hemoglobin (coagulation

factors in hemophilia and platelets in purpura, for instance). Even in anemia of lesser severity it often provides the child with a sense of well-being and permits better appetite and a more active existence. In some forms of anemia it is the only possible method of ameliorating the failure of an inactive bone marrow. The nursing management of transfusion has been considered in Chapter 6.

Anemia which is due to insufficient intake of iron or to loss of the body stores of iron through hemorrhage requires an increase in the iron intake. This supplies the missing element necessary to build new hemoglobin and also stimulates the activity of the bone marrow. Iron may be given by mouth in a number of ways. Ferrous sulfate, ferric ammonium citrate and ferrous glycinate are some of the compounds in common use. In infants particularly, it is desirable to start with a small dose and work up to the desired level gradually, because it sometimes irritates the gastro-intestinal tract, and vomiting and diarrhea may result. When adequate dosage is achieved the stools usually assume a dark-green or black pigmentation. In occasional circumstances iron is given intravenously. Sometimes copper and cobalt salts are added to the iron medication in the hope of augmenting its erythropoietic powers.

Vitamin B complex factors such as folic acid, vitamin B_{12} and liver or liver extracts are essential adjuvants in treating some of the anemias associated with a megaloblastic bone marrow. In scurvy the correction of the deficiency by treatment with vitamin C rapidly helps the associated anemia.

Splenectomy is usually curative in congenital hemolytic jaundice and sometimes is used to advantage in Mediterranean anemia and other forms associated with tremendous enlargement of the spleen. In nursing the older child with anemia, supportive measures are essential. Good general hygiene to build up resistance to intercurrent infections is important. Anorexia is a common symptom, and encouragement is often necessary to help the child to eat foods that are high in vitamins, calories and iron. Observation to note symptoms of fatigue should be made during the meal periods. Often these children are too weak to feed themselves and yet they resent being completely dependent during this routine. Allowing the child to begin feeding himself, giving him help when fatigue is apparent and then, after a rest, giving him an opportunity to finish independently often will influence his acceptance of larger quantities of food and satisfy his desire for independence.

In play, overfatigue must be guarded against. Some children stop playing when they are tired, but more of them become absorbed in play and do not react to fatigue until they become overstimulated. Redirection of play into less strenuous activities, such as doing puzzles or molding clay, should take place before injurious overstimulation develops.

When periodic transfusions require hospitalization, the nurse and the parents should help the child to meet the problem of frequent separations which involve procedures difficult for a young child to face. As a child grows old enough to understand, his interest and co-operation can be won by showing him a blood smear under a microscope and demonstrating to him the way in which a transfusion set gives him blood to increase his ability to do the things that other children are capable of doing. It is not uncommon to see a child with anemia accept his transfusion happily because he has learned from experience that co-operation brings less pain, recognition for his achievement and an increased amount of energy which is necessary to satisfy his need for activity. Emotional trauma produced by necessary blood counts can be lessened if the technician will give the child opportunity to investigate the apparatus, to cleanse the area and to assist in manipulating the equipment.

If an individual child's personality characteristics and interests have become known during hospitalization, helping him to adjust on subsequent admissions is facilitated greatly. When a child is greeted by a head nurse and a doctor who know and understand him, it gives him a sense of security and lessens the discomfort he feels when he returns to the hospital. A favorite toy may be in readiness, and in some instances it may be feasible to allow the child to select his own bed location. Encouraging the child to make his own preparations for the hospital trip may bring satisfactions that compensate in part for the uncomfortable aspects of the experience.

ANEMIA DUE TO BLOOD LOSS

When there is sudden loss of blood from the body as from a severe epistaxis, a freely bleeding wound or a gastro-intestinal hemorrhage, the disturbance in body physiology is not related to the loss of blood cells alone, but in addition there is a loss of the plasma portion of the blood with reduction in the circulating blood volume. Thus, in addition to the effects of anemia, the child also may be suffering from shock. Treatment consists of transfusion and, of course, appropriate measures to terminate the hemorrhage.

The common causes of excessive blood loss vary with the age of the child. In the newborn the common causes are an improperly tied umbilical cord, birth injury from a difficult delivery and free bleeding from the gastro-intestinal tract. In the infant, bleeding from the bowel is most common. In the older child it is more commonly the result of a traumatic accident or a defect in the clotting mechanism of the blood, such as hemophilia or purpura.

When blood loss occurs at a slower rate, as from chronic ulcerative colitis or bleeding from an intestinal polyp, the reduction in blood volume does not take place, and the symptoms are due chiefly to the resulting anemia. Treatment is directed at the underlying cause and may include transfusion as a temporarily supportive measure.

NUTRITIONAL ANEMIAS

Hypochromic or Iron-Deficiency Anemia. The most common form of anemia in infants is that which develops from a failure of the child to take in enough iron in his diet to supply building material for the new hemoglobin which he needs for his expanding size. The anemia is characterized by a relatively normal production of red blood cells. The cells are smaller than normal in size and very deficient in hemoglobin content, so that each may contain less than half the normal quantity. This type of anemia is called hypochromic or microcytic. It occurs between the ages of 9 months and 2½ years. Almost invariably the infant is one who has developed an inordinate fondness for milk, consuming 1 or 2 quarts per day and refusing most other foods. In spite of rather severe degrees of anemia, there is little interference with activity. The child is usually pale, irritable and obstinate about his refusal of solid foods. Treatment consists of the addition of one of the iron preparations to his daily milk ration. This usually produces a rapid improvement in anemia and at the same time increases the appetite for foods other than milk so that gradually the child can be encouraged to accept a diet which is better balanced nutritionally. Restoration of normal blood values can be expected in 4 to 8 weeks' time. If the anemia is so severe that the circulation is embarrassed or if the child is otherwise ill, it may be necessary to effect a more rapid correction by transfusion.

Megaloblastic Anemia. During fetal life the bone marrow contains very large cells (megaloblasts) which are the precursors of the fetal red blood cells. Normally, these large cells disappear from the bone marrow during the last weeks of intra-uterine life and are replaced by a smaller type of cell (erythroblast) which is the precursor of the adult type of red blood cell. Under certain clinical conditions megaloblasts may persist in the bone marrow after birth or may return to it.

Their presence in the bone marrow can be detected only by marrow aspiration, but it may be suspected when the circulating blood contains red cells which are larger than normal (macrocytes) or when anemia is accompanied by a sharp decrease in the number of red blood cells in the circulating blood in addition to the reduction of hemoglobin. In hypochromic anemia, as described above, each red blood cell carries an abnormally small quantity of hemoglobin, but the number of cells is close to normal. In megaloblastic anemia the number of cells is decreased, but each cell may carry a normal quantity of hemoglobin (normochromic) or even an increased quantity (hyperchromic), due to its large size.

A variety of clinical circumstances may precede the development of megaloblastic anemia. These have in common a disturbing effect upon the normal metabolism of folic acid, folinic acid (citrovorum factor), vitamin B_{12} or vitamin C. These disturbances in turn interfere with the synthesis of nucleoproteins which are necessary for the maturation of the red blood cells. The clinical conditions which may result in megaloblastic anemia are not very common. Among them are scurvy, dietary deficiency of folic acid, pernicious anemia, celiac disease and certain varieties of liver disease. Treatment depends upon the exact nature of the metabolic disturbance, but in most instances correction can be achieved by giving liver extract, vitamin B_{12}, folic acid or vitamin C.

ANEMIA OF INFECTION

With repeated acute infections or with chronic infection of long standing, some degree of anemia usually is found. Increased red cell destruction is sometimes a factor, but the more severe effect of infections is on the blood-forming tissues. The formation of hemoglobin is retarded in most instances, with a secondary effect of decreased formation of red cells. In other instances, in addition the blood generative cells are affected adversely, a condition known as hypoplasia when the decreased formation is partial and as aplasia when it is complete. Hypoplasia may outlast the infection. In many instances, the hypoplasia does not affect the generation of white cells; rather, a leukocytosis occurs. A few infections cause deficient generation of both white cells and platelets. If aplasia of granular leukocytes (agranulocytosis) occurs, the condition becomes serious, and death is likely to result. In the case of most of the infections, the anemia is neither severe nor serious.

HYPOPLASTIC TYPES OF ANEMIA

Under this heading are included those forms of anemia in which the *main* abnormality is the inability of the bone marrow to manufacture new red blood cells and hemoglobin at a rate which will support a normal concentration of these substances in the circulating blood.

Anemia of Prematurity. At the time of his birth the premature infant usually has average normal values of hemoglobin and red cells. Likewise, he has a store of iron from his mother which is appropriate for his small size. However, since he grows at a very rapid rate during the first few months of life and since his diet contains very little iron, his bone marrow is frequently unable to keep pace with the demands for new blood cells, particularly with the demand for more hemoglobin. In consequence an exaggerated decline of the red blood cell count and of the hemoglobin level of the blood takes place. This is similar to the fall in values suffered by the full-term infant but is more exaggerated in degree. The smaller the premature at the time of his birth, the more severe his anemia is likely to become during these first few months.

Usually, iron is given to prematures routinely in an attempt to prevent or to lessen the degree of fall in hemoglobin. Success in this type of therapy is not always achieved for it now seems to be true that the premature is not able to absorb and utilize iron very well for the first 6 to 8 weeks of his life. Usually the hemoglobin can be permitted to fall as low as from 6 to 8 Gm. per cent. A more marked degree of anemia may demand transfusion.

Drugs and Poisons. A number of substances which are used in treatment of childhood diseases or are ingested accidentally by children may interfere with the formation of red cells and hemoglobin by the bone marrow. Tridione, chloromycetin, arsphenamines, the folic acid antagonists used in the treatment of leukemia and nitrogen mustards are examples of therapeutic agents which must be controlled with periodic blood examinations. To this list the effects of radiation from roentgen therapy or from the use of radioactive compounds in the treatment of neoplastic diseases must be added. Lead and benzene derivatives are the most common types of poison that may depress bone-marrow activity.

Bone-Marrow Invasion. In leukemia and in some of the tumors of childhood which have widespread metastases (neuroblastoma of the adrenal, for instance) there may be so much replacement of normal marrow tissue that an insufficient quantity remains available to form new blood cells. This type of anemia also is called myelophthisic anemia.

Miscellaneous Causes. Congenital and idiopathic types of hypoplastic and aplastic anemia are known to occur. In the congenital variety the failure to form sufficient red cells is present at birth. In the idiopathic variety the deficiency appears later in life for unknown reasons. Hypoplastic anemia implies that the rate of formation of red cells is slowed; aplastic anemia implies that the formation of red cells has stopped altogether. Usually there is an associated defect in the formation of the other elements of the blood, such as the platelets and the white blood cells. Stimulation of the sluggish bone marrow is sometimes possible through the administration of ACTH or cortisone. Where this fails, repeated transfusions must be given in the hope that a spontaneous remission will occur.

Certain disorders associated with splenic enlargement may be accompanied by anemia. Both the excessive destruction of red cells by the spleen and a depressant effect upon the bone marrow by unknown substances produced in the spleen have been blamed. In some instances removal of the spleen causes improvement in the anemia. In other instances the splenic anemia is part of a more widespread disorder which cannot be treated in this fashion.

✗ Hemolytic Types of Anemia ✗

In the hemolytic varieties of anemia the predominating mechanism is too rapid destruction of the red blood cells. The speed at which excessive destruction takes place determines the nature of the symptoms. Very rapid destruction takes place in the types of hemolytic anemia which are mediated by antibody reactions. These include erythroblastosis fetalis and transfusion reactions. Under these circumstances a large quantity of pigment resulting from the breakdown of hemoglobin from destroyed red cells is presented suddenly to the liver for excretion. Since the liver is unable to clear the blood of this pigment, jaundice develops. The process is acute, often serious and usually limited to a brief time. In congenital hemolytic jaundice a slower degree of hemolysis takes place continuously, with superimposed "crises" during which the rate of hemolysis is accelerated temporarily. A similar but less marked phenomenon may occur with sickle-cell anemia, but in Mediterranean anemia the hemolysis tends to be slow and steady. Jaundice in these latter disorders is ordinarily difficult to detect except during a crisis. However, increased levels of bilirubin are present in the circulating blood. In all varieties of hemolytic anemia the bone marrow responds to the demands for a more rapid production of red cells. It hypertrophies and occupies a larger

than normal share of the inner structure of the bones. Microscopic examination of a sample of bone marrow obtained by aspiration reveals evidence of great acceleration of red blood-cell formation. Reticulocytes and in some cases nucleated red blood cells appear in the circulating blood in increased numbers.

Transfusion Reaction. When mismatched blood is transfused there is rapid agglutination of red blood cells, due to admixture with agglutinins of the same type as the agglutinogens of the transfused cells. Once agglutinated, the red cell masses are destroyed rapidly, and their hemoglobin is released. Jaundice results. No aggravation of the pre-existing anemia takes place, since only the transfused cells are being destroyed.

Erythroblastosis Fetalis. This disorder, also known as acute hemolytic anemia of the newborn, is discussed in Chapter 7.

Congenital Hemolytic Jaundice. This disease occurs only in the white race. The outstanding clinical features are mild jaundice and enlarged spleen. Anemia may be only moderate. In the typical case, the red cells show increased fragility when suspended in salt solution of decreasing concentration in a series of test tubes. Hemolysis normally begins when the concentration has been decreased to 0.42 per cent and is complete with a decrease to 0.32 per cent. In congenital hemolytic jaundice, hemolysis may begin before the salt concentration has been reduced to 0.5 per cent and is complete at concentrations higher than that required for normal blood. The increased fragility in the test tube does not explain the increased fragility in the body, because similar osmotic conditions do not exist. In some instances in which the disease cannot be otherwise distinguished from congenital hemolytic jaundice, the fragility in the test tube is unaltered from the normal. Other evidence that the red cells of this disease are abnormal is shown when a preparation of fresh blood is examined under a microscope. Many of the red cells are more or less spherical in shape (spherocytes) instead of being the usual biconcave disks.

The disease makes its appearance at any time after birth and persists indefinitely. Often the health apparently is unaffected. In other instances, severe anemia may develop. An acute hemolytic crisis may occur abruptly with fever and chill and it may last for several days or weeks. Recovery is usual.

The treatment consists of splenectomy. Removal of the spleen always causes improvement and often apparent cure. Increased phagocytic activity for red cells has been demonstrated in the spleen. Immediately after splenectomy, a major increase in red cells and hemoglobin equivalent to an autotransfusion occurs.

The classic variety of congenital hemolytic jaundice depends upon a hereditarily transmitted abnormality of the red cells. In other members of the child's family, either the full-blown disorder or the laboratory evidence of increased fragility of the red cells and spherocytosis usually can be discovered. When these typical features are present, splenectomy is curative. When hereditary transmission is not apparent or other features are missing, the disorder may not be affected by splenectomy.

Sickle-Cell Anemia. This disorder occurs almost exclusively in the Negro race. The red blood cells tend to assume a crescentic or sickle shape, due to the presence of an abnormal hemoglobin which is designated as hemoglobin S. The tendency of the cells to sickle can be demonstrated by the following test: A drop of blood on a slide is mixed with a drop of normal saline, covered with a thin cover slip which is rimmed with petrolatum and allowed to stand 24 hours at room temperature. The number of cells which sickle depends upon the proportion of hemoglobin S as compared with normal hemoglobin in each cell. When the sickling trait is inherited from one parent and the other parent is normal, it does not cause an anemia. But when it is inherited from both parents, an anemia develops as a result of the rapid breakdown of red cells carrying a large proportion of hemoglobin S, and the child shows all of the signs of a chronic hemolytic anemia, i.e., enlargement of the spleen, jaundice and fragility of the bones which develops as a result of the widening of the marrow spaces. The active disease may have its onset at any time after birth, either gradually or with a febrile crisis. No satisfactory treatment is known.

Mediterranean Anemia (Cooley's Anemia, Erythroblastic Anemia). This is a hemolytic anemia which is both hereditary and racial. It occurs in families whose national extraction can be traced to the races inhabiting the Mediterranean Sea, predominantly Greek, Italian and Sicilian. It is congenital and often familial. Although congenital, the signs of the disease are rarely present in the newborn period but develop within the first few months of life. The anemia progresses slowly and is severe; it is characterized by marked distortion of the shape and the size of the red blood cells and the presence of large numbers of nucleated red cells (erythroblasts and normoblasts) in the peripheral blood. The characteristic feature of the disease is the extreme activity of the blood-forming organs, which produce large numbers of immature and defective red cells which are destroyed rapidly. The distinctive clinical signs—enlargement of the spleen and the liver and thinning of the long bones of the skull and the face—result from the combination of excessive blood formation and destruction. The physical appearance of severely affected children is similar; physical growth is stunted, the pallor is muddy, the faces are broad with high malar prominences and shallow orbits, the abdomen is enlarged, the posture is poor and the musculature is flabby. Roentgenograms of the bones reveal progressive evidence of dilatation of the medullary cavity and atrophy of cortical and cancellous bones. The anemia eventually becomes severe and causes death. No satisfactory treatment is known. Transfusions are necessary to support life but cannot correct the anemia adequately or indefinitely.

Other Types of Hemolytic Anemia. Drugs, poisons and infections may produce an accelerated rate of red blood-cell destruction which eventually leads to anemia. Sulfanilamide, acetanilid, naphthalene and fava beans are examples of substances whose ingestion may lead to hemolytic anemia. During the course of malaria the parasites disrupt the red blood cells and produce hemolysis which eventually leads to anemia. In various types of septicemia, notably that caused by the hemolytic streptococcus, acute hemolysis may occur. Lederer's anemia is a severe acute form of hemolytic anemia seen among children. Its mechanism is not entirely understood but it frequently appears to be the result of an acute infection. Ordinarily it does not recur.

LEUKEMIA

Leukemia in childhood is an acute, rapidly progressive and fatal disease in which the essential pathologic lesion is an overproduction of any one of several types of white blood cells. The most common types seen in children are (1) acute undifferentiated or stem-cell, (2) acute myeloblastic and (3) less commonly, the acute monoblastic type. The subacute and the chronic forms of lymphatic and myelogenous leukemia are extremely rare in children.

PATHOGENESIS

In all of the 3 types of acute leukemia, immature white blood cells or blast forms are produced in large numbers in the blood-forming tissues throughout the body, while the production of normal cells is reduced progressively. The immaturity of the leukemic blasts may limit their identification by any of the specialized hematologic technics, and it is often impossible to distinguish among the different types of cells involved in the acute forms of the disease. However, certain characteristics are common to all of the blast cells typical of leukemia: (1) they multiply rapidly, (2) they fail to develop into the mature cells of the strain which they represent and (3) therefore they are unable to function as mature white blood cells. The factors which stimulate production of these cells and limit their maturity are unknown, but at the present time it is felt that leukemia has many of the features of a neoplasm. The immaturity of the blasts and the infiltration of these cells into tissues outside of the centers of blood formation support this concept of the disease.

Although it is true that an overproduction of a single cell type always occurs in leukemia, the number of leukemic cells which circulate in the blood is not always high. When the white blood count is high, the blasts are present in high percentage, and the blood picture is said to be "leukemic." When the count is low, with a low percentage of blasts, it is spoken of as "aleukemic." In the latter case it may be necessary to confirm the diagnosis by a study of a sample of the bone marrow, which is obtained by aspiration of fluid marrow.

Anemia develops rapidly in the early course of leukemia in children. It is a hypoplastic type of anemia in which the hemoglobin and the red cell count are reduced proportionately, and a low reticulocyte count reflects the failure of red cell formation.

Platelet production is impaired, and the level of platelets in the blood is reduced severely. The hemorrhagic manifestation of the disease is due largely to the lack of platelets and the consequent oozing of blood from the smaller blood vessels.

The lymph nodes throughout the body enlarge, and the liver and the spleen may grow to great size unless the development of the leukemic tissue can be controlled. The bony skeleton may be involved as a result of widening of the medullary spaces and infiltration of the periosteum with leukemic cells.

The age incidence of leukemia shows that the peak incidence in children occurs between 3 and 8 years. This curve is similar to that of the acute communicable diseases. However, no relationship has been demonstrated between leukemia and infections to date. The disease may occur at any age; several cases are recorded of congenital leukemia recognizable at birth. It occurs throughout childhood, adolescence and young adult life. The acute leukemias are rare in people over 30.

SYMPTOMS

In general, the symptoms of the acute leukemias are the same regardless of the cell type involved. The onset may be gradual or rapid. Common first symptoms which date the onset of the disease are low-grade fever, pallor, tendency to bruise, enlargement of the lymph nodes, pain in the legs or joints and lassitude. When pain in the bones occurs early, the condition may be confused with rheumatic fever. The early symptoms must be differentiated from many of the acute infectious diseases which involve the peripheral lymph nodes and the spleen. As the disease progresses, fever of a relapsing type, hemorrhagic manifestations, increasing pallor and enlargement of the liver and the spleen develop. The symptoms vary greatly in individual cases, as might be expected in a disease

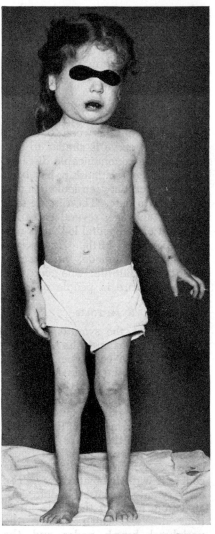

FIG. 65. A child with leukemia, showing parotid and cervical gland swelling, mouth and skin lesions.

infiltration or indirectly by the changes in the blood which is brought to them. In the natural course of the disease, the complications which develop from a lack of normal white blood cells are usually fatal; ulcerations of the mouth and the pharynx form as a result of bacterial invasion of the buccal mucous membrane, and hemorrhages from these sites are common. The low level of blood platelets causes purpuric and petechial hemorrhages in the skin and elsewhere throughout the body (Fig. 65). Intracranial and visceral hemorrhages are not uncommon. Anemia is progressive, and although it can be supported with transfusions temporarily, the child becomes weaker, and death results either from the disease itself or from an intercurrent infection. Prior to 1948, when certain drugs became available for the treatment, the course of the disease averaged 3 months. Death sometimes followed within 3 weeks and rarely was postponed until 6 months following the onset of symptoms.

DIAGNOSIS

Leukemia often is suspected from the combination of weakness, pallor, hemorrhagic manifestations and enlargement of lymph nodes, the spleen or the liver. If immature cells are present in the peripheral blood, the diagnosis is made easily from the differential blood smear. When there is doubt, microscopic examination of bone marrow is usually conclusive. In some instances the suspicion of leukemia may arise through histologic study of a lymph node biopsy.

Sometimes leukemia is confused with other disorders which produce

which affects not only the blood-forming organs primarily, but all of the tissues of the body, either by

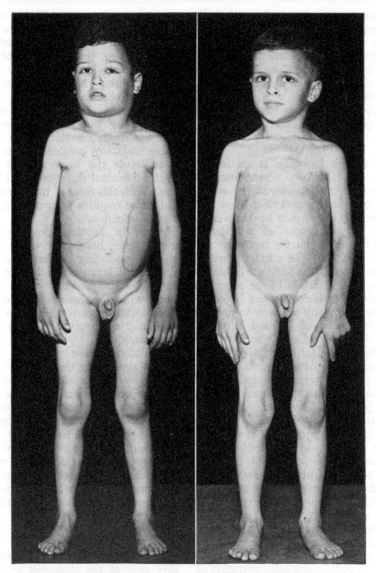

Fig. 66. A child with leukemia before treatment with ACTH. Note enlargement of cervical and inguinal lymph nodes and the penciled outline of liver and spleen.

Fig. 67. Same child after treatment with ACTH, showing decrease in size of lymph nodes of neck and groin.

an increase in the numbers of circulating white blood cells or an alteration of their appearance. Pertussis, severe infections, infectious mononucleosis and occasionally the iron-deficiency anemia of infancy may cause temporary confusion until study of the bone marrow eliminates the possibility of leukemia.

TREATMENT

Although leukemia is an invariably fatal disease, recent medical advances have improved the methods of palliation and offer hope that eventually a cure may be discovered. Two general types of substances which can produce a remission are now available—the adrenal cortical hormones and the folic acid antagonists. The duration of life after the discovery of leukemia has been extended for many children to periods up to and even beyond 2 years. ACTH, cortisone and hydrocortisone all have been found capable of initiating a complete or partial remission of the symptoms, together with a change in the appearance of both the peripheral blood and the bone marrow (Figs. 66 and 67). The duration of improvement is variable, from a few weeks to several months. In some cases a second or third effect can be obtained by retreatment. The usual manifestations of hormone therapy can be expected as side effects when heavy dosage or prolonged administration is used. In addition, these children must be protected from intercurrent infection by continuous administration of antibiotic drugs because of their lowered resistance.

Similar effects may be obtained by the administration of the folic acid antagonist drugs—Aminopterin and A-methopterin. These drugs presumably interfere with the metabolism of folic acid, which is necessary to the synthesis of the nucleoproteins required by the rapidly multiplying white cells. Remissions obtained by these substances are often longer than those initiated by the steroid hormones, but the drugs themselves are quite toxic and may produce severe depression of the bone marrow and gastro-intestinal irritation and bleeding. With this form of treatment the child also requires protection against casual infection.

Recently another drug, 6-mercaptopurine, has proved to be effective in producing remissions of the disease. It acts differently from the folic acid antagonists but also interferes with the metabolism of the nucleoproteins of the leukemic cells by inhibiting their use of the purine, hypoxanthine.

Antibiotics have played a large role in prolonging the course of leukemia by controlling the tendency to intercurrent infections. However, there is no indication that the use of any one antibiotic has been effective against the disease itself.

Transfusions are required to correct severe degrees of anemia when the leukemic process is not in remission or to stem the bleeding which may result from toxic effects of the folic acid antagonists.

NURSING CARE

Bone-marrow aspiration is a necessary part of the diagnosis and the control of the treatment of leukemia. To obtain bone marrow for study, a special Turkel bone-marrow needle is inserted through a nick in the skin into the sternum or the iliac crest.

Procaine is used to anesthetize the area, and pressure is necessary to get the needle into the bone from whence the marrow is aspirated. The procaine anesthetizes the area, but the child feels the drug on his skin, the first injection, the pressure of the needle as it penetrates his tissues and the immobilization which is necessary to carry out the procedure effectively. Therefore, the child needs to have these details anticipated for him. He also should know that the doctor is going to get a tiny bit of tissue and blood from his chest or hip bone to help him find ways to make him more comfortable. He will feel supported if he knows that his nurse will be there to assist him in finding ways to help the doctor. The equipment listed is necessary for a bone-marrow aspiration:

Turkel bone marrow needle, 2 cc. syringe, No. 25 gauge needle and procaine 1 to 2 per cent for local anesthesia, 20 cc. syringe and No. 22 gauge needle to obtain heparin from the vial to prevent clotting, 50 cc. syringe, No. 11 scalpel blade and handle, sponges, iodine and alcohol, an eye dropper, 3 towels, gloves, gauze dressing and adhesive tape.

The symptomatic nursing care of the child with leukemia is not unlike that which is necessary for one with anemia. Frequently, the child with leukemia comes into the hospital not once but many times. He comes in for diagnostic procedures and treatments which are painful. For this reason it is especially important that he have help in making a constructive adjustment to the hospital experience. Many of these children need their mothers with them to alleviate anxiety and to make the

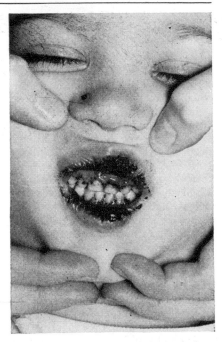

FIG. 68.   The mouth lesions of leukemia.

experience more tolerable. With the nurse's assistance, the mother can help the child adapt himself to routines and to become acquainted with other children and the personnel. With the use of the newer drugs, many children experience long periods of remission. When they are hospitalized during these periods, they need to participate in an activity program which keeps them happy and growing emotionally.

In the terminal stage of leukemia, more intensive nursing care is necessary to give the child the maximum amount of physical and emotional comfort. Often the child with leukemia is miserably uncomfortable. He is irritable and demanding; it is

understandable why he is perpetually dissatisfied with all that is done
for him. His gums may be sore and
bleeding (Fig. 68), his arms and
legs may be painful to touch, he is
dyspneic, and the mucous membrane
of his rectum often is inflamed,
painful and, in some instances, necrotic. He is nauseated, yet thirsty;
he is lonely, yet fatigues easily and
becomes irritated by those who attend him. He is apprehensive and
fearful and is apt to be irritable
when any change in routine is anticipated for him. He acts as if he
senses the advent of danger. Part of
that feeling comes from his parents'
response to his rapid failure and
part from sensitivity to bodily
changes that he cannot help feeling.

Both the child and his parents
need gentleness, sympathy and understanding. Although the parents
have known perhaps for months that
their child could not live, hope usually remains until the last. When
death is imminent, it often seems
unbearable to them. An ability to
feel with the parents and to accept
the way in which they express their
grief is a quality which is needed
in the nurse who must minister to
a dying child and his family.

During the terminal stage of the
child's illness, the nurse gives him a
degree of comfort when she carries
out procedures to keep his mouth
and nose clean, his lips and tongue
moistened, when she administers
sedatives regularly, bathes his feverish skin, changes his position when
she sees that he is becoming fatigued
and stays with him to minimize the
anxiety which he is experiencing.
When the child's parents cannot be
with him, the nurse must remain to
support him when pain is acute and

to give him the security of knowing
that someone is with him.

Although the child may lapse into
unconsciousness, a nurse's presence
is a great comfort to the parents.
They need to see that everything
possible is being done for their
child. They also should have the
sympathetic understanding of the
staff.

Leaving them alone with their
grief communicates disinterest; it
also may be interpreted as rejection
—especially is this true if the parents manifest their grief overtly. The
nurse who possesses the capacity for
empathy can support the parents
and make the experience more tolerable for them.

MALIGNANT LYMPHOMA (HODGKIN'S DISEASE, LYM-PHOSARCOMA, RETICULUM-CELL SARCOMA)

The several types of malignant
lymphoma are closely related neoplastic disorders affecting the lymph
glands and the related lymphatic
tissue. Differentiation among the 3
types is made by the histologic
appearance of the tissue in the enlarged lymph nodes which are characteristic of the disease. All of the
types are progressive but at a variable rate. In Hodgkin's disease the
progression may be very slow; in
reticulum-cell sarcoma, very rapid.

The cause is unknown. In some respects, the lesion appears to be neoplastic in much the same manner as
does lymphoid leukemia, except that
a different type of cell is involved
in the hyperplasia. The disease runs
a much slower course than leukemia
of childhood, from 2 to 4 or more
years, but the outcome usually is
the same.

In the beginning, only a few glands are affected. Often these are in the neck, where the increase in size becomes obvious. Later, other groups of glands are involved. The spleen usually is enlarged. Lymphoid tissue of the bone marrow increases and gradually replaces blood-forming tissue.

SYMPTOMS

At first symptoms are meager or absent. As the various groups of glands enlarge, pressure symptoms are likely to appear. Glands in the mediastinum may press on the trachea and the bronchi, causing respiratory embarrassment. Other groups may press on blood vessels, causing edema or ascites. Many types of pressure symptoms are possible. After the disease has progressed sufficiently, constitutional symptoms appear. Fever of remittent and intermittent type is present. Anemia of hypoplastic type gradually increases. Weight loss occurs. Death occurs eventually from general weakness if it does not occur sooner because of disturbance of some vital function from gland pressure.

DIAGNOSIS

Diagnosis is made with certainty only by histologic examination of a lymph gland and the finding of cells characteristic of the disease.

TREATMENT

In a few fortunate instances the process may be discovered early when it is limited to a few lymph nodes which can be completely removed surgically. More often by the time the diagnosis is made, widespread changes are apparent. Roent-

gen therapy is effective in reducing the size of the nodes, but there is a limit to the amount which can safely be given to any one area or to the body as a whole. Usually, such treatment is given to nodes which are causing pressure symptoms by impinging on adjacent vital structures. The nitrogen mustard compounds are also effective in reducing the size of lymph nodes by destroying the more rapidly growing cells. The frequency and the dosage of administration must be regulated carefully, since these compounds also have a depressing effect upon the bone marrow in general.

INFECTIOUS MONONUCLEOSIS (GLANDULAR FEVER)

This mildly contagious disease presumably is caused by a specific virus, although the agent has not been identified. It is characterized by fever, sore throat and swelling of the lymph nodes in the cervical region. The peripheral blood contains large, atypical white blood cells of the lymphocytic series. For these reasons, the disorder sometimes is confused with leukemia. However, its course is benign and self-limited. No treatment is effective. Diagnosis depends upon the recognition of the abnormal cells in the blood and the appearance of heterophile antibodies during the second week of the disease.

INFECTIOUS LYMPHOCYTOSIS

Infectious lymphocytosis is also a contagious disease, the cause of which is unknown. Symptoms are mild or even absent. Its importance lies in the fact that a very great increase in the number of normal lymphocytes in the blood occurs.

Often it is discovered during the course of routine blood examination and may cause unnecessary concern. No treatment is required.

PURPURA

Purpura is a condition in which spontaneous hemorrhages occur. They are mostly in the skin but sometimes in the mucous membranes, on serous surfaces and in internal organs. The hemorrhages may be minute (petechiae) or up to several centimeters in diameter.

ETIOLOGY

The hemorrhages of purpura occur from blood capillaries. Capillaries are extremely fragile structures, more so than thin paper tissue. The capillaries, especially those of the skin, are subject to injury with almost every motion of the body. When the capillary wall is broken, bleeding into the surrounding tissue would occur were it not for normal and prompt blood clotting. One of the key parts of the clotting mechanism is the blood platelet. Platelets adhere to injured tissue, disintegrate and release thromboplastin, which starts the clotting process and stops the bleeding. Also, platelets tend to agglutinate in the injured capillaries and thus aid the control of bleeding. So it is that purpura may occur in association with any condition which decreases the number of platelets in the blood (thrombocytopenic purpura or thrombopenic purpura). In some instances, the cause of platelet decrease is apparent (symptomatic thrombopenic purpura); in others, the cause remains unknown (idiopathic thrombopenic purpura). Any condition which causes hypoplasia of bone marrow causes platelet decrease. These conditions include certain infections, certain chemical intoxications and leukemia.

In some instances, purpura occurs despite a normal number of platelets. In all such instances damage has been done to the capillary walls in excess of the capacity of the platelets to take care of the situation. In some instances, the platelets seem to be abnormal in structure, in that they appear unusually stable. Even when platelets are normal in structure, their number is very small, and the normal number is only one twentieth that of red cells. The thromboplastin available is inadequate when capillary walls are made defective by disease or when extraordinary stress is placed on them. Defective capillary walls are present in scurvy, in cachectic or wasting states caused by disease and in some toxic states caused by infection. Petechiae occur in some infections in which the organisms are present in the blood and lodge in the capillaries. Petechiae from this cause are common in bacterial endocarditis and epidemic meningitis.

Petechiae occur in association with certain allergic reactions. In these instances, it seems likely that the purpura is the result of a localized specific tissue reaction which causes capillary stress, a reaction comparable in some respects with hives.

CLINICAL SIGNIFICANCE OF PURPURA

Most of the purpuras dependent on defective capillary walls (purpura simplex) are of no great importance clinically. The purpura of cachectic states is mild and is limited to the skin. The condition causing the wasting requires attention, but usually not the purpura. The same can be said for the purpuras of bacterial endocarditis, meningitis and other septicemic states. The management of the symptomatic thrombocytopenic purpuras is largely that of the underlying disease. It is desirable to discuss idiopathic thrombocytopenic purpura and allergic purpura separately.

IDIOPATHIC THROMBOCYTOPENIC PURPURA

This disease has wide variation in severity of symptoms. In the mildest form, the constitutional disturbance is only moderate, and the purpuric lesions are limited largely to the skin. When more severe, the purpura involves both the skin and the mucous membranes. The skin lesions are larger and more extensive than in the milder form. Fever and moderate or great prostration are present. The mucous membrane lesions frequently are the site of hemorrhage (purpura haemorrhagica). Bleeding may occur from the nose, the gums or the mouth. Blood may be vomited or passed in the feces and rarely it may be present in the urine. Rarely, hyperacute purpura occurs (purpura fulminans) with sudden onset, high fever and great prostration, with delirium, stupor, coma and death. Usually, cerebral hemorrhage is present.

Except for the few instances in which death occurs, a single attack of purpura runs a course of from 1 to 5 weeks and gradually subsides. Recurrence of the attacks is common. In the course of an attack, the lesions appear in crops, a phenomenon easily observed in the skin. The color at first is bright red and it does not disappear with pressure, which distinguishes the lesions from erythematous eruptions. The color of the lesions becomes darker and gradually fades. The color changes are familiar to all those who have had a bruise.

Because of the decreased platelets, the bleeding time from a skin puncture is prolonged. When blood is drawn into a test tube, the clotting time is normal, but the clot fails to retract in the normal manner. A tourniquet applied to the upper arm causes petechiae to appear in the skin below the constriction.

TREATMENT

Treatment is not required for the mildest variety of purpura. When the disease is more severe, transfusions are indicated. The adrenocortical hormones may be effective in restoring the platelet level to normal. If the disease is recurrent or chronic and does not respond to hormone therapy, a splenectomy should be done. The favorable effect of splenectomy on the disease is not understood completely, but removal of the spleen is followed in most cases by an improvement in the bleeding tendency and a rise in the level of platelets in the blood. Even if the platelet level of the blood does not rise, the rate of their destruction appears to be retarded, and the disease is made milder.

ALLERGIC PURPURA (SCHÖNLEIN-HENOCH PURPURA)

This is a condition in which purpura is only one of several symptoms, often a minor one. In some instances, a prominent feature is pain in several of the large joints (purpura rheumatica, Schönlein's purpura); in others, acute abdominal symptoms predominate (He-noch's purpura). It is possible for both the abdominal and the joint symptoms to be present in the same child.

The purpura of this condition may be associated with other skin manifestations of allergy, such as urticaria and erythematous allergic lesions. Sometimes the urine contains albumin and at times blood. Bleeding may occur in the intestinal tract. The blood contains a normal number of platelets, and the tourniquet test is negative.

The abdominal symptoms are likely to be severe, and the diagnosis may be difficult. Intense colicky pain is present. The abdominal wall is held rigid. Nausea is common. Fever may be present. The arthritis may be confused with rheumatic fever. Even though the pain is often intense, other local signs tend to be meager. The attacks last several days. Recurrences are common, and at times the interval between attacks is very short.

The responsible allergen is not easy to determine. Skin tests are not often helpful. In some instances, the disease may depend on bacterial allergy and a focus of infection. Perhaps more often food allergy is responsible. In the search for the cause, it is useful to keep a food diary, noting what foods were ingested preceding an attack.

HEMOPHILIA

Hemophilia is an inherited disease in which a congenital defect in blood coagulation leads to a severe bleeding tendency. It is a disease of males only. The genes of the disease are carried by the females and trans-ferred to their male offspring, yet the female herself has no symptoms of disease. A male hemophiliac will transmit the latent form of the disease to his female children, but will not transmit the disease to his sons if he marries a normal woman.

The defect in blood coagulation is demonstrated by the increased clotting time of the blood. Normal blood will clot within 20 minutes after removal from the body. Hemophiliac blood requires a longer time—often from 60 to 90 minutes—for the clot to form. The specific nature of the defect in hemophiliac blood is not known, but it is known that normal plasma free of platelets will correct the deficiency. Bleeding from a cut or an abrasion tends to continue indefinitely. Despite this characteristic of the disease, the bleeding time is normal when tested by the standard technic, the reason presumably being that the test cut is small and smooth-edged, the cut surfaces lie in close approximation and adequate thromboplastin becomes available from damaged tissue cells.

Bleeding from even a small accidental cut eventually may become serious because of the total loss of blood with continued bleeding. At times, hemorrhage may be spontaneous or result from a slight bruise. Common sites for spontaneous hemorrhage are the nose and the knees. Repeated hemorrhage into the knee joints may lead to ankylosis and permanent crippling.

TREATMENT

Treatment consists of use of those measures which stop bleeding. In some instances, compression may be appropriate; in others, the local application of thromboplastic substances. In any case, the bleeding usually will be stopped by transfusion of blood. The effect of transfusion is transitory, though it serves to stop the current attack. It affects coagulation time by supplying those elements which are necessary for the normal coagulation mechanism and are missing from hemophilic blood. In addition, whole blood transfusion helps to correct the anemia which has been suffered from blood loss. When bleeding has been slight, coagulation time may be controlled by administration of frozen or lyophilized plasma or antihemophilic globulin prepared from normal blood. Sometimes orthopedic measures are required for joints that have been crippled badly by repeated hemorrhage.

NURSING CARE

A diagnosis of hemophilia is frightening and evokes resentment in the parents and is potentially crippling for the child. To be faced with the responsibility of raising a child with hemophilia cannot help but evoke some feelings of resentment. An abundance of protection is essential to safeguard the child's health and life. If the diagnosis is made early in life, the infant must be protected with padded crib-sides and toys that are noninjurious. When he begins to crawl and walk, his mother must be vigilant constantly to prevent falls and to restrict potentially dangerous investigative pursuits. The care of a young child with hemophilia is a burdensome task which must be faced. If it is not faced, guilt and overprotection will result. When the child begins to seek play-

mates, the mother's fear of injury becomes manifested in warnings against fighting, running, falling and climbing. Every newly acquired capacity poses a potential crisis situation. Eternally the parents interrogate themselves in a manner similar to the following: "Dare I permit my child to go out to play with the neighbor's children? Will they be too rough or lure him into activities which might be dangerous? Dare I let him go to kindergarten? Should we take a chance and permit him to join the Scouts or let him take a week-end trip which is supervised by the scoutmaster?" If the child is hurt, many mothers blame themselves and feel as if they had been incompetent.

Living in a guarded environment suggested by the above comments poses problems for the child afflicted with hemophilia. Experiences which are necessary for psychological growth often are denied him. He feels his parents' anxiety and overprotectiveness, experiences frustrations unknown to normal children, experiences conflict and anxiety and searches for ways to relieve his discomfort. He may withdraw to lessen his anxiety and meet his parents' need to overprotect or he may use his condition to control his parents. To master his fear of being an invalid or helpless he may defy his parents and do things that are potentially dangerous for him.

The child with hemophilia needs protective nursing care which meets his individual psychological requirements. Often he is faced with many hospital experiences. He comes into the hospital for blood work, transfusions or because he has been injured or has developed a crippled joint from repeated hemorrhage. The nurse needs to understand his background experiences within his family. She also needs to be able to understand his parents and recognize from whence their attitudes have come. When the child has been admitted because he has suffered an injury, his mother may be defensive because she expects to be labeled a negligent mother. The nurse who cares for a child with hemophilia will feel the impact of her responsibility in caring for the child 8 hours a day. She will recognize her need to scrutinize his environment and to institute protective measures to safeguard further injury without making him feel "crippled," inadequate or fearful. Her responsibility is minimal in comparison with that which a mother must face. A mother has the responsibility 24 hours a day, 365 days a year. When a nurse realizes the magnitude of the mother's responsibilities she will be able to feel with her and help her to handle her problems more effectively. It is not easy to protect in a way that eliminates feelings of inadequacy and fear. Nor is it easy to provide experiences that are both growth-producing and safe. Many mothers need help in this area of guidance. The nurse who can help a child face his limitations and find safe constructive activities that bring feelings of inner strength will be able to give mothers the tangible help that many of them require.

SITUATIONS FOR FURTHER STUDY

1. Review fetal hemopoiesis. How does hemopoiesis of a normal infant differ from that of a baby with erythroblastosis?

2. How do you imagine a mother might feel when she discovers her child is a hemophiliac? How might she manifest these feelings?

3. How might hemophilia affect a child's personality development?

4. What guidance does a child with hemophilia require?

BIBLIOGRAPHY

Blackfan, K. D., and Diamond, L. K.: Atlas of the Blood in Children, New York, Commonwealth Fund, 1951.

Blake, F. G.: The expansion of curiosity, in The Child, His Parents and the Nurse, p. 212, Philadelphia, Lippincott, 1954.

Conley, C. L.: The anemias, Am. J. Nursing 52:957, 1952.

Cooke, J. V.: Leukemia in children, Am. J. Nursing 50:353, 1950.

Cooley, T. B.: The anemias of infancy and childhood, in Brenneman's System of Pediatrics, vol. 3, Chap. 16, Hagerstown, Md., Prior, 1948.

Smith, C. H.: Anemias of infancy and childhood, Am. J. Nursing 48: 617, 1948.

Wintrobe, M. M.: Clinical Hematology, Philadelphia, Lea & Febiger, 1951.

Viral and Rickettsial Infections

GENERAL DISCUSSION

The various infectious diseases differ greatly in the ease with which they may be transferred from one person to another. Certain of them cannot be transmitted by contact. To this group belong those diseases which are transmitted by biting insects. The group includes yellow fever, plague, dengue, malaria, relapsing fever, typhus and Rocky Mountain spotted fever.

Those infectious diseases which have their portal of entry by way of the alimentary tract are not easily communicable by contact. The causative agent must be ingested. This group includes cholera, dysentery, typhoid, Salmonella infections and probably poliomyelitis.

More easily, but not highly, communicable by contact are some of the infections of the skin and the mucous membranes. The group includes erysipelas, impetigo, tularemia, syphilis and gonococcus infections.

Some infectious diseases are highly communicable and require only casual contact for transmission. These infections have one feature in common, namely, the causative agent has easy access to the body and easy exit from it. For most of the highly communicable infections the respiratory tract constitutes the portal of entry as well as a channel of exit for the causative agent. The responsible organisms are expelled easily from the infected person by coughing, sneezing or even talking and, as a part of the particles thus propelled into the air, they are inhaled easily by persons in the immediate vicinity. Of course, these same diseases may be transmitted by crude infection instead of by droplets: saliva and discharges may be transmitted grossly.

Thus, the most common means of transmission of the more highly communicable infections is by contact of a susceptible person with one who has the disease or with one who is a carrier of the causative agent.

Certain of the communicable diseases may be transmitted by a third or intermediate person or by means of articles such as books and toys. Diseases that are transmitted more easily in this manner are those whose causative organisms are relatively long-lived, for example, scarlet fever and diphtheria. In the case of such diseases as measles and chickenpox, the virus dies quickly after leaving the body, and transmission by indirect contact is difficult. However, in institutions or in circumstances in which the interval between contacts is brief, indirect contact assumes importance for all communicable infections.

Athough communicable diseases sometimes seem to appear out of nowhere when there has been no known direct or indirect contact with an afflicted person, it is not appropriate to consider these diseases as air-borne. They can be air-borne in only a limited sense. When droplets containing the causative agent are expelled from the mouth, they may be carried several feet by favorable air currents. The water of the droplets may evaporate, leaving an infectious nucleus floating. Such material may be carried somewhat farther than droplets. Contaminated dust may be a similar menace with improper sweeping and dusting. However, these events would not affect neighboring houses and are not within the usual meaning of air-borne infection. When a communicable disease appears without apparent relationship to the same disease in another person, the source is usually an unsuspected carrier or a person having the disease in an exceedingly mild and unrecognized form.

The diseases that are highly communicable by direct or indirect contact have been designated as *contagious diseases.* Since different diseases present all gradations of infectivity by contact, no sharp dividing line exists between the highly contagious diseases and those of low communicability. For practical purposes, it is customary to make such a division in hospital practice by putting persons with certain diseases in quarters separate from the general wards and keeping those with other diseases in the general wards with certain precautions.

The diseases for which isolation is customary are diphtheria, measles, smallpox, scarlet fever, whooping cough, chickenpox, mumps, poliomyelitis, meningococcus meningitis, gonococcus infections, influenza, erysipelas, open tuberculosis and typhoid fever.

No isolation is required for any variety of meningitis other than meningococcic, for closed tuberculosis or syphilis, for malaria or rheumatic fever or for a large group of local infections such as appendicitis and pyelitis.

ISOLATION AND QUARANTINE

A child who is suspected of having a contagious disease should be separated from others until a diagnosis can be made. One who has the disease should be isolated until the danger of transmitting it to others no longer exists. A distinction is made between isolation and quarantine. Quarantine consists of compulsory stoppage of travel or movement from or into the place of confinement. A ship coming into port from another port having a serious disease, such as plague or cholera, is held in quarantine until the port health officer is satisfied that communicable disease is not present. Passengers and crew are confined to the ship, and no visitors are permitted. Such strict quarantine is employed for homes for very few diseases. It is customary to quarantine for smallpox until all contacts have attained the height of a successful vaccination or have shown an immune reaction to vaccination. In the case of diphtheria, the members of the household commonly are quarantined until they are shown not to be carriers. In the case of measles, homes are not quarantined, but quarantine is common for child-caring institutions, dormitories and wards, especially wards for infants. Often, limited quarantine is placed on the home in case of poliomyelitis and scarlet fever. Usually it is limited to those exposed persons who are food-handlers by occupation or those who have contacts with children, such as teachers and school children. For certain other diseases, such as whooping cough and chickenpox, exposed children are excluded from school. In an isolation hospital, the isolation is strict, but quarantine is limited to the exclusion of visitors; nurses, physicians and students go and come with only limited restrictions.

The period appropriate for isolation depends on the duration of communicability of the disease. For some diseases, this period is determined easily by the presence or the absence of the causative agent; in others, the causative agent is identified with difficulty. In this latter group, an arbitrary isolation period is determined on a statistical basis. Statistical studies show that after a certain time has elapsed the child no longer transmits the disease to susceptible persons. By means of such observations, suitable isolation periods have been established for each disease.

NEED FOR IMMUNIZATION

Although there can be no question as to the value of isolation in limiting the spread of communicable diseases, these diseases never can be exterminated by isolation alone. Despite most drastic isolation and quarantine measures, communicable diseases will continue to be spread by (1) carriers, (2) persons with mild illness and (3) persons in the prodromal stage of the disease.

A carrier is a person who harbors the causative agent without showing evidence of the disease. He may or may not have had the disease in the past but in order to be a carrier without showing evidence of the disease he must be immune. The carrier state is recognized in diphtheria, meningococcic meningitis, poliomyelitis, typhoid fever and several other infections and without doubt exists in many more.

Communicable diseases manifest themselves with all degrees of severity. Sometimes the mildness of the disease is due to resistance of the host and sometimes to the low virulence of the causative agent. In either case, the person may not be ill enough to call a physician, or the physician may not be able to recognize the disease in its mildness. A disease acquired from one who is mildly ill is not necessarily mild—often quite the reverse.

Most of the communicable diseases which have a prodromal stage are highly infectious during this stage. The disease is not recognized in this early stage, and isolation is not instituted.

Since it is impossible to prevent exposure of all susceptible persons to communicable diseases, it is desirable to immunize against as many of them as constitute a menace. Methods of immunization are discussed under those diseases for which means of protection are known. Completely satisfactory methods of active immunization exist for smallpox and diphtheria; partially satisfactory methods exist for whooping cough and scarlet fever. Passive immunization is useful for temporary prevention when exposure is known to have occurred. Means for passive immunization exist for diphtheria, measles, chickenpox, mumps and scarlet fever. A very high proportion of deaths from measles and whooping cough occur under 3 years of age. Obviously, it is desirable to protect children, at least until they are past this age period, against those diseases that affect the young so seriously.

Aseptic Technic

It is possible for persons with different communicable diseases to be cared for in adjacent rooms by the same attendants without the transmission of the disease of one patient to another (cross-infection) and without the attendants themselves becoming infected. For such accomplishment a special technic is necessary. The technic employed is known as medical asepsis or aseptic technic. In many respects, this technic is the reverse of surgical technic. When ready for a surgical operation, the patient as prepared is "clean," as are also the instruments and the instrument tables: anyone entering the room unprepared is "dirty" or contaminated as far as the technic is concerned. In the care of persons with communicable disease, anyone entering the room is presumably clean until contaminated by touching the patient or anything which the patient has contaminated.

One may enter a contaminated room and, if nothing is touched, not become contaminated. Minor offices often may be done for the patient with contamination of only the hands, which when washed are again clean.

For prolonged or intimate nursing care, protection of the clothing by a gown becomes necessary. In some institutions, a gown is worn only once. After giving care to a child, the gown is removed and discarded in a special hamper, the hands are washed, and the nurse is again clean. In other institutions, gowns are used for a 24-hour period.

When the nurse must care for patients with contagious disease for long periods, it is preferable that she not only wear a gown while with the patient but that she also exchange her street clothing or usual uniform for a special uniform before entering the sickroom or the isolation ward.

General Rules and Considerations of Aseptic Technic. All floors are considered as being contaminated.

Nothing dropped on the floor should be used again without cleaning. The infant's toys should be tied to his bed. A toy bag should be attached to the head of the older child's crib or bed, and its use demonstrated as soon as the child is well enough to play. The bed, the bedside table and the wall near the patient are contaminated. If gowns are hung to be reused, the place where they are hung is contaminated. The inside of the sink bowl is contaminated, but otherwise the sink is considered as being clean. All other areas are kept clean.

Gown and Mask Technic. A mask is worn over both nose and mouth to prevent the spreading of disease and the inhaling of infectious material. The gown should be long enough to cover the skirt and the apron. The gown should have its opening in the back and should overlap sufficiently to prevent separation. An additional tie at the waistline aids in holding the gown in place when the nurse bends over the bed. When the gown is used only once, the ties are untied, the gown is removed and discarded, and the hands are cleansed thoroughly.

If the gown is used for a 24-hour period, special technic in putting it on, taking it off and hanging it up is required. The gown is folded and hung in the unit with the contaminated side out. For removal of the gown, the waist ties are loosened before cleansing the hands. Cleansing before the gown is removed is necessary to keep the inside clean. After cleansing the hands, the clean neckband ties are loosened, the fingers of the right hand are inserted under the cuff of the left sleeve, and the left sleeve is pulled over the left

hand. The cuff of the right sleeve is grasped on the outside and the sleeve is removed by the left hand still covered by the left sleeve. Next, the clean hands are used to bring the ties of the neckband together. Then the hands are contaminated when they are used to bring the shoulders of the gown together and to hang it over a hook in the child's unit. The gown is hung in such a way that the inside remains clean and so that the attendant's clothing is protected from contamination. Handling the outside of the gown to hang it in the unit contaminates the hands, and another cleansing is necessary to make the attendant clean.

Hand-washing Technic. Facilities in institutions differ, but the equipment always consists of soap, running water, brush and towels. The brush is commonly kept in a disinfectant solution on or near the sink. The hand-operated faucet is kept clean by using the brush to turn it. In the cleansing of the hands, plain but thorough soap-and-water washing (lathering and rinsing at least 3 times) is all that is necessary unless the hands are grossly contaminated with bodily secretions. In instances where there is gross contamination, cleansing the hands and the nail beds with a brush is required. The use of antiseptic solutions in addition is not necessary and certainly should not replace disinfection by washing. The towels, usually of paper, may be kept on a clean shelf above the sink. Keeping the hands free of cuts and abrasions and preventing chapping with the use of hand lotion is important for the nurse not only to protect her own health but also because chapped hands are a deterrent to thorough disinfection.

MISCELLANEOUS TECHNICS

Each patient is provided with his own personal equipment, including a face basin, a soap dish, a toothbrush, a thermometer and other material according to circumstances.

Taking the History. For the younger children, the history is taken from the parents in the admitting room or elsewhere, according to local conditions. For the older patient who gives his own history after he is admitted, the writing is done at the bedside. A gown is placed over a chair near the bed, and the chair thus made clean is used by the physician in making his record.

Physical Examination. A nurse always assists the physician in order to keep as much as possible of the equipment clean. In taking the blood pressure, the arm and the bed are protected by a clean gown or sheet in order to prevent contamination of the instrument. When a flashlight, an otoscope or an ophthalmoscope is used, the instrument is wrapped in a towel (paper) to keep it clean. Any portion which becomes contaminated is cleaned with 70-per-cent alcohol. The stethoscope is placed in the physician's ears by the nurse, and the doctor handles only the tip, which subsequently is removed and immersed in a disinfectant solution. For making a blood count, the equipment is placed on a clean towel on the bedside table. Without contaminating his hands the physician cleans a finger with alcohol. The cleaned finger is placed through a hole in a clean finger sheet, thus providing a clean area

in which to work. A watch used by the physician or the nurse with contaminated hands is pinned inside a towel and handled through the towel.

Feeding Patients. Any necessary preparation of the patient is made in advance. The trays are prepared in the kitchen by a nurse who remains clean. The trays of those who must be fed are served last. After the meal, the trays are collected carefully with contamination of only the hands. No hand washing is necessary in the course of the collection. The contaminated trays are carried to the kitchen and placed on a paper-covered table, the paper preventing contamination of the table. Food remnants are scraped into a garbage can. Paper tray-covers and napkins are placed in a can provided for the purpose. The trays and all dishes and utensils are disinfected by boiling for 20 minutes and then are washed. The disposal of garbage and waste depends on local facilities. With adequate city sewage disposal, no special handling is required. Otherwise, either chemical disinfection or burning in an incinerator is necessary.

The Technic of Discharging a Patient. Discharging a patient from isolation is simple, provided that there are convenient bathing facilities. All contaminated clothing is left in the sickroom, and the patient takes or is given a thorough cleansing bath, washing of the hair included. Then in a clean room he dresses with clean clothing. The use of antiseptic solutions in addition to the bath is unnecessary.

Concurrent Disinfection. This term is used to designate the disinfection which must be carried out more or less continuously while the patient is under care. It includes the disinfection of contaminated materials, such as dishes, eating utensils and bedding, which are to be used again, perhaps for other patients. It includes the disposal of sputum and excreta.

Terminal Disinfection. This term is used to designate the disinfection of the living quarters and of all contaminated material after the discharge of the patient.

Methods of Disinfection. Every article of any kind that is contaminated by its use for the patient either should be made noninfectious before its use for others or should be destroyed. Treatment by heat is always the safest, but it is obvious that many articles, for example, shoes and furs, should not be so treated. It is common practice to use the autoclave for disinfection of letters, cards, magazines and pamphlets. In some institutions, mattresses are autoclaved. Boiling is used for dishes, silverware, trays, feeding bottles, rubber nipples, enamelware, hand brushes and linen. Immersion in a disinfectant solution is used for thermometers and combs. Immersion in 70-percent alcohol is used for surgical knives and scissors and for silver and paper money. Soap-and-water scrubbing is used for furniture, walls, windows and floors. A 3-day exposure to light and air commonly is used for clothing, billfolds, oxygen tanks, croup kettles, electric plates and mechanical suction apparatus. A similar but longer exposure, usually 7 days, is used for radios and books. In some institutions, the mattress is disinfected by exposure rather than by autoclaving. A combination of soap-and-water scrubbing and exposure to light and air is used for rubber sheets, hot-water bottles, ice caps and bell cords.

The terminal disinfection of a room is aided greatly by having very simple furnishings. Rugs, carpets and hangings serve to collect contaminated dust and to make the cleaning of the room more difficult. However, if they have been used, they should be either autoclaved or exposed to light and air for a long period. After disinfection by housecleaning, the room should be aired thoroughly for at least 24 hours before being used again.

Isolation in a Home. Such isolation may offer more difficulties than in a hospital equipped for the purpose. Often running water is lacking in the sickroom, and there are many other similar minor difficulties. Two rooms en suite serve better than one. The anteroom should be kept uncontaminated and may serve many purposes. The nurse may use it as a place in which to have her meals and exchange her contaminated clothing for her street clothing. It also may be used for boiling or soaking linen. The family should be kept out of the sickroom as much as possible. Any member of the family who enters the room should observe the same technic as is prescribed for the nurse. Even though the nurse is unaccustomed to doing the work of a housemaid, it is advisable for her to take the responsibility of keeping the room wiped up daily with a moistened dust cloth. The nurse also should supervise the boiling of the dishes and other disinfection procedures.

In some instances, it is necessary to teach the mother the details of

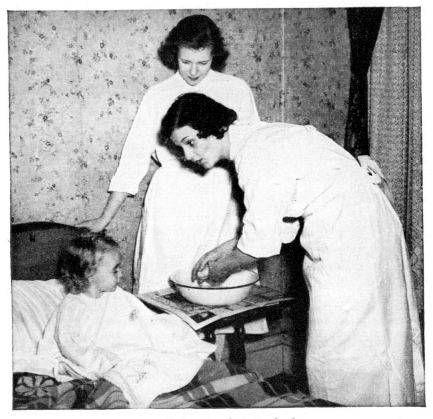

Fig. 69. Isolation technic in the home.

isolation technic (Fig. 69). Some improvising often is necessary. Contaminated material to be carried from the sickroom should be so wrapped or prepared as to permit its being transported without contamination of the person carrying it. Papers can be spread outside the door as a place on which to deposit contaminated linen. Then the linen can be wrapped without contamination of the outside of the paper and can be carried to the place of boiling. The food can be brought on a tray or in a pan and removed to the table for eating, the pan being kept clean for use in carrying away the dishes for boiling after the meal.

It is customary to require other children of the household to remain home from school and not to associate at play with the children of the neighborhood. Such children should remain at home for the entire period of the illness of the patient or should be removed to another home for the incubation period of the disease. Removal of the sick child to a hospital will shorten the stay of the well children at home to the incubation period of the disease.

Hospital Admitting Ward. Institutions for the care of sick children should be provided with facilities suitable for the separate isolation of those newly admitted children who may have a communicable disease. For this purpose, some hospitals have cubicled admitting wards in which isolation technic is carried out. All newly admitted children pass through this ward, even though no indication of communicable disease exists. The need for special admitting wards to accommodate all newly admitted children is much less than formerly, in a large measure because of the greatly decreased number of diphtheria carriers. Usually at present isolation is practiced only for those children suspected of having communicable infection.

VIRAL INFECTIONS

Viruses, which cause a number of our common infectious diseases, are minute submicroscopic particles with certain common properties. In some measure these properties explain the characteristics of virus infections. The general remarks about viruses which follow are not strictly applicable to each of the virus infections subsequently described but they may give the reader a theoretic framework which will aid in the understanding of the symptomatology, the prevention and the treatment.

Unlike the bacteria, viruses cannot survive for long unless they are in intimate relation with living cells. Some viruses are quite precise in their requirements and must parasitize not only a certain type of tissue cell, but even require also a certain species of animal. Virus particles are regarded as incomplete forms of life which must borrow enzyme systems from living cells in order to carry out their metabolic processes and to reproduce themselves. Once furnished with an appropriate environment, many of them will increase at an extraordinarily rapid rate and overwhelm the tissues which they infect. Recent laboratory technics have made it possible to support virus life outside the animal body by supplying the proper living cells in tissue culture media.

In general, viruses enter the body and then remain clinically dormant through an incubation period which is at least a week in length and sometimes much longer. During this period they presumably are migrating toward the cells which they wish to infect. Symptoms of disease do not appear until virus multiplication is well advanced and the favored cells are being attacked. Thus, by the time a clinical diagnosis can be made, the virus already has gained a foothold in the tissues which it seeks to invade.

Treatment of most virus infections is relatively ineffectual in controlling the growth of virus particles which already have entered cells. In this sheltered location it is impossible for specific antibody or antibiotics to affect them. (There are a few exceptions to this statement.) Under natural circumstances the disease is brought to a conclusion when the body begins to produce specific antibody against the infecting virus. This antibody probably does not enter the cells but it limits infection to those cells which already have been attacked and disposes of virus which is circulating among or being released from them. In some instances artificially given antibody or antibiotic may speed this process but in general they have little advantage over natural controlling mechanisms. Clinical recovery is frequently abrupt and probably corresponds to the point at which antibody has gained the upper hand over the infecting virus. For most of the diseases which will be discussed subsequently, the quantity of antibody production is sufficiently great to result in a long period of protection from reinfection—often the protection lasts for the rest of the person's life.

Prevention of virus diseases may be achieved in two ways: (1) by artificially stimulating the body to produce antibody through the administration of a vaccine and (2) by administration of antibodies which have been formed previously by another person who has had the infection. The first method (active immunization) is used before the person encounters the disease in question and is the best method of providing a long-standing protection. Unfortunately, it is not available for many virus diseases. The second method of passive immunization may be used during the incubation period when known exposure has occurred but before the virus has been able to get an irreversible foothold in the tissues.

MEASLES
(RUBEOLA, MORBILLI)

Measles is a disease having symptoms of respiratory infection and a characteristic enanthem and exanthem (Plate 2).

ETIOLOGY

Measles is caused by a virus which, during the active stage of the disease, is present in the nose, the mouth, the throat and the eyes and in the discharges from them. Measles is one of the most highly communicable diseases. It is communicable from the beginning of the respiratory symptoms and before the appearance of the rash. The period of greatest communicability is at the height of the respiratory symptoms and it diminishes as these symptoms subside. Measles occurs chiefly in the late winter and the early spring. Infants under 6 months of age usually do not acquire measles even though thoroughly exposed to it. After this age, the susceptibility at all ages is great. One attack usually protects permanently against a second attack. Second attacks occur occasionally, but in most instances of reported recurrence one of the two illnesses probably was due to some disease other than measles. Relatively few adults acquire measles because of the protection afforded the majority by a previous attack in childhood.

SYMPTOMS

The symptoms of measles begin to appear after an incubation period of from 10 to 11 days. Approximately 14 days elapse between exposure and development of the rash. The invasion is gradual, with fever and coryza. During this early stage, it is difficult to distinguish measles from an ordinary cold. The enanthem appears on the second or the third day and the exanthem on the third, the fourth or the fifth day. The original respiratory symptoms continue and extend. Lacrimation and photophobia are associated with the conjunctivitis. The discharge from the eyes becomes purulent. Sneezing is frequent at the onset, and complaint is made of soreness of the throat. The infection may extend to the ears and cause otitis media. It always extends to the larynx, the trachea and the bronchi, and frequent cough, sometimes modified to a "brassy" sound by the laryngitis, is a distressing symptom. By secondary invasion of other organisms— usually streptococci—bronchopneumonia becomes a relatively common complication. The white count is normal or low throughout the course of measles except when pyogenic complications occur.

The fever reaches its height within a few days of the onset and remains high until the rash is fully developed over the body. In a few instances, a transitory decrease in fever occurs just before the appearance of the eruption. In the absence of complications, the fever either ceases by crisis or decreases rapidly by lysis with full development of the rash. The constitutional symptoms usually correspond in severity and duration with the course of the temperature. Irritability, malaise, drowsiness and often chilly sensations are present. Headache is common, and delirium may occur. As with other infections, the child may be affected mildly, moderately or severely. The illness may be so severe that the child dies before the rash appears, or the rash may be hemorrhagic. Such severe varieties of measles are uncommon, and death seldom occurs as a direct result of measles but as a result of complications.

Enanthem. The most characteristic feature of the enanthem is bluish-white spots, pinpoint size, surrounded by a red areola on the mucous membrane of the mouth. These spots are known as Koplik's spots and are important in the early diagnosis of measles before the rash appears on the skin. Koplik's spots disappear quickly, sometimes by the time the rash has appeared.

Exanthem. The exanthem or rash appears first somewhere on the head and spreads gradually over the body. From 3 to 4 days are required for it to reach its greatest extent and then it persists for from 1 to 6 days longer. The rash consists of small dark-red papules which increase in size and coalesce into groups. Between these groups of papules the skin appears to be normal. The contrast between the blotchy, raised areas of redness and the normal skin surrounding them produces the appearance characteristic of the rash of measles. The character of the rash is thus very different from that of scarlet fever, in which the appearance from a distance is that of diffuse redness with no normal skin in the same area as the rash. Unlike scarlet fever, the rash of measles always involves the face in the same manner as other parts of the body. After the rash has faded, there remains in the same blotchy areas a pigmentation of the skin which persists for several days.

The superficial layer of skin begins to desquamate during the second week in very fine flakes, the desquamated skin never being of the size or the thickness found after scarlet fever. This process lasts from 5 to 10 days. In rare instances when the illness and the rash are unusually severe, petechial hemorrhages occur in the areas of eruption, causing what has been termed "black measles."

COMPLICATIONS

Bronchopneumonia is the most important of the common complications of measles. Otitis media, though frequent, is not so serious. The stomatitis which is a part of measles in the early stage usually causes no difficulty and requires no special attention but it prepares the way for the more serious ulcerative variety which sometimes occurs as a complication. Nephritis is infrequent. Encephalitis, although not common, occurs more frequently than formerly. It is a cause of death in a few instances. Complete recovery may be expected in more than half the cases, residual defects of varying severity persisting in the remainder. Measles is reputed to be an activator of pre-existing tuberculous infection. In severe measles, as in any other severe infection, the intoxication may be great enough to affect the myocardium and cause dilatation of the heart and a rapid feeble pulse. If the circulation fails for this reason during the eruptive stage, the rash fades or even disappears. The popular fear of the "rash going in" has no foundation except as this event may be dependent on circulatory failure. Keeping the rash well out by the use of heavy clothing or a hot room is more of a disadvantage than otherwise.

ISOLATION PERIOD

The isolation period of measles should be for the duration of the catarrhal symptoms. This period is from 1 to 2 weeks after the beginning of symptoms and from 2 to 3 days after the temperature becomes normal. In most instances, 5 days after the appearance of the rash is a sufficient isolation period.

PROGNOSIS

The prognosis in measles is dependent in part on the age and also on the previous condition of the child. The younger the child and the poorer the physical condition, the more likely the disease to result seriously. In the general population, the mortality rate is seldom more than from 4 to 5 per cent and it is usually less. In a hospital where children already are ill, especially in a ward for infants, the mortality rate may be expected to be several times that in the general population.

PREVENTION

Active immunization against measles is at present in the experimental stage and is not yet available. Temporary passive immunity may be conferred by means of convalescents' serum, by means of "immune globulin" prepared from human placenta or by means of gamma globulin extracted from pooled blood plasma. If immune serum or globulin is given parenterally within a few days of exposure to measles, development of the disease will be prevented. If 5 or 6 days are allowed to pass before serum is given, measles will develop, but in a mild and modified form. After symptoms of measles have appeared, serum has no effect on the course of the disease. In the case of young or ill children or children in an institution, complete prevention is desirable, and the serum should be given as soon as possible after exposure. In the case of older and healthy children in their own homes, it is often desirable to give the serum late in order to permit the development of the disease in a controlled mild form, and perhaps confer lasting active immunity. Serum given late tends to prolong the incubation period.

DIAGNOSIS

Typical measles offers little difficulty in making a diagnosis. The rash of measles may be simulated by that of German measles, in which condition respiratory symptoms are mild or lacking, and Koplik's spots never are present. Some drug eruptions may resemble measles for a short time. These rashes may be distinguished from measles by the history of drug ingestion and by the absence of respiratory symptoms.

TREATMENT AND NURSING CARE

The child should be kept in bed as long as fever persists and as much longer as cough and physical signs of lung infection are present. No special diet is indicated, except that in any acute febrile illness the diet during the acute stage should be light and easily digestible, consisting chiefly of liquids. Because of photophobia, the eyes should be protected from light until it is no longer unpleasant. For this purpose, some means other than darkening the room is preferable. The child's bed may be placed in such a position that he does not have to look directly into the light of a window. Wearing an eye shade and placing a screen behind the bed will shield the child's eyes from bright light. Unusually high fever is controlled by hydrotherapy. Cough is controlled by sedatives when severe

enough to disturb sleep and rest. Often "steam" is used in the management of laryngitis or bronchitis. Any itching associated with the eruption may be controlled as suggested for scarlet fever.

All of the complications of measles except encephalomyelitis are the result of bacterial invasion of mucous membrane surfaces which have been debilitated by the infection with measles virus. Antibiotic therapy controls these complications. In some instances antibiotics are given during the febrile period of measles in order to forestall bacterial invasion.

RUBELLA
(GERMAN MEASLES)

Rubella is a contagious disease characterized chiefly by a skin eruption and mildness of constitutional and associated symptoms. It is a relatively unimportant disease because of the slight and fleeting incapacity produced. Its chief importance is from the standpoint of diagnosis because of its resemblance to measles or scarlet fever.

ETIOLOGY

Rubella is caused by a virus which is present during the early stage in the upper respiratory tract. The incubation period varies from 7 to 22 days. The disease does not commonly occur in the first 6 months of life. The immunity produced by the disease is permanent, and recurrences are rare.

SYMPTOMS

Symptoms of invasion are often absent. When present, they consist of slight fever and malaise and mild catarrh. The fever rarely lasts more than 2 days, usually less. The catarrhal symptoms consist of coughing and sneezing. Congestion of the mucous membranes of the nose and the eyes is present. Even though no complaint may be made of sore throat, there is to be seen almost constantly a diffuse redness of the pharynx and often slight swelling of the tonsils. In many cases, there is an enanthem on the soft palate, consisting of red spots pinhead in size. Koplik's spots never are found. Slight general glandular enlargement occurs. Enlargement of the posterior cervical and occipital glands is of some diagnostic importance. The white blood count is normal or low.

Rash. Soon after the onset of the symptoms of invasion or in their absence, the eruption appears on the face and in the course of from a few hours to a day spreads over the body. The first thing calling attention to the disease may be the finding of a rash covering the body. Sometimes the rash has faded from the face and the neck by the time the extremities are involved. The total duration of the rash is not more than from 2 to 4 days, often less. The eruption consists of erythematous spots, slightly papular, which vary in size from that of a pinpoint to several millimeters, and they are usually discrete. In some areas these spots may become confluent and assume somewhat the blotchy appearance of measles. The eruption is subject to considerable variation, even in different cases in the same epidemic. It may be of such a character as to resemble closely the rash of measles in one case and that of scarlet fever in another. A faint desquamation similar to that found in measles sometimes follows the eruption.

COMPLICATIONS

On rare occasions encephalitis occurs as a complication of rubella. The only other complications of importance are certain congenital malformations of the fetus when the mother develops the disease. If rubella affects the mother during the first 3 months of pregnancy, the fetus may develop congenital cataract or malformation of the heart or both. Later in the pregnancy rubella has no effect upon the fetus.

ISOLATION

Isolation is not considered necessary except in institutions if the diagnosis is certain. By the time the diagnosis is made the remaining infective period is brief. The child probably is not a source of infection after the rash has faded.

PROGNOSIS

The prognosis in rubella is good except in those few instances in which encephalitis occurs as a complication. In many instances, recovery from encephalitis is complete.

PREVENTION

Sometimes prevention is attempted when a susceptible woman is exposed during the first trimester of pregnancy. Gamma globulin is used, but its efficacy is not well established.

DIAGNOSIS

Diagnosis is relatively easy in an epidemic but difficult in sporadic cases. The disease can be simulated by various toxic and drug eruptions and by very mild scarlet fever. It lacks Koplik's spots and the more severe catarrhal symptoms of measles.

TREATMENT

Treatment other than brief isolation is not required.

EXANTHEM SUBITUM (ROSEOLA INFANTUM, ERYTHEMA INFECTIOSUM)

Exanthem subitum is a benign, presumably infectious, disease of infancy and early childhood characterized by fever of from 3 to 5 days in duration which terminates by crisis and by a morbilliform eruption which appears as the temperature declines.

ETIOLOGY

The causative agent has not been identified but probably it is a virus. Although direct communicability is not evident and no epidemics have been reported, sporadic cases tend to occur in a community at approximately the same time. The disease occurs predominantly in infancy and nearly always under 3 years of age, though a few cases in older children have been reported.

SYMPTOMS

The onset is abrupt, with fever which rises to between 102° and 105° F. in a few hours. Accompanying the fever may be a moderate amount of restlessness, fretfulness, irritability and food refusal, but these are not constant. Despite the high fever, the child does not appear toxic and even may be playful and apparently comfortable. On examination, no abnormality other than fever may be noted. One constant characteristic of the disease is leuko-penia, with relative increase in lymphocytes. In different cases the white count varies from 2,500 to 7,000, and the proportion of lymphocytes is between 75 and 85 per cent.

A few children present slight redness of the throat. In some groups of cases reported, moderate enlargement of the superficial glands of the neck has been present; in other groups, this has been absent. The glandular enlargement, if present, appears on the second or the third day. The fever continues for approximately 4 days, with some tendency to slight morning remissions. The fever ends usually by crisis, and at the same time the characteristic eruption appears. With the cessation of fever and the appearance of the eruption, any previous indisposition disappears, and the child seems to be as well as ever.

Eruption. The eruption is macular or at times slightly maculopapular. The early individual lesions are pink or pale red and about 3 mm. in diameter. They tend to increase in size and to coalesce, in this respect resembling measles. The color disappears on pressure. As the lesion becomes older, it tends to fade at the center and irregularly acquires a slightly bluish color, similar to some lesions of erythema multiforme. No unanimity exists in published reports as to the site of first appearance of the eruption, and one is led to the conclusion that no uniformity exists. Regardless of where it begins, it spreads rapidly to its maximum extent and when fully out is most extensive and prominent on the trunk or perhaps the trunk and the neck, and the lesions are relatively sparse on the face and the extremities. Usually the eruption reaches its height in 24 hours or less and disappears in another 24 hours or more. Either no desquamation, or at most a very faint branny desquamation, follows.

COMPLICATIONS

No complications or fatalities ever have been reported.

ISOLATION

No isolation is required. Any transmissibility that the disease may have probably is terminated by the time the rash appears and the diagnosis is made.

DIAGNOSIS

The diagnosis cannot be made with certainty before the eruption appears. After it appears, the diagnosis presents no difficulty. The two diseases with which it might be confused are measles and rubella. It does not have the catarrhal symptoms or the Koplik's spots of measles. High prodromal fever is absent in rubella.

TREATMENT

No treatment is needed.

SMALLPOX (VARIOLA)

Smallpox is a highly communicable disease with severe constitutional symptoms and a generalized pustular eruption which tends to leave permanent pitted scars.

ETIOLOGY

Smallpox is caused by a virus which, in the course of the disease, is present in the skin and the mucous-membrane lesions, the nose and the throat, the blood, the alimentary tract, the feces and the urine. The disease is contagious from the beginning of the earliest symptoms and until all lesions are healed. It is transmitted easily by a third person and by fomites.

Smallpox occurs in any exposed person, regardless of age, who is not immune by reason of a previous attack or of vaccination. Were it not for vaccination, smallpox would be chiefly a disease of childhood. Smallpox may occur as a mild illness because of partial but waning immunity from vaccination many years previously. It may occur as a mild illness also because of low virulence of the virus strain. A few epidemics are caused by a strain of fixed and relatively low virulence.

SYMPTOMS

After an incubation period, which averages from 11 to 12 days, the symptoms of invasion appear. The onset is abrupt, with headache, backache and fever, and with the temperature rising to between 103° and 104° F. The sudden rise in temperature often causes a chill or a convulsion. With high fever, delirium is likely to be present. Prostration is severe. Vomiting and constipation are common. After from 1 to 2 days of illness, there appears a rash characteristic of smallpox. This prodromal rash may resemble that of scarlet fever or of measles. It is of brief duration.

Eruption. Approximately 3 days after the onset of symptoms, the characteristic eruption begins. It tends to appear first on the forehead and the wrists. In the next 1 to 3 days it spreads over the remainder of the body, with a greater concentration of lesions on the head, the arms and the legs than on the trunk. Thus the distribution is centrifugal.

The earliest lesion is a small round macule. Rapidly and within a few hours the macule becomes a papule, which enlarges. In approximately 3 days, the papule becomes vesicular with a depressed center (umbilicated). The lesion becomes definitely pustular during the next few days. The course of the lesion is similar to that of vaccinia. The lesion of smallpox is deep-seated in the skin. In the papule stage it feels shotty. The early vesicle is pearl-colored and it never has the clear, watery appearance of an early varicella vesicle. After the pustule has developed fully, it begins to dry, and a firmly adherent crust forms. The crust gradually loosens and falls off in from 4 to 6 weeks after the onset of the disease.

The pustules often become confluent on the face and sometimes on the extremities. Discrete pustules have a red areola. The severe inflammation of the pustule causes edema. Where the lesions are grouped closely, as on the face, the edema may be severe. Usually many pustules become ruptured, and some become infected secondarily with pyogenic bacteria. The odor of the free pus is unpleasant. When smallpox is very severe, blood may extravasate into the skin lesions and thus change their appearance markedly.

Enanthem. The lesions of smallpox may occur on any mucous surface. They are easily visible in the mouth and the throat. When they occur on a surface constantly moist, they lose their covering quickly and appear as ulcers. At times these lesions interfere seriously with the ingestion of food. When they occur on the cornea, careful treatment is required to preserve vision. If they occur in the larynx, tracheotomy may be necessary.

COMPLICATIONS

The most common complications are those caused by pyogenic bacteria which have invaded the pustules. Furunculosis, erysipelas or septicemia may result. Because of the virus infection, myelitis or encephalitis may occur. As in any severe toxic disease, bronchopneumonia may be a complication.

PROGNOSIS

Except in those instances in which the virus is of low virulence, the mortality from smallpox among the unvaccinated is in the range of from 25 to 35 per cent. It is higher among infants and young children than among those older. Most of the deaths occur within the first 2 weeks of the disease.

PREVENTION

Vaccination with cowpox virus is a fully adequate and satisfactory means of prevention. Vaccinia is discussed separately.

DIAGNOSIS

Diagnosis before the eruptive stage is difficult and may be impossible with certainty. If an epidemic is present, the diagnosis may be strongly suspected from the symptoms of invasion. During the eruptive stage, varicella is the chief disease to be considered in differential diagnosis. The lesions of smallpox are more deep-seated in the skin. At no stage do they have the clear, watery appearance of the varicella lesion in its early stage. The lesions of smallpox are more abundant on the extremities than on the trunk. In chickenpox the reverse is true. Varicella lesions appear in crops, and in any one area several stages in the evolution of the eruption are to be found. In smallpox, all lesions of any one area are in the same stage of development. Usually, varicella is a mild disease, and variola is severe. Difficulties in diagnosis arise when smallpox occurs as a mild disease.

TREATMENT AND NURSING CARE

An important phase of the management is isolation. The isolation technic must be far more rigid than for any other communicable disease. A completely separate unit is preferable for the hospital care of those with smallpox. Closed technic is desirable. With such technic, no contaminated article and preferably no contaminated person should leave the smallpox unit before disinfection. Vaccination of everyone in the vicinity is desirable. Isolation should be continued until all crusts are off and should be terminated with a thorough bath.

Discomfort is great during the invasion period and again later during the height of the pustular stage. Sedatives usually are indicated for these periods. An icebag is useful for the headache and a hot-water bottle for the lumbar backache of the invasion period. Soreness of the mouth during the pustular stage may require local treatment. If eating is prevented, fluids must be given parenterally.

The skin lesions usually require no treatment until pustule formation is well advanced. At this stage, many pustules are likely to be rup-tured and many are likely to become infected with pyogenic bacteria. Boric-acid compresses are useful in keeping the skin clean and in minimizing inflammation. They also help to allay itching and subsequently to hasten detachment of the crusts. Infected pustules should be treated by local application of some antiseptic such as 3-per-cent gentian violet. Antibiotic therapy also is useful during the period when infected pustules are present. During the pustular stage, it is desirable to keep the bedcovers away from the skin by means of a cradle. The use of an air mattress also helps to protect the pustules.

VACCINIA

Vaccinia is a local skin lesion produced by the inoculation of cowpox virus for the purpose of protecting against smallpox. Cowpox is a pustular disease affecting cattle and is communicable to man. It is a less virulent and less serious disease for both cattle and man than is smallpox for man. A man who has had cowpox is thereafter immune to smallpox. This view was current among the country folk of England during the life of Edward Jenner (eighteenth century). Jenner was the first to take advantage of this knowledge by making the experiment of inoculating a human being with cowpox (1796). Since then, cowpox vaccination has become customary in many countries and compulsory in some.

Cowpox acquired naturally is a generalized disease, as is smallpox. Inoculation into the skin produces only a local lesion but it gives immunity to both cowpox and smallpox. The virus of cowpox is contained in the pustules of this disease. Early in the history of vaccination, inoculations were made from the pustule of one human to the skin of another. Complications were not uncommon. Sometimes pyogenic and other bacteria were carried along with the virus. Inoculation is no longer made from the human. Much of the virus is obtained from the calf under most carefully controlled conditions. The safeguards are such that complications of the variety mentioned are all but impossible. Some of the available vaccine is produced by growing the virus in the chorio-allantoic membrane of the chick embryo with still further elimination of the hazard of bacterial contamination.

VACCINATION

Vaccination or the inoculation of cowpox virus may be carried out as follows: The skin of the site chosen for inoculation is washed first with soap and water and then with ether or acetone. After drying, the skin is scratched or punctured through a drop of the prepared vaccine. The object is to infect the skin with the virus and with the virus alone. If the scratch procedure is used, 2 or 3 short parallel scratches are made with a needle point, not deep enough to draw blood. If the multiple puncture method is used, the skin is punctured lightly several times with the needle. Usually the needle is held almost parallel with the skin surface in order to control the depth of puncture. After the inoculation, the vaccine remaining is wiped off. No dressing is applied.

Inoculation Site. The inoculation site usually chosen is the left arm at the insertion of the deltoid muscle.

In the case of girls and women, the lateral surface of the calf of the leg is sometimes chosen, or the inoculation may be made on the thigh. (In these areas the risk of secondary infection is greater.)

Course of the Lesion. After the lapse of 2 or 3 days, the inoculation site should appear normal except for slight evidence of the original trauma. On the fourth or the fifth day, a papule appears. This increases rapidly in size and becomes vesicular. The vesicle is pearly gray and surrounded by an area of redness. The vesicle is a pustule or quickly becomes pustular. It increases in size and reaches its maximum extent by the ninth or the tenth day. At this time, there may be some swelling of the axillary glands and constitutional symptoms consisting of fever, malaise and irritability. After the tenth day, the pustule begins to dry and the neighboring inflammation to disappear. The constitutional symptoms subside rapidly. The crust which forms as a result of the drying of the pustule gradually loosens and falls off, usually late in the third week, leaving a scar which later becomes white and depressed and is characteristically pitted.

Management of the Lesion. Many prefer no dressing at any stage of the lesion. Some suggest that gauze be pinned inside the sleeve over the pustule. A very good procedure is to place a plain gauze dressing over the pustule and hold it in place by adhesive tape in such a manner that constriction of the swollen arm by the tape is not possible. The object of the dressing is to prevent secondary infection in case the pustule should be broken accidentally. If the

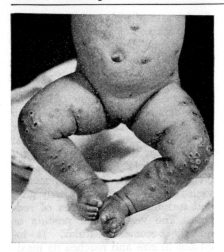

Fig. 70. Generalized vaccinia.

pustule should rupture, the dressing will adhere to it. Then if it is desired to change the dressing, the outlying portions of the gauze are cut away, leaving the small circle of gauze stuck to the lesion. Then a new dressing is applied over the old one. A "vaccination shield" should not be used.

COMPLICATIONS

Complications in vaccinia are uncommon. The most common are those arising from secondary infection of the pustule, such as erysipelas and sepsis. Sometimes a child will rub the freshly vaccinated spot with a finger, then with the same finger rub the skin elsewhere and produce a second lesion. Generalized vaccinia or cowpox is a rare complication but *potentially serious* (Fig. 70). Infants with exuding eczema are particularly susceptible. They should be neither vaccinated nor exposed to others who have been vaccinated recently. Also rare is

encephalitis, a serious complication when it does occur. For the 60 to 70 per cent who survive, recovery is complete. Encephalitis is more rare in infancy than later.

TREATMENT OF SYMPTOMS

Usually the constitutional symptoms are not severe enough to require treatment. For severe symptoms, remaining in bed is sufficient. The treatment of any pyogenic complication is that which is applicable irrespective of vaccinia. The treatment of encephalitis and of generalized vaccinia is symptomatic.

VACCINATION FAILURE

Vaccination may fail to "take" because of faulty performance of the procedure. When properly done, two reasons exist for failure. It will be unsuccessful if the person is immune because of previous vaccination or smallpox. In these circumstances, an immune reaction will appear. This reaction consists of the development of a small area of induration and redness within a day or two of vaccination. More often, vaccination is unsuccessful because the virus used is no longer living. The virus as dispensed commercially will remain living for many months if kept cold and away from sunlight. Continued exposure in a warm room will soon make it useless.

REVACCINATION

Although a single vaccination may protect for life, immunity for so long a period cannot be relied on. Vaccination in infancy and revaccinations from 12 to 14 years and at from 25 to 30 years are to be recommended. When the first vaccination is performed in early infancy, the reaction is much less severe than at later periods of life. After successful vaccination all subsequent vaccinations tend to have milder reactions.

CHICKENPOX (VARICELLA)

Chickenpox is a highly communicable virus disease in which the chief feature is a generalized vesicular eruption (Plate 2).

ETIOLOGY

The virus of chickenpox is present in the nose and the throat, in the vesicles of the eruption and probably in the crusts resulting from the drying of the vesicles. The disease is rare in the first 3 months of life but occurs at the first exposure after this age. It is one of the most highly communicable diseases.

SYMPTOMS

The incubation period is from 14 to 16 days. Prodromal symptoms usually are absent or are limited to a slight fever of which no complaint is made. Rarely, high fever may be present and even convulsions. Commonly, the first thing noted is the rash, which appears first on the face or the trunk and a little later on the extremities. New lesions continue to appear over the entire body for a period of from 3 to 4 days. The individual lesion appears first as a macule, which quickly develops into a vesicle, or first a papule and then a vesicle. The vesicle rapidly increases in size to 3 or 4 mm. in diameter within 24 hours of the first appearance of the macule. The characteristic mature chickenpox lesion is a vesicle with a red areola and filled with clear fluid. The vesicle then dries gradually, first be-

coming depressed at the center, and later becomes a flat crust. The crust falls off in from 1 to 3 weeks.

After the eruption has been present for a day or two, all stages of it may be seen on the skin in the same area. In the same general area may be seen macules, papules, immature and mature vesicles and crusts of dried lesions. The presence of many stages of eruption at the same time is due in part to the development of the lesions in successive crops and in part to beginning retrogression of a large number of lesions before maturity, perhaps because of developing immunity.

The lesions of chickenpox also appear on the mucous membrane of the mouth and the vagina. In these areas no vesicles are seen, but the appearance is as if a vesicle had been present and the top rubbed off, that is, a gray-white spot surrounded by a ring of redness.

COMPLICATIONS

Complications are infrequent. Scratched or traumatized lesions offer a portal of entry for pyogenic bacteria, with resultant local suppuration and sometimes the development of erysipelas. The virus of the disease sometimes causes encephalitis, but complete recovery is the rule. Unlike measles, the small infant obtains little temporary immunity from his mother. At this age the disease tends to be more severe.

ISOLATION PERIOD

An isolation period of from 10 to 14 days is generally considered sufficient, but in institutions that care for children it is preferable that isolation be continued until all crusts are off.

PREVENTION

When chickenpox occurs among children in their own homes, preventive measures other than isolation are not carried out because of the mildness of constitutional symptoms and the rarity of serious complications. On the other hand, the disease becomes important when it occurs in a children's hospital, where it may cause postponement of the treatment for which the child was admitted, for example, of a surgical operation. Other obvious reasons exist as to why an epidemic cannot be allowed to continue in a hospital.

Convalescent serum and gamma globulin are not effective as sources of passive immunity.

DIAGNOSIS

The disease most likely to be confused with chickenpox is smallpox. Usually, smallpox is a serious disease with great prostration but it may be mild and resemble chickenpox. Smallpox has but one crop of lesions in any one skin area, and all are in the same stage of maturity at any one time. Smallpox affects more prominently the exposed parts, the extremities and the face, while chickenpox affects chiefly the trunk, with scattered lesions on the face and the extremities. The vesicular lesions of chickenpox are superficial in the skin, and the early lesions contain obviously clear fluid. Smallpox lesions are more deeply seated in the skin, and the early vesicular lesions have a pearly appearance, never that of containing obviously clear fluid.

TREATMENT

Usually no treatment is required. Scratching and picking at the lesions should be prevented by applying petrolatum, by using elbow restraints and by keeping the fingernails cut short. Itching may be relieved by the application of ointments or lotions containing calamine and antihistaminics.

MUMPS
(EPIDEMIC PAROTITIS)

Mumps is an acute contagious disease affecting chiefly the salivary glands, especially the parotid glands. It causes swelling of these glands, local discomfort and usually moderate constitutional symptoms.

ETIOLOGY

Mumps is a virus disease. It occurs infrequently under 2 years of age and is not common in adults. The period of greatest incidence is between 4 and 15 years. Closer contact is required for the transmission of mumps than for most of the contagious diseases, and only a small proportion of those exposed acquire the disease. One attack usually protects from subsequent attacks. The incubation period varies. It is usually between 2 and 3 weeks, with an average of 18 days.

SYMPTOMS

In most instances there are no prodromal symptoms. When present, they consist of slight fever, malaise, headache and anorexia. These are of short duration before the swelling of the parotid gland begins, associated with local, dull, aching pain. Sometimes both parotids are involved simultaneously, sometimes the disease remains limited to one; but more often one parotid gland is involved first, and after an interval of several days the disease in the other parotid becomes manifest.

The parotid becomes greatly swollen, tender and painful. Much individual variation exists in the amount of local and general symptoms. In the majority, the disease is mild, and most of the discomfort is local. It is difficult to confine such children to bed. Some children have high fever and are prostrated. Opening the mouth may be impossible because of swelling and pain. The swelling begins to subside within 2 or 3 days, and at the same time the constitutional symptoms subside rapidly. By the eighth to the tenth day the swelling and all signs of the disease usually have disappeared.

Frequently, the submaxillary and the sublingual salivary glands are involved coincidentally with the parotid glands. Occasionally, the submaxillary or the sublingual glands alone are affected.

COMPLICATIONS

Although complications occur frequently in some epidemics among adults, they are uncommon in childhood. The most common complication among males past puberty is orchitis. This occurs usually 1 week (sometimes up to 2 weeks) after the onset of mumps, and the local and the general symptoms are severe. The testis becomes greatly swollen and subsequent atrophy occurs in about half the cases. A similar inflammation may occur in the ovaries, the uterus, the breasts or the external genitalia of the female. Certain other complications are observed rarely; these include mumps meningitis or encephalitis and pancreatitis. None of these is fatal, and usually the recovery from encephalitis is complete. Deafness also rarely occurs as a complication, but when it does it is usually unilateral and permanent.

ISOLATION

Isolation of those with mumps should be continued for 2 or 3 days after the swelling has disappeared. Thus, most children can be released by the end of 2 weeks. Any complication prolongs the course of the disease approximately 1 week.

PREVENTION

No proved means for active immunization exists. Convalescents' serum given parenterally within a few days of exposure prevents the development of the disease. An appropriate amount of serum is 10 cc.

DIAGNOSIS

A common error in diagnosis is confusion of cervical lymphadenitis with mumps. The lobe of the ear is at the center of parotid swelling, while the swelling of lymphadenitis is slightly lower in the neck. An aid in diagnosis is redness and swelling of the outlet of the parotid duct in the mouth. The blood leukocytes are normal in number or decreased in uncomplicated mumps and increased in acute lymphadenitis.

Laboratory assistance in confirming the suspicion of mumps is now available by looking for the appearance of specific antibodies in the blood. A skin test with inactivated virus is useful in distinguishing between persons who are susceptible and those who are immune. An inflammatory response at the site of injection of the killed virus indicates immunity.

TREATMENT AND NURSING CARE

Treatment and nursing care are symptomatic. Often no treatment is required. For local pain, the application of heat usually gives relief. It may be necessary to restrict the diet to articles of food which do not require chewing. Acid foods tend to increase the pain. Many children are not sick enough to wish to remain in bed. It is common belief that rest in bed helps to prevent complications. Observation of soldiers in World War I showed that this was not the case, particularly as regards orchitis. Complications usually require treatment in bed.

POLIOMYELITIS (INFANTILE PARALYSIS)

ETIOLOGY

Poliomyelitis is caused by a small virus which, when it gains access to the central nervous system, produces dysfunction or death of nerve cells, particularly those in the anterior horn of the spinal cord and the corresponding regions of the brain, i.e., the cells that supply motor nerves. Three general types of poliomyelitis virus have been separated by immunologic methods. These types are called Brunhilde, Leon and Lansing. In nature, the viruses infect man alone; experimentally, the disease can be produced readily in monkeys and under special circumstances in a few other animals.

METHOD OF INVASION

The manner in which the virus enters the body and gains access to the cells of the spinal cord or the brain has been under study for a great many years but is not understood thoroughly. Entrance into the body is probably through the mouth, the pharynx and the intestinal tract, perhaps occasionally through the nose. For a brief time early in the disease the virus can be recovered from throat swabs, but a more consistent source is the stools. From some time before the onset of symptoms and often until a month after recovery, virus can be recovered from the contents of the lower intestinal tract. This, together with other experimental evidence, suggests that the chief site of virus multiplication is in the intestine. Recently, its presence in the blood has been determined during a brief period of the illness. In experimental infection of monkeys and in examination of tissues of children who have died, the virus is recovered from various parts of the nervous system. The exact pathway from the intestinal tract to the central nervous system is not settled. Originally, it was believed that the spread occurred along the nerve trunks from their branches in the intestinal wall backward to the cord or the brain. Recently, the mediation of the blood stream as an avenue has been demonstrated.

There is reason to believe that asymptomatic infection with the poliomyelitis virus is a common, almost a universal, event among children. During epidemic periods virus is found in the stools of children living in association with poliomyelitis victims, children who themselves show mild or no evidence of disease. It is judged that only 1 out of 10 or 1 out of 100 children who excrete virus in the stools will have evidence of clinical disease. Furthermore, examination of the blood of adults shows that a high percentage have antibodies against poliomyelitis even though they never have had the disease. The belief is growing that most children acquire virus infection early in life but that only a few permit the virus to migrate from their intestinal tracts to their nervous systems. The reasons why some fail to keep it localized have yet to be discovered. Vaccination against poliomyelitis presumably would provide the child with a better defense against the transmission of virus from intestine to nervous system.

EPIDEMIOLOGY

There are some peculiarities about the spread of poliomyelitis which require an explanation before any theory of its epidemiology can be accepted. The disease is of little importance in tropical regions but appears with regularity in both north and south temperate zones during the period of the year when hot weather is prevalent. In small geographic areas it fluctuates in importance from year to year, but some areas have more poliomyelitis than others. In large cities it may run in cycles. It seldom attacks small infants. Formerly, it attacked children from 1 to 5 almost exclusively, but in recent years the incidence among older children, adolescents and adults has been rising steadily. The disease tends to be more severe in older children and adults. It is surprisingly uncommon to have more than one person in a family affected, in spite of the fact that others in the family or in the immediate environment can be shown to harbor virus in their intestines.

An intriguing theory which explains many of these facts but is not yet fully substantiated is the following: tropical regions with their steady warm climate and relatively poor sanitation provide favorable circumstances for maintenance and dissemination of poliomyelitis virus present in the stools. Small infants acquire temporary protection from their mothers by passage of antibodies through the placenta before birth. While still having some protection from this source and during a relatively favorable age period they become exposed to virus and acquire an active immunity of their own without suffering from the paralytic disease. Thus much of the populace in tropical areas grows up immune to poliomyelitis. By contrast, the children in temperate zones are reared in a region where virus is present in the community only during a portion of the year and then is removed carefully by modern sanitary facilities. Such children are more likely to grow up without having any contact with the virus until they reach an older age, at which time they are more susceptible to the paralytic form of the disease.

TYPES OF DISEASE

Infection with the virus of poliomyelitis can result in a great variety of clinical manifestations. For convenience these are usually grouped into the carrier state, abortive infection, nonparalytic and paralytic poliomyelitis. The last category is subdivided into spinal and bulbar forms of the paralytic disease. Since the management of each type is somewhat different, they will be considered separately.

The Carrier State

This merely signifies that the child has poliomyelitis virus in his stools but has no evidence of disease. The condition goes unrecognized except when special epidemiologic studies are in progress. No treatment is required.

Abortive Poliomyelitis

During epidemic periods a large number of children are observed with illnesses which are suspected of being the initial symptoms of poliomyelitis. In some instances this is a correct presumption which can be confirmed by isolation of virus from stools. In other instances it is impossible to be sure what the nature of the illness really is. The symptoms may include brief fever, headache, sore throat, mild diarrhea, abdominal pain, nausea and vomiting. Signs of involvement of the nervous system are lacking, and the spinal fluid is normal. Since the symptoms subside rapidly, no treatment is necessary except limitation of activity and a brief period of observation to be certain that further manifestations are not going to appear.

Nonparalytic Poliomyelitis

This is similar to the foregoing, except that symptoms may be prolonged over several days' time, and in addition there is clinical evidence of meningeal irritation. The latter is manifest by pain in the neck or the back with limitation of flexion of the spine. There may be increased sensitivity of skin or muscles and peculiar sensations such as tingling or transient weakness of muscles. The spinal fluid shows an increase in the number of lymphocytes and a slight increase in protein content. Treatment consists of bed rest and observation until the fever and the other symptoms disappear and it is clear that no paralysis will occur.

Spinal Form of Paralytic Poliomyelitis

Symptoms. In what might be called the average or typical case, the onset is sudden, with fever, headache and prostration, sometimes vomiting, and rarely convulsions. The fever, the headache and the prostration continue. Irritability, general or local hyperesthesia and neck and back rigidity develop. The child may be mentally clear or drowsy. In severe infections, coma may occur. These symptoms constitute the essential features of the preparalytic stage. In most instances, constipation is present, though diarrhea has been a feature of some epidemics. Frequently, the child sweats profusely. Acute upper respiratory infection has been associated with early symptoms in some epidemics.

In many instances, the symptoms enumerated are preceded by a short period of fever with varying minor symptoms, none of which is indicative of the nature of the infection. An afebrile period of from 2 to 3 days intervenes between this vague illness and the more characteristic illness already described. When the disease produces these two "humps" of fever, sometimes it is spoken of as the "dromedary" type (although it is the camel that has two humps).

After the symptoms described have persisted for a variable period, often from 2 to 3 days, paralysis and other phenomena appear. Such true paralysis as occurs is flaccid in type, and the muscle fibers affected cannot function and therefore cannot exhibit spasm. Either the maximum amount of paralysis appears at once or it increases in degree and extent for a period of 3 or 4 days. In the order of their frequency, paralysis occurs in the following parts of the body: one or both legs, one or both arms, combined arms and legs, legs and trunk. The legs are involved in the majority of cases; other parts, to a much less extent.

True paralysis is dependent on the effect of the inflammation on the anterior horn cells and their motor neurons. This effect may be destructive by action of the virus directly on the anterior horn cells, or the effect may be through functional impairment, such as in edema. The indirect effects of the inflammation may be temporary, and in some instances perhap the direct effects may fall short of destruction and be temporary. Usually, not all of the nerve supply of any muscle is destroyed, although for some muscles all the nerve supply may be thrown out of function temporarily. During the period of temporary dysfunction of the nerve supply, the intact muscle fibers are subject to the harmful effects of spasm. The muscle spasm of this condition is reflex. It is painful and usually tonic, but visible twitching and tremors may be noted. The spasm of an affected muscle causes dysfunction of its antagonist. The muscle spasm is aggravated by manipulation of the affected parts as well as by splinting in a fixed position.

The constitutional symptoms characteristic of the early stages of poliomyelitis seldom last more than 6 or 7 days. Sometimes the hyperesthesia and the irritability last longer. After the paralysis has developed fully, it remains stationary from 1 to several weeks. Although no change occurs in the paralysis during this time, those muscles or portions of muscles which already are paralyzed undergo more or less atrophy. After this short stationary period, improvement in power of the paralyzed parts takes place. Some show complete recovery in a few weeks; others will be completely well in 3 months. The most rapid improvement occurs in the first 6 months. After this time, recovery is slow but may continue for as long as 2 years. After 2 years, nearly half of the children will have recovered completely, while the remainder will show permanent paralysis of varying extent. If the permanent paralysis extensively involves a limb, its further growth, in both size and length, is stunted, the skin is cold and mottled from poor blood supply, and unless proper care is given, contractures occur and result in deformity.

Treatment and Nursing Care. In the absence of useful specific therapy, the treatment is symptomatic and supportive. Seldom in childhood is the fever high enough to require relief. When caused by increased intracranial pressure and if severe enough, headache may be relieved justifiably by spinal puncture. Care of the bladder and the bowel is an important part of the early treatment in many cases. Often the bladder overfills, and catheterization becomes necessary. Some advocate irrigation of the bladder several times daily with 1:1,000 solution of Merthiolate to prevent infection from repeated catheterization. Parasympathetic stimulants such as Furmethide may stimulate bladder contraction. Often spasm of the lower back and the abdomen cause difficulty in emptying the bowel. If constipation is present, appropriate measures should be taken for relief. Prostigmin is sometimes effective. There are those who advocate the giving of an effective saline cathartic in all instances and the use of enemas on several succeeding days for the purpose of ridding the bowel of as much virus as possible. Since the stools contain virus, they should be considered as infectious and treated in the same way as the stools of those with typhoid fever or dysentery.

Maintaining good body alignment is necessary to prevent deformities. The child should be placed on a firm, flat mattress. In those instances in which the legs are affected, the mattress may be pulled away enough from the foot of the bed to allow the heels or the toes to extend over the end. A board should be attached to the foot of the bed to maintain the feet at right angles when the feet are resting against it. The position of the child should be changed frequently.

The diet should be that suitable for the severity of the illness. Usually a soft diet is appropriate except when bulbar involvement causes difficulty in swallowing. Although the fluid intake should be maintained, fluids should not be forced.

The older treatment included immobilization of the paralyzed parts in splints or casts and the relief of pain with sedatives. Neither of these measures is now common practice. Immobilization causes normal muscle units to atrophy and delays recovery of paralyzed muscles. Freedom of motion maintains the normal individual muscle units in good condition, and with appropriate treatment these units of a single muscle may hypertrophy to compensate for damaged portions of that muscle, with no loss of total function.

The pain of poliomyelitis is chiefly from muscle spasm, and the spasm is relieved within a short time by hot applications (Kenny treatment). For the first few days, in most instances the application of hot compresses or packs is the chief treatment used. When spasm and pain have been relieved, passive motion is carried out by moving the part gently throughout the normal range of motion 4 or 5 times daily. The passive motion serves to maintain muscle nutrition and joint sense. Active motion is permitted and encouraged when such activity does not increase spasm and tenderness. When conditions permit and if desired, active motion may be carried out under water within a few days. All manipulation, passive or active, must be limited to that which does not cause pain, spasm or fatigue.

The majority of children over 6 years of age suffer from acute anxiety. They have heard about "polio" over the radio and from their peers and parents. They react to their parents' anxiety and they fear that they will be crippled as others have been. Discovering the child's fears is of vital importance in his care. After his fears have been verbalized, he needs to be kept informed about his progress and given help in facing the possible outcomes of the disease.

The next step in the treatment is muscle training and re-education. This procedure begins with the use of active motion. Throughout the early treatment period and for as long as any spasm or tenderness remains, the hot packs are applied regularly every day. For a long subsequent period, overactivity may cause return of muscle spasm and dysfunction.

The kind of treatment described can be carried out best in a hospital and by personnel specially trained in the necessary procedures. With this type of treatment, contracture from muscle shortening is prevented, and, as compared with the older methods, the proportion who recover is higher, and the residual disability is less. If possible, hospital treatment should continue for as long as evidence exists of return of muscle function. In those instances in which the legs are paralyzed and a stage has been reached at which the physician desires the child to attempt walking, braces or splints may be prescribed for support.

The final steps in treatment may require operative procedures to improve the efficiency of permanently paralyzed extremities.

Bulbar Paralysis

Symptoms. When the inflammatory reaction of poliomyelitis attacks the higher portions of the central nervous system, especially the bulb, or medulla oblongata, nervous control of vital functions becomes threatened, and the prognosis for survival is reduced. In favorable instances the muscles of the eye, the face, the jaws or the palate alone may be affected. Recovery is complete in most cases, and no serious effects are suffered from the temporary disability. But when the lower cranial nerves and the upper portions of the spinal cord are involved there may be serious disturbance of swallowing, of respiration or of the central control of circulation. Paralysis of swallowing prevents not only the intake of food but also interferes with the disposition of the normal accumulations of mucus and saliva in the pharynx. Aspiration into the trachea may result in pneumonia or atelectasis. When certain areas of the brain stem are involved there may be serious disturbance of the general circulation with progressive cyanosis and weak, feeble pulse. Disturbances of respiration may be due either to involvement of the respiratory center which governs the automatic effort to breath or to paralysis of the muscles of respiration such as the diaphragm, the intercostal muscles and the pectoral muscles. Most of the fatalities in poliomyelitis are caused by disturbances of the circulation or the respiration.

Bulbar poliomyelitis has had a variable incidence in different epidemics, from 5 to 20 per cent of paralytic cases. It is more common in adults and is particularly prone to affect pregnant women. An increased risk of the bulbar form of the disease is observed in children who have had recent tonsillectomies.

Treatment and Nursing Care. The management of bulbar poliomyelitis is frequently difficult and demands the best medical judgment and skillful attentive nursing. If the child's difficulties are limited to an inability to swallow, repeated gentle suction of the pharynx and postural drainage may be sufficient to protect his airway until his ability to swallow returns. Feeding is accomplished by gavage or by a nasal tube left in place. Parenteral fluids may be required if a satisfactory intake cannot be achieved in this way. When the child has respiratory difficulties in addition, it may be impossible to keep his airway clear without performing a tracheotomy.

Patients who require care in a respirator because of failing respiratory muscles present a complicated problem which is handled best by a staff of doctors and nurses who are specially trained for this purpose. Some of the difficulties which must be met are those of maintaining an airway, preventing aspiration, providing mechanical aids in exchanging air, maintaining nutrition and morale, physiotherapy, prevention of intercurrent respiratory and urinary tract infections and eventually rehabilitation of a patient who sometimes is paralyzed extensively and fearful of being weaned from the respirator.

DIAGNOSIS

The diagnosis of poliomyelitis after paralysis has occurred presents no difficulty. Diagnosis in the preparalytic stage with any degree of certainty is obviously not so easy. The preparalytic symptoms which have been enumerated, together with the results of an examination of the cerebrospinal fluid, will give strong presumptive evidence of a correct diagnosis. The cerebrospinal fluid in poliomyelitis, whether preparalytic or abortive, always shows moderate but definite abnormality. The cells are increased, often up to 100, seldom to 500 for each cubic millimeter, and rarely sufficiently to cause the fluid to be definitely cloudy. The proteins of the fluid are increased, and the colloidal tests (Lange, etc.) are positive.

Poliomyelitis may be confused with other infections of the central nervous system such as Coxsackie virus disease, mumps encephalitis, infectious polyneuritis or the virus encephalitides. Spinal fluid examination usually permits a ready distinction between poliomyelitis and acute meningitis.

ISOLATION PRECAUTIONS

To limit the spread of virus from a hospitalized child with known infection, the same sort of precautions as those taken with typhoid fever are required, namely, careful disposal of stools and aseptic technic. The period during which this must be continued is determined arbitrarily and usually is set at about 2 weeks after the onset of symptoms. The child who is cared for at home already has contaminated his environment with virus by the time his disease is discovered, so that enforcement of such isolation measures is probably futile.

PREVENTION

Active immunization with a satisfactory and safe vaccine would be the desirable method of preventing poliomyelitis. At the present writing such a vaccine is under trial but its value has yet to be determined. Passive protection of exposed children by administration of transfusions, convalescent serum and pooled gamma globulin preparations has been tried in the past, but to date there is no scientific evidence to indicate that these procedures influence the course of an epidemic. Quarantine measures, closing of schools during an epidemic and isolation of children from one another likewise have failed to have any observable influence. Generally it is considered wise to keep susceptible children from entering households which are known to be contaminated and to prevent chilling and overexertion during the polio season.

COXSACKIE VIRUS DISEASE

This peculiar name (pronounced cook-sock-ee) is applied to a recently discovered family of virus agents which often travel with poliomyelitis viruses and may be isolated simultaneously from the same patient at times. Clinical symptoms of infection include meningeal irritation, pain in the muscles of the chest and ulcerative lesions in the mouth. Fever is usually present for a few days. The infections are self-limited, free from complications and are not known to cause death. Their chief importance lies in the confusion with poliomyelitis which they may occasion.

RABIES

Rabies is a uniformly fatal disease resulting from a specific virus infection of the nervous system usually acquired through the bite of an animal afflicted with the disease. Presumably, all warm-blooded animals are susceptible, although in settled communities the dog is the animal most commonly affected. Rabies occurs at any season. The season of "dog days" has no connection either with dogs or rabies, but some increase of the amount of rabies in dogs takes place in warm weather, beginning in April.

The virus of rabies is present in the saliva of rabid dogs and is introduced into the body by means of a bite. The virus travels along nerves, eventually reaching the central nervous system by this route.

The time of travel represents all or most of the incubation period, which is widely variable, depending on the quantity of virus introduced, the virulence of the virus, the nerve supply and the distance of the point bitten from the central nervous system. Rabies from bites about the head has a short incubation period. The incubation period is rarely shorter than 2 weeks and may be as long as 6 or 7 months. The average time is from 1 to 2 months. If the virus is introduced in small quantity in an area poorly supplied by nerves, the disease may never develop. Bites through thick clothing are not very dangerous because of the small quantity of virus inoculated. Only from 15 to 20 per cent of those bitten by rabid animals develop the disease.

SYMPTOMS

Regardless of the length of the incubation period the symptoms are equally severe when they occur. The onset and the course are rapid. An outstanding feature is hypersensitiveness and increased reaction to external stimuli. The hyperirritability may be local at first but it rapidly involves the entire body. One of the early symptoms is convulsive contracture of the muscles of swallowing when ingestion is attempted. Soon the convulsive seizures are general and they may occur at the slightest stimulus. There are periods of excitement in which the child may rage about, become destructive and perhaps attempt to escape. The convulsive and the excitement periods sometimes are interspersed with times of apparently complete normality. Usually the mind is clear throughout this stage of the disease, except during the brief periods of excitement. During convulsions, the child experiences acute agony. Death may occur during the convulsive stage 2 or 3 days after onset of the disease. If the child survives longer, the hyperirritability is replaced by increasing weakness and finally by complete paralysis; death occurs from respiratory paralysis or cardiac failure 3 or 4 days after the onset.

In some instances, the convulsive stage is largely lacking, and in its place a general trembling precedes the paralytic stage. This is spoken of as the paralytic, or in animals the "dumb," type of rabies in contrast with the "furious" type already described. Children with paralytic rabies usually live 1 or 2 days longer than those with the convulsive type.

TREATMENT

Treatment is entirely symptomatic and completely futile.

PREVENTION

The only hope in the management of rabies lies in its prevention. The first step in prevention is proper treatment of the wound, and the second is active immunization. Bleeding from the wound should be encouraged. The wound should be cleansed promptly and thoroughly and then either cauterized with fuming nitric acid or irrigated thoroughly with a 20-per-cent solution of soft soap. Tincture of green soap is as effective as nitric acid and is not tissue-scarring. Such treatment of the wound gets rid of much of the virus and thus tends to prolong the incubation period. It may even prevent the disease. Immunization is delayed pending the diagnosis of

the condition of the dog, unless the dog has escaped and is not available.

If the dog shows undoubted symptoms of rabies, it should be killed and examined. If the dog is apparently normal, it should be confined for 2 weeks. If the dog remains well for 2 weeks, it did not infect the child with rabies. A dog with manifest rabies does not live longer than 4 or 5 days. The dog's saliva is infective for 3 to 4 days before the symptoms appear. The symptoms of rabies in dogs are not very different from those already described for man. First there occurs a change in disposition either to one of sullenness and irritability or to one of unusual affection and desire to be petted. The dog becomes restless and is startled easily. Then occurs either the furious or the dumb type of rabies. In the furious type, the dog runs away and wanders aimlessly, biting whatever animals or humans get in the way. Soon the difficulty in swallowing and convulsions appear, with death in from 3 to 5 days after the onset of the symptoms. In the paralytic type, the dog usually remains at home and is not so much of a public menace. The incubation period in dogs is usually 14 days or less.

The dog should not be killed for examination until the symptoms of rabies are established very definitely, for the reason that satisfactory examination cannot always be made in the early stages. For examination, the dog's head and part of the neck are sent to a suitable laboratory. If the weather is warm and the distance great, the head should be packed in ice for preservation. Rabies is diagnosed by the finding of inclusion bodies, known as Negri bodies, within the cells in smears or sections of material from certain parts of the brain and the spinal cord. If rabies is diagnosed in the dog, immunization of the bitten child should be begun at once.

Immunization. In the procedure advocated by Pasteur immunization is carried out by daily injections of active, living but attenuated virus contained in the spinal cords of rabbits in which it has been propagated. The attenuation of the virus is brought about by drying the cords for periods of from 2 to 8 days. The cords are pulverized and suspended in water for injection. The more attenuated virus is injected first, and virus of increasing virulence subsequently. By this procedure, 3 weeks are required to give all the necessary injections. Another satisfactory procedure is to inject gradually increasing quantities of rabbit-cord virus of known and constant virulence. By this method, the necessary injections may be given in 2-weeks' time. A more recent procedure is to use killed virus for immunization. For all methods, the same doses are employed for children as for adults. From 4 to 5 weeks are required for the development of full immunity, 2 or 3 weeks of this time being occupied by the injections. Death from rabies of persons immunized in the manner described is limited largely to those instances in which the incubation period was short or the immunization delayed. Even with these handicaps, the death rate is less than 0.5 per cent of those bitten by rabid animals in contrast with from 15 to 20 per cent among the unimmunized.

The immunization injections are given subcutaneously in the abdominal wall and are spaced as widely as possible. Usually some local reaction occurs, particularly in the second week, with redness, soreness and itching. Occasionally, a slight constitutional reaction is experienced, including urticaria. The immunization is relatively safe, accumulated statistics ascribing to the injected material approximately 1 death in 10,000 immunizations. The deaths are chiefly among adults and never in young children. The cause of the deaths has not been explained.

INFLUENZA

Influenza is a specific respiratory virus infection caused by a group of closely related virus agents. The symptomatology is well-known—chills, fever, muscular aches, headache and sore throat. A similar train of symptoms may be observed with other acute respiratory infections which are not due to the specific virus of influenza, and differentiation is possible only by special laboratory examination or by suspicion during the course of an epidemic. In general, children are not so seriously affected as adults, and for this reason, prophylactic immunization with influenza vaccine has found little favor. Treatment consists of bed rest, aspirin for relief of symptoms and protection against superimposed bacterial infections.

RICKETTSIAL INFECTIONS

The infectious agents called rickettsia are larger than viruses and barely visible by the ordinary microscope. They are agents which primarily infect ticks, mites, fleas and lice but may be transmitted to man in some instances. Like the viruses they are incapable of surviving unless in close association with living cells. The rickettsial diseases of man are not transmissible from man to man but require the mediation of one of the small parasites mentioned above. The diseases that rickettsia produce have some common characteristics—fever, headache, skin eruption, leukopenia, self-limited course and favorable response to chlortetracycline (Aureomycin), oxytetracycline (Terramycin) and chloramphenicol. Detailed description will not be given because these infections are uncommon in the United States, and each has a rather limited geographic area of prevalence.

ROCKY MOUNTAIN SPOTTED FEVER OR TICK TYPHUS

This is the most severe rickettsial infection seen in the United States. As the names suggest, it is found in the Rocky Mountain area and is transmitted to man by infected ticks. The onset is abrupt with high fever and severe headache followed by a measleslike rash which generally is more marked on the extremities than on the trunk. The prognosis of the untreated disease is rather serious, but rapid response to chlortetracycline or its related antibiotics is to be anticipated. A vaccine is available for active immunization.

MURINE TYPHUS

Murine typhus is transmitted to man by fleas and mites which live on rats. It is seen in the southern part of the United States. The symptomatology is similar to tick fever but less severe. It responds to the same treatment.

RICKETTSIALPOX

This is a new disease which thus far has been observed only in New York City. A mouse mite is responsible for its transmission to children. A local lesion develops at the site of the infecting bite and before the appearance of the general rash. The disease is self-limited and improves under chlortetracycline treatment.

Q FEVER

This is a rickettsial infection which simulates protracted influenza. It is derived from infected cattle; the mechanism of transmission is imperfectly understood. It too responds to chlortetracycline.

SITUATIONS FOR FURTHER STUDY

1. How do symptoms of German measles differ from those of rubeola? Do infants under 6 months of age acquire measles? What is the period of greatest communicability in measles? In what age period is the mortality rate of measles the highest?

2. Compare the lesions of chickenpox and smallpox. How do they differ? What is the difference in the distribution of the lesions?

3. What specific protective measures against communicable disease can be given during the period of infancy?

4. When caring for a child in the acute stage of poliomyelitis, how could you assist in preventing deformities?

5. What is entailed in the convalescent care of a child with poliomyelitis? What problems would he need help in facing during the convalescent period?

6. A child has been bitten by a neighborhood dog. The mother asks you for advice. What suggestions would you make?

7. What should parents teach their children about dogs?

BIBLIOGRAPHY

Chant, H. L.: Rabies, Am. J. Nursing 47:391, 1947.

Lowman, C. L., Siedenfeld, M. A., and Newton, Kathleen: Poliomyelitis. I. The management of poliomyelitis; II. Psychological considerations in poliomyeltitis care; III. The nurse in poliomyelitis, Am. J. Nursing 47:367, 1947.

McKhann, C. F., and Wilson, J. L.: Acute anterior poliomyelitis, in Brenneman's System of Pediatrics, vol. 2, Hagerstown, Md., Prior, 1948.

Parise, C. Di P.: The patient in a respirator, Am. J. Nursing 51:360, 1951.

Rivers, T. M.: Viral and Rickettsial Infections of Man, ed. 2, Philadelphia, Lippincott, 1952.

Stevenson, J. L.: Nursing for the poliomyelitis patient, Am. J. Nursing 48:290, 1948.

Webster, L. T.: Rabies, New York, Macmillan, 1942.

Wright, J.: The respir-aid rocking bed in poliomyelitis, Am. J. Nursing 47:454, 1947.

Nursing for the poliomyelitis patient (pamphlet), 1948, Joint Orthopedic Nursing Advisory Service of the National Organization for Public Health Nursing and the National League of Nursing Education, 2 Park Ave., New York 6, N. Y.

CHAPTER EIGHTEEN

Bacterial, Fungous, Spirochetal and Protozoal Infections

BACTERIAL INFECTIONS

A large number of bacteria are known to produce infection in man. In this text only a few of the more important pediatric conditions will be considered. Some of them are discussed in other chapters—gonorrheal ophthalmia in Chapter 7, bacterial meningitis in Chapter 12 and dysentery in Chapter 25. In contrast with the viral infections, the incubation period tends to be short, and the course of the untreated disease is prolonged. The degree of immunity which is achieved is variable but in many instances does not result in lifelong protection. For most of these diseases some form of antitoxic or antibiotic treatment is available; hence their prompt and accurate recognition becomes important in order to provide optimum therapy. Isolation of the infecting organism is possible in all of them except tetanus.

DIPHTHERIA

Diphtheria is characterized by the growth of the specific bacillus of this disease on an epithelial or mucous-membrane surface with the production of an exudative membrane and with the production and the absorption of toxin which has severe and destructive effects locally and in distant tissues and organs.

ETIOLOGY

The disease is caused by the diphtheria bacillus, *Corynebacterium diphtheriae*. Diphtheria is endemic in all large communities that have not yet suppressed it with programs of mass immunization of infants. It occurs to some extent in all seasons. With the coming of winter the incidence increases, sometimes to the extent of an epidemic, and it declines in late spring. Diphtheria occurs at all ages, but with the greatest frequency between 2 and 6 years. Because antitoxin is used in treatment and because toxin does not produce immunity in the presence of an excess of antitoxin, one attack protects against subsequent attacks in only about one third of the cases.

SYMPTOMS

The characteristic lesion of diphtheria is destruction of superficial epithelium at the site of the infection with exudation of fibrin and pus cells to produce a pseudomembrane by coagulation of the fibrin in a thick layer. The most frequent location of the infection is in the throat, particularly on the tonsils. It occurs also in the nose and in the larynx and the trachea, and sometimes on the skin. It may be limited to any one of these sites or it may affect several of them simultaneously.

FAUCIAL DIPHTHERIA

Diphtheria of the tonsils and the tonsillar region is known as faucial diphtheria and is the variety most frequently observed. It has an incubation period of from 1 to 4 days. In the average or typical case the symptoms consist chiefly of fever, sore throat, malaise, headache, and often general aches and pains. An early throat redness is followed quickly by an exudate which coalesces, becomes thicker and resembles a membrane. The membrane at

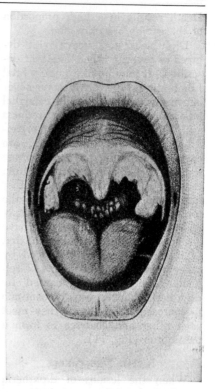

Fig. 71. Faucial diphtheria. Showing a characteristic distribution of membrane.

first is grayish white but later it becomes a dirty gray. The breath has an unpleasant and rather characteristic odor. When the membrane is removed forcibly, a bleeding surface remains. When no treatment is given, the membrane spreads in all directions. It may involve the posterior pharynx, the uvula and the soft palate, and in severe infections the hard palate. The cervical lymph glands are moderately to greatly enlarged, with proportionate visible swelling of the neck. Prostration increases as the disease progresses.

Death results in a high proportion of those who are untreated.

Diphtheria may occur with degrees of severity other than that described. It may be of a rapidly fatal fulminating type or it may never become more than a mild catarrhal inflammation manifest by redness and slight soreness. Other organisms, particularly streptococci, are capable of producing a membrane indistinguishable in appearance from that of diphtheria. On the other hand, the lesion produced on the tonsils by diphtheria bacilli, especially in the early stages, may have an appearance identical with that of follicular tonsillitis produced by other organisms. The points of follicular exudate, when caused by diphtheria bacilli, usually continue to increase in size until they meet each other and coalesce to form a membrane (Fig. 71).

Nasal Diphtheria

When the lesions of diphtheria are limited to the nose, little and often no constitutional disturbance results. Internal examination of the nose reveals areas of membrane. Nasal discharge is present, sometimes thickly purulent, but more often thin and tinged with blood. The discharge excoriates the upper lip. The disease may extend to the pharynx and the fauces. Nasal diphtheria tends to remain chronic over a period of weeks. Because of the relative infrequency of paralyses and other usual complications of diphtheria, it may be concluded that a lesser amount of toxin absorption occurs in nasal diphtheria.

Laryngeal Diphtheria

Diphtheria may occur primarily in the larynx and remain limited to it. More commonly, laryngeal diphtheria occurs in association with and probably as an extension from faucial diphtheria. When the process is limited to the larynx, usually little constitutional disturbance, except that produced by obstruction to the passage of air, is present. The absorption of toxin from this area is relatively poor. Obstruction is caused by inflammatory edema and by membrane and sometimes by an additional factor of spasm of laryngeal muscles excited by the infection. A croupy cough is present, and the voice is lost because of involvement of the vocal cords. Otherwise, the symptoms are chiefly those of respiratory difficulty. The breathing is noisy or stridulous on both inspiration and expiration. The accessory muscles of respiration are brought into use by voluntary effort. Retraction of the tissues of the neck above the clavicle, of the intercostal spaces and often of the abdomen at the chest margin occurs during inspiration. Cyanosis is present, the degree depending on the amount of obstruction. Death from asphyxia is frequent.

The membrane of laryngeal diphtheria frequently extends down the trachea and into the larger bronchi. Symptoms of such extension usually are absent or overlooked because obstruction to respiration is limited to the larynx. The trachea is relatively large, and the laryngeal space between the vocal cords is small. Sometimes laryngeal diphtheria is spoken of as membranous croup, in contrast with catarrhal or spasmodic croup, which has symptoms similar in some respects.

EFFECTS OF DIPHTHERIA TOXIN

The only important damage produced by the diphtheria bacillus is that caused by its toxin. The toxin causes degeneration and death of tissue. At the site of the diphtheria membrane the toxin has killed the superficial tissues. From this site the toxin is absorbed and carried over the body by the blood stream. The effects on the various tissues of the body are proportionate to the amount of toxin absorbed. Certain of the body tissues show the effect more strikingly than others.

Degeneration of the heart muscle (myocarditis) is one of the most serious effects of diphtheria toxin. If myocarditis becomes manifest, it usually becomes evident in the third week of the disease, after all local signs of diphtheria have disappeared. The heart often becomes dilated, the pulse rate changes markedly from the normal, and death from cardiac failure is the usual result.

Diphtheria toxin also causes degeneration of nerves. In cases of faucial diphtheria, the first nerves to show this effect are those of the soft palate. Paralysis of the soft palate occurs in the second week of the disease. It causes a "nasal voice" and difficulty in swallowing, with frequent expulsion of fluid through the nose because of this difficulty.

It is in the third week or later that other paralyses appear. Paralysis may be general or it may be more conspicuous in one part than in another. The most serious paral-ysis is that of the muscles of respiration. Complete recovery from all these paralyses always occurs, provided that interference with vital functions (respiration) is not great enough to cause death. Even with respiratory paralysis, recovery occurs if the child can be kept breathing by means of a respirator.

COMPLICATIONS

The direct effects of diphtheria toxin are a part of the disease rather than complications. Otitis media is not uncommon as a complication. Pneumonia occurs occasionally when the illness has been severe.

ISOLATION

Isolation is maintained until several consecutive cultures of the nose and the throat fail to grow the diphtheria bacillus.

PROGNOSIS

In general, the mortality rate is between 5 and 10 per cent. It is higher with laryngeal diphtheria and lower when the infection is limited to the nose. For those who live, complete recovery is to be expected.

PREVENTION

In the event of known exposure of a nonimmune child, temporary protection can be given by antitoxin, which usually is injected subcutaneously for this purpose. A satisfactory prophylactic dose is 2,000 units. A previously immunized child should be given a booster dose of toxoid.

Active immunization produces long-lasting immunity. It is used extensively and is to be recommended strongly. The procedure is carried out by means of injections of diphtheria toxin which has been modified in such a manner as to make it harmless. Three varieties of preparation are available, namely, a toxin-antitoxin mixture, a toxoid and an alum-precipitated toxoid. Alum-precipitated toxoid is the one in most common use and usually is combined with tetanus toxoid and pertussis vaccine. Although a single injection of this material may give satisfactory immunity, it is preferable to give 3 injections a month apart. The time required to produce satisfactory immunity varies from 2 weeks to 6 months. The majority are immune within 2 months. It is desirable to verify the existence of immunity subsequently by means of the Schick test. If the test is positive, the child should have more immunizing injections. In some cases a program of booster injections every 3 years is carried out arbitrarily without Schick testing.

Schick Test. The Schick test consists of injecting into the skin ⅟₅₀ of the minimum lethal dose of toxin for the guinea pig. This amount of toxin is contained in a volume of 0.1 cc. A positive or nonimmune reaction consists of redness, swelling and later pigmentation. In the performance of the test on adults and older children, it is desirable to make a control injection using material identical with that used for the Schick test except that it has been heated to 100° C. for 5 minutes. Heat destroys diphtheria toxin. Any reaction which occurs with the control solution is due to proteins which it contains and not to toxin. By comparing the test with the control, the amount of reaction due to the toxin can be determined. The reaction from protein reaches its height usually within 24 hours, while that from toxin does not attain a maximum for several days, at which time the protein reaction usually has disappeared.

DIAGNOSIS

The diagnosis of diphtheria is made by means of the clinical features which have been described and by the finding of the diphtheria bacillus in material from the site of the local lesion. These organisms are found with the greatest reliability when inoculations are made from the diseased area onto a special culture medium (Löffler's blood serum) and the culture is incubated for from 8 to 12 hours or longer. The cultural growth is placed on a glass slide, stained and examined microscopically. Certain throat infections may resemble diphtheria closely. These are distinguished from diphtheria by identification of the causative organism by culture.

TREATMENT

The administration of diphtheria antitoxin at the earliest possible moment is of primary importance. It alone can neutralize the effects of free toxin which has not yet become attached to cells. It probably has no effect on toxin which already is combined with cells. A single dosage with antitoxin is to be preferred to repeated small doses, and the common practice is to give 40,000 units intramuscularly. In children who exhibit symptoms of severe toxicity, an additional 40,000 units may be given intravenously. In either circumstance it is imperative to test the child for sensitivity to horse serum first. Unlike toxoid, antitoxin is prepared in horses and

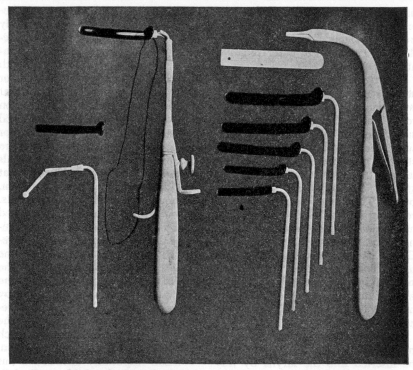

Fig. 72. A set of tubes for intubation of the larynx, together with the instruments used for inserting and extracting the tubes.

is capable of producing a severe or even fatal reaction in a child who is sensitive to it. Testing is done by conjunctival or intracutaneous inoculation of a small amount of the diluted material. An immediate inflammatory reaction appears if the individual is sensitive.

Several of the antibiotics are effective against diphtheria bacilli. The neutralization of the antitoxin should be followed by full dosage with penicillin or one of the broad spectrum antibiotics such as oxytetracycline, chlortetracycline or tetracycline.

In addition to administration of antitoxin and antibiotics, certain other treatment measures are important. The child should be kept in bed until afebrile in all cases—for at least 2 weeks in cases of moderate severity and for at least 3 weeks in cases of greater severity. Cleansing gargles or similar appropriate measures add to the comfort of the child. The diet should be modified according to the amount of soreness of the throat and the degree of prostration. If myocarditis should develop, absolute rest in bed is the chief therapeutic measure of importance. Confinement to bed should be maintained until the child has recovered entirely and for several weeks thereafter. The necessary inactivity should be aided by full doses of morphine or other sedative at short intervals.

Laryngeal Stenosis. If laryngeal stenosis is present, the breathing of warm moist air (croup tent or steam room) and the administration of such drugs as antipyrine and ipecac will relieve whatever part of the stenosis is caused by spasm of the larynx, but will have no effect on stenosis due to edema and membrane. The several possible ways of relieving stenosis due to edema and membrane require special equipment and a certain amount of skill. Cotton swabs passed into the larynx may dislodge and remove membrane sufficiently to allow adequate passage of air. Similarly, aspiration by means of a suction tube may accomplish the same purpose.

Intubation and Tracheotomy. A tube shaped to fit the larynx may be inserted into the larynx by way of the mouth (intubation) and left in place until the inflammation has subsided sufficiently to permit satisfactory breathing without it (Fig. 72). A tube may be placed in the trachea through an incised opening in the neck (tracheotomy).

The choice between intubation and tracheotomy depends chiefly on the availability of expert medical care. Intubation is the procedure of choice whenever expert care can be obtained promptly. It does not require incision and it permits the child to warm and moisten the air he breathes. The mortality from tracheotomy in diphtheria is higher than that from intubation, due chiefly to the greater frequency of pneumonia.

For either intubation or tracheotomy, the child is wrapped securely in a sheet ("mummied"). For tracheotomy the child is always recumbent. Intubation may be done with the child in either a recumbent or a sitting position. The recumbent position is preferable for the reason that one less assistant is required and the child is in a position for tracheotomy, should this procedure become necessary. All materials needed for tracheotomy should be at hand before undertaking intubation, as should also emergency stimulants. The silk thread which is attached to the head of the tube for convenience during intubation usually is removed after it is certain that the tube is in place in the larynx. If the thread should be left attached, the free end is secured to the cheek by adhesive tape and the hands are restrained to prevent removal by the child. The restraint should be such as not to interfere with respiration.

When respiratory obstruction has been relieved, the child usually falls asleep immediately and seems to be entirely comfortable. After intubation, some care in feeding must be exercised in order to prevent aspiration of food and consequent choking. Usually, some position in which swallowing can be achieved without difficulty can be found for the child. If it cannot, gavage must be used.

The intubation tube usually is removed after from 2 to 3 days. If respiratory difficulty recurs, the tube is replaced and allowed to remain for an additional 2 to 3 days. In the majority of cases, the tube is not needed longer than from 4 to 5 days and in many cases not so long. It is important to remember that when the tube is removed or when it is coughed out accidentally, no respiratory difficulty is to be expected for anywhere from several minutes to an hour or more, after which time evidence of the return of edema may become manifest. If tracheotomy has been done, special nursing care is required.

DIPHTHERIA CARRIERS

Individuals who are found to harbor diphtheria bacilli in their throats without being ill themselves are known as carriers. They are a potential menace to the community and should be isolated until freed of their organisms. Penicillin in full dosage for from 1 to 2 weeks is usually effective. If it fails, one of the broad-spectrum antibiotics should be used. If this too fails, removal of tonsils and adenoids or thorough drainage of infected sinuses may be required.

TETANUS

Tetanus (lockjaw) is a disease characterized by tonic muscular spasm, either local or generalized, the spasm being a manifestation of toxic effects on the nervous system produced by the exotoxin of the tetanus bacillus. Unlike diphtheria, it is not contagious or transmissible by contact. It resembles diphtheria in that symptoms are due to a soluble exotoxin which disseminates from the infecting bacilli.

The tetanus bacillus (*Clostridium tetani*) commonly is found in the soil and in the fecal discharges of man and animals. It is a spore-forming organism and in its spore stage can live for an indefinite period of time in dust and under other unfavorable conditions. It is harmless in the alimentary tract. When introduced into the body by way of a wound, it frequently finds conditions favorable to its growth. The organism is anaerobic. An anaerobic environment often prevails in injured tissue. Its growth produces no identifiable local tissue damage and therefore no characteristic lesion. Its growth is accompanied by the production of an exotoxin. The toxin has a special affinity for nervous tissue and finds its way to the central nervous system along the various motor nerves.

Motor nerves of the region of the wound may carry the earliest and largest supply of toxin in some cases, thus accounting for the occasional occurrence of local tetanus. However, usually the toxin reaches the blood by way of the lymph channels and is carried to all the motor nerves of the body, entering them presumably by way of the motor end plates. The interval between the time of infection and the development of symptoms depends on the rate of toxin production, which in turn depends on whether conditions in the wound are favorable for growth of the organism, on the number of organisms introduced and on their virulence or ability to produce toxin. Thus it is that the shorter the incubation, the more severe the disease and the more likely it is to prove fatal. Incubation periods vary from 3 days to 1 month or more, falling between 7 and 14 days in a high proportion of cases. It has been stated as a rule, not strictly true, that the prognosis is bad when the incubation period is less than 9 days and relatively good when the incubation period is longer than this.

SYMPTOMS

Sometimes the earliest symptom is twitching of the muscles in the

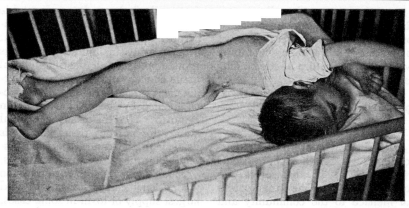

FIG. 73. Opisthotonos of tetanus.

neighborhood of the wound. More often—in fact, usually—the first symptoms are in association with the shortest motor nerves of the body, namely, those of the head. Thus a stiffness of the muscles controlling the jaw, a condition known as trismus, is the outstanding first or early symptom. The jaw is held tightly closed and it cannot be opened. Involvement of the muscles of the throat and the tongue causes difficulties in swallowing and in speech. Soon the muscles in the distribution of the spinal nerves are affected, first those supplied by the shorter nerves (the trunk) and then those supplied by the longer nerves (the extremities).

All the voluntary musculature of the body becomes affected and is in a tonic state. Superimposed on this state of continued tonicity are to be observed paroxysms of increased muscular spasm. These paroxysms are termed convulsions, though they differ considerably from the cerebral type of convulsion. Consciousness is not lost or impaired, unless through asphyxia

from spastic fixation of the thorax. The convulsions are precipitated by relatively small external stimuli, such as noises, bright lights or jarring of the bed. When all the muscles of the body are in strong contraction, the position of the body is determined by the strongest muscle groups. The characteristic position is one of opisthotonos, often extreme, with the head drawn back and the back arched. (Fig. 73). Such strong muscular contractions are very painful, and pain is felt particularly in the back and the head. During the severe paroxysms, the thorax is held immovable, so that the respiratory movements are feeble or absent. This results in cyanosis and anoxia and in many instances in death by asphyxia.

The disease in its most characteristic form runs a course: first it increases in severity and then, in those who recover, it gradually decreases in severity. During the stage of increasing severity, the convulsions usually are preceded by twitchings which become more frequent and more severe and gradually merge into the convulsive stage. The convulsions increase in frequency and violence, and the continued tonicity between convulsions becomes greater. The interval after the onset of symptoms required for the full development of the convulsive stage varies from a few hours to 2 days, with an average of about 24 hours.

In the children who survive, the symptoms remain unchanged for a period of from 5 to 10 days or more, after which time they gradually subside, their complete disappearance requiring from 2 to 3 weeks or longer. The temperature may be normal throughout the course of the disease or it may rise to 104° or more. In those who die, terminal pyrexia is common. Death may occur from exhaustion or from aspiration pneumonia. The most common cause of death is asphyxia from fixation of the respiratory muscles. Bad prognostic signs are a short incubation period, early complete trismus, rapid general development of spasms and high fever. Without treatment by antitoxin the average mortality from tetanus was as high as 80 to 90 per cent. With antitoxin and modern methods it has been reduced to 20 to 50 per cent.

Prevention

Passive Immunization. Tetanus may be prevented by parenteral administration of antitoxin soon after the injury which permitted the introduction of the tetanus bacilli. The antitoxin is similar to that used in diphtheria and is prepared in the same manner in horses. Testing for sensitivity to horse serum is essential before it is used. The usual prophylactic dose is 1,500 units. If the wound is large or grossly contaminated, it is sometimes desirable to repeat the dose within a week or 10 days. Decision as to which wounds require antitoxin administration and which do not is sometimes difficult. In cases of doubt the antitoxin should be given. Burns, compound fractures, wounds from explosives (e.g., Fourth-of-July accidents) and any wound in which soil contamination is likely require tetanus prophylaxis.

Active Immunization. Immunity produced by injection of tetanus toxoid (alone or in combination with diphtheria toxoid) produces a long-lasting immunity which may be more or less permanent. At least 2 doses of toxoid are required, spaced from 1 to 3 months apart. The basic immunity thus established may be reactivated within 4 to 6 days if a booster injection is given. Thus in children known to have basic immunity, toxoid rather than antitoxin is given as prophylaxis. No test for horse serum sensitivity is necessary when toxoid is used.

Isolation

Isolation is not necessary, since the infecting organisms are harmless unless inserted into a deep wound.

Treatment

The treatment of tetanus, once the symptoms have appeared, may be considered as having 3 phases: (1) the performance of any necessary surgery; (2) antitoxin treatment; and (3) symptomatic treatment.

Surgical Treatment. The indications for surgical treatment of the causative wound are the same as for a similar wound in the absence of tetanus. Any foreign body should be removed, any cellulitis or inflammation treated appropriately. The existence of tetanus does not call for radical or emergency operative measures, for the reason that antitoxin will neutralize any toxin that is present or that will be formed in the wound. In most instances, the wound will be healed and require no attention by the time tetanus develops.

Antitoxin Treatment. Various dosages of antitoxin and schedules for its administration have been proposed. In the past, multiple and daily dosage has been customary, and intrathecal administration has been practiced commonly. Intrathecal antitoxin may have irritating effects, and use of this route is unnecessary and not to be recommended. Rather than give multiple injections of antitoxin, it is far more logical and efficacious to give in a single dose all the antitoxin that is to be administered. When a single dose of from 60,000 to 70,000 units is given intramuscularly to a child, such toxin as is present in the body and not fixed is neutralized promptly, and large and amply protective amounts of antitoxin persist in the body for a considerable number of weeks. Any toxin newly formed in the wound is neutralized at once at the site of formation. The advocacy of a single injection has the support of successful clinical use, as well as the reasonableness of the procedure.

Symptomatic Treatment and Nursing Care. The most important factors in the symptomatic treatment of tetanus are those measures which are effective in decreasing the frequency and the severity of convulsions. The convulsions are dependent on changes in the nervous system pro-

duced by toxin which has been "fixed" in the cells. Antitoxin has no effect on the fixed toxin and, consequently, no effect on convulsions. Further fixation of toxin in the cells is prevented by the antitoxin administered. The effect of fixed toxin on the nervous system will continue unaltered for a period of from 5 to 10 days or more, during which time the convulsions will continue to recur unless brought under control by medication. It is important that convulsions be controlled as completely as possible. It is because of the convulsions that many of these children die, and the importance of their control has not been stressed sufficiently. When a child is brought under care for tetanus, the duty of first importance is to carry out the measures necessary for control of convulsions. This procedure takes precedence over antitoxin administration and all other nursing and medical procedures.

For the control of convulsions it is necessary to employ sedatives in large dosage and in addition to have the child in such a location that he will not be disturbed by noises, bright lights or anything else that is irritating to him. The sedative used will depend on the preference of the physician in charge, but could be chloral hydrate, Amytal, Avertin, one of the barbituric acid derivatives or some other drug. With such a drug as Avertin it is possible not only to prevent convulsions but also to maintain a state of relaxation which in the milder illnesses will permit the ingestion of food with relative ease and comfort. Relaxation usually can be obtained well within the toxic limits of the drug and in some cases without disturbing appreciably the consciousness of the child. Some of the drugs mentioned have only a small margin of safety between the therapeutic and the toxic dose. If the child is conscious, an anesthetic should be used for any painful procedure.

The ideal sedative management includes the giving of a dosage which maintains the child continuously in a relaxed state but is no larger than is required for this purpose. Avertin lends itself well to this kind of management. Avertin is given by rectum. When this drug is used, the rectal tube should be kept constantly in place, ready for injection at any time. The Avertin fluid is kept in a constant-temperature water bath at body temperature ready for immediate use. After the initial large dose and after relaxation has been attained, subsequent doses of Avertin should be small and given frequently, if necessary, rather than large doses given infrequently. An even level of sedation is desirable. Various criteria may be used as indications for further sedation, but the recurrence of rigidity of the abdominal muscles serves well.

The life of the child, particularly when tetanus is severe, depends in large measure on meticulous nursing and medical attention. A nurse should be with the child constantly, and the presence of both a nurse and a doctor is desirable. Without constant watching, suddenly the child may develop a convulsion and die. When the tetanus is severe, the amount of sedative required is sufficient to make the child unconscious, and in some instances the state of unconsciousness must be maintained for a week, or even 2 weeks, con-

tinuously. An unconscious child requires many things not needed by one whose reflexes are intact. The food must be given by gavage, and the fluid intake requires special attention. Parenteral fluid administration is often necessary. Bowel and bladder retention must be watched. Accumulated mucus must be kept aspirated from the throat. The development of pneumonia is always a danger to be feared. The pneumonia that occurs in these circumstances is extremely severe and is very likely to cause death. Frequent respiratory stimulation with a breathing mixture of carbon dioxide and oxygen is desirable. The only use for a respirator would be when an overdose of sedative had been given inadvertently; it has no place in the treatment of asphyxia from muscle spasm.

Frequently, the management of pharyngeal and laryngeal spasm and of mucus accumulations is made easier if a tracheotomy is performed early in the disease. The nursing care required has been described previously.

PERTUSSIS
(WHOOPING COUGH)

Whooping cough is characterized by paroxysms of coughing and a crowing sound with each quick intake of air during the course of the paroxysm.

ETIOLOGY

Whooping cough is caused by a bacillus, *Hemophilus pertussis,* described originally by Bordet and Gengou. The disease commonly occurs under 6 years of age and rarely after 10. Very young infants are susceptible, for immunity is not conducted across the placenta as in measles. It occurs in epidemics and endemically. One attack may be expected to confer lifelong immunity, though it does not do so in all instances. Second attacks of the disease occasionally occur.

SYMPTOMS

The incubation period varies. It is between 7 and 14 days. The disease begins as an ordinary bronchitis with only slight fever and little or no prostration. The cough becomes increasingly severe and finally assumes the peculiar paroxysmal nature characteristic of pertussis. The early stage is known as the catarrhal stage. Its duration is about a week but it may vary from 2 days to 2 weeks. The stage of severe cough is known as the paroxysmal or spasmodic stage. The duration of this stage also is variable but is usually from 2 to 3 weeks.

The typical paroxysm of pertussis consists of a series of explosive coughs rapidly repeated on a single expiration with no time for a breath between them. When the breath is expired to such an extent that no more coughing is possible, there is a rapid intake of air, and the coughing continues. This procedure may be repeated 3 or 4 or even more times.

Each inspiration during the paroxysm is accompanied by a peculiar crowing sound or whoop. The sound is produced by a spasm of the glottis. A severe paroxysm is a serious and terrifying ordeal for the child. Due to inability to breathe over such a long period, there is a feeling of impending suffocation. At first the face becomes red because of the coughing effort. As the attack progresses, the face becomes darker

in color, the eyes and the veins of the neck become prominent, the tongue protrudes with each cough, and tears, saliva and perspiration flow freely.

The paroxysm continues until the mucus which was the immediate exciting cause is dislodged. Toward the end of the paroxysm this mass of ropy mucus may be expelled a considerable distance from the mouth. Vomiting is frequent immediately after a paroxysm, often making the nutrition of the child a serious problem. The paroxysms vary in number, from only a few up to 50 or 60 in 24 hours. They are more frequent at night.

Unless the child suffers from loss of sleep because of frequent cough and from loss of food by vomiting, he passes through the paroxysmal stage with unimpaired nutrition and in apparent good health. In the absence of complications there is no fever. As in other infectious diseases, pertussis occurs with varying degrees of severity. Sometimes the paroxysms are infrequent and mild, and no doubt there are many instances of pertussis infection in which the symptoms are so mild that the condition is not diagnosed.

After the paroxysmal stage comes the stage of decline, lasting from 2 to 3 weeks. The attacks decrease gradually in severity and frequency. The development of simple bronchitis may prolong the paroxysmal cough indefinitely. Sometimes bronchitis acquired several weeks after complete recovery from whooping cough will cause paroxysmal cough and even whooping. The second attack is not pertussis; the peculiar cough is the result of habit or neurosis. The total duration of pertussis is from 6 weeks to several months.

COMPLICATIONS

The most frequent serious complication of pertussis is bronchopneumonia. Moderate bronchitis, which is a part of pertussis, produces increased susceptibility of the lower respiratory tract to secondary infection. Infants especially are likely to develop pneumonia, and as a consequence the mortality of pertussis in infancy is high. When pneumonia is present, the cough loses its paroxysmal character.

Hemorrhage is common in whooping cough but usually it is not serious. Hemorrhage from the nose is frequent. Hemorrhage beneath the conjunctiva occurs occasionally. Brain hemorrhage is infrequent. Hemorrhages are caused by the intense congestion incident to severe paroxysms of cough.

Convulsions, paralyses, coma and other cerebral symptoms sometimes occur. Occasionally, these are caused by gross brain hemorrhage, but more often they are not. The exact cause is not always easy to determine. These symptoms may be due to edema of the brain from passive congestion or vascular changes. Sometimes petechial hemorrhages are present as a cause, and occasionally inflammation of the meninges.

When paroxysms of cough are severe, the increased abdominal pressure may cause hernia. In some instances it may cause rectal prolapse. The dragging of the tongue over the lower incisor teeth during the cough may cause traumatic ulcer of the frenum of the tongue.

ISOLATION

Usually isolation is continued until whooping has ceased, which is from 2 to 3 weeks after the beginning of the paroxysmal stage.

PREVENTION

Active immunity is produced by injections of vaccine, which are given in a series of 3 injections at weekly or longer intervals and in a total dose of at least 80 billion bacilli. The immunity thus produced may be of relatively short duration, modified whooping cough sometimes developing after exposure a year after the injections. Even though immunization is not so satisfactory as that for diphtheria and smallpox, it is to be recommended for the infant and the young child because of the seriousness of the disease at this age. Frequently pertussis vaccine is combined with diphtheria and tetanus toxoid and given as a "triple vaccine."

Passive immunity produced by injection of convalescent serum or by hyperimmune human or rabbit serum is effective in prevention if given soon after exposure to the disease. This procedure is useful in controlling epidemics in institutions and in deferring the disease in the infant and the young child.

DIAGNOSIS

Diagnosis is usually easy after the cough has become typically paroxysmal and difficult before this period. By the time the cough has become paroxysmal, the white cells of the blood are increased definitely and often markedly, with relatively large predominance of lymphocytes. When the child is caused to cough onto a culture plate containing an appropriate medium, the organisms of the disease will grow and can be identified.

TREATMENT

No specific means of treatment now available seems to be entirely satisfactory, although good results are claimed from the use of large doses of hyperimmune serum and antibiotics. Hyperimmune serum is produced by giving a series of injections of vaccine to adult humans who have had whooping cough. A similar serum may be prepared in rabbits. Reliance must be placed largely on symptomatic management. No treatment is required when the disease is mild. Confinement to bed is unnecessary except as required by complications. Living or playing out of doors diminishes the frequency and the severity of paroxysms and is to be recommended when weather permits.

Sulfadiazine, oxytetracycline, chlortetracycline and chloramphenicol all have been useful in lessening the severity of pertussis, although they do not always stop the symptoms completely.

Much dependence is to be placed on sedative drugs for the control of paroxysms. Ether dissolved in oil and given by rectum is preferred by many for severe whooping cough. The barbiturates are useful, as also is codeine.

NURSING CARE

Intelligent, careful nursing is of the greatest importance in the management of a child with severe whooping cough, especially if the patient is an infant or a young child. Expert attention is needed during a severe paroxysm. During a parox-

ysm, an infant should be turned on his side to prevent aspiration of vomitus or mucus. An abdominal support gives comfort and when suitably applied helps to prevent hernia. When an older child coughs, the nurse should support his abdominal musculature with one hand and hold his forehead with the other. Keeping the child's nose free of secretion is of value, especially in preparation for the night. Such management tends to lessen the paroxysms. The throat should be kept free of mucus. Sodium bicarbonate mouthwashes cleanse and dissolve the mucus that may initiate coughing.

The vomiting associated with coughing paroxysms is not associated with nausea. After an infant or a child has vomited, he should be given a meal that contains approximately as many calories as he has vomited. The child's diet should be an easily digested, bland type. Supplying the necessary fluids between meals rather than with meals tends to lessen vomiting. Because pressure on the diaphragm stimulates coughing, distention should be prevented.

After a paroxysm, the child's skin should be dried and care taken to prevent chilling. Rest periods prior to meals and during the day prevent overstimulation and emotional reactions which increase the frequency and the severity of the paroxysms. The nurse attending the child with whooping cough should not give him an exaggerated amount of sympathy during the paroxysms. A child whose affectional needs are not satisfied may learn quickly that coughing brings him the attention he misses and craves. To prevent undue attention from being associated with the paroxysms, one must give the child the support he needs with poise and serenity.

STREPTOCOCCAL INFECTIONS

GENERAL CONSIDERATIONS

The Streptococci

The streptococci are a large and ubiquitous family of bacteria which have in common the properties of round shape, positive staining by Gram's method and a tendency to form chains during the process of reproduction. They are of great importance in human disease, particularly in pediatric infections. Unlike the typhoid bacillus, there is not one single variety of streptococcus but rather a large family, the members of which have widely differing abilities to create disease. Some are natural inhabitants of the body; others are harbingers of important disease. A general understanding of the classification is desirable in order to interpret bacteriologic reports.

To differentiate among the streptococci it is first necessary to discover what type of hemolysis the growing colony produces on a blood agar plate. Streptococci that are productive of alpha or gamma type of hemolysis are common inhabitants of the upper respiratory and the gastro-intestinal tracts, and their presence does not indicate disease in these locations. On the other hand, if found in blood cultures or in urine cultures, they assume pathogenic importance. The streptococci that are of major importance in pediatric disease produce a type of hemolysis that is known as beta hemolysis. The more exact term

"beta-hemolytic streptococcus" often is shortened to "hemolytic streptococcus" in everyday usage. Actually, there are about a dozen groups of beta-hemolytic streptococci which can be identified by immunologic methods. Only those in Group A are important in human disease. However, few laboratories actually test the grouping of the streptococci but assume that a beta-hemolytic streptococcus isolated from a person with an illness is probably a member of Group A. Occasionally, this assumption is wrong, and the streptococcus that is isolated turns out to be a harmless member of one of the other groups (B to N).

Group A beta-hemolytic streptococci can be subdivided further into some 40-odd types by a different immunologic procedure. Determination of these types has utility in the investigation of certain aspects of epidemiology but is not practiced commonly in clinical medicine. Group A streptococci produce a number of substances which exude from the bacterial cells and have a bearing upon the type of disease which results. Among these substances are erythrogenic toxin (or Dick toxin), streptolysin O and streptolysin S, streptokinase (or fibrinolysin) and hyaluronidase. As a result of streptococcal infection the body may produce antibodies against these substances which are known respectively as streptococcal antitoxin, antistreptolysin, antistreptokinase and antihyaluronidase. Fuller discussion of these substances can be sought from the bibliography.

Types of Streptococcal Disease

The most common site of infection with Group A beta-hemolytic streptococci is the upper respiratory tract. Many of the infections discussed in Chapter 9 (pharyngitis, tonsillitis, cervical adenitis, otitis media) are initiated by these organisms. The same sort of infection by a strain that produces a large amount of erythrogenic toxin and happens to affect a person who has no antitoxic immunity will result in scarlet fever. These upper respiratory infections constitute the common form of beta-hemolytic streptococcus infection in childhood.

In another group of disorders, the hemolytic streptococcus infection is not a primary one but is favored by previous illness such as measles, pertussis or diphtheria. Secondary streptococcus infection of this sort is particularly troublesome after the virus infections.

The skin may be invaded by hemolytic streptococci in 3 characteristic ways: erysipelas, impetigo and cellulitis. Erysipelas will be described below. Impetigo has been discussed in Chapter 13. Cellulitis usually results from the invasion of a break in the skin by beta-hemolytic streptococci. It is a diffuse erythema and edema of the skin which surrounds the local wound. It may be accompanied by lymphangitis and local adenitis.

The Group A beta-hemolytic streptococci have an additional role in human disease. Glomerular nephritis, rheumatic fever and perhaps some other systemic diseases are preceded regularly by hemolytic streptococcus infections. The resultant disease is not due to direct streptococcal invasion of the organs affected but is rather a secondary phenomenon associated with the development of antibodies during the

recovery from the local streptococcal disease.

Hemolytic streptococci also may be responsible for pneumonia, septicemia, osteomyelitis, pyogenic arthritis or meningitis. Fortunately, these are rare varieties of infection.

Epidemiology

Streptococcal disease is endemic in most areas of the United States. It tends to become more prevalent during the winter and the late spring, probably due to the collection of children indoors during the school year and during inclement weather. It is most prevalent in those who are in the first or the second year of schooling and presumably in the process of having their first contact with such organisms. In families where there are several children the school-age children may be responsible for introducing the infection into the family and transmitting it to preschool siblings or even infants. In the latter the disease is likely to be more severe and persistent. Younger children who suffer from repeated infections over many months sometimes are said to have "streptococcosis" analogous to the first infection with tubercle bacilli.

In addition to infected school contacts, children may acquire the infection from carrier adults who are well or suffer only minor symptoms in spite of the fact they harbor virulent streptococci in their noses and throats. Search for and treatment of such carriers is often essential before the recurring infections of the child can be terminated.

The density of streptococcal infection varies in a given community from one winter to the next. Usually the incidence of scarlet fever, nephritis and rheumatic fever parallels the amount of general streptococcal infection in any given year.

SCARLET FEVER
(SCARLATINA)

ETIOLOGY

Scarlet fever is an upper respiratory infection with Group A betahemolytic streptococci accompanied by a generalized erythematous skin eruption and toxic manifestations due to the effects of erythrogenic toxin upon a susceptible person. In occasional circumstances the initial streptococcal infection is in a wound or a burn rather than in the upper respiratory tract.

The disease occurs rarely in the first year. The incidence is at its height between 5 and 8 years, after which time it decreases. The disease occurs chiefly in the fall and the winter months, only rarely in summer.

The incubation period varies from 1 to 7 days; most frequently it is from 2 to 4 days. The period of greatest communicability is during the height of the febrile period, the first 3 to 5 days. The causative streptococcus is abundant in the throat and in all discharges from this site. Streptococci gradually decrease in number and may be expected to have disappeared within 5 weeks of the onset.

SYMPTOMS

The onset of scarlet fever is sudden, with sore throat, vomiting, prostration and fever. The onset is so sudden that the mother often can state an exact time. The appearance of the throat is that of acute tonsillitis. Within from 24 to 36 hours both an enanthem and an exanthem appear, and the fever reaches its height. This period is marked by restlessness, great thirst and often delirium. Also, the pulse rate is high and out of proportion to the temperature. After reaching the maximum, the temperature remains elevated continuously for several days, then gradually declines, reaching normal in from 10 to 14 days after the onset.

Enanthem. The enanthem consists of closely packed, minute, dark-red macules on the palate and the fauces, which later spread to the cheeks and the gums. The macules may fuse to a diffuse redness. The tongue in the beginning is coated, then first the edge and finally the entire tongue becomes clean. As the tongue clears, a swelling of its papillae is apparent. Very early in the disease, usually after the third or the fourth day, the tongue assumes the appearance known as "strawberry tongue," due to the general redness and the papillae swollen above the surface. Although strawberry tongue occurs in most cases of scarlet fever, it occurs also in other diseases and is not characteristic of any disease. The changes in the tongue are a part of the enanthem.

Exanthem. The exanthem, or rash, starts about the neck and the upper trunk, spreads over the body and attains its maximum in from 12 to 24 hours. It lasts from 3 to 7 days and gradually disappears. It is followed by desquamation, which begins about the eighth day or later and lasts 4 or 5 weeks. The rash from a distance looks like a diffuse red blush but on closer inspection is seen to consist of small points of redness, closely grouped. The appearance on the face is that of a diffuse blush, with the exception of a narrow area about the mouth, which by contrast appears to be white. When the rash is fully developed, the entire surface of the body is red except for the small area of pallor about the mouth. When the disease is mild, the skin, especially of the extremities, may be involved incompletely by the eruption.

The extent of skin desquamation is dependent on the severity of the eruption preceding it. If the eruption was mild, there is little desquamation. The desquamation on the body is usually in fine flakes ("branny") and involves the skin only superficially. On the hands and the feet it is more extensive and involves thicker layers of skin. In no case is the entire thickness of the skin involved in the desquamation, there being left an intact and adequate skin covering. These scales are not infectious, except as they have been contaminated by discharges from the throat. The duration of the desquamation is not a criterion of termination of isolation.

Variations in Severity

The preceding description of scarlet fever corresponds to a case of average severity. Great variations in the severity of scarlet fever are to be observed. In one instance, the disease may be so mild that it is difficult to recognize and in another, so severe that the child succumbs within a few days, sometimes before a rash has appeared.

Complications

The most common complications are otitis media, cervical adenitis and nephritis. Less common are arthritis, carditis and pneumonia. The otitis and the adenitis are extensions of the process in the throat. Although nephritis may appear earlier or later, it starts most commonly in the third week. Carditis and pneumonia may be expected to occur only when the illness is severe.

Isolation

The isolation period should be based on the persistence of streptococci in the throat. With the occurrence of complications with suppuration, such as otitis media, mastoiditis or empyema, the child remains a source of infection for a longer period than with the uncomplicated disease. Often the child is a source of infection for as long as discharges from these lesions continue.

Prognosis

In general, scarlet fever as it occurs at the present time is less severe than that of former years, and few deaths result directly from the toxic effects of the disease. Children nearly always recover from the nephritis of scarlet fever. The infectious complications tend to be more serious than the toxic effects.

Phases of Scarlet Fever

Scarlet fever may be divided into two distinct parts. One part consists of an infection with specific hemolytic streptococci; the other is a reaction to erythrogenic toxin produced by the streptococci. Perhaps some immunity to streptococcic infection exists, but the chief immunity to scarlet fever consists of immunity to the toxin of the bacterium. Thus, one may have a streptococcic infection of the throat or

PLATE 2

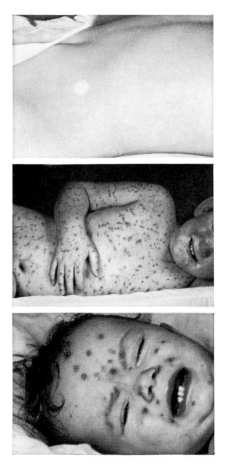

(Top) The rash of scarlet fever, showing a positive Schultz-Charlton reaction. *(Middle)* The rash of measles. *(Bottom)* The rash of Chickenpox.

elsewhere without having the rash of scarlet fever. If a person susceptible to scarlet fever is given an injection of the toxin, he develops a rash without having an infection. The conditions due directly to the infection are the sore throat and the accompanying malaise, fever and leukocytosis. Such complications as otitis, mastoiditis and cervical adenitis are dependent also on the infection. The phenomena caused by the toxin include fever, the initial vomiting, slight general glandular enlargement, the enanthem and the exanthem.

Toxic Filtrate

When scarlet-fever streptococci are grown in a broth medium and the bacteria subsequently are filtered out, the filtrate, though sterile, is toxic for some people. The toxic material is considered by some to be a toxin analogous to the toxin of the diphtheria bacillus. Other clinicians consider the toxic material to be an allergen, the rash of scarlet fever being an allergic response in one who previously had been sensitized by streptococcic infection. The distinction between these two concepts is of considerable academic interest but of no great practical importance.

Dick Test

The Dick test consists of the injection of a small amount of the toxic filtrate into the skin. If a local reaction occurs, the result is positive and the person is susceptible to scarlet fever. The amount used for injection is that which will produce a moderate local reaction in a person known to react to this material. This amount is known as a skin-test dose. A positive reaction to the Dick test begins to be evident in from 4 to 6 hours after injection and proceeds rapidly to its maximum. It should be read in 24 hours. The Dick test gives information as to susceptibility to the rash and associated phenomena of scarlet fever, but none as to susceptibility to streptococcic infection.

Diagnosis

Eruptions similar to the rash of scarlet fever may be produced by certain drugs. In such instances, sore throat and other characteristic symptoms are likely to be absent. Sometimes erythematous eruptions from other causes are distinguished from the rash of mild scarlet fever with some difficulty. In such instances, the Schultz-Charlton test is of value.

Schultz-Charlton Reaction. The injection of immune serum into the skin in an area of scarlet-fever eruption, if made early in the course of the eruption, will cause a blanching of the rash in the area surrounding the site of injection (Plate 2). No other rash responds in this manner.

Prevention

Active immunization against scarlet fever has been accomplished in the past by repeated injections of toxin. It has not been accepted generally because the resulting immunity is only against the toxin and does not prevent hemolytic streptococcal infection and because the reactions to the injections are frequently quite uncomfortable. Children known to be exposed to scarlet fever or other hemolytic streptococcus infections can be protected in many instances by prophylactic administration of a small dose of sulfadiazine, penicillin or other antibiotic given early during the incubation period.

TREATMENT AND NURSING CARE

In most instances the treatment is the same as that for any hemolytic streptococcus respiratory infection. Penicillin is the antibiotic of choice unless the child is sensitive to it. Sulfadiazine, oxytetracycline, chlortetracycline and tetracycline are also effective. Occasionally, a child with severe symptoms of toxicity may benefit from convalescent serum or antitoxin administered intramuscularly. During the second and the third weeks of the disease urinalysis is generally desirable to discover the child who occasionally develops nephritis as a sequel.

ERYSIPELAS
(ST. ANTHONY'S FIRE)

ETIOLOGY

The causative hemolytic streptococci gain entrance to the skin through a wound or other skin lesion. It affects people of all ages. In childhood, it is more common in infancy than later.

SYMPTOMS

The lesion of erysipelas is red and tender. The edge is demarcated sharply and raised above the level of the neighboring normal skin because of swelling. The inflammation spreads by way of the skin lymphatics. Streptococci are present in the skin in large numbers at the edge of the advancing lesion. The speed and the extent of spread of the lesion vary. In a few instances it may migrate over a considerable portion of the body, clearing up behind as it advances. The affected areas subsequently desquamate.

The constitutional symptoms include fever, which tends to be high and irregular. Very young or weak babies may have no fever. Varying degrees of intoxication are present. Appetite is lost, at least some drowsiness is present, and loss of strength occurs. Leukocytosis is nearly always present. The disease is self-limited and with the older methods of treatment lasts from 6 to 9 days.

PROGNOSIS

Erysipelas used to be feared as a serious disease, particularly in debilitated infants. It seldom is seen in recent times and is controlled readily by antibiotic therapy.

TREATMENT

As with any other hemolytic streptococcus infection, prompt response to penicillin or another suitable antibiotic can be anticipated. No local treatment is required.

TYPHOID FEVER

Typhoid fever is an acute infectious disease which in its most typical form is characterized by fever, prostration, stupor, enlarged spleen and inflammation of the intestine.

ETIOLOGY

The causative bacterium is the bacillus typhosus, *Salmonella typhosa*. The portal of entry is the alimentary tract. In areas where water supplies are supervised and sewage disposal is adequate, typhoid fever is uncommon. In such areas, the infection is acquired chiefly from persons who have the disease or are carriers of the typhoid bacillus. Typhoid fever has its greatest incidence in late childhood and early adulthood (15 to 25 years). It is uncommon, though not rare, in infancy and early childhood.

SYMPTOMS

The incubation period is variable and because of the insidious onset it is difficult to determine. In general, it may be stated as being from 1 to 2 weeks.

The symptoms vary greatly with the age of the child. The younger the child, the less severe the disease. As children approach the age of puberty, the disease occurs with a severity approaching that observed in the adult.

The prodromal symptoms may be malaise, anorexia, headache and thirst. In a few cases in childhood, the disease develops abruptly without prodromal symptoms. In the more severe case, the fever is high and usually remittent. It reaches its peak within the first week. Prostration is severe. The mental state is affected sometimes by delirium, sometimes by stupor. It is the stupor that gives rise to the term typhoid state.

The infection is implanted first in the intestinal tract, and the greatest anatomic damage occurs at this site, but the organisms also reach the mesenteric lymph glands and the blood stream and are distributed throughout the body. The organisms are found in the blood during the first week of the disease but usually not subsequently. It is the lymphoid tissue (Peyer's patches) of the intestine that is affected most severely. The patches of lymphoid tissue become swollen and then ulcerated. The ulcerations may cause hemorrhage within the intestine, or

an ulcer may extend entirely through the bowel wall into the peritoneal cavity and cause peritonitis. The inflammation of the intestinal mucosa, other than in the lymphoid tissue, is only moderate but it is sufficient in most instances to cause diarrhea. In a few cases, constipation is present. Abdominal distention is the rule, often requiring special treatment measures. The pulse rate is low, out of proportion to the fever. The white cells of the blood are not increased and frequently are decreased. The spleen becomes palpable during the first week of the disease and remains enlarged throughout the illness. Late in the first week an eruption (rose spots) appears on the abdomen in a large proportion of cases. The rash disappears within a few days. When the disease is severe, degenerative changes may occur in the liver, the heart and the kidneys. Albuminuria may be present.

In the young child, the disease is less severe. The onset is often indefinite and ill-defined, and the disease is of shorter duration, often only from 2 to 3 weeks. The nervous symptoms may be more marked than the gastro-intestinal but they are less severe than in the adult. A few children have meningismus. Severe typhoid states are seldom seen, although apathy and sometimes slight nocturnal delirium may be present. Many children show no prostration, remain comfortable and scarcely have the appearance of being ill. Others are fussy and irritable. Gastro-intestinal symptoms often are negligible. Either constipation or diarrhea may be present. Even with diarrhea, the stools are not passed involuntarily, as they frequently are in adults. Usually only moderate abdominal distention is present. Vomiting, especially at the onset, is sometimes a feature of typhoid fever in children, while it occurs seldom in adults. In infants, typhoid fever may manifest itself chiefly by vomiting and diarrhea and resemble in every way, except duration and response to dietary therapy, a gastrointestinal disturbance due to improper food or to parenteral infection.

Anatomically also the disease is more mild in the infant and the young child. The younger the child, the less the ulceration in the intestine, the process often being limited to simple hyperplasia of Peyer's patches. Intestinal hemorrhage occurs almost exclusively after the age of 10 years. Intestinal perforation also is unusual and is limited chiefly to late childhood. The symptoms of perforation in childhood are more indefinite, and the diagnosis is more difficult than in adults. The temperature curve is similar to that of adults, except that in children the fever is of shorter duration and is less likely to be markedly remittent. Occasionally, it ends by crisis. Bronchitis is frequent. Relapse, although infrequent, occurs about as often as in adults.

COMPLICATIONS

Intestinal hemorrhage and perforation are the usual complications and are the cause of most of the deaths in childhood.

ISOLATION

Isolation should be continued until several successive stool cultures fail to grow the typhoid bacillus.

PROGNOSIS

The mortality in children is less than half that in adults because of the relative mildness of the disease and the infrequency of complications.

PREVENTION

Typhoid vaccine is as useful for children as for adults. It is to be recommended especially if the family is sojourning in places where the food and the water supply may be subject to poor sanitation. The vaccine is used in the same manner as for adults in fractions of the adult dose proportionate to the weight of the child. Children have less reaction to the vaccine than do adults. Seldom does it cause inconvenience. Protective immunity may be expected to last for from 2 to 3 years.

DIAGNOSIS

Diagnosis in the young child may be difficult because of the lack of characteristic symptoms. At any age a diagnosis can be made if the organisms are found by culture in the blood, the urine or the stool. An agglutination test (Widal) is useful. A positive result may be expected by the end of the first week, with subsequent increase in titer. Both agglutination tests and cultures are useful in diagnosing Salmonella infections and undulant fever, diseases that may simulate typhoid fever. Dysentery also may be excluded by stool culture.

TREATMENT AND NURSING CARE

To the symptomatic treatment of typhoid fever there has been added recently an effective antibiotic—chloramphenicol. The child should be kept in bed regardless of the mildness of the illness or how well he feels. The diet should be complete, with high energy value but with little rough residue. Foods should be finely divided and of a character which will not aggravate existing diarrhea. Milk, eggs and puréed fruits and vegetables should be prominent in the diet. The sugars may be used to increase energy value. Hydrotherapy for nervous symptoms and for fever is not indicated as often as in adults. When children are found to react poorly to hydrotherapy it should be discontinued. Special mouth care is indicated in the care of children.

When diarrhea is present, specific nursing care is indicated (see Diarrhea). Dehydration is especially likely to occur in infants. Moderate anemia is common with severe typhoid fever. Sometimes transfusions are desirable to promote quick recovery. When a child is confined to bed for a long period, especially if he is in a state of stupor, special nursing care is required to keep the skin free from pressure areas. Nursing measures to prevent distention are required for the older child.

When the disease is severe, the nurse should be alert for symptoms that indicate intestinal hemorrhage or perforation. Restlessness, rise in rate and change in quality of the pulse, abdominal pain and distention are symptoms of perforation that require immediate attention.

Chloramphenicol is highly effective in shortening the course of typhoid fever. Administration in high dosage (50 to 100 mgm./kg. of body weight per day) usually will produce reduction of fever and sterilization of the blood stream in from 24 to 48 hours. Treatment is continued for at least 3 weeks in order to assure the eradication of organisms from all recesses of the intestinal tract.

The principles of aseptic technic previously described for communicable diseases apply also to typhoid fever, but it should be borne in mind that the alimentary tract is the portal of entry and the chief exit of the typhoid bacillus. The stools contain an abundance of the organisms. For a short period early in the disease, the organisms are present also in the urine in many instances.

SALMONELLA INFECTIONS

The Salmonella group of organisms is a very large family that has characteristics similar to the typhoid bacillus. Unlike the latter, infection generally is spread to man from contact with the products of infected animals. The resultant disease is in some instances quite similar to, although usually milder than, typhoid fever, requiring the same sort of diagnostic measures, isolation precautions and treatment. Occasionally these organisms produce acute food-poisoning. In small infants there may be insidious infection with unexplained fever and mild diarrhea. As long as the infection remains confined to the intestinal tract it tends to be mild, albeit often protracted. If a heavy infection of the blood stream occurs, there may be more serious consequences, such as osteomyelitis or meningitis, which are more difficult to eradicate.

BRUCELLOSIS (UNDULANT FEVER, MALTA FEVER)

Brucellosis is a generalized infection by organisms of the genus

Brucella. The disease is characterized chiefly by intermittent fever without definitely pathognomonic symptoms.

Three different strains of the causative organism are recognized, namely, the bovine (cow) strain *Brucella abortus,* the porcine (swine) strain *Brucella suis,* and the caprine (goat) strain *Brucella melitensis.* The caprine strain is the cause of Malta fever. It is the most highly infective strain for man but it is not common in this country. Both the bovine and the porcine strains have wide distribution, and their prevalence in this country is extensive. *Brucella abortus* is the cause of infectious abortion in cattle. For man it is the least infectious of the 3 varieties when ingestion is the means of transmission. Cattle may become infected also with *Brucella suis.* The Brucella organisms are present in the milk of infected cows, and humans may be infected with either strain through the medium of cow's milk. Apparently, large numbers of organisms must be ingested by man in order to produce an infection. The infection is transmitted much more easily through an abrasion and by contact. Consequently, brucellosis in this country is commonly an occupational disease of handlers of meat and milk. Brucellosis is relatively uncommon in childhood, partly for reasons just stated and perhaps also because of an assumed relative immunity in the young. Nevertheless, the disease does occur in the young, and unless the possibility of its presence is considered in relation to fevers of obscure causation, a correct diagnosis cannot be made.

SYMPTOMS

The incubation period varies from 1 to 3 weeks and occasionally it is longer. The onset of the disease is insidious and indefinite. As the illness gradually becomes definite, the symptoms most likely to be present are irregular fever, with chills or chilliness, malaise, general weakness and loss of appetite. There also may be general aches and pains, often migratory. In some cases sweating is profuse during sleep. The symptoms usually are sufficiently severe to cause the child to be confined to bed, although the illness may be mild and the child ambulatory. Examination of the child reveals little of significance. Often evidence of weight loss is apparent. The spleen may be enlarged. Blood examination shows slight anemia and usually moderate leukopenia. A red macular eruption is found at times on a few children, but this may be merely miliaria or "sweat rash." Fever is the only constant symptom and this has its remissions. The temperature may be nearly normal in the morning and high in the afternoon. The disease runs a variable course, from a few weeks to many months. An average duration is approximately 2 months for the older person and somewhat shorter for the younger. Eventually, the disease subsides, usually without serious complications or sequelae.

DIAGNOSIS

The diagnostic aid of first importance is the obtaining of the causative organism in blood culture. A special medium is used, and a period of from 10 days to 3 weeks or more is required for the organism to grow sufficiently for recognition. A positive blood culture makes the diagnosis certain but does not appear early in the course of the disease. Agglutination and skin tests are available to aid in diagnosis but must be interpreted cautiously. Conclusive proof of brucella infection is often difficult to obtain.

TREATMENT

The prognosis for life in cases of brucellosis always has been good, but chronic forms of the disease were attended by prolonged or recurring periods of fatigability and vague symptoms. Chlortetracycline now appears to be able to terminate these symptoms if given in full dosage for a period of from 2 to 3 weeks. The efficacy of the newer "mycin" drugs has not yet been established, but presumably oxytetracycline, chloramphenicol and tetracycline also will be effective. Nursing care is mainly symptomatic and should include rest in bed until the fever has been brought under control.

TULAREMIA (RABBIT FEVER)

This disease is acquired from contact with infected animals, usually wild animals such as rabbits, squirrels, skunks, deer and woodchucks. The bacterium responsible (*Pasteurella tularensis*) is able to penetrate skin and mucous membrane surfaces rather easily, so that mere handling of infected animals may be sufficient to produce human infection. Symptoms develop in from 2 to 5 days' time after exposure and depend upon the site at which the organisms enter the body. In one form a local skin ulcer appears, associated with enlarged and painful lymph nodes (ulceroglandular type); in another form (oculoglandular) the portal of entry is through the conjunctiva, so that conjunctivitis and enlargement of lymph nodes about the eye are the presenting symptoms; in another type entry occurs through the tonsil and the cervical lymph nodes; in some instances the site of entry is obscure and the symptoms may simulate typhoid fever. The diagnosis can be confirmed by isolation of the specific organism from the blood or by detection of agglutinins which appear in the blood in the second week of the disease. Thus far, streptomycin, chlortetracycline and chloramphenicol have been demonstrated to be effective in treatment. Complications are unusual, and fatalities are rare even in the absence of treatment. Since spread from man to man is unknown, isolation is necessary only if open discharging lesions are present.

TUBERCULOSIS

Tuberculosis is the result of infection by the tubercle bacillus (*Mycobacterium tuberculosis*). The most frequent source of this infection is human, and for the child this source is most often the home. Infection may occur also from more casual human contacts or from tuberculous animals. The common animal source is the cow, and the infection is conveyed by means of contaminated milk. With present-day precautions in inspecting dairy herds and in the handling and the treatment of milk, relatively few infections occur from this source in this country. The infection is communicable at all ages. At no age is susceptibility to the primary infection greater than at any other age.

Often it has seemed that young infants are more susceptible, but this impression may be due largely to the fact that when an infant is exposed at all, he is likely to be exposed constantly and to massive doses of the organisms. It may be also that susceptibility to primary infection is greater than that to reinfection because of moderate immunity conferred by the first infection.

INCIDENCE

The general frequency of tuberculous infection varies widely between different communities and different countries. The skin tuberculin test, when positive, means that the person has a tuberculous infection, although not necessarily tuberculous disease. Surveys by means of this test have shown that in some communities 10 per cent or less of the children have been infected by the time they have reached adolescence. In other places, the incidence of positive tests at this age has been 50 per cent, and in still others, 90 per cent. Regardless of how low the incidence may be in a community, it is high in a tuberculous family. Tuberculosis is a family disease, and when one member develops the disease in an infectious form and remains in contact with the family, the other members will be infected in the course of time in a high proportion of instances.

PRIMARY INFECTION

Tubercle bacilli gain entrance to the body by way of either the respiratory or the alimentary tract. Because the common source is human, the most frequent portal of entry is the respiratory tract, and the primary lesion is most frequently in some part of the lung. The initial lesion often is small and relatively insignificant, especially if the dose of tubercle bacilli was not large. In these circumstances, it usually causes no symptoms and presents no physical signs. On the other hand, especially if the exposure has been intimate and prolonged, the primary focus may be more extensive and sometimes, when in the lung, it may involve the whole lobe in an exudative process. Organisms from the primary infection site travel along the lymphatics to the lymph glands that drain the region. Here the tissue reaction and change are often more marked than at the primary focus. Part or all of the gland undergoes necrosis, and the necrotic area has the consistency of certain varieties of cheese (caseation).

If the number of organisms is not large and the body defenses are reasonably good, the disease progresses no further and ultimately undergoes healing. In the process of healing, often calcium is deposited in the necrosed areas, and the primary infection site and the regional glands become the seat of dense calcium deposits. Roentgenograms of the chest frequently show a solitary calcified tubercle (Ghon tubercle) in the parenchyma of the lung and calcium deposits in the regional glands. With more massive infection, the essential lesions are the same, although they involve a larger area and the organisms are not so easily confined to the site of infection. If they filter past the lymph glands, the organisms pass on through the lymph channels into the blood stream and are distributed to other organs or, depending on the numbers, to the entire body, thus giving rise to miliary tuberculosis or to tuberculous meningitis or to various lesions of bones and joints. An attempt is made to distinguish between clinical tuberculosis and tuberculous infection without clinical disease. Tuberculous disease is present when the evidences of activity are revealed on examination. When those evidences are not apparent and the presence of tuberculosis is shown only by a positive result of a tuberculin test or a calcified pulmonary or gland tubercle, the condition is referred to as tuberculous infection. The dividing line between disease and infection is entirely artificial and is based on the limitations of diagnostic ability. Frequently, there are found at necropsy foci of active infection which were entirely unsuspected and in such locations that they could not be demonstrated during life.

Role of Allergy

The majority of infected persons survive the primary infection, but accompanying this initial infection there develops a state of specific allergy which affects the future of these persons. The allergy is produced in response to the proteins of the tubercle bacillus. The skin tuberculin test gives evidence of this allergy and is a means of testing for it. A positive tuberculin reaction may be obtained 4 weeks or more after the primary infection. Because of the existence of allergy, the body behaves differently to later infections than it does to the primary infection. Sensitized cells tend to fix the tubercle bacilli and not to let them pass on to the regional glands. The tissue reaction at the site of the primary infection tends to be nonspecific, that is, the tissue reacts as it might to a number of different irritants, while the reaction at the site of a later infection is specific. By then the cells have become sensitized to this particular irritant and react in a more violent inflammatory manner. Long ago Koch observed that if tubercle bacilli are inoculated subcutaneously in an animal previously infected, the inoculated area rapidly sloughs out and subsequently undergoes healing. Thus, along with the violent and destructive allergic response is associated a certain degree of immunity.

First and Later Infections

From the preceding discussion it is apparent that tuberculosis associated with the first infection differs much from that resulting from later infection. Both the first and the later infections are predominantly pulmonary in initial location. The resultant pulmonary disease differs strikingly in the two instances. In the later infections, the disease tends to be confined to the lungs, while with the first infection the regional glands always are involved, and occasionally from these sites organisms are carried to other parts of the body. Thus, glandular tuberculosis, miliary tuberculosis, bone and joint tuberculosis and tuberculosis of other locations are associated almost entirely with primary infections and only rarely with later infections. The confinement of the disease chiefly to one location in the late infection is perhaps indicative of increased resistance.

Pulmonary infection as it results from infection subsequent to the primary infection is observed chiefly in late adolescence and adult life. It will not be discussed here except in comparison with the first infection or "childhood type." The childhood type has a strong tendency to heal without much loss of tissue, while the reinfection or "adult type" tends to slough out, leaving cavities. Healing in the childhood type is by resorption of exudate and calcification of the necrosed areas, while in the adult type healing is largely by means of scar tissue (fibrosis). In the adult type, the regional glands are not involved. The pulmonary lesion in the adult type is nearly always in the apex, while the primary lesion may be located in any part of the lung.

SYMPTOMS

Pulmonary tuberculosis as it results from the primary infection has been described to some extent in the preceding discussion. The area of inflammation about the original focus may be so small that it is missed easily by the most careful and complete examination or it may extend throughout an entire lobe. The extension beyond the original focus is in the nature of a consolidation brought about by exudate. Necrosis usually occurs only at the original focus, and not always even there. Upon healing, the exudate resorbs, leaving no trace of its former existence. Only the caseous area of the primary focus becomes calcified. With moderate involvement of the lung no symptoms are associated, and often a frank and progressive lesion gives rise to no symptoms whatsoever. In the more extensive infections, one may encounter cough, fever and loss of weight or the symptoms of mild pneumonia. In the average case, physical examination is of little help, although an extensive consolidation may present the signs of pneumonia. Besides the skin tuberculin test, a roentgenogram of the chest gives the most important and conclusive diagnostic evidence. In primary tuberculosis, usually little or no exudative material is free to be coughed up, yet frequently tubercle bacilli are carried up to the pharynx and swallowed. Thus tubercle bacilli may be found in material washed from the stomach after a brief fast.

TUBERCULOSIS OF THE LYMPH GLANDS

This is the predominant type of tuberculous disease during childhood. The tracheobronchial and the hilum glands are the ones most frequently affected. The development and the course of hilum-gland tuberculosis have been discussed already. The symptoms are vague or entirely lacking, though in infants the enlargement of the tracheobronchial glands may give rise to an expiratory stridor. Frequently, the glands are not discernible in a roentgenogram. Their presence may be diagnosed by this means only when they show some calcification or when they form a mass large enough to encroach on the lung field. Thus, tuberculosis in the hilum glands may be active and progressive without giving conclusive evidence of its presence and location.

Tuberculosis of the Mesenteric Glands. This is not so frequent as that of hilum glands in this country. It is to be found particularly when the portal of entry has been the alimentary tract.

Fig. 74. Tuberculous adenitis, cervical. Showing also a strongly positive tuberculin reaction of the forearm.

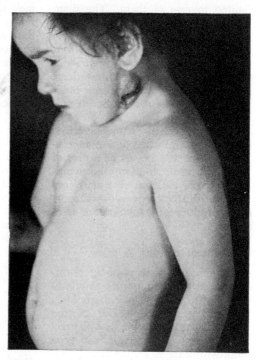

Fig. 74. Tuberculous adenitis, cervical. Showing also a strongly positive tuberculin reaction of the forearm.

Tuberculosis of the Cervical Glands. This infection occurs when the portal of entry is the upper respiratory tract or the tonsils. The clinical course of the disease in the glands of the neck is observed more easily than that of the disease in glands elsewhere. In the neck, the swollen glands are palpable, and the swelling is visible externally (Fig. 74). The chronicity of the disease, as well as the great variability of the course, is apparent. In cases of more severe involvement, the process extends beyond the glands and involves the skin; the skin becomes red, and an area of softness is felt in the center of the indurated mass. Finally, the necrosis may extend to the surface, and a discharging sinus may result from it. Tuberculous sinuses tend to remain open with drainage for long periods. In other cases, after a time the process recedes before it has become extensive and finally heals with calcification.

MILIARY TUBERCULOSIS

This is a condition in which tubercle bacilli have been disseminated in large numbers by way of the blood stream, usually from the breakdown of infected glands. Thus many foci are set up, and the disease runs a rapid course, so rapid that by the time of the death of the child the tuberculous lesions are still very small. The distribution may be in both the pulmonary and the general circulations or it may be limited to one of them. The diagnosis of miliary tuberculosis often is difficult because of the lack of characteristic symptoms. Fever, weight loss and increasing prostration may be the only manifestations. In the systemic form, the spleen enlarges. When the distribution is pulmonary, lung signs are few or lacking, though a roentgenogram is definitely diagnostic. When meningitis (Chap. 12) occurs as a part of the general distribution, the symptoms of this localization usually are sufficiently prominent to overshadow those produced by tuberculosis elsewhere.

TUBERCULOUS PLEURISY

Tuberculous pleurisy of the fibrinous adhesive type occurs regularly with the adult type of tuberculosis, particularly near the site of the apical disease. The kind of pleurisy that occurs with the childhood type of tuberculosis is exudative. It seldom occurs before 5 years of age and is not frequent in childhood. This type of pleurisy usually represents a state of marked allergy. The onset is with pain, which stops quickly as the pleural surfaces are separated by exudate. The exudate is a clear serous fluid that usually is resorbed within a short time, especially if the child is kept at rest. Although one might expect the pleurisy to have its origin in a lesion of the adjacent lung parenchyma, such a lesion is not always found by available methods of examination.

TUBERCULOUS PERITONITIS

Tuberculous peritonitis may be of the same exudative type as that described for pleurisy and it may have the same favorable prognosis. In other instances, the exudate is fibrinous, and the peritoneal surfaces tend to become adherent. In this latter type, the prognosis is not so favorable, but a large proportion of the children recover when well cared for.

TUBERCULOSIS OF BONES AND JOINTS

Tubercle bacilli transported by the blood stream may lodge in bones and there set up tuberculous disease. In the long bones, the site of the lesion may be in the shaft but most frequently it is near an epiphysis, in which case the line of least resistance for extension is toward the neighboring joint. It is in this manner that tuberculosis of the joints most frequently originates. The weight-bearing joints are affected most frequently, possibly because resistance is lowered by trauma. Joint tuberculosis is characterized clinically chiefly by pain, muscle spasm, limitation of motion and early muscle and bone atrophy. The prognosis as to life is good, especially in childhood. The outlook for function depends somewhat on the adequacy and the promptness of treatment. In some instances good function results, but in most a stiff joint may be expected.

The spine is a common site for bone tuberculosis, and the thoracic spine is the part most frequently affected. The disease always arises in the anterior portion of the vertebra and erodes the vertebral body. The erosion soon permits a kyphos, which is the characteristic deformity. Muscle spasm and referred pain are constant when the spine is not at rest in a good position.

TUBERCULOUS ABSCESSES

Tuberculous abscesses are common in bone and joint tuberculosis. These usually progress slowly and may burrow for considerable distances before coming to the surface. Often they are referred to as "cold abscesses" because of the lack of heat characteristic of the usual pyogenic abscess. With good treatment of the bone and joint tuberculosis, the abscesses often are resorbed without having been drained. The treatment for bone and joint tuberculosis consists of the general care suitable for a child with any type of tuberculosis and, in addition, mechanical or surgical measures which fix the parts at rest in proper positions.

TUBERCULIN TEST

This is a test for allergy to the proteins of the tubercle bacillus. With a few exceptions, a negative reaction to a test properly performed indicates that the person does not have a tuberculous infection. In order to have a positive reaction, a person must have had an infection with the tubercle bacillus. There is a tendency to believe that a positive reaction has more significance for a child than for an adult. The infection in a young child cannot be very old and therefore may still be active or latent. However, in the adult the infection may have been in the distant past and may be well healed, the allergy only remaining. Thus one encounters the belief that in the adult and the older child a tuberculin test gives little information of value. On the other hand, it is possible that the allergic state gradually disappears as the original infection becomes completely cured, in which case a positive reaction would mean that some focus is still more or less active. If this is true, a positive tuberculin reaction is of real significance at any age. Whatever the merits of these concepts, a highly allergic state at any time may be considered a menace if the person should be exposed to tuberculosis, despite some degree of immunity that accompanies this state.

Several methods are available for performing the tuberculin skin test. By one method (Pirquet), scarification of the skin is made through a drop of undiluted tuberculin. Because of unavoidable variations in the degree of scarification and the consequent variations in the amount of tuberculin absorbed, the Pirquet test is not reliable when the test is negative unless it is repeatedly negative. Another method is known as the patch test, in which tuberculin-impregnated material is attached to the skin by adhesive without scarification. This method has a high degree of reliability but it is not as dependable as the Mantoux test. The Mantoux, or intradermal, test consists of the injection into the skin of a measured amount of tuberculin. The dose most commonly employed for intradermal injection is 0.1 mg. of tuberculin contained in 0.1 cc. of diluent. For greater certainty in excluding the presence of tuberculosis, a negative intradermal test should be followed by the injection of a larger dose of tuberculin, e.g., 1 mg. The tuberculin referred to is called old tuberculin (O.T.). A somewhat purer preparation known as purified protein derivative (P.P.D.) is now available. It is prepared in two strengths, the first of which can be used to detect sen-

sivitity of a high degree. A negative response to the second strength
offers conclusive proof that allergy
is lacking.

DIAGNOSIS

The diagnosis of tuberculosis is
based on the factors already discussed, namely, positive skin tuberculin reaction, roentgen-ray examination in suitable cases and finding
tubercle bacilli. The history of exposure and the previous course of
the illness often are helpful, but the
symptoms in some varieties of
tuberculosis are useless for diagnosis in that they do not differentiate between tuberculosis and other
infections.

PROGNOSIS

The prognosis in tuberculosis has
been described to some extent under
the various forms of tuberculosis
which have been discussed. The
ability of the body to overcome the
primary infection is usually good at
all ages. When exposure to extrane-
ous infection has been discontinued,
the majority of persons with a first
infection will recover from their disease. The mortality during infancy
and adolescence is much higher than
during the preschool and school
years. Case fatality rates as high as
50 per cent have been reported in
infants before antibiotic therapy was
available. When exposed, the infant
usually suffers repeated and heavy
exposure from close contact with
the infectious person. In the adolescent and the young adult the reinfection type of tuberculosis in the
rapidly growing person carries a
high mortality rate unless specific
treatment is instituted.

PREVENTION

General Measures. In the prevention of tuberculosis it is clear that
the factor of greatest importance is
the avoidance of exposure. Much
already has been accomplished in
this direction. Accomplishment has
been noteworthy in elimination of
tubercle bacilli from the milk supply.
Dairy herds are tuberculin-tested,
and the reactors are eliminated. A
high proportion of the milk supply
is pasteurized. It is chiefly because
of these measures that abdominal
tuberculosis has almost disappeared
in this country.

Another fruitful field of activity
is the attempt to prevent tuberculous
disease when tuberculous infection
is present. This objective is to be
accomplished by special care and
observation of those who have been
infected. In many communities,
special schools and facilities have
been established for this purpose.
In these schools, extra food and
hours of rest, as well as medical
supervision, are provided. It is to
be remembered that tuberculosis,
especially of the glands, may remain
latent for many years or even a
lifetime, despite the fact that some
calcification may have taken place.
Infected persons should be kept
under observation and their nutrition and general health maintained
as well as possible. A latent focus
may have its activity renewed by
some illness, such as measles, pertussis or influenza, or by any factor
that greatly lowers resistance. Another predisposing factor is over-
crowded living quarters with insufficient light and fresh air.

In the public-health field, "case-
finding" measures have been useful.
These measures include tuberculin

testing in the schools and x-ray examination of the reactors. They include also the examination of members of a household in which a tuberculous person has been found. So that these measures may be effective, appropriate care must be given to those found to have infection or disease.

Immunization. By propagating bovine tubercle bacilli through successive transplants on artificial media for many years, Calmette produced a strain (*Bacillus Calmette-Guérin* or BCG) of low virulence with which he claimed to be able to produce immunity of perhaps several years' duration. He advocated its use especially for infants of tuberculous parentage. The vaccine was given in 3 doses by mouth on alternate days in the first 10 days after birth. Currently in the United States this vaccine is administered by multiple puncture, scarification of the skin or intracutaneously. The infants are isolated from the tuberculous parents for at least 4 weeks. If a positive skin tuberculin reaction does not develop or if the skin reaction later becomes negative, vaccination is repeated. The procedure is used extensively in Scandinavian countries and elsewhere, not only for infants but also for older persons who have negative tuberculin tests. It has had only limited and experimental use in this country, where there has been a steadily declining tuberculosis rate despite the absence of an immunization program. Although the vaccine is believed to be relatively safe, its value as an immunizing agent remains controversial. It should not be regarded as a substitute for approved hygienic measures or public-health practices.

If it is to be used, use should be restricted to selected groups of nonreactors most likely to be exposed to tuberculosis.

TREATMENT AND NURSING CARE

General Measures. Removal of the child from continued contact with his source of tuberculous infection is the first requisite of adequate care. When this cannot be accomplished, an attempt to control the amount of exposure by the use of appropriate isolation precautions should be made. The diet ought to provide a liberal intake of calories and of protein of high biologic value. The tuberculous child should be shielded from intercurrent infections (measles in particular) which may have an adverse effect upon his disease. The use of cortisone and ACTH generally is contraindicated, since these hormones lower the resistance to infection.

Rest in bed is often desirable over long periods of time, whether specific drug therapy is being used or not. If hospitalization is necessary, continuous constructive relationship experiences are imperative to prevent anxiety and to provide the experiences that the child needs for psychological growth.

Drug Therapy. A number of drugs are now available which are able to impede the multiplication of tubercle bacilli. Unfortunately, no one of these substances is capable of serving as an ideal therapeutic weapon. Each of them creates toxic reactions in the patient under treatment; each must be used over a long period of time, and some of them lose their effectiveness because of the emergence of strains of tubercle bacilli that are resistant. In spite of these disadvantages the treatment of major tuberculosis has been improved to the point where a large fraction of children suffering from meningitis can be saved (see Chap. 12), and most of those with miliary tuberculosis survive. In combination with newer surgical technics, many of those with cavitational tuberculosis also can be salvaged, although the effectiveness of drugs is impaired somewhat by mechanical factors in this type of disease.

Ordinarily drug therapy is reserved for the more severe types of tuberculosis and is not used in primary infection of the usual severity. The logic of this attitude is still under debate, for in many ways it would seem better to attack the organisms during the earliest possible form of the disease.

Streptomycin and dihydrostreptomycin given intramuscularly are effective agents. They have the disadvantage that they produce toxic damage to the eighth cranial nerve when used over long periods of time in heavy dosage. Deafness or loss of equilibrium may result. In addition, the strain of tubercle bacillus under treatment gradually may become resistant to their antibiotic effects. For these reasons, streptomycin usually is used in conjunction with another tuberculostatic drug. Promizole (or other sulfone compounds) or para-aminosalicylic acid is used for this purpose. A third group of substances which is effective against the tubercle bacillus is the isonicotinic acid compounds, of which isoniazid appears to be the most useful. The sulfones and the isonicotinic acid derivatives are given orally.

The drug treatment of tuberculosis is still in the experimental stage, and many regimens are being tested to discover the most effective one. Generally speaking, at least 2 and sometimes 3 of the effective agents are employed in order to reduce the likelihood of toxic reactions and to prevent the development of drug resistance. Prolonged treatment for 6 months to a year is considered necessary for any of the extensive manifestations of disease.

Some of the toxic reactions to which the nurse should be alert can be listed as follows:

Streptomycin and dihydrostreptomycin—deafness, dizziness, ataxia, exfoliative dermatitis, fever, peculiar sensations.

Promizole and other sulfones—anemia, red pigmentation of the urine, goiter, enlargement of the breasts.

Isonicotinic acid derivatives—excitement, convulsions, dizziness, difficulty in starting the urinary stream, increased sensitivity to drugs such as adrenalin and ephedrine.

FUNGOUS INFECTIONS

The common varieties of fungous infection in man are superficial invasions of the skin (epidermophytosis) or the oral cavity (monilia). A few varieties of fungus are capable of producing systemic disease. Both coccidioidomycosis and histoplasmosis are similar to tuberculosis in their clinical manifestations.

COCCIDIOIDOMYCOSIS (SAN JOAQUIN VALLEY FEVER)

This disease is confined to the southwestern portion of the United States where the climate is hot and arid. The fungous spores are disseminated with the dust and gain entrance into the body either through the respiratory tract or through cuts and abrasions of the skin. The initial invasion may be accompanied by an influenzalike illness or it may be unrecognized. Roentgen examination of the chest reveals enlargement of hilar lymph nodes, soft patches of infiltration in the lung fields and occasionally cavities. Allergy to the fungus may be demonstrated by a skin test similar to the tuberculin test. Erythema nodosum is present in some instances during the onset of allergy. Widespread dissemination of the fungus takes place in a small fraction of infected persons. Manifestations similar to those of disseminated tuberculosis, including meningitis, may occur. No specific therapy is available. Ordinarily, the disease is self-limited, but the uncommon generalized form carries a significant mortality.

Differentiation from tuberculosis may be difficult on clinical grounds but usually can be achieved through skin test reactions and immunologic procedures.

HISTOPLASMOSIS

Histoplasmosis is the result of infection with a fungus that occurs widely in the Mississippi Valley and to a lesser extent in areas along the eastern seaboard of the United States. It too is confused frequently with tuberculosis but generally is discovered accidentally through roentgen examination of the chest. The early lesions simulate primary tuberculous infection, and the healed lesions calcify. Differentiation is made through the use of skin tests which demonstrate allergy to the protein of the fungus.

In most instances the disease is asymptomatic and presents purely academic interest. In a few children the infection may be heavy and produce severe pulmonary disease with cavitation or a generalized blood stream involvement which is progressive and usually fatal. No effective treatment is known for this latter type of disease.

OTHER FUNGOUS INFECTIONS

In rare instances children may be infected with other types of fungus such as actinomycosis, blastomycosis and sporotrichosis. The characteristics of these infections are not distinctive in children, and their rarity makes them unsuitable for discussion in a brief text. Reference should be made to the standard treatises on internal medicine.

SPIROCHETAL INFECTIONS

SYPHILIS

Syphilis is a chronic infection with a motile spirillum, *Treponema pallidum*, which may persist over many years. It has acute, subacute and latent phases.

ETIOLOGY

Although syphilis is looked upon as a venereal disease and its victims are thereby stigmatized, it must be recognized that by most children and many adults it is acquired innocently. The organism gains entrance to the body before birth by way of the placenta, and after birth by way of a lesion of the skin or orificial mucous membrane. The infection is easily communicable from a superficial lesion containing spirochetes to the skin or the mucous membrane of another person. The infection is not conveyed easily through a dry, healthy, intact skin.

A baby with active syphilis of the skin can be handled without danger of infection if the hands are washed immediately afterward and if it is certain that no breaks in the continuity of the skin are present. Because it is impossible to be sure of this latter condition, it is safer to wear gloves. The *Treponema pallidum* dies quickly on exposure and lives for only a brief period on such surfaces as doorknobs and toilet seats. On contaminated linen it is quickly killed by drying or by ordinary washing.

Syphilis in children acquired after birth is relatively rare, and the initial lesion in most instances is extragenital, often on the lips. Acquired syphilis in children runs essentially the same course as it does in adults.

PRENATAL TRANSMISSION

Transmission of syphilis to the infant before birth presents many interesting aspects and some unsolved problems. Usually syphilis is brought into the family by the father and usually after the father has had treatment and his infection is in a latent stage and presents no clinical evidence of its presence. In these circumstances, it is highly probable that the spirochetes are present in the testes without producing dysfunction or manifest disturbance. From this site they find their way into the semen and are discharged with it. By this means, the mother becomes infected. Relatively few mothers of syphilitic children have any symptoms or knowledge of their infection. Why the disease treats them so kindly is one of the questions not completely answered. It is known that pregnancy exerts a favorable influence on the course of

this infection, but this does not seem to be a sufficient explanation. Several explanatory hypotheses have been advanced but not proved. The evidence that all mothers of congenitally syphilitic children are syphilitic seems to be entirely satisfactory. It is based on serum reactions and the finding of spirochetes in certain groups of mothers who were subjected to special study. The infection of the fetus is accomplished by the implantation of spirochetes at the placental site and their growth into the placenta. From this location they are distributed to all parts of the fetus by way of the blood stream.

Effects of Syphilis Prenatally Transmitted

Fetus. The effects of syphilis on the fetus are variable. Both miscarriages and premature births are 2 or 3 times as frequent in syphilitic as in nonsyphilitic families. Infection of the fetus apparently does not occur before the fifth month of fetal life. Perhaps in the majority of instances the infection of the fetus takes place late in the pregnancy. A severe infection is likely to lead to the death of the fetus before birth. Thus, syphilis is a rather common cause of stillbirth. In other instances the baby, though infected, is born alive, and a living syphilitic child is the result.

Infant After Birth—Early Lesions. On rare occasions an infant will show evidences of syphilitic infection at birth, but more commonly it is between the third and the eighth weeks that such evidences appear. As a rule, the earlier they appear the more severe the infection. Syphilis is capable of producing many different lesions, but never do all of them occur in one infant. Therefore, the average or typical case cannot be described.

RHINITIS. Of the various lesions, rhinitis ("snuffles") is the most frequent. The inflammation in the nose, together with the discharge, interferes with breathing. The condition often resists treatment rather obstinately. If it is severe and continues over a long period, growth of the nasal bones is disturbed and results in the deformity known as "saddle nose."

RASH. Skin eruptions are frequent. Often these are of the copper-colored macular variety seen in the secondary stage of acquired syphilis. In a high proportion of cases, the palms and the soles become reddened and thickened, with later desquamation. This same type of inflammation may occur in the skin about the mouth. When it does, it is accompanied by fissures that radiate in all directions from the mouth (Fig. 75). Untreated, these fissures tend to remain for a long period and finally to heal with permanent scarring. The radiating scars are known as rhagades and are considered as pathognomonic of a former syphilitic infection.

BONES. Syphilitic inflammation at the ends of the long bones is a common occurrence. Often it becomes severe enough to cause pain to the extent that the part is not moved voluntarily. This pseudo-paralysis of syphilis occurs almost exclusively in the first 6 months of life. The lesion is commonly designated epiphysitis, but the term osteochondritis is more nearly accurate.

NEUROSYPHILIS. Syphilitic infec-

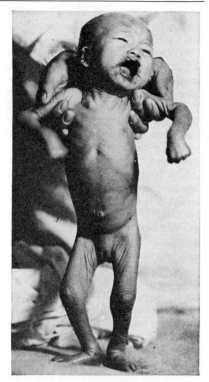

FIG. 75. Illustrating some of the skin manifestations of syphilis.

tion of the central nervous system occurs in approximately one third of all syphilitic infants, but it is manifest in less than 10 per cent. In those without external evidence, the diagnosis is made by examination of the cerebrospinal fluid. These babies are candidates for later development of manifest neurosyphilis.

OTHER CONDITIONS. Syphilis of the eye is relatively uncommon in infancy, although in the older child it is the most common of all lesions. A high proportion of babies with syphilis have enlargement of the spleen, and approximately one third

582   Nursing in the Care of the Sick Infant and Child

have fever in some degree during the acute stages, but this usually is not high.

SEVERITY. The severity of syphilis in infants varies markedly. In some, the infection is so mild that the baby appears to be in excellent health, and the examination reveals no abnormality except a positive Wassermann reaction. In others, especially with severe visceral involvement, prostration is obvious, weight loss is rapid, and the baby dies in the course of a few weeks. Between these two extremes all degrees of severity are encountered.

COMPARISON WITH ACQUIRED SYPHILIS. The symptoms that have been enumerated as occurring in the infant correspond to those which occur in the secondary stage of acquired syphilis. Since the infant with inherited syphilis has had no primary lesion, these secondary symptoms are referred to as constituting "early" or "infantile" hereditary or congenital syphilis. Except for the primary stage, the inherited and the acquired diseases go through precisely the same stages, but with certain differences in severity and in the type of manifestations. In the early or secondary stage the high infant mortality has no counterpart in the acquired syphilis of adults. Certain developmental defects (e.g., Hutchinson's teeth) occur as a result of infantile syphilis. These could not occur in a person fully developed. Skin inflammation in infantile syphilis is often much more severe than that ever seen in the adult. The presence of rhagades about the mouth is evidence of this fact. In infantile syphilis, the metaphyses of the long bones are commonly affected,

whereas in syphilis of the adult this does not happen. Most of the differences between inherited and acquired syphilis are in the early or secondary stage. Only two other later events are outstandingly different. These are the frequent occurrence of interstitial keratitis and the relative absence of cardiovascular syphilis as a result of the inherited infection, in contrast with the opposite state of affairs as the result of acquired syphilis.

Infant and Young Child—Late Secondary Lesions. After the subsidence of the secondary or early symptoms, a group of lesions known as late secondary lesions sometimes develop. To this group belong condylomata, mucous patches and skin syphilides. These are most frequent in the second or the third year of life but they may occur earlier or later. Condylomata are wartlike growths which appear about the mucocutaneous junctions, most often at the anus. Mucous patches are seen chiefly in the mouth. Both these lesions contain large numbers of spirochetes and are potential sources of contagion.

The Child—Late Lesions. After the secondary stage, the infection becomes quiescent. The period of latency before the development of some late lesion varies widely with different children. During this latent period, except for possible scars of preceding activity, the only evidence of the presence of syphilis is a positive Wassermann reaction.

At about 6 or 7 years, sometimes sooner, often much later, there begin to appear lesions which are of a type usually very different from those characteristic of the infection in infancy. In the inherited infection, this group of symptoms constitutes the "late" stage of the disease, which corresponds to the tertiary stage of the acquired infection.

EYES. The most frequent lesion of late congenital syphilis is interstitial or parenchymatous keratitis. This condition develops soon or late in fully half of all syphilitic children. Clinically, it is seen as a clouding of the cornea with prominence of the blood vessels immediately round the cornea. Vision is impaired greatly and remains so as long as the cornea is clouded. Photophobia is present in the acute stage. Keratitis responds slowly to treatment, but with early and vigorous treatment vision eventually is unimpaired. In cases of neglect, more or less permanent clouding of the cornea may cause even complete blindness.

Other affections of the eyes occur but with far less frequency than keratitis. Choroiditis causes impairment of vision in proportion to the extent of the lesion. Loss of all useful vision is not rare. Choroiditis does not respond to treatment, chiefly for the reason that by the time the child is brought to the physician with complaint of impaired vision, the damage that has been done to this specialized tissue is irreparable. Loss of vision through atrophy of the optic nerve is considered in this text with lesions of the nervous system.

NEUROSYPHILIS. As stated previously, approximately one third of all syphilitic infants have changes in their cerebrospinal fluid which show that the central nervous system has been infected. The infection of the nervous system of most infants is latent, but it is these

babies who are candidates for later development of manifest neurosyphilis. Examination of the cerebrospinal fluid of older syphilitic children reveals evidence of infection in approximately one fifth of them. The difference in incidence among infants and older children may be due to the infant mortality in this group. As those who survive become older, an increasing proportion develop manifest signs of neurosyphilis. Neurosyphilis is second in frequency among the syphilitic manifestations of older children. Any one or several of a number of conditions may develop. Some of the more common occurrences are altered pupillary reflexes, optic atrophy, various paralyses and dementia. Tabes and general paresis, if they occur, are more likely to be found in late childhood or early adulthood. Most of the conditions mentioned are the result of inflammation of the meninges and their blood vessels, which in turn affects the underlying structures. Destruction of nervous tissues causes permanent damage; repair is impossible. Little can be expected from treatment after neurosyphilis becomes clinically evident, except the arrest of its progress. Thorough treatment before these conditions develop usually will prevent their occurrence.

BONES. Third in frequency among the syphilitic lesions of older children are those of the bones. Although any bone may be involved, the tibia is the one most frequently affected. Usually the lesion is bilateral. The lesion most commonly encountered is periostitis. The periosteal thickening is detected easily by a roentgenogram, and often the swelling is visible and palpable externally. The chief symptom is pain, and this symptom causes the seeking of medical attention. Pain is relieved quickly by treatment, and the bone eventually becomes normal. Sometimes the inflammation extends much deeper into the bone than the periosteum. The bone gumma thus produced may be extensive enough to cause pathologic fracture or it may break down to the surface and give rise to a draining sinus. Bone gumma also responds to treatment, although sometimes surgical measures are necessary in addition.

JOINTS. Of the various joints that may be affected in syphilis, those at the knees are involved most often. The common lesion is synovitis, which produces chronic swelling of the joints from excess of fluid within them, with little or no pain and with only moderate loss of function. Less commonly, the joint lesion causes acute pain, with consequent complete loss of function. The painful variety responds to treatment rapidly, while arthritis of the other type usually persists for many weeks after treatment is started.

GUMMAS of the skin and the mucous membranes occur in the same manner as in the acquired infection of adults, but less frequently. These may give rise to perforations of the nasal septum or the palate, or to chronic ulcerations of the skin. They heal rapidly with treatment.

DIAGNOSIS

Some of the lesions of syphilis are so characteristic that the diagnosis can be made with reasonable certainty when they are present. Other lesions require corroborative evidence for diagnosis. When the infection is latent, the diagnosis can be made only by serologic reactions, but the diagnosis may be suspected when such stigmata as Hutchinson's teeth, rhagades and corneal or retinal scars are present. Any early lesion contains large numbers of spirochetes, and the diagnosis may be made definitely by the finding of spirochetes in material from an accessible lesion. However, this method of diagnosis is applicable in only a small proportion of cases. Examination of the serum by means of the Wassermann test or one of the flocculation tests is the diagnostic measure most universally to be depended on.

The Wassermann reaction (or other serologic test for syphilis) is not positive in all newborn syphilitic babies but it becomes so in the course of 2 months. In a few instances, a syphilitic mother transmits to her infant the positive Wassermann reaction without transmitting the infection. In all such instances, the reaction quickly becomes negative in the baby. Thus, without interpretation the Wassermann reaction is not wholly reliable in the first 2 months of life. However, after this time all syphilitic babies have a strongly positive reaction, and all uninfected babies have a negative reaction. The reliability of the Wassermann reaction continues throughout childhood. Only in later childhood, and then but rarely, will be found a child with an active lesion of syphilis and a negative Wassermann reaction. Syphilis should be diagnosed in a child with a negative Wassermann reaction only when the evidence for this infection is otherwise indisputable and proved.

During the course of several diseases the serologic tests for syphilis may give "biologic false positive results." Thus a positive serology cannot be taken as conclusive evidence of syphilis in the older child. The presence or the absence of syphilis in an infant or a child cannot be determined by examination of the parents. While it may be expected that syphilitic parents will transmit the infection to their children, they do not always do so. On the other hand, a child may be syphilitic by heredity when the parents have negative serologic reactions. In fact, in more than 40 per cent of the fathers of syphilitic children the infection has become latent to the extent of a negative Wassermann reaction by the time the disease is recognized in the child.

PROGNOSIS

With the exception of neglected cases and those discovered after the occurrence of neurosyphilis, the general statement may be made that with adequate treatment the prognosis for the syphilitic child is good. In some instances, treatment must be continued for several years, but ultimately cure is effected, although the child may bear scars of the former presence of the disease. Even in cases of manifest neurosyphilis, the child often may be cured of the infection, but because of dementia or convulsions there can be little pride in the accomplishment. Certain children are spoken of as being "Wassermann fast," because long-continued intensive treatment has not affected the strongly positive Wassermann reaction. Children with neurosyphilis contribute the greatest proportion to the Wassermann-fast group, and it is in the latent-neurosyphilis group especially that treatment should be persistent in order that manifest neurosyphilis may be prevented, even though treatment over many years is required.

PREVENTION

It is easy to prevent transmission of syphilis to the child if the infection is discovered in the mother. Even though treatment of the mother is given late in the course of her pregnancy, it is highly effective in protecting the infant. Many states now have laws which require serologic testing of pregnant women in order to discover infection of the mother before the birth of the child. Where such programs are enforced properly, the occurrence of congenital syphilis can be virtually eliminated.

TREATMENT

The older methods of treatment with heavy metal injections have been superseded completely by penicillin given in a dose of 100,000 to 1,000,000 units per kilogram of body weight over a period of 3 to 5 days. With the possible exception of spirochetes which have long been entrenched in the central nervous system, this treatment can be expected to kill all the organisms present in the body. Of course, it cannot be counted on to undo the scars of previous damage. Although the need for additional therapy is remote, generally it is agreed that children should be kept under surveillance for 1 to 2 years after treatment. Reversal of the blood serology from positive to negative occurs in all but a small fraction of the cases.

The broad-spectrum antibiotics are generally effective against the spirochete of syphilis when penicillin sensitivity makes its use inadvisable.

OTHER SPIROCHETAL INFECTIONS

In the United States there are few other infections in which spirochetes play a part. In one form of ulcerostomatitis (Vincent's infection) a spirillum is found which is thought to be at least partially responsible for the symptoms. It responds readily to penicillin therapy. Rat-bite fever is an uncommon infection with a specific spirochete which, as the name implies, is transmitted to the child by the bite of an infected rat. It too is terminated by penicillin treatment. Leptospirosis is a spirochetal disease also acquired from rats but usually transmitted by way of well or sewage water which has been contaminated by the urine of infected rats. In addition to general symptoms of infection there may be jaundice or meningitis. Penicillin is of doubtful value in the treatment.

PROTOZOAL INFECTIONS

A few of the ailments of children are due to infection with protozoa. Amebiasis is considered in Chapter 25. Malaria is still present in some of the southern portions of the United States. Toxoplasmosis is a form of granulomatous encephalitis which probably is transmitted to the infant at the time of birth and may lead to hydrocephalus and mental retardation and usually is accompanied by a characteristic type of lesion in the choroid layer of the retina.

SITUATIONS FOR FURTHER STUDY

1. If respiratory difficulty were observed in a child with diphtheria, what emergency equipment would you assemble? What care would a child with a tracheotomy require?

2. How can tetanus be prevented? If you were notified that a 3-year-old child with tetanus was coming into the children's ward, what preparation for his care would you make? What equipment should be in readiness for his medical and nursing care?

3. Study the mortality rate of whooping cough. At what age is the mortality rate the highest? Why? How could the rate be reduced? What help would a mother require to give adequate care to her 3-year-old child with whooping cough?

4. What are the common complications of scarlet fever? How can they be prevented?

5. How do the symptoms of typhoid fever differ in infancy and in childhood? How does nursing care differ in infancy and in childhood?

6. To confirm a diagnosis of tuberculosis, sputum examination often is desired. How would a sputum specimen be obtained from a 2-year-old child? What equipment would be necessary? How would you help a child meet the experience?

7. What supervision would a child with tuberculosis require? How can tuberculosis be prevented?

8. What care would an infant born of a tuberculous woman require?

9. What care would an infant with syphilis require?

10. Is the Wassermann reaction wholly reliable during the first 2 months of life?

11. How can congenital syphilis be prevented?

BIBLIOGRAPHY

Brennan, Florence: Brucellosis, Am. J. Nursing 50:358, 1950.

Du Bos, René: Bacterial and Mycotic Infections of Man, ed. 2, Philadelphia, Lippincott, 1952.

Harris, Isabel, and Shapiro, S. K.: Tetanus, a challenge to nursing, Am. J. Nursing 50:362, 1950.

Jeans, Philip, and Cooke, J. V.: Prepubescent Syphilis, New York, Appleton, 1930.

Kohn, Jerome, and Olson, Elsie: Whooping cough, Am. J. Nursing 50:1723, 1950.

Lapin, J. H.: Whooping Cough, Springfield, Ill., Thomas, 1943.

Siegel, P. T.: More about B.C.G., Am. J. Nursing 49:753, 1949.

Shapiro, Charlotte: Diphtheria, Trained Nurse & Hosp. Rev. 118-119:416, 1947.

————: Typhoid fever, Trained Nurse & Hosp. Rev. 120-121:118, 1948.

Stimson, P. M.: A Manual of the Common Contagious Diseases, ed. 4, Philadelphia, Lea & Febiger, 1947.

Tebrock, H. E., Fisher, M. M., and Mamlok, E. R.: The new drug—isoniazid, Am. J. Nursing 52:1342, 1952.

Thirlaway, Jean: The new look in typhoid fever, Canadian Nurse 46:729, 1950.

Other General Diseases

◇◇

THE COLLAGEN DISEASES

The term collagen disease is applied to a group of disorders which have as their common feature destruction and degeneration of the supporting connective tissue of the body. The name collagen refers to the fibers that can be seen under the microscope. There is evidence too that the ground substance between and among fibrils also is disturbed. The etiology of each of these disorders is obscure or at least under debate at the present time. They all improve under the influence of adrenal cortical steroid therapy. In general their symptomatology is sufficiently distinctive to permit sharp grouping into diagnostic entities, but in a few cases it may be difficult to decide which diagnosis to apply to an individual child. In pediatric medicine, rheumatic fever is much the most common representative of the group; rheumatoid arthritis and disseminated lupus erythematosus are uncommon; der-matomyositis, scleroderma and periarteritis nodosa are distinctly rare.

RHEUMATIC FEVER

Rheumatic fever is a systemic disease that causes characteristic involvement of many organs and tissues, most important of which is its effect upon the heart. The common manifestations are migratory joint pains, various skin eruptions, subcutaneous nodules, chorea and carditis. The acute and the chronic effects of rheumatic fever upon the heart have been considered in Chapter 10.

Etiology. The causative mechanism in rheumatic fever is the subject of controversy. The facts seem to be sufficient to warrant certain tentative conclusions. The primary underlying factor is infection in the throat with Group A beta-hemolytic streptococcus. As a result of chronic infection or repeated acute infections, the body becomes sensitized to the organism. Continued infection or repeated infection after sensitization leads to allergic response, the response varying in nature and degree according to the degree of sensitization. Before sensitization, the throat infection has apparent effects only locally. After sensitization, the systemic phenomena consist of certain proliferative and exudative changes with their accompanying symptoms (carditis, arthritis, skin eruptions, rheumatic nodules).

Incidence. The stated cause of rheumatic fever explains its age incidence. Rheumatic fever is rare in the first years of life, not because infections are uncommon, but because the development of allergy requires time. The curve of incidence of onset gradually rises. It has reached a fair height by 5 years of age and is at its peak between 7 and 10. After this time it declines. Rheumatic fever is most prevalent in those parts of the world (temperate zones) and in those seasons of the year in which respiratory infections are most frequent. Rheumatic fever has a relatively high family incidence. A hereditary predisposition to the disease is recognized. The environment and the living conditions are often such that respiratory infections are induced easily, and the causative organism is transferred easily. It is well recognized that rheumatic fever is more frequent in the low-income than in the high-income levels. No doubt this difference is explained in part by living conditions, but nutritional status also is known to be important.

Symptoms. The symptomatology of rheumatic fever is extremely variable in its type and severity. Some children are affected so mildly that the symptoms are vague, and even the most careful and extensive study by laboratory methods leaves some doubt about the validity of the diagnosis. Other children are assailed by a severe, fulminating disorder that rapidly threatens life.

Unlike many of the infectious diseases, the medical problem in rheumatic fever involves more than the management of a single episode of disease, for the child who has experienced one attack is vulnerable to recurrences. Each return of rheumatic activity carries with it the threat of additional cardiac damage. Consequently, it is very important to know which children have suffered from rheumatic fever in order to shield them from additional attacks, even though the first one may have been mild. Conversely, it is undesirable to classify a child as rheumatic unless good evidence is available, for in many instances this leads to unnecessary anxiety and restriction of activity, which hamper normal physical and emotional development.

The symptoms of rheumatic fever may be grouped into major manifestations and minor manifestations. If present in characteristic form, any one of the major manifestations is presumptive evidence of rheumatic fever. The minor manifestations may or may not be due to rheumatic fever, but when several of them are present alone or in conjunction with a major manifestation they add to the suspicion. The major manifestations are polyarthritis, carditis, chorea and subcutaneous nodules. In the young child carditis is apt to be the presenting manifestation, with polyarthritis present in mild degree. In the older child polyarthritis and chorea are more common as presenting complaints.

POLYARTHRITIS. The arthritis of rheumatic fever tends to involve the larger joints such as the knee, the elbow, the ankle, the wrist and the shoulder. However, it may be present in any joint, including the spinal articulations and the mandibular joint. Pain, tenderness and restriction of motion are present. In the young child these symptoms tend to be mild and to endure for only a few days but they may return in a different joint. More severe joint manifestations usually are seen in older children, in whom the part may be swollen, visibly inflamed and exquisitely tender to touch or manipulation. Spontaneous subsidence within a few days even without treatment is characteristic, but migration to other joints may persist over a period of weeks.

The arthritis of rheumatic fever has two distinctive characteristics—it is rapidly relieved by salicylates and it never results in permanent deformity of the joint. The pathologic changes are those of exudation of fluid into the joint and inflammation of the surrounding structures.

The problem of differentiating rheumatic pains from "growing pains" is often a difficult one. Usually the latter are limited to the night hours after the child has fallen asleep. They seldom interfere with his daytime play or provide visible evidence of pain or restricted motion. They tend to recur nightly for long periods of time and are not associated with other manifestations of the rheumatic state.

CARDITIS. Acute rheumatic carditis is discussed in detail in Chapter 10. The pathologic changes consist of exudation and proliferation. In the pericardium the early changes are those of acute inflammation with exudation of fibrin between the two layers. When healing takes place the exudate may be converted into pericardial adhesions. In the myocardium there is swelling and degeneration of muscle fibers and the appearance of minute granulomas called Aschoff bodies. During healing these areas are converted into microscopic scars. Some of the cardiac muscle fibers are lost in the process. In the endocardium there is at first an acute inflammatory reaction which later becomes an organizing fibrinous exudate. On the valve leaflets this may result in warty growths called vegetations. During healing the scar tissue which forms tends to contract and deform the valve orifices and the adjacent structures. Such scarring may leave the valves unable to close completely, so that blood regurgitates back past them, or the orifices may be narrowed abnormally, so that blood cannot pass through them at the accustomed speed. The maximum effects of the contracting scar tissue are not apparent until several years after the original acute inflammation. These late complications are responsible for the manifestations of chronic valvular heart disease which are discussed in Chapter 10.

CHOREA (SYDENHAM'S CHOREA). Chorea is characterized by involuntary, purposeless, irregular movements commonly involving all the voluntary musculature, but occasionally affecting one side of the body more than the other.

The greatest incidence of chorea is between the ages of 6 and 15 years. It is much more frequent in girls than in boys and more frequent in the spring than at other seasons. It has been suggested that a nervous tendency is necessary in addition to an infectious cause. Chorea is said to be more frequent in neurotic families, and it has been assumed that heredity plays a role.

The most prominent symptom in chorea consists of peculiar body movements. These are jerking, spasmodic, in-co-ordinate and without regularity. They cannot be suppressed by volition; in fact, they are made worse by attempts at repression, as well as by the mental stress of excitement or embarrassment. In severe chorea, these movements may be so extreme that the child will be bruised and injured by tossing and jerking against the sides of the bed unless the bed is padded. Such children cannot walk, talk, sit or feed themselves and are incontinent. Fortunately, in most instances the disease is not so severe. To be seen are all grades of severity from that described to such mildness that recognition of the condition requires close observation. Frequently, one half of the body is affected so much more than the other half that the condition is spoken of as hemichorea.

All attacks begin gradually, with signs of increased nervousness. Difficulty in the finer movements such as writing or buttoning clothing is evident early. The child stumbles easily and often drops articles being handled. Food is spilled, and soon, because of the jerky movements, self-feeding becomes impossible. The involvement of the muscles of the face causes grimaces. In-co-ordinate movements affecting speech make speech difficult or impossible. When one part of the body is involved more than the remainder, as in hemichorea, the chief complaint often is stated as "paralysis." The paralysis is apparent and not real and is due to inability to use the parts purposefully. Choreic movements are absent during sleep.

Children with chorea often are very emotional. Little or nothing obvious is required to produce a fit of giggling or of weeping, and the mood may shift rapidly from one extreme to the other. These children are irritable and fretful. The appetite usually is poor, the sleep disturbed, headaches are common and the child is easily fatigued. Fever is a feature only in the more severe disease.

Spontaneous recovery is to be expected in from 1 to 2 months. Relapse and second attacks are frequent. Relapses may prolong the illness to 4 months or longer. Complete recovery is the rule, and attacks never recur after puberty except during the course of a later pregnancy. When the disease is extremely severe, death may result from exhaustion. However, death is rare unless due to associated cardiac disease.

SUBCUTANEOUS NODULES. Nodules are not a very common manifestation of rheumatic fever but when they do occur they are almost certain confirmation of the diagnosis. They consist of accumulations of fibrous tissue proliferation which are located beneath the skin near the larger joints or along the spine or in the scalp. Small ones are difficult to find and are easily missed unless careful palpation is carried out. The larger ones are often visible through the skin (Fig. 76).

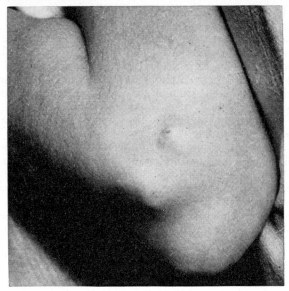

FIG. 76. Rheumatic nodules at the elbow.

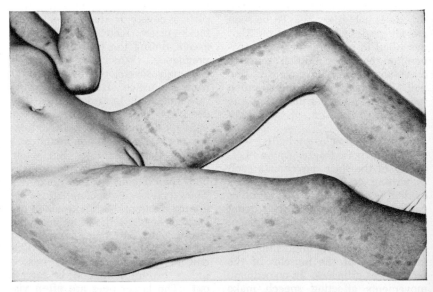

FIG. 77. The rash of rheumatic fever (erythema marginatum).

They are painless and persist for weeks or months before they disappear gradually.

MINOR MANIFESTATIONS. Rheumatic fever is accompanied by a number of other symptoms which by themselves are not necessarily rheumatic. Lassitude, pallor, fatigability and loss of appetite are seen frequently.

Fever is usually present, but its degree may be very variable. In severe rheumatic fever it is regularly present and may be high. Sometimes it is present only during the period when arthritis is evident. At other times it may appear as a low-grade protracted elevation which extends over many weeks during the activity of the rheumatic process. However, absence of fever cannot be regarded as equivalent to absence of rheumatic activity, for the two features are not always parallel.

Muscle pains which are transient or mild may or may not have a rheumatic basis.

Nosebleed is a traditional but actually not very frequent symptom that may be present during activity. The amount of bleeding is usually mild and creates no significant problem in management.

Abdominal pain is an important symptom because it may be severe enough to lead to the diagnosis of appendicitis and an exploratory operation. The exact mechanism of such pain is poorly understood but is attributed ordinarily to peritoneal inflammation or mesenteric lymph node enlargement.

Erythema marginatum is a faint, changing skin eruption which consists of small red circles, wavy lines or portions of circles which appear and disappear rather rapidly on the trunk and the abdomen (Fig. 77). The characteristic eruption seldom is seen except during the progress of rheumatic fever and is regarded by many people as being a clear evidence of rheumatic activity. It creates no symptoms and is not necessarily associated with fever.

Laboratory Aids to Diagnosis. Very often the clinical task of deciding whether an individual child does or does not have rheumatic fever is a difficult one. It would be highly desirable to have a specific laboratory test which indicated the presence of the disease and the degree of its activity. Unfortunately, no specific test is yet available, although several give useful nonspecific information. Each such test requires interpretation in the light of the patient's entire clinical picture.

An increase in the sedimentation rate of the red blood cells indicates the presence of an inflammatory reaction or a disturbance of the plasma proteins. It is a relatively simple procedure which is widely used as a means of following the course of rheumatic activity after the diagnosis has been established by other means. Of course, it can be influenced by inflammatory processes that have nothing to do with rheumatic fever.

Determination of the C-reactive protein of the blood is a similar indicator of the presence of an inflammatory reaction.

Leukocytosis also indicates inflammation but is a less sensitive index than the other tests named.

Since it now is believed that rheumatic fever almost invariably follows beta-hemolytic streptococcus infection, the detection of evidence of such an infection adds weight to the suspicion that symptoms are being produced by rheumatic fever. Usually the streptococcal infection is sufficiently distant or has been treated adequately, so that the organisms are not present in the throat culture at the time that rheumatic symptoms appear. However, certain antibodies may have been formed against the streptococcus products; by laboratory means it is possible to detect *antistreptolysin, antifibrinolysin* or *antihyaluronidase*. Of course, their presence merely proves that the person has suffered a streptococcal infection and does not indicate the presence of rheumatic fever specifically.

The *electrocardiogram* provides valuable evidence of the presence of carditis. This is discussed in Chapter 10.

Course and Prognosis. The prognosis for children with rheumatic fever depends entirely upon the effect that the disease has upon the heart. Except for the carditis, none of the other manifestations is likely to be lethal or to leave any permanent after-effects. The common form of first attack (monocyclic) consists of a period of activity which lasts from 1 to 4 months and during which about half of the children will have evidence of cardiac involvement. More serious is the polycyclic form of the disease in which continuing waves of activity keep the disease process going for many months or even a year or two. It appears as though treatment is able to suppress the activity temporarily but not to shorten the course of the disease.

Once the child has passed through an initial attack he is a candidate for a recurrence if he suffers another beta-hemolytic streptococcal infection. Studies indicate that the risk of recurrence is greatest during the first 5 years after an initial attack and that it declines rapidly thereafter. Each attack or period of prolonged rheumatic activity carries with it the threat of additional heart damage from carditis.

Prophylaxis. Once the child has been identified as a rheumatic subject it becomes very important to prevent future episodes of infection. Since recurrence will depend upon reinfection with beta-hemolytic streptococci, this objective can be attained if he is protected adequately against these organisms. It now is recognized that children with rheumatic fever may be so protected by administering a small daily dose of sulfadiazine or penicillin by mouth. The administration must be continuous so that the child has a constant low level of the drug present in his tissues to protect him from the very first minimal exposure to streptococci. Many clinicians feel that such prophylactic drugs should be taken during the 5 years following the first attack.

Treatment and Nursing Care. GENERAL CONSIDERATIONS. In the main, the treatment of rheumatic fever is the treatment of acute rheumatic carditis, which is discussed fully in Chapter 10. Even when the child has little or no evidence of cardiac involvement during a first attack, usually he is given suppressive treatment with salicylates or hormones in the hope of warding off any important cardiac damage, and at the same time he is kept relatively inactive until it can be demonstrated that his stage of rheumatic activity has passed.

TREATMENT AND NURSING CARE OF CHOREA. The treatment of chorea is largely palliative and symptomatic. Neither the salicylates nor the hormones have any effect upon this aspect of rheumatic fever. As soon as the disease is recognized, the child should be confined to bed, all excitement avoided and the nutrition guarded carefully. In the milder attacks, no specific care is required. When the disease is more severe, sedative drugs are required. Prolonged warm baths often are useful as a sedative measure. Some degree of success has attended the use of hyperthermia, whether produced by injection of foreign protein such as typhoid vaccine, by short-wave radiotherms or by other means. Hyperthermia applied several times a week tends to shorten the attack but it must be used with caution and not at all if cardiac damage is present.

In the later stages of chorea, especially if the attack has been prolonged and if at the time the manifestations are only moderate and if all laboratory evidence of infection has disappeared, often children will do better if they are allowed out of bed and have a fair amount of liberty.

Children with chorea have uncontrolled body movements, often to the point of helplessness, but they do not feel ill. Until they can do things for themselves, everything must be done for them. Not only must all their needs be supplied by others, but also in many instances their needs must be anticipated be-

cause they have lost their ability to talk. They must be fed, and the process must be a slow and safe one because of the in-co-ordinate movements of the head, the mouth and the muscles of swallowing. If movements are severe, a fork never should be used in feeding the child with chorea.

Children with chorea need physical and emotional rest. Usually they rest best if they are in a room by themselves where protection from stimuli can be provided. However, occasionally an isolated child will show increased restlessness and a need for the companionship of another child. Reaction to his environment should be noted and his needs supplied as the physical condition warrants.

Observation as to reaction to and behavior after parental visiting should be noted. The onset of chorea is gradual and often the acute symptoms are preceded by symptoms of nervous instability. In this period, when the child's family was unaware of his disease, behavior changes may have initiated unfortunate forms of discipline. In the period preceding the onset of choreiform movements, the child may have shown this increasing instability by frequent quarreling with siblings, less attention to schoolwork, recurrence of tantrums and fears, or by fretfulness and willfulness which tried the patience of those with whom he lived and played. If a poor parent-child relationship developed during that period, visiting periods may have to be shortened until a good relationship has been re-established.

Special attention must be given to

the skin of the elbows, the knees and other points of contact which are constantly being rubbed and chafed because of the many purposeless movements. Massaging the skin over the joints with zinc-oxide ointment and keeping the extremities covered with flannel pajamas will protect these areas from irritation. When chorea is severe, continuous nursing is desirable in order to prevent self-injury and to perform the many duties required by a helpless but mentally active child. He should be cared for in a crib bed with padded sides, and those toys which might prove injurious should be eliminated.

These children often are malnourished. Their constant movements use energy, and though their appetites are usually good, they are underweight and anemic. Frequent feedings should be provided. These should be high in protein, calories, vitamins and iron.

Understanding the instability of the child with chorea will help the nurse to exercise patience, consideration and insight in all her relations with him. When chorea develops in an intelligent, sensitive child, personality changes often manifest themselves. At the onset of the disease, he does not understand his inability to concentrate and to control the expression of his emotions. Often, too, he does not feel that his parents have responded fairly to his uncontrolled behavior. Tendencies toward introversion and introspection develop, and often it is with these personality characteristics that the nurse first sees the child.

A nurse who is poised, unhurried, thoughtful of the child's needs and sensitive to the origin of the personality traits can do much toward building up the child's confidence that perhaps was shattered when he did things that were so annoying to himself and to those in his immediate environment. Listening intently to his defective speech, reading his favorite stories, playing records that soothe and delight him, placing appropriate pictures and pots of growing plants where he can see them, talking calmly of things that interest him—all help him to sense a genuine interest in his well-being. It is the nurse who gradually can increase the child's understanding of his parents' previous reactions to his uncontrolled behavior. She can help, too, in eliminating the parents' feeling of guilt when they realize the situation and reflect on their attitudes and behavior in the prodromal stage of their child's illness. In this way, wholesome relationships can be re-established and compensating overprotection lessened.

During convalescence, when movements are controllable, play materials appropriate to the child's needs should be provided. At first, materials that require use of the larger muscles should be provided. Then, as improvement manifests itself, materials that require fine coordination, such as drawing, clay modeling, sewing or airplane construction, can be presented. In this period, the child needs materials to work with so that he again may do well those things of which he was capable before he became ill. Feelings of self-esteem can be restored through well-directed activity programs.

RHEUMATOID ARTHRITIS

Rheumatoid arthritis is a chronic systemic disease which has as its distinguishing feature protracted and deforming inflammation of the joints. It is not very common among children but may be seen at almost any age. The onset may be with joint swelling or may be in a nonspecific fashion. Fairly high fever with splenic and generalized lymph node enlargement is common in the acute stage. The small joints of the body are attacked most regularly, but the larger joints and the spine also may be involved. In contrast with rheumatic fever the disease has no apparent relation to streptococcal sensitization; the arthritis is not readily relieved with aspirin; the symptoms remain in the joints originally involved; the inflammation runs a protracted course and may result in permanent disability of the joint. Although the course of the disease is ultimately self-limited, the spontaneous subsidence of symptoms usually does not take place until the person has been sick for several years. During this period, joint deformity and muscle atrophy may progress to a point where complete restoration to normal cannot be expected. Occasionally, the heart is involved during the course of rheumatoid arthritis, but this is the uncommon exception rather than the expected complication that it is in rheumatic fever.

Before the steroid hormones were available for treatment, a great many measures were used in an attempt to relieve symptoms and terminate the disease. None of these measures was regularly successful. Cortisone, ACTH and compound F will suppress the manifestations of the disease, as in rheumatic fever, by controlling fever and reducing the inflammatory reaction in the joints.

(Sometimes compound F is injected into the joint cavity to relieve acute inflammation.) However, administration of these substances must be continued for very long periods of time, and the appearance of toxic reactions to them limits their effectiveness. However, they are tremendously superior to the older methods of treatment.

The symptomatic nursing care of rheumatoid arthritis includes shielding of joints from unexpected motion during the time they are acutely inflamed. This is achieved by the use of splints or bivalved lightweight casts which are applied at night while the child sleeps. During the acute stage of the disease the child may need to be fed, dressed and bathed by the nurse because of the restricted usefulness of his hands. For those with the severer forms of the disease there may be long periods of hospitalization during which the nurse and the occupational therapist can do much to keep the child constructively occupied, growing socially and emotionally and to maintain his morale. The importance of emotional stress as a factor in rheumatoid arthritis is recognized, and not infrequently exacerbations of the disease are related to psychic disturbance. Whether such emotional stress is the primary cause or merely a secondary product of the protracted illness is a debated question.

DISSEMINATED LUPUS ERYTHEMATOSUS

Disseminated lupus is an uncommon disorder seen mainly in adolescent and young adult females. It is a slowly progressive and invariably fatal disorder, and the multitudinous symptoms depend upon a widespread abnormality of the vascular tree. Prolonged fever, recurring arthritis, pleurisy, erythematous skin eruptions upon portions of the body exposed to the sun, chronic nephritis, endocarditis and hypersplenism are some of the features that may be present clinically. Diagnosis usually is suspected from the combination of some or all of these findings in a girl. The skin eruption and a persistent leukopenia are the features which most often direct attention to the correct diagnosis. Confirmation is obtained by finding characteristic polymorphonuclear leukocytes that contain large masses of amorphous substance (L. E. cells). These cells may be found in bone-marrow preparations or in leukocytes which have been incubated with the patient's serum. The underlying disturbance is thought to be an abnormality of protein metabolism which affects nucleic acid in particular. Accumulation of the same sort of material as that seen in the typical L. E. cell takes place beneath the endocardium to create a verrucous endocarditis and beneath the endothelium of small vessels anywhere in the body, resulting in occlusion of such vessels.

Treatment with steroid hormones is temporarily effective in obtaining remission of symptoms. Unfortunately, these persons tend to become easily sensitized by sulfonamides and other substances, including the hormones. Eventually, therapy becomes less effective or progression of the renal disease takes place and the child succumbs to it. Nursing care is that of any protracted and ultimately fatal illness.

OTHER COLLAGEN DISEASES

Other collagen diseases which are seen very infrequently among children are *dermatomyositis, scleroderma* and *periarteritis nodosa.* The reader is referred to the bibliography for full description and discussion of these disorders which, like lupus, involve widespread changes in many tissues with a progressive and usually fatal course.

ALLERGY

The term "allergy" is used to designate an altered or abnormal degree of sensitivity to various materials which act as antigens or substances having the power to cause the production of counteracting substances or antibodies. The altered susceptibility is caused by the presence of antibody to the antigen. In practically all instances the antibody is present because of response to previous introduction of antigen. Thus, antigen causes production of antibody to the antigen, and thereafter, whenever antigen is present, a symptom-producing reaction takes place between the antigen and its antibody. The responsible antigen most frequently is a protein, but it may be a nonprotein chemical substance which combines in the body with protein to form an antigen.

If a material such as horse serum is given parenterally, antibody to the foreign protein* may develop. If a large amount of serum has been given, antibody may develop in quantity before all the foreign pro-

---

*"Foreign protein" emphasizes its origin from a different animal species. Horse serum and rabbit serum are foreign proteins for man, but human plasma, convalescent human serum and gamma globulin are not.

tein has been excreted or destroyed. In such an instance, the period required to develop antibody in quantity is from 8 to 13 days. Thus, an allergic reaction may develop as a result of a single injection. The reaction thus produced is called a delayed reaction. Subsequent injections of serum are likely to produce an immediate or early reaction because of the presence of antibody at the time of injection. Smaller initial injections may produce no symptoms, but subsequent injections may cause a reaction because of the antibody produced by the first injection. This type of reaction is not limited to serum; serum is used as an example. When the allergic state develops as the result of a previous introduction of antigen in a person whose capacity to become susceptible is not a hereditary constitutional trait, the allergic response to further introduction of antigen is known as anaphylaxis. Often the term "atopy" is used synonymously with allergy, but it is more nearly correct to restrict its use to certain allergies present in those with a hereditary constitutional capacity to develop allergy. In the restricted atopic group belong hay fever, asthma, some urticarias (hives) and certain of the eczemas.

Another type of allergy is that associated with certain infections. For example, in tuberculosis the body becomes sensitive to tuberculoprotein in approximately 30 days after the initial infection. Thereafter a positive skin reaction is obtained with tuberculin, the reaction being an allergic one. Positive skin reactions are obtainable in a similar manner in other infectious diseases, including undulant fever, syphilis, rheumatic fever and scarlet fever.

The allergy is not only manifest by a skin reaction, but in these and other infections the subsequent course of the chronic infections and the course of the acute illness of recurring infections are also altered importantly because of the allergy. The adult type of tuberculosis differs from the childhood type (primary infection) because of the allergic response of the body. The tertiary lesions of syphilis differ from the earlier lesions because of allergy. Primary pneumococcus pneumonia of the child and the adult differs from the same disease in the young infant because of allergy in the older person.

Allergic phenomena occurring spontaneously are usually caused by sensitivity to either foods or materials inhaled or in some instances to both. Hay fever (allergic rhinitis) and allergic asthma commonly are caused by inhalants. The general principles which should underlie the management of allergy to inhalants are discussed under asthma. The general principles of the management of allergy to foods are discussed under eczema. Certain of the allergies in these two groups lend themselves to complete or partial desensitization; others do not. In any case, the desensitization is a slow and tedious process, and in many instances, especially in the case of foods, it is easier to avoid the offending material. Desensitization in the case of inhalants is carried out by hypodermic injections of extracts of the material in gradually increasing doses, with less than the amount which produces symptoms always being given. Food desensitization is accomplished by giving the material by mouth in gradually increasing amounts but in amounts which do not cause reactions.

SERUM DISEASE

An allergic illness which does not occur spontaneously as the result of fortuitous ingestion or inhalation of offending materials, and the one most frequently encountered, is that caused by the prophylactic or therapeutic injection of various sera. All manufacturers of commercial therapeutic sera refine their products in such a manner that the final product contains only the pseudoglobulin portion. Such sera are much less allergenic than the original raw sera. In addition, some therapeutic sera are partially digested in the final stages of the preparation and by this process have lost much more of their allergenic property.

It already has been pointed out that allergic illness from serum may occur with the first injection as a delayed reaction or with subsequent injection as an immediate or early reaction. These reactions are anaphylactic. In certain constitutionally atopic persons, immediate illness may result from the first injection. It is most important to recognize constitutional atopy, since it is probably only persons with this condition who are likely to die as a result of serum injection.

Serum sickness occurs with various degrees of severity. In the most common variety, the illness is mild. One may expect moderate fever, local redness and itching or pain at the site of injection and a generalized skin eruption which most commonly is urticarial but may be morbilliform or scarlatiniform. The child is uncomfortable but not particularly ill. A more severe and less common variety includes also several or more of the following symptoms: malaise, albuminuria, joint pains, swelling of the mucous membranes with hoarseness and cough, vertigo, nausea and vomiting. A rare and still more severe variety produces extreme weakness approaching collapse; the temperature may be subnormal and the pulse weak; catarrhal or hemorrhagic enteritis may be present. The most rare type of reaction is that which produces immediate shock, usually fatal. Usually the duration of the common varieties of serum sickness is 3 or 4 days. The more serious effects of serum sickness may be controlled to a large extent by the administration of epinephrine or ephedrine, which must be repeated from time to time as indicated by the recurrence of the symptoms. Urticaria also responds to epinephrine and to cortisone, but usually the skin lesions may be managed adequately by the application of antipruritic lotions.

Serum is used frequently in the prevention and the treatment of various diseases. Therefore, it becomes important to know the proper approach to its administration. It is customary and appropriate to make sensitivity tests as a preliminary procedure, but it is well to remember that these may be misleading. The chances of death from serum administration are extremely small. It has been estimated that not more than 1 in 70,000 injections has caused death. Practically all the deaths have occurred in association with the first injection of serum, when no previous sensitizing dose had been given. From this point of view, the fact that the child has had a previous injection of serum gives good assurance that death will not occur from a second or subsequent injection, regardless of the result of sensitivity tests. In fact, a few deaths have occurred among those with negative sensitivity reactions. Because of the possibility of sudden death, foreign serum should not be given or should be given with the greatest caution to those with hay fever and allergic eczema and particularly to those with allergic asthma.

If the child has no history of atopic disease, a suitable skin-test procedure is to give intracutaneously 0.1 cc. of the serum to be used. If no wheal results or if the wheal is no larger than ¾ in. within 20 minutes, the full dose of serum may be given. If a greater degree of hypersensitiveness exists, as shown by a larger wheal, the first dose of serum should be from ¼ to ½ cc. If no systemic reaction has occurred within 20 minutes, the full dose may be given. Small amounts of serum, such as would be used for a customary dose of diphtheria antitoxin, are safe for nonatopic children, even though the skin test is positive. Serum sickness may develop, but the reaction will not be fatal.

If the child has a history of atopic disease, the sensitivity test should be made with greater caution. A suitable procedure is to give 0.05 cc. of a 1:100 dilution intradermally or to place one drop of this same dilution into the conjunctival sac. If a reaction occurs, further serum is contraindicated. In some instances, as in the case of diphtheria, the decision to give no serum is difficult to make. Desensitization sufficiently rapid to permit the administration of serum in the treatment of

acute illness probably is impossible. One may decide to risk giving the serum in minute doses serially, starting with 0.1 cc. In such case, epinephrine should be in a syringe ready for use. It is probable that most of the severe reactions could be managed by prompt and appropriate use of epinephrine.

ACRODYNIA (ERYTHREDEMA, PINK DISEASE)

Acrodynia is a peculiar disorder which is seen sporadically in infants during the first 2 years of life. It is characterized by a prolonged course during which there is swelling, itching and peeling of the fingers, combined with general irritability and evidence of irritation of the sympathetic nervous system.

Etiology

Until recently the cause of acrodynia was obscure. The finding of mercury in the urine of nearly all infants who suffer from the disease and the successful treatment with BAL, which is an effective agent in some heavy metal poisonings, has demonstrated that mercury poisoning is an important aspect of the disease. Since a child who has contact with mercury appears only rarely to suffer from acrodynia, it is presumed that an individual sensitivity to mercury is necessary or that some additional factor which has not yet been recognized must be involved.

Symptoms

Usually the onset is insidious, and it is often difficult to determine from the history the relative time of onset of the various symptoms. When the disease has developed sufficiently for identification the symptoms are numerous. Perhaps the one pathognomonic feature and the one without which the diagnosis is uncertain consists of the changes that take place in the hands and the feet (Fig. 78). In the outspoken disease, the palms and the soles are bluish red and slightly swollen. Associated with this change is an annoying or painful itching or stinging which causes frequent or nearly constant rubbing and scratching. As the disease becomes older, the thickened skin of the palms and the soles begins to desquamate. The redness of the hands fades gradually at the wrist into the normal color of the arm, and there is no sharp line of demarcation such as is found in pellagra.

One finds that the disposition and the behavior of the child have changed. Early in the disease there is hyperesthesia of the skin and the muscles, which results in resentment at being handled and contributes to fretfulness and irritability, which are usually present. As the disease advances, the deep reflexes diminish, and a progressive muscular weakness becomes apparent. The result is decrease of such activity or effort as is represented by sitting, standing or walking. The most characteristic attitude is to lie in a knee-chest position, usually on the front, sometimes on the side, with the face buried in the pillow or the bedclothes. Covering of the face is to be accounted for by photophobia, which is present in the majority of cases. Insomnia is often a conspicuous feature. Partial or complete loss of appetite is usual.

In the early stage, an acute exanthem often is to be noted. The rash is a diffuse erythema and more often than not is associated with

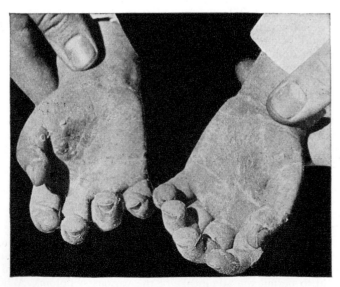

FIG. 78. The hands in acrodynia.

profuse perspiration, in which case the rash is chiefly miliaria. Acute upper respiratory infection is common. At least a moderate amount of fever usually is present. Tachycardia and elevation of the blood pressure are common. The white blood count may be normal or increased considerably.

As the disease progresses, weight loss becomes increasingly apparent, with a resultant poor nutritional state. Perspiration frequently becomes excessive. Salivation may be conspicuous. In many of the more severe illnesses stomatitis develops, with swollen tender gums and loosening or even loss of teeth. In a few cases, a patchy alopecia is to be observed. In some cases, a profuse nasal discharge persists throughout most of the course of the illness.

In severe illnesses the course is slow, and in a few instances the disease has persisted for as long as a year. The duration of the milder illnesses may be as short as 6 weeks. Despite the severity and the persistence of this disease, the mortality is low, and death, when it occurs, usually is due to some intercurrent infection such as pneumonia.

TREATMENT

Intramuscular injection of BAL every 4 hours during the acute stage of the illness and then at decreasing intervals as the symptoms subside is reported to be effective in acrodynia. Symptomatic treatment includes control of respiratory infections which are often present, sedation and general nursing care.

NURSING CARE

The child with acrodynia presents a picture of abject misery. He rarely smiles, is irritable, negative, temperamental and prone to exaggerated emotional responses. However, at times he is apathetic and withdrawn. At other times he is hyperactive; he may chew on his fingers and pull out his hair. He perspires profusely and shows symptoms of excessive thirst because of fluid loss through the skin. At times he shows complete disinterest in food.

An understanding of the behavior pattern that characterizes the child with acrodynia is necessary to provide the kind of nursing care that he requires. The child with this disease is difficult yet challenging to nurse. He is difficult to nurse because results are slow and discouraging, and his responses to thoughtful, kindly given care are different from those of the usual child. He is so miserable that he can give little in return for all he gets. He is challenging to nurse because expert nursing care assists him in adjusting to a disease that deprives him of normal satisfactions. Expert nursing care does not bring rapid and dramatic results but it lessens the severity of his discomfort. Symptoms of nervous instability can be minimized with poise, insight and kindness. They will be magnified if the nurse fails to accept his behavior. If she does not understand him, he will feel unloved as well as physically uncomfortable. Although the child may seem to be uninterested in everything and everyone within his environment, efforts to relieve his anxiety and physical discomfort never must cease.

Physical nursing care consists of protective measures, good skin and mouth care and the provision of thoughtful, patient feeding experiences. Padded cribsides are frequently necessary to protect the child from injury. Elbow restraints to prevent finger chewing and hair pulling are indicated in periods when the child cannot have the constant attention of his nurse. Baths twice daily are necessary to keep the skin clean and free from pyogenic infection. If sponge baths bring discomfort, tub baths should be given. The child should be lifted carefully and held securely to prevent his slipping in the tub. When the illness is severe, teeth drop out or become loosened, and the gums are swollen, red and spongy. Good mouth care will keep the teeth free of food particles and prevent stomatitis. In cleansing, care must be taken to prevent traumatization of the delicate buccal mucosa. Protection from bright lights should be provided. If sun treatments are ordered, the child should be provided with goggles.

Attention to nutrition might be considered one of the major factors leading to recovery. The child with acrodynia presents many problems in relation to food intake. Because he loses much fluid through the skin, he needs high-vitamin, high-caloric fluid drinks at frequent intervals. Since the child with acrodynia has little or no appetite, patience and ingenuity are needed to encourage an adequate intake of food. Often he cannot handle feeding utensils because his hands are painful, his muscles are hypotonic and he fatigues easily. He requires feeding and kind firmness to help him to understand that he is expected to take the small amounts of food that are offered at short intervals.

Gavage feedings may be necessary. Many times gavage feeding is preferable to forced feedings because invariably the resistance they evoke causes hyperirritability and vomiting.

Sedatives are often necessary for wakefulness, which may last for long periods of time. Often the child falls asleep from sheer exhaustion. When he does, he should be covered lightly to prevent chilling. He has poor resistance, low vitality and is unusually susceptible to respiratory infections. Every possible precaution must be taken to protect him from cross-infection.

LEAD POISONING

In the adult, lead poisoning usually results in a chronic illness marked by abdominal colic and weakness due to peripheral neuritis and anemia. The infant or the young child who suffers from lead intoxication is more likely to present a medical emergency because of the rapid appearance of cerebral edema with vomiting, headache, stupor, convulsions or coma. Early recognition of the disorder is highly important, for the longer the symptoms of encephalopathy persist the more certain it is that the child will suffer irreparable damage to the brain.

Etiology

The infant or the small child may ingest or inhale lead in a variety of ways. In the past, small infants have been poisoned by lead derived from lead nipple shields or from ointments containing lead which were used on the mothers' breasts. Teething powders, drinking water which passed through lead pipes and food contaminated by paint are other sources. One of the most common mechanisms of lead poisoning is that of pica, or perverted appetite, which leads the small child to chew on any and all objects, including painted toys, furniture, household fixtures and plaster. In the course of time he consumes a significant amount of lead if these objects are coated with lead-containing paint. In the United States all children's toys and furniture now must be painted with lead-free paint by the manufacturers. However, this does not control the type of paint used by the amateur in his home. Lead also may be derived from inhaled gases such as burned storage battery casings or from the fumes of gasoline containing tetraethyl lead.

Lead that is taken into the body is deposited and stored in many tissues. In the bones it accumulates at the rapidly growing epiphyseal lines, where it is visible on roentgen examination. Its deposition in the brain leads to edema and signs of increased intracranial pressure. It is released slowly from the tissues when the blood level begins to fall and is excreted by the urine.

SYMPTOMS

The symptoms of lead poisoning vary with the degree of cerebral irritation that is produced. Sometimes there will be warning signs of loss of appetite, periodic unexplained vomiting, irritability, changed disposition or ataxic gait. More frequently the encephalopathy appears abruptly with persistent major convulsions which are very difficult to control and may be followed by stupor or coma. A small fraction of children suffer from a more chronic form of the disease with anemia, weakness, colic and peripheral neuritis as the chief symptoms.

DIAGNOSIS

The diagnosis is suspected from the history of lead exposure in combination with the appearance of symptoms as above. Several laboratory tests aid in its confirmation. An anemia is usually present which is associated with basophilic stippling of the red blood cells seen on the smear. There may be a mild degree of glycosuria. The spinal fluid ordinarily has an increased quantity of protein without much or any increase in the number of cells. It is under high pressure when encephalopathy is present. X-ray examination of the bones will demonstrate a band of increased density at the epiphyseal line. The width of this band gives some indication of the length of time that the lead ingestion has been in progress. Conclusive diagnosis can be reached by measuring the level of lead in the blood or the amount that is being excreted in the urine. Precautions are necessary in obtaining specimens in receptacles which are scrupulously freed of lead, for the amounts to be determined are minute, and contamination may result in a wrong interpretation.

TREATMENT

The main problem in treatment is to get the lead out of the tissues, particularly out of the brain, and have it transported through the blood for excretion by the kidneys. To be effective this must be engineered in such a way that additional lead is not taken up by the brain during the process. In the past it was customary to give large doses of vitamin D and sodium phosphate in the hope of removing lead from the blood stream and depositing it in the growing bones. The more recent approach is to give some substance that will tie up the lead in a chemically inactive form in the blood stream while it is being transported to the kidneys for excretion. Sodium citrate has been used in this manner and more recently BAL. A new type of chemical known as a chelating agent is now under study. This substance is called Versene or Ca E.D.T.A. (calcium ethylenediaminetetra-acetate).

In addition to such attempts to immobilize lead in the blood stream, measures must be taken to terminate or prevent the convulsions that accompany encephalopathy. The usual sedatives such as phenobarbital are less effective than under ordinary circumstances and must be used in large dosage. Magnesium sulfate given intramuscularly in the same fashion as for hypertensive encephalopathy may aid in the control of cerebral edema. Surgical measures of decompression have been tried but are usually ineffective. Once the acute phase has passed, it is desirable to shield the child from acute infections that may reactivate his disease. Months are required to complete the process of de-leading the tissues and thus removing the threat of recurrence.

Nursing Care

The specific nursing care is that of a child with convulsions from any cause. Avoidance of unnecessary handling is desirable in order to give a minimum amount of stimulation to the central nervous system.

In protracted coma it may be necessary to resort to gavage feedings and the skin care that is accorded to any unconscious patient.

Prognosis

In general the prognosis following lead poisoning is not very good. The mortality from acute encephalopathy even with early treatment is significantly high—around 25 per cent —and of those who survive, a high percentage will show evidence of neurologic disturbances, including mental retardation. How many of these victims were retarded children before the acute onset of encephalopathy is always hard to judge. The retarded child is more likely to be one who develops a perverted appetite for lead-coated objects, but pica certainly is not confined to the retarded group. Children who do not have acute encephalopathy, whose lead intoxication can be terminated early in its course, have a much more favorable prognosis for full recovery.

Prophylaxis

Because of the generally unsatisfactory results of treatment it is most important to try to prevent lead poisoning. The approach has been made through the passage of laws which forbid the use of lead paint on articles designed for use by children and through public education calling attention to the dangers of lead intoxication and indicating the common sources from which the child obtains lead. The nurse visiting a home can do much to discover and point out such potential dangers to the parents.

RECURRENT VOMITING (CYCLIC VOMITING)

Recurrent vomiting may be considered a metabolic disturbance characterized by recurrent attacks of vomiting and associated with ketosis, each attack having a duration of from 3 to 5 days and terminating in spontaneous recovery.

ETIOLOGY

Recurrent vomiting occurs more frequently in the upper than in the lower economic levels. The causative mechanism is not well understood. The hypoglycemia which accompanies the condition may well be the cause of the symptoms. It is not clear in most instances why the hypoglycemia should occur. In some cases, the illness is preceded by an infection, often mild; in others, by emotional disturbance. In some children who are unusually labile in regard to the sugar content of the blood, attacks are precipitated apparently by even short periods of fasting. Liver damage, probably functional in most instances, has been assumed to be the cause of the hypoglycemia. One reason for this assumption is that in those rare instances in which the illness is severe enough to cause death, the liver is greatly enlarged and shows marked fatty infiltration and also that in acute infections liver function is impaired for sugar utilization.

It has been reported that recurrent vomiting may be prevented and its recurrence stopped by abdominal support, which at the same time acts to correct poor body posture and body mechanics. Recurrent vomiting occurs chiefly among those who are classed as nervous children.

Children so designated usually have a poor appetite and consequently are malnourished. The poor body posture would seem to be the direct result of malnutrition with its associated inadequate musculature. Such children have little reserve and are easily fatigued. The fatigue may be one of the factors in producing the poor appetite. The breaking of this cycle at any point would tend to promote better health and greater robustness in the child.

It has been pointed out that this disease may occur only once and need not be recurrent. Most of the deaths apparently have occurred in the first attack. Also, the illness may be typical in all other respects but lacking in vomiting. The criticism has been made that the disease is named after a symptom which is not necessarily present. The term "spontaneous hypoglycemia" has been proposed to designate the disease.

SYMPTOMS

In its most common form, the individual attack manifests itself by a period of vague abdominal discomfort, which is followed quickly by severe vomiting. All food and drink are vomited as soon as swallowed. Prostration increases rapidly. In cases of moderately severe illness, somnolence is present and in the most severe this may increase to coma. Some children have convulsions at the beginning of the attack, although this is not frequent. Severe thirst is a constant feature. Acetone bodies are found in the urine in large amounts. The ketosis has been reported as occurring in some instances before the onset of vomiting. The formation of acetone bodies may be sufficient to produce definite and sometimes severe acidosis. Although the child is alarmingly ill, the symptoms begin to subside spontaneously within a few days, and with the retention of nourishment recovery is very rapid. The child is free from symptoms between attacks, which occur at intervals of weeks or months. Attacks usually become less frequent as adolescence approaches, ceasing entirely at that time. Some observers associate migraine in adults with this condition.

TREATMENT

Dextrose and fluids are indicated in the management of the attacks. These materials may be given by any effective route. Because of the vomiting, oral administration is inadequate. The intravenous route is the most certain and consequently the most effective. The administration of dextrose must be repeated, preferably at short intervals in submaximum amounts. Ordinary degrees of acidosis respond quickly to the treatment with fluids and dextrose, but severe acidosis may require some alkali therapy in addition.

A certain degree of success in aborting attacks has been attained by the administration of extra sugar or sugar and alkali at the earliest indication of indisposition. Any chronic focus of infection, usually the nose and the throat, should be attended to. Every effort should be made to raise nutrition to a good standard for the individual child. Preferably, the diet should be definitely antiketogenic at all times. Usually, long intervals between meals are to be avoided, and to this end it may be advisable to offer a bedtime lunch.

ACIDOSIS AND ALKALOSIS

GENERAL CONSIDERATIONS

The reaction of all the body fluids during life is very slightly alkaline. The exact degree of alkalinity is maintained within very narrow limits. Any marked deviation is incompatible with life. Life processes are associated constantly with the production of acid and alkali. Food substances, when utilized in the body, leave acidic or basic residues. The excess of acid or alkali must be eliminated. Its transport through the body before elimination must be accomplished with only minute changes in the normal reaction of the fluids used in transport. Normally, this is accomplished. However, in certain conditions, acidic or basic substances preponderate in the body. The terms "acidosis" and "alkalosis" are applied to these conditions. (See Chap. 6 for additional discussion.)

Food Sources of Alkali. The chief food sources of alkali in the body are fruits, vegetables and milk. Fruits and vegetables contain salts of organic acids which are oxidized in the body to bicarbonates and therefore are essentially basic. However, certain organic acids, such as oxalic and benzoic acids, cannot be oxidized in the body and must be excreted.

Sources of Acid. The chief sources of acid in the body, aside from carbonic acid, are the protein foods, especially meat, and the cereal foods. The sulfur and the phosphorus of the protein molecule are changed in the body to sulfuric and phosphoric acids. The cereals contain a relatively large amount of phosphorus.

Other Acids. Under certain abnormal conditions other acids are formed in the body. If fat is incompletely burned, as in uncontrolled diabetes, acetone bodies result. These consist of acetone, acetoacetic acid and hydroxybutyric acid. The last two substances are strongly acid. When for any reason the oxygen supply to the tissues is insufficient, lactic acid accumulates.

Role of the Kidneys. All these acids, except carbonic acid, must be excreted through the kidneys. They must be neutralized before they can be transported from the tissues to the kidneys and they must be at least partly neutralized, that is, in the form of acid salts, to be excreted. Neutralization requires base, and if an excess is not available the kidney conserves base by excreting the most acid form of salt. For example, a molecule of disodium phosphate contains 2 atoms of sodium and 1 of hydrogen, and the kidney is able to excrete the most acid form of this salt, which contains 1 atom of sodium and 2 of hydrogen, thus saving to the body 1 atom of base. Ammonia can be formed in the kidney from amino acids and is used to neutralize part of the acids, thus conserving what are known as the fixed bases—sodium, potassium and calcium. The ability of the kidney to manufacture ammonia is limited, and if a large amount of acid is to be excreted, a depletion of body base will result.

Carbonic Acid. The metabolic products formed in the body in largest quantity are carbon dioxide and water, which together constitute carbonic acid. These substances are the only residues from the breakdown of carbohydrates and normally of fats. Unless the diet is very alkaline, carbonic acid is excreted wholly through the lungs. The amounts of carbonic acid which must be transported and excreted are so large that if all were carried as carbonic acid the blood would be about 1,000 times too acid. If all were carried as bicarbonate, the blood would be much too alkaline. A definite proportion of each must be carried in order to preserve the correct alkalinity of the blood. Sufficient base must be provided to form the bicarbonate needed.

Buffers. Maintenance of the normal reaction of the blood is aided by buffer substances present. A buffer substance is one which in solution is able to take up extra acid or base without any marked change in its original acidity or alkalinity. The buffer substances of the blood are the salts of the weak acids and consist of the alkali salts of the proteins, especially oxyhemoglobin and reduced hemoglobin, bicarbonates and phosphates. The reactions entering into the acid-base equilibrium of the blood are complex and will not be discussed.

ACIDOSIS

Under all ordinary conditions and by means of the mechanisms which have been discussed, the body is able without harm to itself to excrete the acids present in excess beyond its needs. Under certain abnormal or unusual conditions these mechanisms become inadequate. When as a consequence the available base is decreased below the normal limits, the condition is known as acidosis. The common types of acidosis will be enumerated and discussed briefly.

Acetone-Body Type. Whenever acetone bodies are formed in such amounts that their combination with base lowers the alkali reserve (available base) below normal levels, the resultant condition is known as the acetone-body type of acidosis. It is necessary to distinguish between acidosis and ketosis without acidosis. The term "ketosis" signifies merely an increased production or the presence of abnormal amounts of the acetone bodies. Sufficient base may be ingested, or the kidney may be able to form sufficient ammonia to neutralize these for excretion without depleting the body appreciably of fixed base. Ketosis has been observed even in the presence of alkalosis. Acetone bodies result from incomplete combustion of fats. This event occurs when the available sugar in the body is decreased greatly or when the body becomes unable to use properly the sugar that is present. Thus, ketosis may occur in diabetes, in acute infections and in recurrent vomiting. Starvation, anesthesia and toxemias are other causes of ketosis.

Lactic-Acid Type. Excessive formation of lactic acid to the extent of producing acidosis is the result of insufficient oxygenation, which in turn is usually the result of impairment of circulation or of pulmonary function. The decrease in available oxygen causes incomplete combustion of carbohydrates, with lactic acid as one of the combustion products. Lactic-acid acidosis usually is associated also with an accumulation of carbonic acid in the body, for the reason that carbon dioxide

leaves the body by way of the lungs approximately in proportion to the amount of oxygen absorbed. Pneumonia is an outstanding example of pulmonary disease that impairs oxygenation of the blood. In cases of circulatory failure, the fault may be in the heart, in the vessels or in the blood. Thus, it may arise in cardiac failure and also in conditions of shock in which capillaries are dilated and the resultant stasis makes proper circulation impossible. Loss of fluid in large amounts from the body operates similarly.

Renal Type. In certain varieties of kidney disease, the ability of the kidney to form ammonia is decreased greatly, as is also its ability to conserve base by excreting acid salts rather than neutral salts. Thus, very important mechanisms for excreting acid are impaired or cease to function, and a marked base deficit may occur as a result. Also, in severe nephritis a retention of phosphates and sulfates occurs, and the binding of base by these lowers still further the base available for carbon dioxide transport.

Loss of Base by Bowel. Acidosis is often a result of severe diarrhea, especially in infancy. The dehydration that accompanies diarrhea produces impairment of circulation and consequent accumulation of lactic acid because of poor oxidation. The dehydration also reduces urine output with resultant decreased excretion of phosphates and sulfates. More important than either of these mechanisms in producing acidosis is loss of base in the stools. Alkaline salts are a part of the normal digestive secretions of the upper part of the intestine. These salts are largely absorbed in the lower intestine and the colon. With diarrhea, the salts are washed out and lost, producing a base deficit.

Therapeutic Acidosis. It is possible to produce acidosis by the administration of acids which cannot be oxidized or of salts which in the body are metabolized with acid production. Ammonium chloride is such a salt, the ammonium radical being converted to urea, leaving hydrochloric acid to combine with fixed base. Moderate acidosis sometimes is produced intentionally by this method for therapeutic purposes.

Symptoms. Obvious symptoms of acidosis may be slight or absent in cases of moderate alkali deficit. With more severe acidosis, stupor or coma is usually present, and the type of breathing is altered greatly from the normal. When the available base is lowered, carbon dioxide is carried from the tissues at a decreased rate. The excess of carbon dioxide in the tissues about the respiratory center serves as a stimulus to this center, and respiration is increased in both rate and depth. The consequent increased aeration in the lungs permits larger amounts of carbon dioxide to be excreted and thus serves as a compensatory mechanism. The type of breathing characteristic of acidosis is called Kussmaul breathing and is spoken of as air hunger. It is not associated with cyanosis except in the presence of circulatory impairment. In the acetone-body type of acidosis, some of the acetone is excreted by way of the lungs, imparting to the breath a fruity odor. Neither the fruity breath nor the finding of acetone bodies in the urine is diagnostic of acidosis, although these findings suggest such a diagnosis.

Diagnosis. The diagnosis of acidosis is often difficult without chemical examination of the blood to determine the amount of available base. The amount of base available is known as the "alkali reserve" or "carbon-dioxide capacity" of the blood. Normally, the carbon-dioxide capacity is from 50 to 75 cc. of carbon dioxide for each 100 cc. of blood plasma, usually designated as volumes per cent. The alkali reserve also may be expressed in millimols of carbon dioxide per liter. The normal range is 22.5 to 34. In infants and young children, the normal value may be from 5 to 10 volumes per cent lower than that stated. A carbon-dioxide capacity of less than 40 (=17.5 mM./L.) is interpreted as indicative of moderate acidosis; from 30 to 20 (=13−9 mM./L.), of severe acidosis; below 20, of an acidosis which will prove fatal unless relieved within a short time. A carbon-dioxide capacity above 75 volumes per cent (34 mM./L.) represents alkalosis.

This method of rating the severity of acidosis can be used only when the disturbance is created by a metabolic disorder rather than a respiratory one.

Prognosis. The prognosis in acidosis is largely dependent on the cause. The acetone-body type yields readily to treatment. The lactic-acid type also does if adequate circulation and elimination of carbon dioxide are made possible. Acidosis associated with nephritis is more serious, because so little can be done to restore renal function, and the salt elimination through other channels is inadequate. When severe acidosis occurs in association with diarrhea and anhydremia it is frequently fatal.

Treatment of acidosis is designed primarily to correct the underlying cause. In all types except that due to cardiac failure, the administration of fluid in large amounts through a channel which will ensure proper assimilation is indicated. Substances given by mouth may be vomited or may not be absorbed or passed on from an atonic stomach. Intravenous administration is of great value. In infants, fluid frequently is given intraperitoneally. Unless the infant is moribund, the fluid will be absorbed rapidly, and the injection may be repeated in a few hours if indicated. If the child is able to take fluids by mouth, their ingestion should be encouraged. A glass an hour is not too much for a large child. Fruit juices to which sugar is added serve also for nourishment.

In acidosis associated with ketosis, carbohydrates should be given in relatively large quantity. Fruit juices and candy are useful, but in severe acidosis, dextrose solutions should be given intravenously in amounts according to the size of the child and should be repeated after an hour or two as often as needed. In diabetes an equivalent amount of insulin should be given simultaneously. At times the insulin is added to the dextrose before injecting, one unit for each gram of dextrose being used. The treatment should be continued vigorously until the acidosis is well controlled.

ALKALI. Occasionally, alkali is needed in cases of severe acidosis in which the alkali reserve has been greatly depleted.

SODIUM BICARBONATE may be given by mouth, from 1 to 5 Gm. an hour, until signs of improvement are shown. Intravenously, it may be used in 4-per-cent solution. Such a solution should not be boiled, because boiling will convert the bicarbonate to carbonate, which is strongly alkaline. It is to be remembered that an excess of alkali in the body may be produced by soda administration, and that this condition is fully as serious as acidosis and more difficult to remedy. Generally, it is unwise to use alkali unless blood-chemical estimations of alkali reserve can be made frequently. In most instances, alkali is not necessary.

HARTMANN'S SOLUTION (sodium lactate—Ringer's solution) also may be used for intravenous administration of potential alkali. This solution has certain advantages over sodium bicarbonate in that the sodium lactate is converted into sodium bicarbonate rather slowly, allowing time for excretion of any excess which might be formed. For this reason, less caution is necessary in its administration than when sodium bicarbonate is given, and alkalosis is less likely to develop. Its administration seems to be safe, even without frequent control examinations of the blood.

In lactic-acid types of acidosis, correction of the underlying condition is the treatment of choice. Bleeding may be beneficial in cases in which cardiac failure is the underlying cause; 500 cc. may be withdrawn from an adult and proportional amounts from children. In anhydremia, restoration of body fluid is indicated. Alkali should not be given or at least should be given cautiously for acidosis due to lactic acid.

Children with renal acidosis should receive treatment similar to that for lactic-acid acidosis in general, together with support and relief for the kidney.

ALKALOSIS

Alkalosis is characterized by a relative preponderance of base in the body, the ratio of bicarbonate to carbonic acid being greater than normal. The alkali reserve is greater than 75 volumes per cent (34 mM./L.). Values as high as 120 volumes per cent (54 mM/L.) have been observed. Alkalosis interferes with normal cell activity. In many ways its effects are similar to those produced by acidosis.

Causes. Alkalosis may be caused by excessive loss of acid from the body. It may occur in association with prolonged vomiting, as in pyloric stenosis, in which condition gastric juice is lost with consequent depletion of chlorides, especially hydrochloric acid.

An excess of carbonic acid may be lost from the body by labored breathing. This type of breathing sometimes may be caused by irritation of the central nervous system, such as may occur with encephalitis.

Alkalosis may be caused also by an excessive intake of base. Some of the drugs commonly used in the practice of medicine may lead to accumulation of base, particularly the citrates and the bicarbonates. These drugs have been responsible in some instances for the production of severe alkalosis. Alkalosis may be caused by deficient excretion of base. In severe nephritis the kidney loses its ability to concentrate salts. Sometimes alkali is given in moderate amounts for the purpose of correcting an existing acidosis. Unless sufficient fluid is given to permit excess base to be excreted, alkali administration may lead to accumulation of base in the tissues.

Diagnosis. Recognition of alkalosis is based primarily on chemical estimations of the alkali reserve of the blood. Prostration and other symptoms, with the possible exception of the type of breathing, are not particularly helpful in the diagnosis. With the exception of that produced by overbreathing, alkalosis is associated with decreased respiratory effort. The slow, irregular, shallow breathing often observed serves to decrease the excretion of carbonic acid, and thus some compensation is achieved. Tetany may be present at times as a result of alkalosis and thus may be a symptom leading to the diagnosis.

Treatment. Excess base must be excreted by the kidney. For this purpose a large volume of urine is necessary, because the kidney cannot excrete a very alkaline urine. It is much more difficult for the body to compensate for alkalosis than for acidosis. When alkalosis has been caused by prolonged deep breathing, the acid-base balance will be restored promptly when a more normal rate of breathing is established. If alkalosis has been the result of alkali administration in the presence of nephritis with poor elimination of salts by the kidneys, the giving of large amounts of fluid should be a satisfactory method of treatment, because thereby excretion of excess base is permitted. In some cases it may be necessary to administer some acid-producing substance, such as ammonium or calcium chloride. From 20 to 100 mg. of ammonium chloride for each kilogram of body weight may be given, depending on the degree of alkalosis. If alkalosis occurs because of excessive alkali administration and at the same time the kidneys are functioning normally, the excess of alkali will be eliminated on the administration of sufficient water.

The type of alkalosis most commonly observed in pediatric practice is that which results from severe and prolonged vomiting without diarrhea. In such cases, not only is hydrochloric acid lost, but also considerable quantities of sodium chloride. Dehydration often is marked because of vomiting, lack of fluid intake and lessened water-holding capacity of the tissues from loss of salts. The dehydration leads to decrease in functional capacity of the kidneys. The excess of alkali cannot be excreted because of the dehydration. Even if an abundance of water be supplied, the alkali will not be excreted in appreciable amounts unless sodium chloride is given at the same time, for the reason that the body tends to hold onto its salts, even though alkaline, in order to maintain osmotic equilibrium. In these cases it is necessary to supply both water and salt and to do this repeatedly until the water and the acid-base balances are restored. The administration of ammonium chloride is seldom necessary in alkalosis due to vomiting if free diuresis can be obtained by means of salt or Ringer's solution.

If present because of alkalosis, tetany will be relieved by the return of the alkali reserve to a normal level. Magnesium sulfate will relieve the tetany promptly, but without affecting the alkalosis.

In alkalosis, as in acidosis, the fluids and the drugs used in the emergency treatment should be administered by such routes that absorption is assured.

SITUATIONS FOR FURTHER STUDY

1. What early symptoms are indicative of rheumatic fever? What are the common manifestations of rheumatic fever? How can recurrences of rheumatic fever be minimized? What does convalescent care of the child with rheumatic fever include?

2. What are some of the problems that you have encountered in nursing the child with rheumatoid arthritis? What problems do you think the child with rheumatoid arthritis experiences?

3. How can a child become desensitized to foods that produce an allergic reaction?

4. How does acrodynia differ from pellagra?

5. If a child with acrodynia were being cared for at home, what guidance would the child's mother require to understand his nursing needs?

6. What are the dangers of lead poisoning? What measures are necessary to prevent it?

7. What symptoms are produced by hypoglycemia?

8. If a child has attacks of recurrent vomiting, what observations would you want to make in planning his nursing care?

9. What diseases tend to produce acidosis? What are the symptoms of acidosis? What produces these symptoms? What treatment is required for acidosis?

10. What diseases might produce alkalosis? How do the symptoms of acidosis differ from those of alkalosis?

BIBLIOGRAPHY

Afremow, M. L., and Odenal, Josephine: Lupus erythematosus, Am. J. Nursing **51**:383, 1951.

Bivings, L.: Acrodynia, a summary of BAL therapy reports, J. Pediat. **34**:322, 1949.

Bland, E. F., and Jones, T. D.: Rheumatic fever and rheumatic heart disease; a twenty year report on 1,000 patients followed since childhood, Circulation **4**: 836, 1951.

Coburn, A. F.: The Factor of Infection in the Rheumatic State, Baltimore, Williams & Wilkins, 1931.

Cohn, A. E., and Lingg, C.: The natural history of rheumatic cardiac disease, J.A.M.A. **121**:1, 131, 1943.

Ennis, J. M., and Harrison, H. E.: Treatment of lead encephalopathy with BAL, J. Pediat. **5**:853, 1950.

Hench, P. S., Slocumb, C. H., Polley, H. F., and Kendall, E. C.: Effect of cortisone and pituitary adrenocorticotropic hormone (ACTH) on rheumatic diseases, J.A.M.A. **144**:1327, 1950.

Paul, J. R.: The Epidemiology of Rheumatic Fever, New York, Am. Heart A., 1943.

Rantz, L. A.: The Prevention of Rheumatic Fever, Springfield, Ill., Thomas, 1952.

Warkany, J., and Hubbard, D. M.: Adverse mercurial reactions in the form of acrodynia and related conditions, Am. J. Dis. Child. **81**: 335, 1951.

Wilson, M. G., and Schweitzer, M. D.: Rheumatic fever as a familial disease, J. Clin. Investigation **16**:555, 1937.

Unit Five

NUTRITION AND THE NUTRITIONAL DISEASES

The Essential Constituents of the Diet and the Amounts Required

⬥⬥

PROTEIN
FAT
CARBOHYDRATE
ENERGY METABOLISM

WATER
MINERAL SALTS
VITAMINS
SITUATIONS FOR FURTHER STUDY

The essential components of the diet are protein, carbohydrate, fat, mineral salts, vitamins and water. In addition to the requirements for these dietary components named, the body requires also a fairly definite amount of food calories or energy. When all these various requirements are fully met, the diet is referred to frequently as being "complete."

PROTEIN

Protein is an essential part of all living cells. In the processes of cell function, protein is used up, and replacement becomes necessary. During growth, still further supplies of protein are required. Plants can form protein from simple substances absorbed from the air and the soil. Man and the animals are unable to build protein from any nonprotein material which may be ingested; it must be supplied in the food. In the process of digestion, the ingested proteins are split into less complex unit structures. These, when absorbed, are rebuilt into proteins specific for the species. Thus proteins become indispensable as a part of the diet. Neither man nor the animals can live for any considerable length of time without them. When protein is present but insufficient, growth is retarded, the muscles are feeble, resistance to infection is lowered, and anemia develops.

COMPOSITION

Proteins are alike in that they are all made up of amino acids in various combinations. At least 22 amino acids are known to be constituents of proteins. The possible combinations of amino acids to form proteins are almost infinite, each combination having its own special characteristics as a protein. Ten of these amino acids are essential in the diet, in that the body must have them and cannot construct them. Others are useful to the body, though they are not essential. Proteins are said to be complete when they contain all the essential amino acids. Many proteins are incomplete. In order to be useful in meeting the protein need, they must be supplemented by other proteins which contain the remainder of the essential amino acids. Most animal proteins are complete, e.g., those of milk and meat. Relatively few vegetable proteins supply all the essential amino acids adequately when taken alone. One of the constituents of protein is nitrogen. It occurs in all proteins in approximately the same proportion. The amount in the diet in materials other than protein is quantitatively unimportant. Consequently, the determination of the amount of nitrogen in foods constitutes an easy method of estimating the amount of protein. From the amount of nitrogen in the urine may be estimated the amount of protein which has been split in the body to its physiologic end products for excretion. After growth has ceased, the amount of nitrogen (protein) ingested and the amount excreted should be equal, a condition known as nitrogen equilibrium. If the amount excreted is greater than the amount ingested, body protein is being burned. If ingestion exceeds excretion, protein is being stored. During growth, protein is being added to the body constantly, and the amount of nitrogen ingested is in excess of that excreted. One who is growing requires more protein in proportion to size than one fully grown.

Protein Requirement of the Infant

Estimates of the protein requirement of the infant have been based largely on the amounts of protein received when infants are breast-fed and thriving. In these circumstances the amount of protein ingested is from 2 to 2.5 Gm. daily for each kilogram of body weight. When human milk is unavailable, cow's milk is the customary substitute. It is a widely accepted concept that cow's-milk protein is biologically inferior to human-milk protein because of the difference in relative proportions of essential amino acids. On the basis that it may be inferior by approximately 20 per cent, the protein requirement when cow's milk is fed is from 2.5 to 3 Gm. for each kilogram. When cow's milk is fed to infants in customary quantities, the protein intake is at least 3.5 Gm. for each kilogram, sometimes as much as 4.5 Gm. The excess over the theoretical requirement is well utilized and produces increased growth. Infants tolerate well any amount of protein it is possible to give them as undiluted milk provided that some means has been used to adapt it to their digestion. Sometimes, when babies are allergic to cow's milk, vegetable preparations, such as soybean "milk," are used in substitution. Soybean protein is complete, but a much larger quantity must be fed in order that all essential amino acids be present in sufficient amount. The amount of soybean protein fed is commonly 50 per cent more than that of cow's milk.

Protein Requirement of the Child

The total amount of protein required by the child increases with the age, but the amount for each unit of body weight gradually decreases. The requirement is met amply by 3 Gm. daily for each kilogram at from 1 to 3 years of age, 2.75 Gm. at from 4 to 6 years, 2.5 Gm. at from 7 to 9 years, 2 Gm. at from 10 to 14 years, 1.5 Gm. at from 16 to 20 years, 1 Gm. for adults. These values have been computed on the basis of a mixed diet in which some of the protein is not of high biologic value. Of the foods supplying a good type of protein in abundance, the more important are milk, eggs, meat, cheese and the legumes. The animal proteins are to be emphasized particularly, and special emphasis is to be placed on milk. A quart of milk supplies most of the protein requirement of the young child and half the requirement at 12 years. Without milk, a satisfactory protein intake for the child is not possible when only customary diets are considered. Protein deficiency among children is much more common than is generally recognized. Insufficient protein leads to impairment of growth, often in ways undetectable by physical examination. For example, the amount of muscle in the body, as determined by creatinine excretion, is commonly less than that which may be considered normal and is easily attainable by ingestion of the stated protein allowances.

FAT

Fats consist of a chemical combination of glycerin and fatty acids. They differ from each other by reason of the differences in the fatty acids. Certain fatty acids (linoleic and arachidonic) have been found essential for some animals on which experiments were made. It is possible that they may be important also for the human, but the necessity for them has not been proved. In fact, young children have been maintained in an excellent state of nutrition for long periods with negligible amounts of fat in the diet. Aside from the possibility that certain fat components may be essential, fat does not appear to be a necessary constituent of the diet, and so no fat requirement exists. The chief nutritional function of fat in the diet is to supply energy, and in this respect it can be replaced completely by carbohydrate. However, certain fats are highly desirable in the diet because they contain fat-soluble vitamins which are essential, though these vitamins may be supplied by special preparations if necessary. Fats are desirable also because they furnish considerably more energy for each unit of weight than protein or carbohydrate, thus conserving the functions of digestion and absorption and distributing the burden of energy production among a greater number of body functions. Also, fats contribute materially to the palatability of the diet, and without them insufficient total food is likely to be ingested if the amount is left to choice.

CARBOHYDRATE

The chief function of carbohydrate is to supply energy. It is an essential constituent of the body. Carbohydrate becomes available through the breakdown of protein and, to some extent, of fat. While it is theoretically possible to derive sufficient carbohydrate from these sources, it is much more practical to consider that a carbohydrate requirement exists. A certain amount of energy must be derived from sources other than fat in order to spare fat combustion. The capacity of the body to burn fat completely is limited. When the energy requirement demands amounts of fat in excess of that which can be burned completely, ketone bodies are formed as a result of incomplete combustion. The minimum requirement for carbohydrate may be considered as that amount which supplies sufficient energy to prevent fat combustion in excess of capacity. This amount is that which supplies 20 per cent of the combined calories from fat and carbohydrate in the diet. During health, and with customary diets, the amount of carbohydrate ingested is much in excess of any theoretical requirement at all ages. The young baby, whether breast or artificially fed, commonly receives from 10 to 12 Gm. of carbohydrate for each kilogram of body weight; 60 per cent of the carbohydrate of the milk formula is that which has been added.

ENERGY METABOLISM

In the functioning of living cells certain substances are consumed. More complex substances are converted into simpler ones. For example, body sugar may be broken down into carbon dioxide and water, which may then be excreted. These processes are necessary to the life and the function of the cell and are continuous. With increased cell activity, as, for example, increased muscular activity, a larger amount of material is consumed. The breaking down of these substances is associated with liberation of heat, very much as if the same materials were burned outside the body. This heat is radiated from the body and is easily measurable.

From the measured amount of heat given off from the body the amount of materials being consumed in the body can be estimated. It is obvious that materials consumed must be replaced by way of the food, otherwise the body would consume not only all its reserve food but also its own more vital tissues. From the measurements of the amount of heat given off from the body under various conditions of rest and muscular activity, it is possible to estimate approximately the amount of food necessary for replacement of the material being consumed under the same conditions. The unit of heat measurement is the calorie (large), which by definition is the amount of heat required to raise 1 liter of water 1° Centigrade. One who radiates heat from the body to the extent of 1,500 calories in 24 hours must ingest an amount of food which, when used by the body, will liberate this amount of heat.

The food constituents which are used by the body with the liberation of heat are fat, carbohydrate and protein. Fat and sugar will liberate 9 and 4 calories, respectively, for each gram, whether oxidized inside or outside the body. Protein, which is not broken down in the body to the same end products as result from combustion, has a physiologic value of 4 calories for each gram. The caloric value of any food is easily determined when the amounts of fat, carbohydrate and protein are known.

The amount of food energy required by the body depends on several factors. First, that required for basal metabolism must be supplied. This represents the materials con-

APPROXIMATE ENERGY AND PROTEIN REQUIREMENTS FOR CHILDREN

Age (Yrs.)	Approximate Height (Ins.)	Approximate Weight (Lbs.)	Average Protein (Gms.)	Average (Total Calories)
1	30	22	30	1000
2	34	27	32	1100
3	37	32	35	1250
4	40	36	37	1375
5	43	41	41	1500
6	46	48	48	1600
7	48	52	52	1750
8	50	58	58	1900
9	52	64	64	2050
10	54	71	71	2200
11	56	78	78	2400
12	58	87	87	2600
13	60	95	95	2800
14	63	110	100	3000
15	65	120	100	3300
16	67	130	100	3500

sumed and the energy liberated when the subject is in complete repose but awake. Food materials are required for replacement and repair even when the body is at rest. Bodily activity increases the energy requirement in proportion to the amount of activity. Growth occurs only when food is supplied in addition to the basal and activity needs. The energy equivalent of this food must be taken into account in computing the energy requirement. The small amount of unutilized food lost in the stools must be considered also. Among these various factors which determine the energy requirement, the one showing the greatest variation is bodily activity. It is obvious that a very active infant or child requires more food than a quiet, placid one.

The energy requirement is proportional to the amount of body tissue which is actively consuming food.

Certain tissues, such as fat and bone, are relatively inert and have no relationship to the energy need. Though it is customary, for lack of a better simple means, to express the energy requirement in terms of calories for each pound or kilogram of body weight, it is apparent that such a statement of need can be only approximate. One who has good muscular development and little fat requires as much total food as one of the same age and development but with an abundance of fat. However, the requirement for each unit of weight is very different. The energy requirement should be estimated on the basis of what the weight should be were the infant or child entirely normal or average.

In the first 3 weeks of life, the energy requirement is relatively low, but for the remainder of the first few months it is approximately 120 calories for each kilogram (55 for each pound) for the average infant. After the first few months, the energy requirement for each unit of weight gradually diminishes. By 6 months, it is approximately 110 calories for each kilogram (50 for each pound). By the end of the first year, it is approximately 100 calories for each kilogram (45 for each pound). In terms of total calories, the average baby should be receiving 500 calories at 1 month, 800 at 6 months and 1,000 at 1 year.

The energy requirement for each unit of weight gradually decreases from infancy to adulthood. After the period of infancy it is more commonly customary to refer to the energy requirement in terms of total calories rather than as calories for each unit of weight. Approximate energy and protein requirements for children are shown in the accompanying table. An important fact not brought out by the table is that during adolescence the total energy requirement is much higher than later. A boy of 16 years often will take more food than a man doing heavy labor. Another fact not shown in the table is the slightly larger energy requirement for girls than for boys which begins at about 11 years, and the smaller requirement for girls than for boys which begins at about 14 years. After 16 years, the energy intake of boys increases for a time beyond the values shown in the table, while the intake of girls decreases rapidly to the adult level.

WATER

Water is an essential, the need for which is manifest by thirst. Because of thirst, the older healthy child may be expected to satisfy his requirements without supervision. Closer attention to the water requirement is necessary for infants and young children and for the sick at all ages.

An infant needs from 100 to 150 Gm. of water daily for each kilogram of body weight, in marked contrast to an average requirement of from 30 to 40 Gm. for each kilogram for adults. The requirement for water is not so nearly constant as that for other nutritional essentials because of variations in the need dependent on external temperature and other factors not easily controlled. The quantity of water required by the infant is proportionately larger because of the higher rate of metabolism and the relatively larger surface area. Water is required for storage of food, combustion of food and excretion of waste products. All these processes take place at a greater rate than in the older child or adult.

The body of the infant contains a much higher proportion of water than does that of the older person. Most of this increased proportion of water is present as interstitial fluid; that is, fluid outside of and between cells. The chief component of interstitial fluid besides water is sodium chloride. Neither of these two components can exist without the other as a part of interstitial fluid; loss of either means loss of both. It is largely because of the high proportion of interstitial fluid that the water content of babies is relatively unstable. Infants become dehydrated much more easily than those older, either from water deprivation or from excessive losses, as from diarrhea. Dehydration to a degree sufficient to cause death is not rare in infancy.

Although children require water,

no fixed rule can be given as to the amount needed or to be allowed. It varies with the weather, the kind of food and the activity of the child. In general, it may be said that the child needs from 3 to 5 glasses of water daily in addition to milk and other food sources of water. It may be taken at or between meals. Water is not harmful at meals; in reasonable amounts it even aids digestion. However, water should not be allowed to replace milk at meals, nor should liquids be used to wash down improperly chewed foods. Children in a hospital often get too little water. It is not easily available and children often hesitate to ask strange adults for a drink.

MINERAL SALTS

Numerous minerals are essential for life and growth. Most of them are present in customary diets in ample amount. Only those likely to be deficient will be discussed.

In the case of the infant, all the essential minerals are supplied by either human or cow's milk with the exception of iron and possibly copper. Normally, at birth the liver contains a small store of iron and copper. The store of iron is increased considerably in the first 2 months by the breakdown of hemoglobin in the change from the high level of hemoglobin at birth to the lower level normal for infancy. During good health, this store is not exhausted for several months. In order to maintain the store, the addition of iron to the diet is necessary at 2 or 3 months of age. Although it is not essential that the store be fully maintained, the addition of iron is desirable before the store is exhausted. Iron-containing foods

should be given not later than 4 months of age. Special attention to copper seems to be unnecessary.

Infants born prematurely are handicapped in numerous ways, among others by small stores of iron and calcium. The percentage of hemoglobin is the same as for babies born at term and the total amount of blood is proportionate to body size, but the size is small, and the infant is expected to grow rapidly to overcome his size handicap. Thus proportionately larger amounts of iron are required and they are needed earlier than for the baby born at term. A somewhat similar situation exists in regard to calcium. Almost all the calcium of the body is present as a part of bone structure. Most of the prenatal calcification of bone occurs in the last 3 months of fetal life, and about one half of it occurs in the last 4 weeks. In order that prematurely born babies may maintain normal bone structure, it is necessary that special consideration be given to the calcium content of the food.

For the child over 2 years of age, the minerals requiring discussion are chiefly calcium and iodine. Deficiency of iron is not common. Iron is supplied by meat, liver, eggs and green vegetables. Iodine is present in sufficient amounts in foods grown and produced in regions where iodine exists in the soil and the water. Sea foods are excellent natural sources of iodine. Iodine is lacking in the soil of a large area round the Great Lakes and in the Pacific Northwest. Since iodine is an essential, the small amounts necessary should be supplied to those living in iodine-deficient regions. The most convenient method of obtaining satisfactory, though minimum, amounts is the use of iodized salt. Iodine is discussed further under Simple Goiter.

Sufficient calcium is obtained by those children who receive at least 1½ pints of milk up to adolescence and a quart during the rapid growth period of adolescence. Milk, including milk products, is the one good food source of calcium. A quart of milk supplies from 4 to 6 times as much calcium as all the remainder of the day's diet. Calcium deficiency of some degree is extremely common because for one reason or another many children do not receive their quota of milk. These same children are very likely also to be receiving insufficient protein and certain other nutritional essentials. Deficiency of calcium is one of the factors responsible for tooth decay. It also causes osteoporosis, a condition of undermineralization of bone which is independent of rickets.

VITAMINS

Vitamin is a term applied to certain organic substances which are essential in minute amounts and cannot be synthesized in the body. A few of the vitamins have a somewhat similar function but most of them are entirely unrelated, and their inclusion in a single group is a result of historic development. One vitamin cannot replace another. Each must be supplied in the required amount in order to ensure good growth and health. As a part of the historic development of our knowledge, the vitamins have been divided into fat-soluble and water-soluble groups. The fat-soluble group includes vitamins A, D and

K; the water-soluble group includes the vitamins of the B complex and vitamin C. The designation of the vitamins by letter resulted from the recognition of the existence of the materials by identification of their functions before their chemical structures became known. Most of them have been identified chemically and have been synthesized. Gradually, the chemical names are replacing the letter designations. When vitamins were known only in terms of their function, they were measured quantitatively in terms of biologic units. Now that most of these materials have been identified chemically, units are being replaced gradually by weight. The present mixture of letters and chemical names and of units and milligrams represents a stage in the development of knowledge.

Vitamin A

Vitamin A is a term usually applied to both vitamin A itself and certain carotenoid pigments which are converted to vitamin A in the liver. Vitamin A is colorless; carotene or provitamin A is yellow. Most of the vitamin A of the usual diet is present as carotene. Its chief sources are the leafy and the yellow vegetables. Vitamin A is present along with carotene in milk and products prepared from milk fat and in egg yolk. Liver is an excellent source, the fish-liver oils being the richest natural source. Vitamin A is utilized more efficiently than is carotene. Neither material is affected to an important degree by the usual processes of cooking. Vitamin A is stored in the body, chiefly in the liver, and a goodly store is to be considered normal.

The functions of vitamin A, as of other vitamins, have been studied first with animals by depriving them of it. It is not known whether all the findings of experiments apply to the human, as, for example, defective ovulation in the mature animal and the occurrence of certain congenital malformations (cleft lip and palate) in the offspring when the mother has been maintained in a state of partial deficiency. Vitamin A is essential for growth, for the formation of normal teeth and bones, for ability to adapt quickly to vision in a dim light from that in a bright light and for the maintenance of a normal state of epithelial structures. The epithelial changes in the conjunctiva characteristic of vitamin-A deficiency lead to xerosis and subsequently to xerophthalmia. The changes in the conjunctiva are such that bacterial invasion occurs and the usefulness of the eye may be lost as a result. Similar changes in the epithelium of the nose constitute a factor predisposing to upper respiratory and sinus infections. The changes in the skin are those of hyperkeratosis, in which the skin is dry and rough, with papules.

The vitamin-A requirement varies with the size or the weight of the body. The requirement of the young infant is met easily by the content of either human or cow's milk when these are average. The customary additions to the milk diet as the infant becomes older increase the intake to maintain it at a level fully adequate. In fact, at all ages any reasonably good diet supplies adequate vitamin A without resort to special preparations of this material. Important deficiency of intake occurs only with diets which depart markedly from a satisfactory pattern. Even with a good intake of vitamin A, deficiency may arise from poor utilization. Utilization becomes markedly impaired by illness, particularly acute infection. The allowance of vitamin A recommended has been placed at 2,500 units at from 4 to 6 years, 3,500 units at from 7 to 9 years, 4,500 units at from 10 to 12 years and 5,000 units at all periods after 13 years, except in the case of women during pregnancy and lactation and of boys from 16 to 20 years of age, when it is larger.

Vitamin D

Vitamin D is produced in the body by the action of ultraviolet rays from sunshine on cholesterol in the skin. Ultraviolet is that portion of sunshine or other source with rays shorter than visible light. Visible light has wave lengths from 770 (red) to 390 (violet) millimicrons. A millimicron ($m\mu$) is one millionth of a millimeter, and is the equivalent of 10 angstrom units. The amount of ultraviolet reaching the earth from the sun varies with the season, inclination of the sun and atmospheric conditions. The shortest waves are the easiest filtered out by clouds, dust and the air layer. The amount is more constant at clear, high altitudes. The shortest waves reaching the earth from the sun are 293 $m\mu$. Waves longer than 320 $m\mu$ have no effect in producing vitamin D, the most marked effect being produced by waves of 300 $m\mu$ or less. Ordinary window glass filters out all waves shorter than 334 $m\mu$. The mercury vapor arc quartz lamp, often used as a source of ultraviolet, gives off rays from 630 down to 200 $m\mu$ or less. The very short waves of radium or x-rays have no effect in producing vitamin D. Vitamin-D deficiency is more common in winter than in summer because of the smaller amount of effective ultraviolet from the sun and because of less exposure to that which is present. Daily exposure of the body for 15 minutes to the direct rays of midday summer sun or for 2 minutes to the mercury vapor lamp produces sufficient vitamin D for protection against deficiency.

Vitamin D is present in ordinary foods in only unimportant quantities. It is present naturally in small amounts in milk, butter and egg yolk. Liver is a good source, the liver oils of fish being the richest natural source. Vitamin D is prepared artificially by irradiation of cholesterol, an animal product, or ergosterol, a vegetable product. Activated ergosterol, when purified to contain only vitamin D, is known as calciferol. Inconclusive evidence indicates that activated cholesterol and naturally occurring vitamin D may be somewhat superior to activated ergosterol in effectiveness for humans, but the difference, if any, is small. Vitamin D is relatively stable and resists destruction in the various processes of cooking food. Vitamin D may be stored to some extent, chiefly in the liver.

The function of vitamin D is to improve and regulate the utilization of calcium and phosphorus of the diet. Vitamin-D deficiency is known to lead to rickets and tetany in the infant and to osteomalacia in the adult. It leads also to subnormal mineralization of teeth and bones in the growing child, even though rickets may not be clinically evident.

At least during the fall, the winter and the spring seasons, vitamin D should be supplied from special sources throughout the growth period. In many instances it should be given during the summer season also. For the young infant, 50 units daily for each kilogram of body weight are ample for maximum utilization of calcium and phosphorus. At no period during infancy or childhood does the requirement exceed 350 units daily when it is given in an unconcentrated state. Vitamin D is not utilized so efficiently from concentrates as from products in which it is held in a dispersed state. Cod-liver oil long has had extensive usage as a source of vitamin D and has the advantage of containing adequate vitamin D in relatively small bulk, yet in a concentration not great enough to affect utilization adversely. The cod-liver oils available on the market vary in potency from 310 units (U.S.P. minimum standard) to 900 units to the teaspoonful. Thus the required amount of vitamin D may be obtained from one teaspoonful or less of most of the oils. The common practice of giving infants 2 or 3 teaspoonfuls of cod-liver oil daily, regardless of potency, is to be regarded as detrimental, in that the resultant larger intakes of vitamin D cause decreased appetite and lessened food intake when they have been continued for several months.

The chief disadvantage of cod-liver oil is that it may be aspirated into the lungs by extremely weak and prematurely born babies. In the lungs it causes severe pneumonia which frequently is fatal. To such babies it is necessary that oils be given with great caution. Often concentrates are used, but it would seem preferable to disperse the vitamin D in the milk formula. Milk fortified with vitamin D is available in most large communities, or it may be prepared for the special needs of an infant by adding to the formula vitamin D which has been dissolved in a dispersible medium. Several such products are available. Most evaporated milk is fortified.

VITAMIN E

Vitamin E (tocopherol) deficiency in animal experimentation leads to sterility in both sexes, and when females have received only minimum amounts their young have muscular dysfunction similar to muscular dystrophy of the human. It is believed that vitamin E may be necessary for muscle development. Satisfactory evidence of deficiency in the human has not been presented. Vitamin E has a distribution so wide that any mixed diet contains an abundance. It is present in foods of animal origin—less abundant in those tissues rich in vitamin A, more abundant in muscle. It is present in green vegetables and vegetable oils, and it is particularly abundant in wheat germ oil. It is relatively stable, though it may be destroyed under conditions which produce rancidity.

VITAMIN K

Vitamin K as found naturally in food is a fat-soluble material, chemically a naphthoquinone which has been given the name *menadione*. Other and synthetic derivatives of naphthoquinone have vitamin-K activity, and some are water-soluble. Vitamin K is found in many foods and also is synthesized in the intestinal tract by fecal bacteria. Deficiencies occur in the newborn infant

before abundant implantation of bacteria in the intestine and at any age when absorption is impaired by absence of bile. Vitamin K is necessary for the formation of prothrombin, a material essential for blood coagulation. Deficiency leads to a tendency to bleed, a condition discussed under Hemorrhagic Disease of the Newborn.

VITAMIN B COMPLEX

Vitamin B complex includes thiamine (B_1), riboflavin (B_2 or G), niacin (nicotinic acid) and many other components. These substances are found in the same foods, though the proportion of each to the others varies in different foods. Deficiency of only one B vitamin is rare, but often one may be more deficient than others. Thiamine, riboflavin and niacin, and probably other members of the complex, are components of enzymes necessary for cell respiration.

Thiamine. Thiamine deficiency, when severe, causes beriberi. Deficiency of lesser degree may cause certain varities of neuritis and neurosis (see Beriberi). Thiamine is necessary for normal appetite and gastro-intestinal function and for successful lactation. Impairment of growth may result from poor appetite. Thiamine has been synthesized on a commercial scale and is available abundantly in crystalline form. In nature it is found in important amounts in whole-grain cereals, peanuts, yeast and lean meat, especially pork and liver. It is found in smaller amounts in many foods, including milk, eggs, vegetables and fruits. It has been added in small amounts to enriched flour and bread. Despite its fairly wide distribution, it is the

B component most likely to be deficient in the average diet. It is easily destroyed by heat, the usual cooking processes resulting in an average loss of 25 per cent or more. It is water-soluble and often is discarded with the water of cooking. Thiamine is necessary for the combustion of carbohydrate, and the requirement is proportional to the nonfat calories of the diet. Recommended allowances vary from 0.4 mg. in the first year to 1.5 mg. at 15 years for average diets, or 0.05 mg. for each 100 calories of the diet.

Riboflavin. Riboflavin deficiency in the human, when severe and chronic, produces characteristic changes in the eyes and about the mouth. The eye changes show first in the conjunctiva about the cornea, where small blood vessels become enlarged and visible. These changes are associated with photophobia, lacrimation, burning sensation and dimness of vision known as twilight blindness. Subsequently, interstitial keratitis may develop. In the mouth, the tongue becomes inflamed, and inflammatory fissures and maceration appear in the skin and the mucous membrane at the corners of the mouth (cheilitis). More severe effects have been observed in experiments on animals. Riboflavin is necessary for growth, and probably also for successful lactation. Riboflavin is a yellow pigment, stable to the heat of cooking but destroyed by exposure to light. The best source in the daily diet is milk. The customary milk formula supplies the requirement of the infant, and a quart of milk supplies most, if not all, of the requirement of the child.

Riboflavin is present in important amounts also in liver, egg yolk, meat, whole-grain cereals and green vegetables, but the requirement is not likely to be met from these sources without the inclusion of milk in the diet. The appropriate allowance for riboflavin is approximately 50 per cent greater than that for thiamine, namely, 0.6 mg. in the first year, increasing to 2.0 mg. at 15 years.

Niacin (Nicotinic Acid). Niacin deficiency causes pellagra. This vitamin exists commercially both as the acid and as its amide. No common food is a rich source of this material, but liver, lean meat, eggs, whole-grain cereals, enriched bread, wheat germ and yeast have it in important amounts. The amount in milk is small, both human and cow's, approximately 1 mg. to the liter. However, it is well established that the dietary requirement for niacin decreases when milk is contained in the diet, presumably because of bacterial synthesis in the intestine. The appropriate allowance of niacin is 10 times that of thiamine in all age groups. The material is stable to usual food handling.

Other B-Complex Factors. Other B-complex factors exist which are known to be essential for experimental animals and are presumably important in human nutrition. Folic acid under ordinary circumstances is produced in the intestine by the bacteria that dwell therein. After heavy antibiotic therapy this source of supply may be cut off because the bacteria are destroyed. Folic acid normally requires an adequate amount of vitamin C to convert it into folinic acid (citrovorum factor) which in turn is essential in the formation of nucleic acids. Disturbance of this complicated chain of chemical events may result in megaloblastic anemia because of inadequate formation of red blood cell protein. Pyridoxine (B_6) is also essential in human metabolism but can be lacking from the average diet only under very special circumstances. A few instances of convulsions in infants have been traced to its destruction during the preparation of commercial canned milk formulas. The remaining members of the B-complex are choline, biotin, inositol and pantothenic acid. Their essentiality in human nutrition has not been proved. The incompleteness of our knowledge about the details of vitamin requirements emphasizes the wisdom of depending upon a mixed diet for nutritional essentials rather than on special preparations of the known vitamins.

ASCORBIC ACID (VITAMIN C)

Ascorbic-acid deficiency causes scurvy. Vitamin C probably is necessary for all living cells. It is found most abundantly in actively growing cells. The effects of deficiency are most apparent in bones, teeth and small blood vessels. Capillary hemorrhages are characteristic of severe deficiency, the hemorrhages presumably being caused by defective growth of connective tissue supporting structure about the capillaries and loss of cement substance between the cells of capillary walls. Ascorbic acid is essential for growth of connective tissue and consequently for normal wound healing. Ascorbic acid is destroyed easily by oxidation in neutral or alkaline media, less easily in an acid medium. Destruction is hastened by heat, and cooking often destroys a high proportion. In view of these facts, the importance of fresh foods in the diet becomes apparent. Ascorbic acid is present in many fruits and vegetables. The citrus fruits are relatively rich sources. The juice of ripe oranges may be considered to contain an average of 50 mg. of ascorbic acid to 100 cc. Canned frozen orange juice retains nearly all of this vitamin C activity but should be used soon after thawing and diluting. Tomato juice, fresh or canned, is a good source of vitamin C, although it has a content smaller and more variable than orange juice. The vitamin C content varies with the soil and the region in which the tomatoes are grown. It varies with the amount of sunshine during the ripening stage. Some tomato juices contain approximately 25 mg. of ascorbic acid to 100 cc., while other samples contain only half as much. When the poorer varieties are used, the volume required to meet the needs of an infant are excessive. Fresh cow's milk contains approximately 20 mg. to the quart, pasteurized milk about one third less. Reconstituted dried milk contains 12 mg., and reconstituted evaporated milk 6 mg. to the quart. The amount in human milk depends on the diet of the mother. With a good intake of vitamin C the milk may contain as much as 75 mg. to the quart. However, average human milk contains much less, possibly from 40 to 50 mg. to the quart. The requirement of the young infant may be considered to be 20 mg. daily. Such an amount cannot be received by the artificially fed baby without supplementing the milk formula. At birth the amount of ascorbic acid in the blood is proportionately greater than that in the mother's blood. The amount decreases rapidly and by the tenth day in artificially fed babies it reaches a level that would lead to scurvy if allowed to persist. Thus vitamin C supplements should be given to artificially fed babies much earlier than is customary. The recommended allowance for ascorbic acid increases with size or age from about 30 mg. in the first year to 80 mg. at 15 years.

MULTIPLE VITAMIN PREPARATIONS

A great many preparations are now marketed for the purpose of ensuring protection against deficiency of any of the known vitamins. For infants such preparations are prepared as drops that may be squirted into the mouth or admixed with formula; for older children they take the form of capsules or palatable liquids to be given by spoon. The virtue of the daily administration of such preparations has been grossly overstated by the advertising campaigns of the manufacturers, and it is undoubtedly true that many children take quantities that are superfluous, particularly when they are receiving adequate well-mixed diets. If carried to extremes the lavish use of some of the vitamins may result in toxic reactions. It is doubtful if any but economic harm results from the practice of giving 2 or 3 times the calculated daily requirement.

SITUATIONS FOR FURTHER STUDY

1. What food factors are essential in the diet of an infant?

2. What is the protein requirement of the infant? What is the protein requirement of the child?

3. How does the water requirement of the infant for each kilogram of body weight compare with the requirement of the adult? Why is there a difference in the need?

4. How many cubic centimeters of water would a child of 5 years require daily on the third day after appendectomy? What methods could you use to encourage fluid intake?

5. At what age should orange juice be added to an infant's diet? By what method should it be given? How much should an infant be ingesting by the end of the fourth month?

6. When should cod-liver oil be added to an infant's diet? How much should he be receiving by the end of the third month of life? What group of infants usually are given an increased amount of vitamin D? What other products contain vitamin D? Are concentrates of vitamin D superior to cod-liver oil? How do they differ in cost?

BIBLIOGRAPHY

Meyer, H. F.: Essentials of Infant Feeding for Physicians, Springfield, Ill., Thomas, 1952.

Lanman, J. T.: Modern Trends in Infant Nutrition and Feeding, Scientific Report Series No. 14, New York, Sugar Research Foundation, 1952.

CHAPTER TWENTY-ONE

Nutrition of the Normal Infant— Digestion

DIGESTION IN INFANCY

DIGESTIVE EQUIPMENT

The digestive equipment of the infant is adequate for its task, but only when the food is appropriately chosen, prepared and administered. The expected rate of growth of the infant is far in excess of that which occurs at any later time. Consequently, in proportion to his size, an infant requires several times as much food as does an adult. Because of the immaturity of the digestive functions, the infant's food must differ from that of the older person in quality as well as relative quantity. Even with the simple diet that babies customarily receive, the amount of food necessary approaches closely the digestive capacity. Digestive capacity is decreased by illness, particularly by certain common infections, with the result that digestive disturbances are much more common in infancy than at any other age period. Such disturbances, when they occur, are more serious for the infant than for the older person. By them he is deprived of much or all of his food through vomiting, diarrhea and food refusal. When deprived of food, the infant uses his body stores at a much greater rate than an older person, and serious consequences are more quickly evident. In order to prevent or to manage the digestive and nutritional disturbances of infancy, more detailed knowledge and attention are required than for feeding older children or adults.

SALIVARY DIGESTION

Salivary digestion is concerned only with the digestion of starch. Even when starch is fed as part of a young infant's diet, the extent to which it is digested by saliva is small. Whatever importance salivary digestion may have is attained at a later age.

GASTRIC DIGESTION

The important factors in gastric digestion are hydrochloric acid and the two enzymes pepsin and rennin. The pepsin enzyme acts on protein, breaking it down to simpler products, which are further digested later by other enzymes in the intestine. No digestion of sugar or starch occurs in the stomach and little if any of fat. Hydrochloric acid serves several useful purposes. When in sufficient concentration, it inhibits bacterial growth, activates the pepsin enzyme and to some extent influences the pyloric reflexes. The amount of acid present at birth is small, but it increases progressively. It is decreased by any illness and by severe malnutrition. When human milk is fed, the gastric acidity finally reached is optimum for peptic digestion. Although cow's milk is neither acid nor alkaline, it has the property of binding small amounts of acid without changing its reaction. To bring about the same degree of acidity it is necessary to add 3 times as much acid to cow's milk as to human milk. Modifications of cow's milk which have proved more or less uniformly successful in infant feeding have the common property requiring relatively small amounts of acid to bring the acidity to a point optimum for peptic digestion. They also have in common the production of a fine curd in the stomach.

Soon after the ingestion of milk the casein is precipitated by the en-

zyme rennin. Because of the small amount of casein in human milk, the precipitate is divided finely. Unmodified cow's milk, because of the larger amount of casein, gives rise to a large rubbery curd which may resist complete breaking up, and parts of it may be passed eventually in the stool as tough lima-beanlike masses. Cow's milk which has been boiled or has been subjected to heat incident to evaporation or drying gives rise to a curd resembling that of human milk, although usually somewhat coarser. When cow's milk is fed to an infant, less difficulty is encountered if the milk has been heat-treated than if it has not been modified in any way. Milk to which acid has been added in such a manner and quantity as to make a fine curd is better tolerated than either plain-boiled or raw milk. The fineness of the curd undoubtedly contributes to the ease of digestion, and it is probable that this factor is of greater importance than the degree of acidity reached in gastric digestion.

Practically no absorption takes place from the stomach. The stomach may be expected to be empty in from 2 to 3 hours when human milk is fed, and in from 2½ to 3½ hours with customary modifications of cow's milk. Emptying of the stomach is delayed by a high proportion of fat in the food and by illness of the infant.

DIGESTION IN DUODENUM AND SMALL INTESTINE

Although much has been said in the preceding discussion concerning gastric digestion, it is in the duodenum and the small intestine that the greater part of digestion is accomplished. Protein that escapes gastric digestion is acted on by the pancreatic secretion, and the resultant products are further broken down into amino acids by an enzyme secreted by the mucous membrane of the intestine. The amino acids are absorbed and either converted to body protein or burned. Fats are changed into soaps and glycerin by pancreatic secretion and bile. These are absorbed from the small intestine to be reconstructed into body fat or burned. Another enzyme of the pancreatic secretion converts starch into sugar. Complex sugars are changed to monosaccharides (dextrose, levulose and galactose) by the secretions of the small intestine before absorption. The ability to digest starch is relatively feeble at birth, but it increases rapidly. If starch is fed in the very early months of life, a large proportion of it is likely to pass through the intestinal tract unchanged. Usually this does no harm and only occasionally are fermentative processes set up. Ability to digest starch is usually adequate by 6 months of age, earlier if starch has been fed.

Chief Function of Large Intestine

The chief function of the large intestine is to absorb water. Though it is capable of absorbing amino acids, salts and simple sugars, it is seldom called on for this purpose. Before reaching the large intestine, practically all the protein and its products will have been digested and absorbed. Sugars reaching the large intestine are fermented quickly by the bacteria present in enormous number. Some soaps remaining from fat digestion pass into the colon, though little or no digestion or absorption takes place.

The period required for food to pass through the gastro-intestinal tract varies from 8 to 36 hours, depending largely on the degree to which different food substances stimulate peristalsis.

Bacteria are not present in the intestinal tract at birth, but gain entrance soon thereafter. They are not present in important numbers until food is given. In the presence of food they multiply greatly. The prevailing type of bacteria present depends on the type of food that the baby receives. With human-milk feeding the bacteria are predominantly gram-positive; with customary formulas of cow's milk they are gram-negative. That one of these two types is more beneficial to the baby than the other has not been shown. The gram-positive types are associated with the slightly acid stools of low protein-high sugar feeding; the gram-negative types with the alkaline stools of relatively high protein feeding. Certain bacteria which grow in an alkaline medium are the cause of ammoniacal excoriations of the skin of the diaper region, a condition which may occur in an otherwise normal baby; it is discussed under Ammonia Dermatitis. Only under abnormal conditions do acid excoriations of the buttocks occur. Their cause is discussed under Diarrhea. Bacteria are unevenly distributed in the intestinal tract. Under normal conditions few are found in the stomach, the duodenum and the upper jejunum. The number increases progressively down the tract, the greatest number being in the colon. Their abnormal presence in the duodenum is discussed under Diarrhea.

STOOLS

MECONIUM

Meconium is the term applied to the first stools passed after birth. Meconium consists of partially dried intestinal secretions which have gradually accumulated in the lower tract. It is dark brownish-green in color, semiformed, and is usually passed from 4 to 6 times daily. The stools continue so until food is ingested. About the third day, with the ingestion of food the stools begin to change, and by the fourth or the fifth day they have assumed the characteristics that persist for the subsequent months.

CHARACTER OF STOOLS

The character of the stools is determined by the type of food. Normal stools of infants fed milk are composed of approximately 20 per cent solids, chiefly soaps, and 80 per cent water.

Human Milk. When human milk is fed, the stools may be passed only once or twice a day or may occur after every feeding. Characteristically, such stools are unformed but not watery; the color is bright or golden yellow or occasionally light green; the odor is unobjectionably aromatic; the reaction is acid. After the initial adjustment to breast feeding, some infants will have soft stools that are passed very infrequently, e.g., only every third or fourth day.

Cow's Milk. When cow's milk is fed in customary formulas, the stools are firmer than those from human milk and are passed less frequently, usually from 1 to 3 times daily. Although yellow, they seldom have the bright yellow color of the stool from human milk. The reaction is neutral or slightly alkaline, and the odor is more or less foul. The differences between the stools from human and from cow's milk are due to the differences in the composition of the food. A high-sugar, low-protein diet (human milk) tends to cause more frequent stools, which are acid in reaction. A low-sugar, high-protein diet tends to cause the reverse condition.

COLOR OF STOOL

The color of stools when milk is the principal food is influenced chiefly by the rate at which the food passes through the intestinal tract. A diarrheal stool usually is green; a soft stool, yellowish; and a firm pasty stool, light yellow or almost white. These variations are due to the fact that the bile pigment in the upper intestine is green, but after it has remained for some time in the intestinal tract chemical action occurs which changes the green to yellow, and after further stay in the tract the yellow pigment is changed to a colorless pigment. When diarrhea occurs, the green bile coloring passes through the intestine so rapidly that it is not changed. A yellow stool, if exposed to the air for some time, often turns green on the surface, due to a process of oxidation. This change of color is of no significance. The feeding of cereals, malt preparations or skimmed milk may lead to stools which are less yellow or even of brownish color. Certain drugs, such as bismuth and iron, may color

the stools black. With atresia of the bile-ducts the stools are gray or clay-colored because of the absence of bile (acholic stools). (See Plate 3.)

MUCUS, PUS AND BLOOD

A slight amount of glairy mucus may be seen normally in the stools, especially those from breast-fed infants. A larger amount of mucus in the stools of either breast-fed or artificially fed babies is an indication of irritation of the intestinal tract, and is often seen when diarrhea is present. Pus does not normally occur in stools. When it is found, it indicates an inflammation of the intestinal wall (ileocolitis or dysentery). When severe inflammation of the wall of the intestine occurs, blood as well as pus may appear in the stools. The blood may be bright, or, if its source is higher in the intestine, it may be altered to a brownish or black color. It is mixed in streaks in the stool, or the whole stool may be bloody. Bloody stools also occur in association with intussusception. Small streaks of blood occurring on the outside of constipated stools usually mean nothing more than a slight crack or fissure at the anus.

CURDS

Curds occurring in stools are of three varieties: soap, casein and mucus.

Soap curds are most frequent. They are small and soft and are easily mashed with a spatula. They occur normally in the stools of breast-fed infants and are seen also in loose stools of artificially fed babies. The presence of soap curds indicates that peristalsis has been rapid, and that there has not been sufficient time for the absorption of

water and the compression of curds into firmer masses. The occurrence of soap curds does not necessarily indicate that too much fat is being fed. They occur in the stools no matter what causes the increased looseness.

Casein curds are seen in the stools only of infants fed raw or pasteurized cow's milk. They are hard, tough, usually yellowish, and about the size and shape of a small lima bean.

Mucus in the stool in excess may become dry and rolled up in the form of small balls or stringy curds. Parents sometimes mistake the mucous strings for intestinal worms.

SITUATIONS FOR FURTHER STUDY

1. Describe diarrheal and meconium stools, as well as those of the breast-fed infant. What influences the color of the stools?

2. Why does an infant with atresia of the bile ducts pass an acholic stool?

3. Describe a stool passed by an infant with intussusception. What gives it its characteristic appearance?

4. How would incomplete absorption of fat influence the appearance of the stool? Would there be any difference between the stool of an infant with cystic fibrosis of the pancreas and that of an infant with celiac disease? What differences in digestion are there in these two conditions?

5. How would dysfunction of the pancreas influence digestion?

6. What type of stool does the infant with pyloric stenosis have before operation? After operation, how will his stools change in appearance? What produces the change?

CHAPTER TWENTY-TWO

Nutrition of the Infant—Breast Feeding

GENERAL DISCUSSION

Human milk remains the ideal food for the young infant despite all advances in the knowledge of artificial feeding. Infants fed human milk have fewer illnesses and have better chances of survival than those artificially fed. When well supervised, artificial feeding has a high degree of success, but breast feeding is likely to be successful with little or no supervision. Human milk contains no harmful bacteria, whereas cow's milk must be guarded carefully in this respect. Human milk requires no modification. It contains all the nutritional essentials in adequate, even though minimum, amounts, with the exception of vitamin D and iron. However, additional iron is not needed by the baby in the first 2 or 3 months, and sunshine can void the need for vitamin D.

Unfortunately, mother's milk is not adequate in all instances. Dairymen realize that the health and the food of the cow influence the quality and the quantity of the milk, and these same factors influence the milk of the human mother. Mothers cannot secrete into their milk vitamins which they do not ingest in sufficient amount. Mothers in poor health or with nutritional deficiencies cannot be expected to secrete either an abundance of milk or a milk of good quality. Appropriate attention to the health and the diet of the mother is conducive to and often essential for successful breast feeding.

The mother's conscious and subconscious attitudes toward breast feeding have a very important bearing upon her ability to produce milk. Several trends in modern American culture contribute subtle influences which are making it more difficult for women to accept and enjoy the process of natural feeding. Factors such as advanced education, professional training, out-of-the-home employment and the hectic, highly organized pace of life in our large cities frequently interfere with the mother's ability to relax and they make her impatient over the inefficiencies and the uncertainties of breast feeding. Delivery of milk to the infant will be impeded by maternal worry over the adequacy of her supply or by the necessity for haste in the completion of the feeding so that she can get on to something else. In addition, some women have a distinct aversion to nursing which is rooted in unwholesome or prudish attitudes toward sex and the maternal role. These attitudes are the product of their own upbringing; they are not easily modified but generally must be accepted as valid reasons for giving up breast feeding after a preliminary exploration.

CONTRAINDICATIONS TO BREAST FEEDING

Few absolute contraindications to breast feeding exist.

TUBERCULOSIS

If the mother has active open tuberculosis, not only should the baby be kept from the breast, but also he should be isolated from the mother completely because of the communicability of the infection. If the mother's tuberculosis is not transmissible (closed) but active, breast feeding causes undesirable strain. If the disease is latent or presumably healed, no contraindication exists. Tuberculosis is not transmitted by way of the milk.

CHRONIC DISEASE

A mother who is ill from a serious chronic disease which keeps her in poor physical condition should not be subjected to the strain of breast feeding. The milk in such cases is likely to be of poor quality. Psychosis, frequent convulsions or uncontrolled insulin reactions may prevent breast feeding because of potential danger to the infant.

ACUTE ILLNESSES AND SURGICAL OPERATIONS

Severe acute illnesses on the part of the mother and major surgical operations constitute valid reasons for temporary weaning. During the period of temporary weaning, effort should be made to maintain the milk secretion by periodic emptying of the breasts.

Menstruation, should it occur during lactation, is not an indication for weaning, even though during the first day or two the baby may be somewhat disturbed. The occurrence of pregnancy is not an indication for sudden weaning. Although weaning is desirable because of the strain on the mother, it should be accomplished gradually. Medication of the mother is not usually a contraindication to breast feeding. It is probable that no commonly used drug given mothers in customary amounts would be secreted in the milk in sufficient quantity to affect the infant deleteriously.

Syphilis in either the mother or the baby is not an indication for weaning, except for the rare occurrence of acquisition of the infection by the mother so late in pregnancy that the infant is not infected. Breast feeding is especially important for the syphilitic infant.

MASTITIS

In the event of the mother's developing mastitis, use of the affected breast should be discontinued. If both breasts become inflamed, complete weaning is necessary. Lesser degrees of nipple disorders require management, as discussed later in this chapter. Inverted, cracked, fissured or painful nipples often can be restored to service by proper attention. A mother who has an unmistakable aversion to breast feeding should not be forced to continue.

CLEFT LIP AND PALATE

An infant with cleft lip and palate is usually unable to suckle at the breast. If the deformity involves the lip only and can be repaired early, it is possible to feed the baby satisfactorily at the breast, provided that the milk supply has been maintained.

PREMATURITY

Prematurely born infants or those very small and weak at birth may be physically unable to obtain sufficient food from the breast. In such cases, an attempt should be made to maintain the mother's milk supply by periodic emptying of the breasts mechanically.

HYGIENE AND DIET OF THE MOTHER

If a mother is to supply sufficient milk, it is desirable that she remain in good physical condition and be free from worry. She should have plenty of sleep. Exercise in the open air is desirable, but it should stop short of fatigue. The greatest stimulus to milk supply is frequent, periodic and complete emptying of the breasts. If the breasts are allowed to fill tightly (to "cake") and remain so, the secretion will diminish and eventually cease. Even after almost complete disappearance of milk because of weaning, the secretion can be stimulated again by periodic emptying of the breasts.

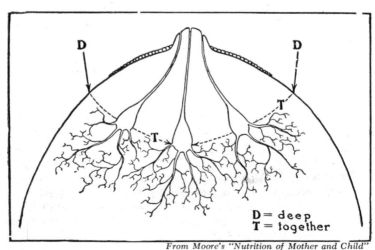

From Moore's "Nutrition of Mother and Child"

FIG. 79. Schematic representation of the breast.

EMPTYING THE BREAST

For one who has mastered the technic, the most effective method of emptying the breast is by manual expression. The principle of this method is indicated in Figures 79 and 80. The thumb and the finger are placed on the opposite sides of and about 1 inch from the nipple; then while in this position they are pressed deeply into the breast. Then the thumb and the finger are brought toward each other with sufficient pressure to empty the underlying milk sacs. Sometimes better success is attained when the bringing together of the thumb and the finger is followed by a forward motion. This series of motions is repeated with a frequency found most efficient in the individual case. There should be no movement of the fingers on the skin; the skin and the fingers should move together. The milk should flow from the nipple in streams, not drops, during the period of pressure.

Breast Pump. The cheapest, simplest and most commonly used type of breast pump is that shown in Figure 81. A negative pressure is obtained by applying the pump with the bulb compressed and then allowing the bulb to expand. The nipple and the areola are drawn into the conical glass with resultant compression of the milk sacs and a consequent flow of milk. The negative pressure must be released by pressure on the bulb to allow the milk sacs to refill and then be reapplied. This process is repeated over and over until the breast is empty. This method is slow and not highly efficient. A similar but more efficient method uses this same principle of intermittent negative pressure, but the suction is produced by an electrically operated machine pump (Fig. 82). Also, suction may be ob-

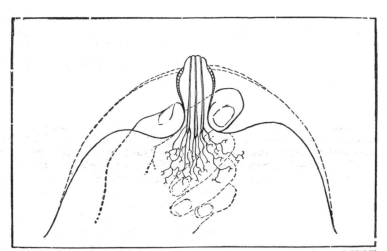

From Moore's "Nutrition of Mother and Child"

FIG. 80. Schematic representation of the manual expression of milk from the breast.

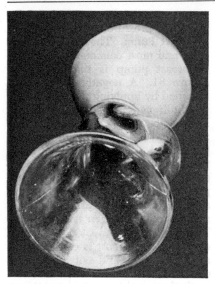

Fig. 81. The common type of breast pump.

tained conveniently by the use of the common laboratory water pump, the continuous suction being made intermittent by finger control on a rubber tube used as a third outlet of the milk bottle.

Diet

The diet of the lactating mother need differ qualitatively in no way from that which is suitable for her at other times. No food will have an ill effect on the milk if it does not cause a disturbance in the mother. For example, the prejudice against "acid" foods is unfounded.

A mother who is secreting from a pint to a quart of milk daily, with an energy value of from 400 to 700 calories and with the accompanying protein, minerals and vitamins, must eat at least that many more calories than her customary allowance in order to supply a good quality of milk

without depleting her own body supplies. Some mothers who are ingesting a restricted diet and secreting little milk secrete more when the diet is improved. Too often the diet is incomplete irrespective of lactation, and during this period it is especially important that all the essential food materials be included in adequate quantities. Although the milk may contain calcium from the body stores (bones) it cannot contain vitamins unless they are ingested regularly by the mother. Allowances recommended for the mother during lactation are as follows: 3,000 calories, 100 Gm. of protein, 2 Gm. of calcium, 8,000 units of vitamin A, 1.5 mg. of thiamine, 150 mg. of ascorbic acid, 3 mg. of riboflavin, 15 mg. of niacin and 400 units of vitamin D. In order to obtain these amounts of nutrients, it is necessary to include in the diet at least 1 quart of milk, preferably more. The daily diet also should contain 1 or 2 eggs, 1 serving of meat and an abundance of fruits and vegetables.

PROPERTIES OF HUMAN MILK

The milk that is secreted during the first few days after the birth of the baby is small in amount and differs much from that secreted after lactation is established. This early milk is known as colostrum. It is of a lemon-yellow color and consequently looks "rich" as compared with later milk. It has a relatively high protein content, and much of the protein consists of globulin. The globulin is considered to have a biologic and immunologic importance for the infant.

On about the third or the fourth day the amount of secretion increases greatly. The breasts become distended and often tender. A gradual transition takes place in the appearance and the composition of the milk. Most of the transition occurs within a week or two, and by the end of the first month it has been completed. After lactation is established, the milk contains approximately from 3.5 to 4 per cent fat, 7.5 per cent sugar, 1.25 per cent protein and 0.2 per cent mineral salts. It has an energy value of 20 calories to the ounce. The composition remains practically constant throughout the period of lactation. At any one withdrawal the first milk that comes from the breast is low in fat, and the last milk relatively rich in fat. Thus any sample taken for analysis should be an entire breast content. Milk analysis usually gives little information of value in determining the difficulty when a breast-fed baby is not thriving. The differences between human and cow's milk are discussed elsewhere.

TECHNIC OF BREAST FEEDING

The time at which a newborn infant is first placed at the breast varies in different hospitals. In some the babies are put to breast as soon as the mother and the baby indicate a readiness to be together; in others,

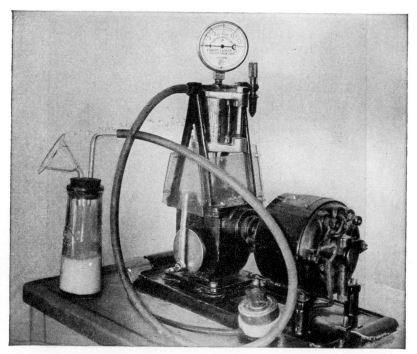

Fig. 82. An electrically operated machine breast pump, using the principle of intermittent negative pressure.

babies are not put to breast until 6 to 12 hours after birth. During the first few days, the infant gets very little from the breast. To supply fluids and a few calories, 5-per-cent sugar solution is offered approximately every 3 or 4 hours.

The object of placing the baby at the breast is to stimulate the flow of milk and to establish a mutually enjoyed experience for the mother and the baby. For this reason, it is important that the mother be prepared for the experience, that the baby be awake and ready to participate in finding his source of supply of milk and that the nurse remain to help make feeding time a pleasant and comfortable experience for both of them (Fig. 83).

SCHEDULE

Regularity in following a feeding schedule seems to be necessary in some nurseries for the newborn. In others, more flexibility exists, and the babies are taken to their mothers whenever they show a need for closeness or food. At home or under the rooming-in type of hospital care, the feeding schedules can be governed by the infant's spontaneous demands for food. By observing the infant, his own regularity in the need for food will become apparent. As he grows and matures his shifting

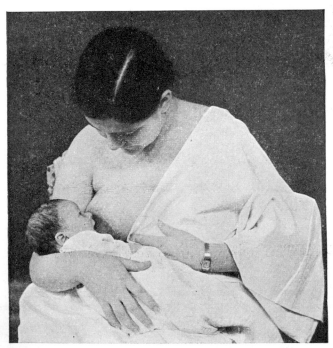

FIG. 83. A suitable position of a baby at the breast. The head is supported, and the nose is free from the breast.

requirements will be signaled promptly to his mother. It is possible to plan a schedule which maintains flexibility in accordance with the individual infant's demands without interfering with the mother's plan of work or freedom to carry on desired activities.

Establishing irregular eating habits or "spoiling" the baby does not result when a schedule has evolved from observation of his needs; rather, it aids in prevention of poor food habits and anxiety by supplying food when he really feels a need for it. When an infant is allowed to cry with hunger because the clock does not indicate the time for feeding, he becomes emotionally overwrought. When food finally is given, he relaxes and falls asleep from fatigue without his nutritional needs being satisfied or he eats so hastily that digestion becomes impaired.

Many infants handled in this fashion will select schedules that closely follow the traditional 4-hour intervals. Some of the smaller ones or those who are tense or insecure or are attempting to make rapid increments in size may require feedings at 3-hour or even 2-hour intervals for a time. During the first week of life a period of constant demand for food is quite common. In most instances, once the mother recovers from her own excitement and begins to understand her infant's needs, a regular feeding pattern emerges. The intervals between nursing periods may not be exactly equal—often there is a relatively brief period of satisfaction in the late afternoon and the early evening. During the 24-hour period, few infants will require less than 5 feedings; most of them desire 6, 7 or 8. In some cases even more frequent feeding is desirable for brief periods. When the latter behavior persists over protracted periods it may be necessary to enquire into the adequacy of the mother's milk supply.

To substitute one bottle feeding for a breast feeding each 24 hours is frequently of great advantage. Such a plan serves several useful purposes. It allows the mother greater freedom, without which in certain cases she would find nursing too great an obstacle to her social routine. It also keeps the infant accustomed to the bottle, so that if weaning suddenly should become necessary or when the normal time comes for weaning, the infant will accept the new method of feeding without serious objection.

In most instances, the supply of milk is abundant enough so that the infant may obtain sufficient from a single breast, and it is desirable to offer alternate breasts, one at one nursing and the other at the next. By satisfying the infant at one breast, that breast is emptied more thoroughly and the production of milk is encouraged. Often when both breasts are given at a single nursing the infant is much overfed, and the result is intestinal disturbance and discomfort, unless the feeding interval is long. In some instances when a 4-hour schedule is selected, the baby may be put to both breasts in order to get sufficient milk. When this is done, the breasts should be alternated in being offered first.

LENGTH OF TIME AT BREAST

The average time for an infant to remain at the breast is about 15 minutes. The time depends on the sucking need and strength of the infant, the amount of milk available and whether the breasts are difficult to empty. Some infants will obtain sufficient and be satisfied in 10 minutes or less. When there is little milk, in a very few minutes the infant may give up the attempt to obtain it. The only method of deter-mining with certainty whether the infant has obtained a sufficient amount is to weigh him before and after feedings. In general it is un-wise to recommend this procedure to the mother, for the information obtained may be inaccurate and it is more likely to stimulate anxiety than to reassure. The flow of milk is much more rapid at the beginning

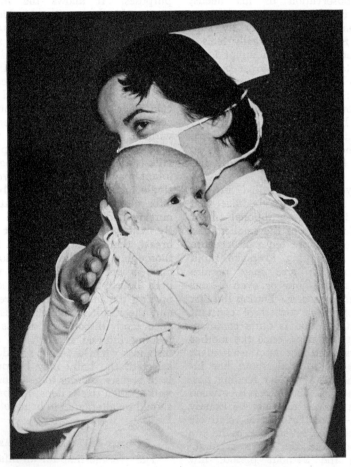

Fig. 84. Holding an infant for "bubbling."

of a feeding than later; about half or more of the total quantity is taken by the infant in the first 5 minutes, more than a quarter during the next 5 minutes, and very little after this time. Many infants who remain at the breast for long periods swallow air in considerable amounts and this may lead to vomiting, colic and fretfulness.

Every infant swallows some air during feeding, and for this reason it should be the custom to hold an infant upright and pat him on the back until the air is belched (Fig. 84). The infant always should be so held after each feeding and many infants before feeding as well. Occasionally, for young infants it is desirable to allow opportunity for eructation during the course of the feeding.

CARE OF THE MOTHER'S NIPPLES

It is desirable to pay attention to the mother's nipples and also to the baby's mouth. Both should be clean and healthy at the time of nursing in order that neither may affect the other. Mouth washing as it often is carried out in infants is likely to do more harm than good because of the trauma associated with the process.

FISSURING OF NIPPLES

The most common and serious difficulty with the mother's breasts is fissuring of the nipples. This condition is analogous to chapping of the hands in its cause, symptoms and treatment. It occurs most frequently in the early days of lactation. The cause is frequent or fairly constant wetting, with production of maceration and depletion of the natural

oils that protect the skin. The cracks in the skin are painful, especially when the skin is manipulated by the suckling of the baby. Often the pain is such that breast feeding cannot be endured. The cracks in the skin may serve as a portal of entry for pyogenic bacteria, with mastitis or breast abscess as a result. The occurrence of mastitis or abscess makes feeding at the involved breast not only inadvisable but impossible.

PREVENTION OF FISSURING

For the prevention of fissuring of the nipples it is important to keep the nipples dry to the extent possible. Exposure of nipples to the air is a simple and effective means of keeping them dry. It may be desirable also to keep them soft with some simple ointment. If the nipples become tender, the application of alcohol is useful in addition to the other measures. When fissures are present, it is usually desirable to take the baby off the involved breast. The milk can be expressed and fed from a bottle. Only occasionally will feeding through a nipple shield be satisfactory. The healing of the fissures may be hastened by an application of a 1- or 2-per-cent solution of silver nitrate.

RETRACTED NIPPLES

Retracted nipples preferably should receive attention during the later months of pregnancy. Sufficient protrusion usually can be obtained by use of a breast pump or by repeated manual traction.

DIFFICULTIES ENCOUNTERED IN BREAST FEEDING

The difficulties encountered in breast feeding are to be explained chiefly by either overfeeding or underfeeding, and the diagnosis of the difficulty is made largely by the application of common sense.

OVERFEEDING

Overfeeding of breast milk is a rather uncommon source of difficulty. Occasionally a mother may produce so much milk that the infant easily takes more than he can digest properly. Vomiting, distention and restlessness may result. Ordinarily, the milk supply adjusts itself within a few days, and the symptoms subside. All-night feeding with the baby sleeping in the mother's bed should be discouraged because of the risks of overfeeding, mutual disturbance of rest and the danger of the mother's rolling onto the infant during sleep.

UNDERFEEDING

The intensity of the signs and the symptoms of underfeeding depends on the degree of deficiency of the diet. There may be a slow gain, no gain or a loss in weight. The stools may remain yellow, may be varying shades of brown or, with complete starvation, will be dark green. The stools are more commonly infrequent but they may be loose and green, similar to stools of overfeeding. There may or may not be excessive crying and if there is, it is due to hunger rather than to colic. If the underfeeding is marked, there is usually disturbance of sleep. There may be some difficulty in differentiating the colic of overfeeding from the hunger of underfeeding, especially in the presence of loose green stools. Parenteral disease may be the cause of weight loss when the milk supply is normal.

The investigation in a case of suspected underfeeding can begin properly with the determination of the amount of milk received by the infant, and this is accomplished best by weighing the baby before and after feeding. Since the amount of milk obtained at different feedings may vary, it is well to take the average of several feedings or, better, to determine the actual amount taken over a 24-hour period. If the infant has received an inadequate amount of milk, the fault may be with the mother or the baby. The next logical step is to determine how much milk remains in the breast. If little or none can be obtained, then the supply is inadequate. If the supply is adequate, the difficulty may be that the nipples are inverted or small or it may be that the infant is unable to suckle properly. Inverted nipples may be drawn out sufficiently by manipulation or by the suction of a pump. Nipples too small or too much inverted for successful breast feeding seldom are encountered. Feeding the baby by means of a nipple shield may be successful, although there is a tendency for the milk to diminish gradually with this procedure. The infant may be too feeble to suckle. He may suckle for a short time and then fall asleep exhausted. A baby with an occluded nose cannot obtain his food satisfactorily; he will grasp the nipple as if hungry, suckle for a brief time and then cry. Many new mothers do not know how to hold the infant in a comfortable position for feeding, or the breast may be allowed to occlude the infant's nares.

The treatment of these various causes of underfeeding is obvious once the cause is determined. A baby should not be weaned from the breast merely because of insufficient milk but should be given milk from a bottle in addition to that obtained from the breast. Often sufficient milk may be obtained by giving both breasts at each feeding. At the same time, measures which have been mentioned previously—improving the diet of the mother and shortening the feeding interval— should be undertaken to increase the supply of milk. Occasionally, because of such measures the supplementary feedings may be discontinued.

Vomiting associated with the signs of underfeeding in the early weeks of infancy may be caused by pyloric stenosis. Weaning the baby because the "milk disagrees" is a serious error; it is uncommon to find milk which seriously disagrees with the infant. When such is the case, it is most often found that the mother is of the highly strung or nervous type. Such mothers also are likely to have a deficient supply.

INANITION OR DEHYDRATION FEVER

It is appropriate to consider in connection with starvation a condition known as inanition fever. This name is given to a febrile illness occurring in the first 5 days after birth. The temperature usually does not rise above 102° F., and no evidence of local disease is present. The condition is associated with loss in weight, often rapid, and a persistence of the meconium character of the stools. The degree of prostration is directly proportionate to the duration of the illness, and its general nature is that of progressive weakness. In the milder forms, there is much crying and restlessness; in the more severe forms, the infant is limp and apathetic, with perhaps a feeble whine. The condition always is associated with dry or nearly dry breasts and always is relieved within a few hours by the administration of food or even an abundance of fluid. The symptoms are due to dehydration. The treatment is to supply fluid primarily and food secondarily, the effect being rapid disappearance of the fever and prostration and recovery of the lost weight.

MIXED FEEDING

Mixed feeding means that an infant is fed in part at the breast and in part artificially. Such a method of feeding may be used from necessity because of inadequate supply of milk or it may be used as a convenience to the mother in order that she may have liberty for social engagements or be relieved of night nursing. When started early it also gets the infant accustomed to the bottle, so weaning from the breast will be accomplished with fewer difficulties. An older infant who has been fed only at the breast frequently will starve himself seriously rather than take his milk in any other manner than that to which he is accustomed. If the infant is gradually accustomed to the bottle early, the difficulty is avoided.

When artificial feeding is chosen only for the convenience of the mother, usually a bottle feeding is given in place of a single feeding at the breast. When it is employed from necessity, the same plan may be used to a limited extent. However, it is to be remembered that if an infant is fed less than a certain minimum at the breast—usually 5 feedings—the supply of milk tends to decrease. If it becomes necessary to give considerable amounts of supplemental food, the mother's milk supply is conserved best by having the baby feed regularly at the breast and by giving the necessary amounts of supplemental food immediately after each breast feeding.

ADDITIONS TO THE DIET OF THE BREAST-FED INFANT

Certain supplements to the milk diet of the infant are required whether he is fed artificially or at the breast. These supplements are discussed more fully in the chapter on artificial feeding. The only noteworthy difference between the requirements of the breast-fed baby and the one artificially fed is in the need for additional ascorbic acid. When the mother is ingesting appropriate amounts of ascorbic acid, her milk contains a supply of this vitamin adequate for her infant. Although orange juice or other food containing ascorbic acid is unnecessary for the breast-fed infant, the giving of such foods serves a useful purpose. An adequate supply of ascorbic acid is made more certain, and the infant has desirable early experience with variety in the diet. Other food needs of the breast-fed baby are the same as those of the baby who is fed artificially.

WET NURSING

At one time, now many years ago, artificial feeding of infants was so universally unsuccessful that when a mother could not nurse her infant it was essential that the baby be fed at the breast of another mother. Human milk is no longer a necessity. Often it is used by preference in certain situations, for example, for feeding prematurely born babies. Human milk for such purposes is obtained by expression. In maternity wards or hospitals are to be found mothers who have an excess of milk beyond the needs of their babies. Often this excess is collected, sterilized and dried or frozen for preservation.

A few cities have established "breast milk dairies" which serve as distributing centers. Many healthy lactating women are able to supply enough milk for two infants. Such mothers should be selected for their ability to give a good supply of milk. They should be healthy and free from communicable disease. Their own infants should be thriving and thus reflect the quality of the milk. The age of their infants makes little difference, since the qualitative changes in milk during the course of lactation are small and unimportant. Women supplying milk require careful training in methods of collecting the milk.

WEANING

There are many reasons why weaning is indicated during the first year of life. The more important reasons for weaning on account of disease or abnormality in the mother or the infant have been discussed. Even when the mother is well and the baby is thriving, a time comes when breast feeding is no longer advantageous. It is pointed out elsewhere that milk is deficient in certain essentials. When these deficiencies are provided by proper food additions and when total food is ingested, infants may be fed successfully at the breast well into the second year. However, the infant begins to indicate readiness for a change in method of feeding before the end of the first year. In the latter part of the first year, also, the infant's ability to digest foods more complex than milk is increased greatly.

From observation of infants and from practical experience, it seems to be a wise rule that all infants, with certain exceptions to be noted, be weaned from the breast at from 6 to 10 months of age, and that cow's milk be substituted. If the infant must be weaned before 6 months of age, bottle feeding is the usual substitute; if late in the first year, feeding from a cup is to be recommended. Babies accustomed to a formula usually can take undiluted milk at from 6 to 8 months of age. However, if they have not been accustomed to whole milk, a sudden change to undiluted milk may cause a digestive disturbance. In these instances, diluted milk should be presented. When weaning at any age, the formula at first should be weaker than is customary for the age. The dilution need not be continued for more than a few days. Preparation for weaning, signs of readiness for learning news ways of drinking and a method of weaning are discussed in Chapter 3.

If a breast-fed baby comes under observation because of acute illness at an age when normally he should be weaned, weaning usually is not advisable until the infant is well. If the illness is due to food, it is more likely to be caused by improper food other than the milk.

More than at present, summer formerly brought many serious digestive disturbances to babies. With excellent reason, weaning in the summer was avoided, and the second summer was feared. When heat is retained by an infant through mismanagement of his hygiene in regard to bathing, clothing and ventilation, digestion and absorption of food are impaired, and gastro-intestinal disturbances develop. Improper food or food contaminated with bacteria aggravates these disturbances or becomes a primary cause. With the application of our present knowledge of the proper choice and preparation of foods, with present methods of sterilization and refrigeration and with good hygiene, the average infant has no more difficulty if weaned in the summer than at any other time. If circumstances are such that these various conditions are not likely to be satisfactory, weaning may well be deferred.

SITUATIONS FOR FURTHER STUDY

1. If a woman has delivered a prematurely born infant so immature that feeding at the breast is contraindicated, would you encourage her to maintain her breast-milk supply? How would you approach her? What would be your objectives?

2. Observe a normal infant of from 2 to 3 months of age to determine times when he indicates a need for food. How does he express it? How can you differentiate between behavior that indicates hunger and behavior that indicates a need for affection or social stimulation? Keep a chart showing periods when food was demanded. Is the time between periods regular?

3. If when her baby was 6 months of age a mother asked you how to prepare her infant for wean-

ing from the breast, what suggestions would you give her?

4. What are the contraindications to breast feeding?

5. If a newly delivered mother asked you if she should breast feed her baby, what would you do?

6. How can the nurse function to make breast feeding an enjoyable experience for both the infant and the mother? What are your attitudes toward breast feeding? What attitudes toward breast feeding have you encountered in mothers? In fathers?

7. What signs would indicate that a baby is being underfed?

8. How would you proceed to help a mother learn to give her baby orange juice and a vitamin D product?

BIBLIOGRAPHY

Barnes, G. R., Jr., Lethin, A. N., Jr., and Jackson, E. B.: Management of breast feeding, J. A. M. A. **151:** 192, 1953.

Nutrition of the Infant— Artificial Feeding

The successful feeding of infants without milk has been shown to be possible, but in order to maintain nutrition adequately the diet must be arranged by one who has special technical knowledge of the composition of foods and the needs of the infant, and unusual mineral additions must be made. It seems best to consider that milk forms the basis of the infant's diet. When human milk is not available, the milk of some animal must be substituted. Because of its easy commercial availability, the milk of the cow is employed almost universally for this purpose. Occasionally, goat's milk is used. Goat's milk is approximately of the same composition as cow's milk and may be used in the same manner.

COW'S MILK—COMPOSITION AND PROPERTIES

The milk of all cows may be considered to be practically the same except for variations in the fat. Certain breeds of cows, such as Jersey and Guernsey, produce milk with a fat content of from 5 to 6 per cent.

Other breeds, such as Holstein, give milk with from 3 to 3.5 per cent fat. The fat content of milk of other breeds falls between these extremes. The ordinary grade of cow produces milk with approximately 4 per cent fat. The combined milk of a large mixed herd may be expected to contain about 4 per cent fat, and this amount usually is considered as the average fat content of milk. The milk from commercial dairies rarely contains more than 4 per cent fat, especially if the legal requirement is below this amount.

Composition of Cow's Milk

The approximate average composition of cow's milk may be stated as follows: fat, from 3.5 to 4 per cent; sugar, 4.5 per cent; protein, 3.5 per cent; and mineral salts, 0.75 per cent.

Comparison of Human and Cow's Milk

Human milk and cow's milk are similar in many respects. Qualitatively, the constituents are the same, although the proportions are different. The energy value is the same. Despite these similarities, experience has demonstrated that the majority of young infants have digestive difficulties when unmodified cow's milk is fed, thus indicating an essential difference between the two milks. The sugar of both milks is lactose and is qualitatively the same. Certain qualitative differences exist in the fat of the two milks. The fat of cow's milk is not so well tolerated as that of human milk. Fats are glycerides of fatty acids. Cow's milk fat contains a larger proportion of glycerides of the lower fatty acids (e.g., butyric acid). These acids are

more irritating than the higher ones (e.g., oleic acid). The proteins of both milks consist of casein and lactalbumin but in different proportions. Lactalbumin constitutes more than half of the protein of human milk, but only one seventh of that of cow's milk. It seems probable that for the infant this difference in the protein is the most important difference between cow's milk and human milk.

Fresh Milk

Milk constitutes an excellent medium for bacterial growth, and all milk is contaminated even when produced under strict precautions. The cleanest and freshest milk contains from 100 to 1,000 bacteria to each cubic centimeter. By the time the milk has reached the consumer the number has increased usually to from 10,000 to 50,000. When milk is not collected or preserved carefully, the number of bacteria often is several million. Depending on the kind of bacteria, milk so badly contaminated may or may not be sour to the taste and may or may not cause gastro-intestinal disturbance, but such milk should be considered as unfit for use in infant feeding. Market milk often is designated by grades, such as Grade A, B, etc., in accordance with local requirements, which vary greatly. The grading is based on conditions of production and handling from the standpoint of bacterial count, cleanliness and quality.

Pasteurized Milk

Pasteurized milk usually is milk which has been heated to 150° F. and kept at this temperature for 30 minutes. A few dairies employ a "flash" method, using a higher temperature and a short period of heating. Pasteurization destroys practically all bacteria capable of causing disease. Even though milk has been pasteurized, it is essential that it be kept cold and free from subsequent contamination. Because much of the commercially pasteurized milk is contaminated after its heat treatment, it is safer to boil it before feeding it to infants, and this is especially important during hot weather.

CERTIFIED MILK

This milk is produced under the supervision and the control of a commercially disinterested committee or group which grants "certification" when the requirements of the committee are met. It is the product of tuberculin-tested cows known to be healthy and is obtained under strict conditions of cleanliness. It is cooled quickly after milking and is kept cold until delivery. It has a guaranteed low bacterial count and sometimes is fed raw to infants. Such milk is preferable to ordinary raw milk, but serious epidemics have resulted from the feeding of raw milk even though it has been certified. Many certified dairies now pasteurize their milk. Even the best grade of certified milk should be boiled before being fed to infants.

SOFT-CURD MILK

This milk produces an easily friable casein curd on coagulation. A few cows produce milk with a natural soft curd. Such milk has soft-curd properties because it is low in total solids and is no different from ordinary milk diluted with water.

Homogenization gives soft-curd character to milk when the pressure and the temperature employed in the process are appropriate. Many dairies now homogenize at least a portion of their milk. The commonly used process consists of pumping the milk past a tightly fitting valve at a pressure of 2,500 or more pounds to the square inch. Homogenized milk has the further property of maintaining an even distribution of the milk fat throughout the milk. Milk that produces a soft curd in the stomach leaves the stomach more quickly and is digested more readily than ordinary milk.

VITAMIN-D MILK

This milk contains increased and specified amounts of vitamin D. It may be produced by ultraviolet irradiation of the milk, by feeding irradiated yeast to cows or by the direct addition of vitamin D to milk. Irradiated milk when it was on the market contained either 135 or 400 units of vitamin D to the quart; other varieties contain 400 units to the quart. At present, probably no irradiated milk is produced. The 135-unit variety prevents rickets in infants but does not supply an optimum amount of vitamin D for best nutrition and growth. The 400-unit variety satisfies the need for vitamin D when customary amounts of milk are fed to infants and when children receive the amounts of milk recommended.

EVAPORATED MILK

Evaporated milk is milk which has been concentrated to slightly less than half its original volume, sealed in airtight containers and sterilized.

It may be preserved for long periods but will spoil as does any other milk after the container has been opened. Homogenization and the heat treatment incident to evaporation and sterilization cause the casein to be precipitated in fine curds when acted on by the rennin enzyme. Evaporated milk is a standardized product, regardless of brand. It is prepared from milk with a fat content of 3.8 per cent and when diluted with equal parts of water it contains 4.1 per cent fat. The 1:1 dilution supplies 22 calories to the fluid ounce and is appreciably richer than average fresh milk, a fact often overlooked in infant feeding. It is used successfully and to an increasing extent in infant feeding even when fresh milk is available.

Dried Milk

Dried milk is whole or skimmed milk from which practically all the water has been removed. Milk is dried either by spraying it into a heated low-pressure chamber or by passing it in a thin layer over the heated rollers. That which is prepared by the spray process goes into solution much more easily than that prepared by the roller process. The process of drying is carried out with such a short period of heating that the vitamin content is little affected, and not all bacteria are killed. Pasteurization is customary prior to drying. Both whole dried milk and skimmed dried milk have been used extensively and satisfactorily in infant feeding. A fine curd results when the casein of dried milk is precipitated.

Summary

It may be stated that cow's milk is available in several forms suitable for infant feeding. The acceptable forms are (1) boiled fresh milk, which for the young infant is modified by dilution, acidification or both, (2) evaporated milk, brought back to its original volume, and (3) dried milk. If the dried milk represents whole milk, it may be brought to its original volume and used in the same manner as fresh milk; if it represents skimmed milk, allowance must be made for the decreased energy value. The method of using dried skimmed milk is described subsequently.

Other Forms

Other forms of milk also are available, for example, malted milk and sweetened condensed milk. Both these products have been used for infant feeding in the past, but neither is well suited for routine use for this purpose. Both have high sugar values out of proportion to the amount of milk.

MODIFICATION OF MILK

Boiling

When unmodified raw cow's milk is fed to young infants, a large proportion develop digestive difficulties. One of the major causes of the digestive disturbances is the formation of a large tough curd in the stomach. One of the objects of modification of milk is prevention of such curd formation.

One method of modifying the milk curd is to boil the milk. The boiling of milk accomplishes a double purpose: the milk is made more readily digestible, and most of the bacteria and all the harmful ones are destroyed. From 1 to 2 minutes of active boiling directly over a flame is sufficient.

None of the objections which have been raised to boiling milk for infant feeding has a sound basis, especially when one weighs against the objections the increased safety and digestibility of the milk. The nutritive value is not affected in ways which are not overcome by recommended dietary supplements, and infants are less likely to have gastro-intestinal disturbances. The advantages of boiled milk so greatly outweigh its possible disadvantages that it now has become a custom to boil all cow's milk before feeding to infants.

DILUTION

Another method of preventing the formation of a coarse curd is to dilute the milk. With sufficient dilution the casein, when precipitated, is in a finely divided state. A diluent commonly employed is plain water. Sometimes 3-per-cent cereal (usually barley) water is used. Considering only the formation of a fine curd, barley water possesses certain advantages over plain water in that the colloidal solution of starch aids in preventing agglutination of the casein curd. Most babies can safely ingest starch in excess of their ability to digest it. In a few, distention and colic result. Gelatin water has been suggested as a diluent from time to time. Although gelatin forms a colloidal solution, its effect in reducing curd size is almost negligible when customary dilutions are used. Another diluent more commonly employed in the past than at present is lime water, which, when added to milk in the proportion of 1 to 20, will prevent the formation of a coarse curd. A substance having a similar physical action, though it

cannot be considered as a diluent, is sodium citrate, and the usual addition is 1 grain to each ounce of milk. Each of these various additions has its advocates, but probably the most universally employed diluent for the feeding of young infants is water.

It is important to know that the water used in infant feeding is entirely sanitary, particularly when used in the larger amounts required for the preparation of evaporated and dried-milk formulas. Rural wells frequently are contaminated by surface drainage. Water from such a source is unsafe, even though all harmful bacteria have been killed by boiling. Unsanitary water is likely to contain a relatively large amount of nitrates. Nitrates may be converted to nitrites by intestinal bacteria in early infancy. After absorption, nitrites convert hemoglobin to methemoglobin, and the result often is extreme cyanosis in young infants.

ACIDIFICATION

The acidity from the growth of lactic-acid-producing bacteria in boiled milk causes a fine curd which is not changed in size after ingestion. Milk soured in this manner has proved to be an excellent infant food. The product is equally satisfactory when the milk has been soured by the direct addition not only of lactic acid but also of acetic and citric acids. Citric acid may be used in its purified state or in the form of orange or lemon juice. Boiled milk appropriately acidified may be fed without dilution or other modification if desired. Dried lactic acid milk is available on the market.

CARBOHYDRATES USED IN INFANT FEEDING

The time-honored method of preparing artificial formulas for infant feeding considers a carbohydrate addition as essential in order to meet the energy requirement of the baby. Carbohydrate is readily assimilable and aids the absorption of soaps and minerals by altering the reaction of the intestinal tract toward the acid side. The common substances used are lactose, sucrose, starch and derivatives of starch (such as dextrin, maltose, dextrose and combinations of these compounds). Some physicians now believe that the addition of carbohydrate to whole milk or evaporated milk formulas is unnecessary for most infants. The presumptive advantages of unsweetened formulas are simplicity of preparation and satisfaction of the infant's appetite by giving more calories derived from protein rather than a high proportion of carbohydrate.

LACTOSE

Lactose is the natural sugar of milk. It has been used in the past more extensively than it is at present. Lactose does not supply any physiologic need that is not supplied by any other sugar.

SUCROSE

Sucrose (saccharose, cane sugar) has proved to be a satisfactory sugar for infant feeding, although it has the slight disadvantage of being very sweet.

STARCH

Starch, when well cooked, frequently is added to formulas for infants. The amounts used for this purpose are small and add relatively little energy value. The cereal waters are considered in this text more appropriately with the milk diluents.

DEXTRIN-MALTOSE MIXTURES

When starch is acted on by malt diastase, it is broken down first to various dextrins and finally to maltose. The conversion process is not uniform, and at any one time all these products are to be found in the mixture. Commercial preparations vary in the relative content of dextrins and maltose, depending on the extent to which the conversion process has been permitted to go. These are sugars used extensively in infant feeding.

CORN SYRUP

Corn syrup is produced by the action of mineral acid on corn starch and differs from the dextrin-maltose mixtures in that the conversion process produces dextrose as the end product, and the commercial mixture contains dextrins, maltose and dextrose. It is commonly marketed as a syrup. The canned table syrups commonly used in infant feeding consist of corn syrup, 85 per cent, and either cane sugar syrup or refiner's syrup, 15 per cent.

DEXTROSE

Dextrose (corn sugar), the end product of starch conversion by acid, is used therapeutically in infant feeding much more often than as a routine addition to the formula.

CHOICE AMONG THE SUGARS

The chief differences among the sugars lie in their activity in the intestinal tract. All the sugars mentioned serve the nutritional needs of the infant equally well after absorption from the intestinal tract. In general, sugars have a laxative effect, but some much more than others. Dextrose is easily fermentable but it is absorbed so quickly and so high in the intestinal tract that diarrhea usually does not result even when relatively large amounts are fed. Therefore, dextrose is an excellent sugar to use when diarrhea is present. Lactose presents the other extreme. It is broken down slowly in the intestinal tract before absorption. A greater opportunity is offered for bacterial decomposition of the sugar, and a greater laxative effect is obtained. The different proprietary malt sugars vary considerably in their laxative effect. The variation probably is due in part to a varying content of vegetable extractives and in part to the addition of potassium carbonate to some of the preparations.

Conversion Table for Materials Used in Infant Feeding

Volume is measured best in a graduate or a medicine glass. However, 2 level tablespoonfuls may be considered as 1 ounce by volume (fluid ounce). One ounce by weight (28.4 Gm.) has a volume in fluid ounces approximately as follows:

Cane sugar 1
Lactose 2
Dextrose .2
Dextrin-maltose mixtures, dry. . .2
Flour, wheat 2
Rolled oats 2.25
Dried milk, packed measure. . . .1.75

One ounce of flavored corn syrup (table syrup) by volume contains 1 ounce of sugar by weight.

PROPRIETARY MILK FORMULAS

From the foregoing discussion it is apparent that the chief food of the young infant who is fed artificially is a mixture of cow's milk, some variety of sugar and possibly a diluent. Such a mixture could be prepared, freed from some or most of its water and preserved in suitable airtight containers. Then it would be ready for use in infant feeding after the addition of an appropriate amount of water. Several proprietary synthetic mixtures for infant feeding are marketed. In the preparation of some of them, an attempt has been made to simulate human milk. Others are more simple mixtures of milk and some variety of sugar. Whatever advantages such mixtures may have, perhaps the chief one is convenience.

OTHER INFANT FOODS

The number of proprietary infant foods is large. Some of them serve a useful purpose for special indications; others are merely a convenience; a few are completely unnecessary. All those adapted for routine use are easily classifiable in a simple scheme of infant feeding. A few of the proprietary foods are mentioned in connection with the diseases in which they are useful.

MILK SUBSTITUTES

Milk substitutes are used for babies allergic to milk or for a trial period for babies suspected of being allergic to milk. Three types of such products are commercially available. One depends on the soybean to supply protein; another uses a hydrolysate of casein; a third contains meat as the protein source. To these basic ingredients have been added nutritional essentials to make the formula more nearly a "complete" food. The additions include minerals, fat, sugar and in some instances vitamins of the B complex. In using these formulas careful check must be made to determine whether or not supplementation with vitamins and iron is necessary.

PRESCRIBING A FORMULA WHEN DILUTION IS EMPLOYED

Because unmodified cow's milk is so likely to cause digestive disturbances in the young infant and because dilution is a method of modification that makes milk better tolerated, modification by dilution is commonly employed. The greater the dilution, the better it is tolerated. However, dilution beyond certain limits will not permit an adequate intake of milk.

The first question to decide is how much milk an infant needs. The protein needs of an infant are supplied when 1½ ounces of milk for each pound of body weight are given in each 24 hours. However, infants grow better and build active tissue faster with a larger milk allowance. The illustrative formula calculation given subsequently is on the basis of 1¾ ounces for each pound for the first half year. In a few instances, when the baby is hungry, 2 ounces to the pound may be indicated.

ENERGY REQUIREMENT

Although the amount of milk specified will supply the protein and certain other needs of the infant, additional energy-producing food must be supplied. The energy requirement is met by additional sugar. The amount of sugar required varies from 1 to 2 ounces for each 24

hours. Those fed less than 1 ounce are not likely to gain satisfactorily, and those given much more than 2 ounces may develop gastro-intestinal disturbances.

DILUENT

Diluent is added to the milk-and-sugar mixture in an amount that will bring the total volume of the food to the quantity easily taken by the infant in 24 hours.

CALCULATION OF A FORMULA FOR A WELL BABY

The newborn infant has an energy requirement somewhat less than later, and at the same time his digestive capacity is easily exceeded. Therefore, it is well to be cautious and start with a formula containing a little less food than would be given according to the requirements stated subsequently for a baby somewhat older. Probably it is never necessary to give a greater dilution than half milk during the first 2 weeks, and most infants will tolerate well a dilution containing two thirds milk.

An infant's food requirements should be calculated on the basis of what he should weigh, rather than on actual weight. A poorly nourished infant of 4 months might weigh as little as 8 or 9 pounds, but his total daily requirement would be the same as if he were of average or expected weight for his age.

A normal healthy infant under 6 months of age usually takes at each feeding a total volume of food in ounces equal to the age in months plus 2 or 3. A baby at 1 month of age usually takes a feeding of 3 or 4 ounces, and in the case of a large baby even 5 ounces. The increase in volume of the formula continues until it has reached from 32 to 35 ounces in the 24 hours. Usually from 5 months onward a baby will want 5 feedings of approximately 7 or 8 ounces each.

The younger baby usually wants from 6 to 8 feedings per day. An older infant usually wants approximately 5 feedings per day. Much depends on the capacity and the needs of the individual baby. As the baby lengthens the interval between feedings, he will take more at each feeding in order to get sufficient food.

In illustration of a method that may be used in calculating a formula, prescription will be made for a baby 4 months old weighing 14 pounds (6.3 kg.). It is assumed that the infant is of average weight for his age. It also is assumed that his energy requirement is 50 calories for each pound or 110 calories for each kilogram for each 24 hours.

Twenty-four ounces of milk (1¾ ounces for each pound) will supply the protein, the calcium and several other needs, as well as a portion of of energy required. The amount of energy thus supplied is 480 calories. The total energy requirement is 700 calories. The difference between the requirement and the amount supplied by the milk is 220 calories, which is to be supplied by additional sugar. One and three-fourths ounces of sugar (120 calories to the ounce) will furnish 210 calories. Thus, with 24 ounces of milk and 1¾ ounces of sugar, all the needs of the infant intended to be supplied by the formula have been met with the exception of water. The formula needs of the 4-month-old baby might be 6 feedings of 5 or 6 ounces each or 5 feedings of 6 or 7 ounces each.

The addition of from 6 to 12 ounces of water will be required.

The prescription will be as follows:

Whole milk . . . . .24 oz.
Sugar . . . . 1¾ oz.
Water . . . . 9 oz.
    5 feedings of 6½ oz. each or 6 feedings of 5½ oz. each.

The total volume of a feeding is not increased appreciably by the addition of a dry sugar in such amounts as are discussed here. However, if a syrup is used, an equal volume of water should be subtracted from the amount stated in the prescription.

With all the rules that have been discussed, it is apparent that considerable latitude of interpretation is allowed. This is necessary. Each baby is an individual and must be so treated. The prescription that has been given is based on theoretical considerations and may not meet the exact needs of the individual infant. Necessary adjustments are to be made after a brief trial. It may be that slightly more total energy is required for satisfactory growth or weight gain or that the baby is somewhat constipated. In either event the amount of sugar should be increased.

A well baby is not likely to develop colic or loose stools with the feeding prescribed, but if he should do so it may be advisable to decrease the amount of sugar or change the kind that is used. These alterations are discussed in greater detail under other topics.

The amount of milk to be given increases with the age of the infant, until at approximately 6 or 7 months he is receiving a quart of undiluted milk daily. No increase beyond this point is indicated, because by this time other foods are being given. A quart of milk is a suitable intake for the remainder of infancy, and also preferably throughout childhood.

USE OF UNDILUTED MILK IN INFANT FEEDING

Milk dilutions have been employed extensively in infant feeding because a dilution helps to modify milk in such a manner that it is tolerated better by the infant and because sufficient milk usually can be supplied in this way to satisfy the nutritional needs.

It has been demonstrated abundantly that a young infant can digest and utilize undiluted milk, provided that certain of its characteristics have been modified sufficiently. It has been demonstrated also that the greater food intake thus permitted causes more rapid growth of the infant. It is not known whether this more rapid growth is more ideal growth, but there is some support for believing that it is.

Certain infants have a relatively small gastric capacity. For such infants, concentrated foods are desirable in order that sufficient food may be ingested. The undiluted milk formulas are particularly suitable for this type of infant.

The variety of modification for undiluted milk formulas that has had the most extensive use in this country is acidification of milk which previously has been boiled. The method of preparation is discussed subsequently. Any sugar desired may be used in these formulas.

There is no objection to feeding acidified milk and sugar mixtures throughout the first year. If the

baby is malnourished or sickly, this is often preferable. A well baby should be able to take undiluted boiled sweet milk from 6 to 8 months on if it is desired to feed him in this manner.

FEEDING OF NORMAL INFANTS WITH DRIED MILK

Some of the dried milks are prepared from whole milk, some from partially skimmed milk, and some from skimmed milk. Of the dried skimmed milks prepared for infant feeding, the greatest usage is of products prepared from milk containing 1.5 per cent fat and thus only partially skimmed. Subsequent discussion is of this product. When dried milks represent whole milk, they may be diluted to their original volume and used in the same manner as has been described for fresh milk. Acid additions usually are unnecessary, but if made, the amount of acid should be much less than that recommended for fresh milk. Each ounce by weight (3½ packed level tablespoonfuls) of dried whole milk is equivalent to 8 ounces by volume of the original milk; each ounce of dried skimmed milk is equivalent to approximately 10 ounces of the original milk.

It is customary to use dried skimmed milk in larger quantity than dried whole milk because of the lower energy value. Each weighed ounce of dried skimmed milk has an energy value of 125 calories. One method of using dried skimmed milk commonly recommended is to prescribe one third of an ounce (10 Gm.) for each pound of body weight for each 24 hours. When used in this manner, relatively little additional sugar is required to satisfy the energy needs. The amount of milk prescribed is diluted to the volume that an infant would be expected to take in 24 hours.

FEEDING OF NORMAL INFANTS WITH EVAPORATED MILK

Evaporated milk, when diluted with an equal volume of water, is approximately equivalent to whole fresh milk and may be used in the same manner. For acidification, only about two thirds as much acid as for fresh milk is required. Evaporated milk has been fed with good results without acidification in a dilution equivalent to fresh whole milk. Digestive difficulties from overfeeding are encountered sometimes under 2 months of age when evaporated milk diluted with only an equal part of water is fed.

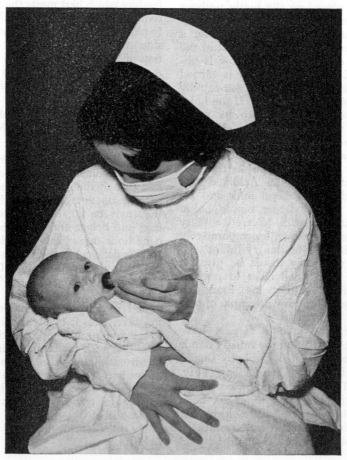

Fig. 85. Position of a baby for feeding.

TECHNIC OF FEEDING

At feeding time the milk is taken from the refrigerator and warmed to body temperature by placing the bottle in a container of warm water. If a sweet-milk formula is overheated in this process, it can be cooled, and no harm is done. However, if acidified milk is overheated, the curd is likely to clump and separate from the whey.

After warming the milk, the nipple is placed on the bottle without contamination of the tip, the temperature is tested by sprinkling a few drops on the inner aspect of the wrist, and the speed of flow is observed. When the bottle is turned up, the milk should drop out rapidly but not run in a stream. If the holes are too small, they can be made larger with a hot needle.

The size of the nipple holes must be geared to the type of formula that is being fed and to the needs of the individual infant. Acidified milk is thicker than sweet milk and requires slightly larger nipple holes. Sick infants with lowered vitality require a nipple with comparatively large holes. The hungry infant who sucks vigorously should be given a nipple with small holes to prevent him from getting his food too rapidly and to provide ample opportunity for sucking.

After the infant's diapers have been changed and the nurse's hands have been washed, the baby should be held during his feeding (Fig. 85). The infant's need for emotional warmth at feeding time has been cited in Chapter 3. If holding the baby for feedings is contraindicated medically, the bottle should be held throughout the feeding unless the infant is desirous of holding it himself.

After feeding, the young baby should be "bubbled," cuddled until he is ready for sleep and placed in bed. If he does not seem to be comfortable after being put down to rest, he should be "bubbled" again. Some babies need to be "bubbled" before, during and after feeding. It takes time to discover the way of feeding which best meets the infant's requirements. It is usually advisable to place the young, sick infant on his side after feeding to prevent aspiration if regurgitation should occur. A rolled bed pad usually is necessary to maintain the side position.

ADDITIONS TO THE MILK DIET OF THE INFANT

Clinical experience has shown that babies fed milk exclusively, whether human or cow's, or milk and carbohydrate mixtures for many months do not do well. Although they may be fat, they become anemic, and rickets and other abnormal conditions are likely to develop. Milk is deficient in several essentials, especially iron and vitamin D, and, in the case of prepared cow's milk, vitamin C. The iron store is depleted sooner in some babies than in others, and it is advisable to follow a routine in supplementing the milk diet with foods containing iron at an early age. Also, the addition of various foods serves the useful purpose of accustoming the baby to variety in texture and flavor, an accomplishment important in the later development of good eating habits.

FRUIT JUICES

Orange juice is traditionally the first thing to be added. It is given chiefly for its vitamin C content. The juice from ripe oranges is tolerated well in the early weeks and should be given early, certainly before the end of the first month. An ounce a day is a satisfactory amount up to about 3 months of age, at which time an increase to 2 ounces is desirable. Often orange juice is diluted with an equal amount of water. It is customary to give it about an hour before one of the morning feedings. Other fruit juices or tomato juice may be substituted for orange juice. Allowance must be made for the smaller vitamin C content of most of these juices. If no fruit juice is fed for any reason, ascorbic acid should be given in the amount of at least 25 mg. daily. When a polyvitamin supplement is being given daily, orange juice is not necessary.

VITAMIN D

The need for vitamin D exists from the time of birth and this should be supplied not later than 2 weeks of age. Vitamin D is available in many forms. Cod-liver oil is the oldest of these and is very satisfactory. The dose can be started at 15 drops once or twice daily and increased rapidly until a teaspoonful (approximately 120 drops) is being taken each day in either a single or divided dose. An amount of cod-liver oil that contains approximately 400 units of vitamin D is an appropriate amount regardless of the volume in teaspoons. This amount is sufficient throughout the period of infancy. An equivalent amount of vitamin D should be given if one of the concentrates is employed.

Many communities are supplied with milk fortified with vitamin D; all evaporated milk is so fortified. Standard fortification is 400 units to the quart or to the reconstituted quart. When such milk is used for the baby, additional vitamin D is unnecessary if the baby is taking most of a quart per day.

IRON

At 6 months of age or less, even normal and apparently healthy babies have a decrease in hemoglobin if the diet has not been supplemented previously with iron or some iron-containing food. Presumably the iron stores have been exhausted. Since it is normal for all humans to have a store of the minerals necessary for hemoglobin formation, it would seem advisable to supply these before the store is exhausted. It is natural to expect an infant to be able to satisfy his nutritional needs from foods rather than from drugs. However, a hesitancy is found in some quarters in administering the iron-containing foods at an early age. In this connection it is to be noted that the soluble iron salts, such as iron ammonium citrate or ferrous sulfate, are not only well tolerated in reasonable dose but are also utilizable in hemoglobin formation. The usual commercial iron preparations contain traces of copper which is useful also in hemoglobin formation. Five ml. of a 1-per-cent iron ammonium citrate (9 mg. of iron) will satisfy fully the iron requirement for most of the first year, as will also 5 ml.

of a 1 per cent solution of ferrous sulfate.

EGG YOLK

Egg yolk is a fairly good food source of iron as well as of other nutritional essentials. In some places it has been customary to feed cooked egg yolk as early as 2 or 3 months of age. It is well tolerated at this early age.

VEGETABLES

The most popular of the iron-containing foods for infants are certain of the vegetables, which are served well cooked and finely sieved in small quantity. The tendency has been to feed vegetables at increasingly earlier ages, many advocating their use at from 1 to 3 months of age. Beginning with small amounts, vegetable purée may be given at one of the regular feeding times. It has been shown that iron and other minerals are not well utilized from spinach, presumably because of the oxalic-acid content. However, spinach is an excellent source of vitamin A and other nutrients and should be retained in the dietary.

MEATS

Meats are difficult to prepare in the home in a manner suitable for feeding young infants. However, commercially prepared meats and meat soups are available and suitable for this purpose. Liver is useful in hemoglobin formation. If it is prepared properly and given in small quantities, it causes no digestive difficulties in the infant.

FRUITS

The strained pulp of certain cooked fruits is offered as the next step after the feeding of vegetables. Fruit may be given at from 1 to 2 months of age. Among the fruits that may be permitted are prunes, apples, apricots, pears and peaches. Some fruits are of value for their ascorbic-acid content, but fruits in general serve other useful purposes. Apricots, peaches and prunes are fairly good sources of iron and copper.

CEREALS

It is a general custom to give cereals early, many physicians advising their use at 2 weeks to 1 month of age. They are well tolerated at this age, but a question arises as to whether the nutritional needs of the baby are served as well by such early use of ordinary cereal preparations as they are by giving some of the other foods first. The baby's needs at this age are particularly for iron and some of the B vitamins. Farina, so commonly fed, has little of these materials. Even whole-grain cereals supply less of them than do the foods previously discussed. From the nutritional point of view the cereals are relatively unimportant, and their use has been overemphasized. The more important foods are likely to be too much restricted if an abundance of cereal is fed. The proprietary cereal preparations have overcome these objections. If cereals are to be fed in the first 6 months, they should be either whole grain or of the fortified variety.

COMPLETE DIET

When the milk formula has been supplemented with the foods that have been discussed, the diet presumably is complete: that is, it con-

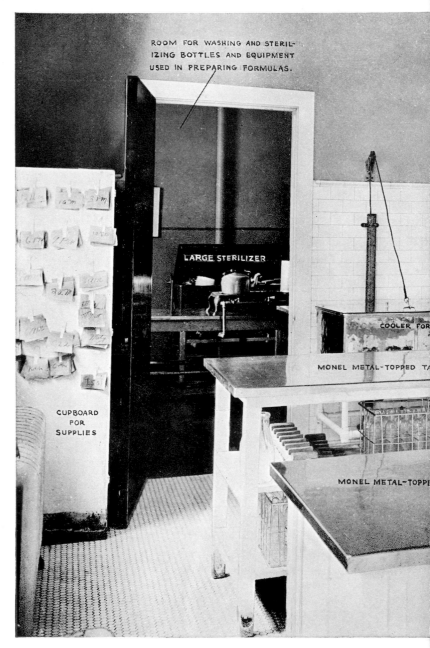

ROOM FOR WASHING AND STERIL-
IZING BOTTLES AND EQUIPMENT
USED IN PREPARING FORMULAS.

LARGE STERILIZER

COOLER FOR

MONEL METAL-TOPPED TA

CUPBOARD
FOR
SUPPLIES

MONEL METAL-TOPPE

FIG. 87. Illustrating milk room equipment not sho
bottles and utensils not in view. In some sit

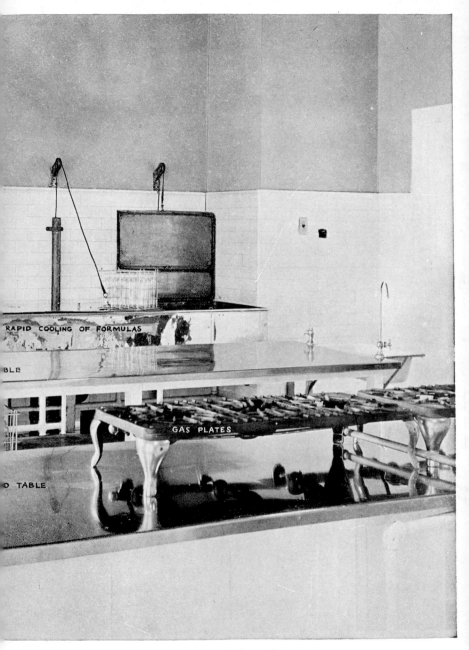

RAPID COOLING OF FORMULAS

BLE

GAS PLATES

D TABLE

wn in the view on the reverse side. Large sink for washing
uations a cream separator may be needed in addition.

tains all the food materials essential for normal growth and development during the first year. Special vitamin preparations other than those mentioned usually are not necessary for the normal infant. Methods of introducing supplementary foods into the infant's diet are discussed in Chapter 3.

HOSPITAL MILK ROOM

Every hospital caring for infants must have some place where milk formulas can be prepared in a satisfactory manner. The room assigned for this purpose is usually referred to as the milk room. Figures 86 and 87 illustrate one type of milk room.

The location of the milk room is frequently a subject for controversy. It is the opinion of some that this room should be attached to the infants' ward and be supervised by the graduate nurse in the ward. The chief argument in favor of this location is that thus a direct correlation between the infant and the formula is made easy. However, it is probable that the disadvantages of such location and supervision outweigh the advantages. Wherever the room is located, it should be a separate room and used for nothing else than the preparation of infants' formulas. When it is convenient to the ward it is likely to be used for other purposes.

The milk room may be located conveniently near the kitchens and supervised by a dietitian or a specially trained nurse. In order to correlate the formulas with the infants, the nurse may be sent to the infant ward in the afternoon after all formula work is completed. She may be assigned a definite problem, such as feeding certain infants,

making calculations of their intakes and drawing up a report of how these observations compare with the theory that she learned in the classroom.

EQUIPMENT

The equipment of the room depends entirely on the type of work being done. A minimum list follows:

Cupboards for supplies
At least 2 tables
Sink
Refrigerator
Cooler
Pitchers or milk containers
Graduates
Scales
Hot plates
Teakettles or water sterilizer
Utensil sterilizer
Pans (long-handled)
Covers for pans
Bottles
Bottle caps
Bottle crates
Funnels
Strainers
Large spoons
Teaspoons
Knives
Egg beater
Bowls
Double boiler
Bulletin boards for posting formulas
Clean gowns and caps for workers

"CLEAN" TECHNIC

The nurses working in the milk room should be considered "clean" at all times and should not go to the ward and handle infants or do anything in the ward while they are engaged in preparing formulas. "Clean" technic is not "sterile" technic, and a clear differentiation should be made so the nurse will not carry this over to situations where true sterile technic is used.

ORDER OF PROCEDURE

The nurse should change from her uniform to a clean milk-room gown, mask and cap. The gown and the cap should not be worn outside the milk room except to the dressing room to change. The hands should be scrubbed thoroughly before beginning work.

Assembling Materials. All utensils and bottles should have been washed previously so that they are ready to be boiled and used. All supplies should be at hand.

Labeling Bottles and Pans. A lead pencil and small pieces of adhesive or metal tags with numbers should be used to mark the bottles. A colored glass marking pencil is not satisfactory because the marks blur and disappear when the formula is heated.

Weighing. All dry ingredients should be weighed on an accurate balance. A spring scale is inaccurate.

Measuring. All milk should be stirred thoroughly each time any is taken from a container. Milk should be measured accurately in a glass graduate. When syrups are used, the measuring should be done in a small graduate, and a knife or a spatula should be used to remove that which adheres to the sides of the glass, or a 50-per-cent solution of the syrup, which will pour easily, should be prepared.

Boiling. All feedings should be stirred well before being placed over the flame. The flame should be turned high. Heating should be accomplished as quickly as possible, with constant stirring. One should not attempt to heat more than 2 pans at a time, or more than 2 or 3 quarts of milk in a single container. To boil 1 minute, the milk may be allowed to foam at the top of the pan 3 times. To boil more than 1 minute, the feeding should be boiled briskly for the number of minutes required.

Pouring. Boiled feedings should be poured at once. After thorough stirring, the feeding should be distributed evenly among all the bottles by pouring through a fine tea strainer placed in a funnel. If any remains in the strainer, it should be pressed through. None of a feeding should be discarded because there seems to be more in each bottle than is specified. Bottles are not as accurately labeled as the graduate used in measuring. For this reason the amount recorded on the bottle will not always be the same as the amount in the bottle.

Capping Bottles. Bottles should be capped immediately after they are filled. Paper caps like ordinary milk bottle caps may be used. Rubber caps which cover the tops of bottles are more satisfactory. Improvised covers of folded paper and rubber bands are not to be used as they become broken, and the milk is easily contaminated. Sometimes in the home cotton plugs are used or cellophane held on tightly by rubber bands.

Cooling Feedings. Any milk formulas that are hot when distributed into individual feeding bottles should be cooled promptly and rapidly in a suitable cooler to 10° C. before being placed in the refrigerator. Some care and judgment are necessary in order to avoid breaking the hot bottles.

CHOICE AND CARE OF BOTTLES AND NIPPLES

Any type of nursing bottle whose every part can be reached easily with a bottle brush is satisfactory. Any nipple which can be turned inside out, scrubbed and boiled is suitable. In the hospital it is taken for granted that a bottle is provided for each feeding in the 24 hours, but in the home mothers sometimes attempt to make 1 or 2 bottles and nipples suffice. The latter cannot be considered good practice, and if such an attempt is made, the bottle and the nipple should be scrubbed and boiled each time before use.

The bottles and the nipples should be washed thoroughly with hot soapsuds and a brush, rinsed and boiled for 5 minutes. Then the bottles are ready for filling. After boiling, the nipples should be kept in a clean dry covered jar. As soon as the baby has taken the feeding, the bottle and the nipple should be rinsed, and the bottle should be left filled with water until the time for the preparation of the next day's feedings.

Some of the newer detergent soaps are poisonous. If they are used in cleansing nursing bottles, great care must be exercised to see that no detergent remains in the bottles before use.

PREPARATION OF VARIOUS TYPES OF FORMULAS USING "CLEAN" TECHNIC

Fresh Milk Feedings

The dry ingredients should be weighed and placed in a pan. Then the measured liquids should be added and the whole stirred well.

The feeding should be heated rapidly to boiling while being stirred constantly and should be boiled for the length of time ordered and brought back to volume with boiled water. The feeding should be poured at once.

Evaporated Milk Feedings

The dry ingredients should be weighed and placed in a pan. The required amount of water should be added and the whole boiled for 2 minutes. Then the prescribed amount of evaporated milk should be added, the mixture stirred thoroughly and poured.

Dried-Milk Feedings. The dry ingredients should be weighed and placed in a pan. The measured boiled water should be added slowly, a paste being made first. The mixture should be beaten with a Dover (rotary) egg beater and then poured.

Lactic-Acid Milk Feedings

Preparation by Bacterial Growth. The milk should be boiled for 3 minutes and cooled to 37° C. Two or 3 cc. of a pure culture of *Streptococcus lacticus* or other culture as desired is added. The milk should be well covered and incubated at room temperature overnight. The top of the tube of culture always should be flamed before the culture is poured into the milk. Every precaution should be taken to keep the milk free from contamination. After the milk has soured, it is made up into individual feedings by the addition of the required amount of sugar or any other material that may be ordered. The preparation of acid milk by means of growth of lactic-

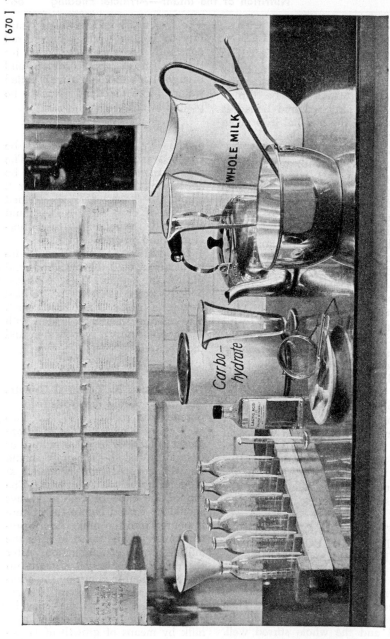

Fig. 88. Materials for the preparation of a lactic-acid-milk formula in the hospital.

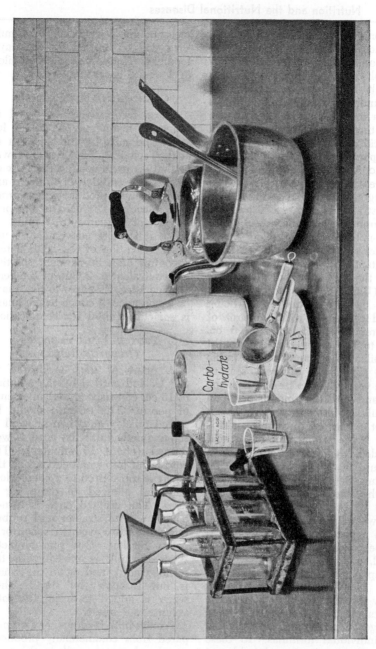

FIG. 89. Materials for the preparation of a lactic-acid-milk formula in the home.

acid-producing bacteria is entirely satisfactory when it can be done in a laboratory or under laboratory control. However, in the home, it is difficult to prevent contamination with undesirable organisms. For this reason it is often safer and at the same time more convenient to add the acid directly to the milk.

Preparation by Acid Addition. LACTIC ACID. The equipment that is necessary to prepare this type of feeding in the hospital and the home is illustrated in Figures 88 and 89. The formula should be mixed as for sweet-milk feedings, boiled for 3 minutes and cooled to 10° C. It is important that the milk be cold when the acid is added. The lactic acid (U.S.P. 85%) is added slowly, drop by drop, the milk being stirred constantly. The amount of acid required is from 4 to 5 cc. (100 to 125 drops) for each quart of milk. The amount desirable varies slightly in different seasons of the year with the freshness of the milk and with the amount of fat in the milk. It also seems to vary with the lot of corn syrup, if this sugar is used. If the proper amount of acid is added, the mixture will have a fine curd that does not settle out on standing. Separation of the curd and the whey indicates an excessive addition of acid or the addition of acid while the milk is still warm. When a great excess of lactic acid has been added, the curd is redissolved, and the mixture may have the appearance of a suitable formula. However, such a mixture is highly toxic for the infant. In some hospitals lactic-acid milk is prepared in large quantities and later divided into individual formulas. In these circumstances it is advisable to measure out 1 quart more of milk than will be needed for the day's feedings. The milk should be boiled in 2- and 3-quart lots.

CITRIC-ACID MILK FEEDINGS

These feedings are prepared in the same manner as described for lactic-acid milk by the addition of acid. Technical difficulties are fewer in that errors in cooling the milk or in speed of addition of the acid are not so likely to produce a poor product. Citric acid is used in the proportion of 2 grams to 1 quart of milk. It is more convenient to use a stock solution of the acid; 2 teaspoonfuls of a 25-per-cent solution are equivalent to 2 Gm. of the acid. Orange juice, 2 ounces to the quart, or lemon juice, ¾ ounce to the quart, is sometimes used for acidification.

PROTEIN MILK FEEDINGS (ALBUMIN MILK)

A quart of milk is heated to 37° C. and curded by the addition of 15 cc. (3 teaspoonfuls) of essence of pepsin. The mixture should be stirred quickly and then allowed to stand quietly until the curd is well formed (about 15 minutes). The curd is cut into small cubes, and the whole is transferred to a cheesecloth bag and allowed to drain for 1 hour. The drained curd is turned out on a wire strainer and rubbed through with a wooden spoon or a potato masher. One pint of lactic skimmed milk is mixed with the strained curd, and again the whole is put through the sieve. Then water is added to bring the total volume to 1 quart.

Protein milk feedings may be prepared from commercially produced powdered protein milk in the same manner as described for dried-milk feedings.

THICK FEEDINGS

Thick feedings are prepared by the addition of from 8 to 10 per cent of flour or fine cereal to the regular prescribed formula. Sometimes part of the sugar of the formula is omitted.

Sample thick feeding:

Whole milk	700 cc.
Water	100 cc.
Wheat flour	80 Gm.
Sugar	60 Gm.

The water is added to the flour in such a manner as to make a thin smooth paste. Then the starch paste is stirred into the milk, which has been heated in the top section of a double boiler. Then the top part of the boiler is removed from the water and heated directly over the flame until the milk mixture is thick (about 5 minutes). It again is placed over the water in the double boiler and cooked for 15 minutes. The water lost by evaporation should be replaced after transferring the food to a graduate. Then the food is put through a fine strainer and distributed in wide-mouthed feeding bottles.

ADDITION OF EGG YOLK TO FEEDINGS

Sweet-Milk Feedings. The egg yolk is beaten well and moistened with a very small quantity of cold boiled water. To the beaten yolk are added several spoonfuls of the hot feeding. Then the egg mixture is added to the entire feeding. The feeding is boiled up once briefly over the flame to coagulate any egg white that may have adhered to the yolk. The egg should not lump if it is added properly.

Acid or Powdered-Milk Feedings. The egg is hard-cooked, and the white is removed. The yolk is pressed through a fine strainer. To the yolk is added a small amount of the feeding to make a smooth paste. Then the yolk is stirred into the entire formula.

TERMINAL STERILIZATION OF FORMULAS

Formulas prepared by "clean" technic may be expected to be safe bacteriologically. A somewhat greater assurance of safety can be attained by sterilization of the formula after it has been bottled and capped. In many instances the procedure is supplemented by placing a nipple and a nipple cover or cap on the formula-filled bottle before sterilization. The milk-room procedure is the same as that described for "clean" technic except that the formula usually is not boiled.

Terminal sterilization may be carried out in any one of several ways. One is by autoclaving the loosely capped bottles at 230° F., 7 pounds to the square inch, for 10 minutes. The same result may be achieved in the home by means of a pressure cooker. A third procedure is to boil in a covered basin containing water; the bottles should be held in an atmosphere of steam for a minimum of 15 minutes. After heating, the bottles are cooled rapidly in water and placed in the refrigerator after tightening the caps.

Sterilization of acidified formulas makes them unfit for use. Preparation of an acidified formula can be accomplished by injection of the acid through the cap or the nipple with a needle while shaking the bottle, using sterile technic; this procedure is done after cooling the sterilized formula.

Terminal sterilization destroys a larger proportion of the heat-labile vitamins than does the quick boiling of "clean" technic. This fact should be kept in mind when dietary supplements are considered for the baby. Usually vitamin C is supplied separately and need not be of concern. The thiamine content of quickly boiled milk approaches closely the minimum requirement; thiamine supplementation may be considered an advantage to babies receiving sterilized milk. Occasional clogging of the nipples with scum may be expected with terminal sterilization of ordinary milk formulas. This depends on undetermined factors which too often limit the usefulness of the method in the home.

PREPARATION OF OTHER INFANT FOODS

VEGETABLES

The following are among the vegetables that may be used: tomatoes, spinach or other greens, carrots, green peas, string beans, beets, asparagus tips, cauliflower and turnips. The vegetables should be washed and cut into small pieces. Then they are cooked in such an amount of water that practically all the water will have evaporated when the vegetables are tender. Any water remaining should be retained. A little salt may be added. The vegetables should be passed through a fine tea strainer for young babies and mashed for those older. It is not necessary in the home to cook vegetables especially for the baby; some of the family vegetable can be sieved for him.

FRUIT SAUCE

Apples, prunes, apricots, peaches or pears may be used. The fruit should be cooked until tender. It may be sweetened lightly. It should be pressed through a fine sieve for young babies, mashed for older infants.

EGGS

Eggs may be hard-boiled and broken into particles or soft-boiled or poached. It is desirable that all the white be coagulated.

LIVER

Liver should be boiled in water until tender and seasoned with salt. It should be ground in a food chopper and then pressed through a fine strainer. The resultant liver powder may be added to vegetables or other foods if desired.

Suitable preparations of all varieties of supplementary foods are now available in small cans and are very convenient for home use.

SITUATIONS FOR FURTHER STUDY

1. Compare human milk and cow's milk. What are the differences in composition? How can cow's milk be modified to approximate the composition of human milk? What are the differences in the proteins of the 2 milks? Can they be made similar?

2. What is the caloric value of human milk? Of cow's milk?

3. How many calories for each kilogram of body weight does an infant of 4 months require? Does this need vary? How does it vary during the period of infancy?

4. If you were a nurse in a well-baby clinic and had the opportunity

to prepare mothers for giving supplementary foods to their infants, how would you proceed? If the doctor had recommended that vegetables be introduced into an infant's diet, what behavior would you anticipate that the mother would encounter? How would you help the mother to know when the infant was ready to begin to learn to eat cereal?

5. Describe the process of preparing an evaporated-milk feeding in a home.

6. If an expectant mother who planned to feed her infant an artificial formula needed suggestions concerning necessary equipment for the preparation of food, what would you include as requirements?

7. What help would a mother who wished to prepare her baby's formula with terminal sterilization require?

BIBLIOGRAPHY

Rouke, A. J.: Infant formulas. No. 1. Study of methods now used, Hospitals 21:67, 1947.

————: Infant formulas. No. 2. Preparation techniques, Hospitals 21:66, 1947.

Smith, F. R., Finley, R. D., Wright, H. J., and Louder, E. A.: Terminal heating of infant formula, J. Am. Dietet. A., 24:755, 1948.

Nutrition of the Child

◇◇◇

IMPORTANCE OF PROPER FOOD
NORMAL DIET
MILK
OTHER IMPORTANT FOODS

PREPARATION OF THE DIET
SERVING THE DIET
DIETARY HABITS
SITUATIONS FOR FURTHER STUDY

IMPORTANCE OF PROPER FOOD

The rate of growth of the child is determined to a considerable extent by the kind and the amount of food he is given. Defects in the diet may cause malnutrition and sometimes serious illness; they may lead to lowered resistance to infection and to intellectual inertia. A lack of knowledge even of general dietary principles and the mistaken belief that whatever satisfies hunger is suitable food often are reasons why mothers permit children to make their own food selection. Thus, a most important factor in physical development is left to chance. Even when opportunities for food selection by the child are minimal, it so often happens that the food habits of the family do not permit the ingestion of a complete and adequate diet. That the average diet of the people of this country is incomplete in several essentials has been pointed out many times by various observers. Much nutritional educa-

tion still is needed. However, over the years diets of children have improved with increase and spread of knowledge of nutrition and with improved economic status. When diets of children are deficient, they are likely to be low in calcium, protein, ascorbic acid and vitamin A more often than in other nutrients. Older children tend to have poorer diets than those younger, and girls poorer diets than boys even in the same family. Adolescent girls tend to fare worst of all; many girls, distressed at rapid changes in size, try to remain slender by decreasing their food. On the other hand, adolescent boys tend to eat heartily.

NORMAL DIET

The nutritional requirements and the fundamental principles of nutrition have been discussed in a preceding chapter. Certain practical applications remain to be considered. The kind of food required by children of different ages varies little, but the amount and the form vary somewhat according to the activity and the age of the child. One third of the energy value of the child's diet may well be derived from carbohydrate. The best sources of carbohydrate are fruits, vegetables, milk and the cereal grains. It is desirable to avoid excessive use of refined products, such as unenriched white bread and cane sugar, and to supply carbohydrate by means of those foods which furnish also essential food constituents. From 40 to 50 per cent of the child's total caloric requirement may be obtained from fat, and milk, butter and eggs should be the chief sources. Fats that melt at low temperatures (butter, beef fat, lard) are digested more readily than those that melt at higher temperatures (mutton fat).

MILK

Much has been said concerning the desirability and the usefulness of milk. In fact, the prescribing of a proper diet is extremely difficult unless milk is included. A commonly accepted standard amount is 1 quart daily. A number of physicians of considerable experience assert that this amount is excessive for many children, because it removes the appetite for other and equally necessary foods. However, it would seem best to retain 1 quart as the standard, and to make exceptions, if necessary, when nutritional prob-

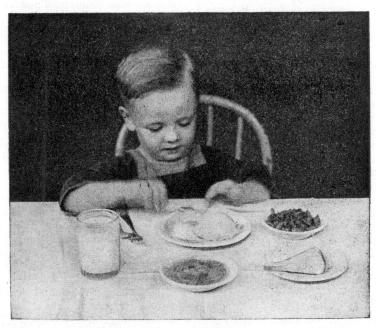

Fig. 90. Noon meal for the normal child of 3 years, in this instance consisting of milk, apple sauce, green beans, bread and butter, mashed potato and poached egg.

lems are encountered. Milk is the only good food source of calcium. The calcium requirement may be met up to the period of adolescence by 1½ pints daily; during adolescence a quart is required. Except for liver, which never is eaten daily, milk is the best food source of riboflavin. The riboflavin recommended allowance may be met by 1½ pints of milk only under 8 years of age. Milk is an excellent source of high quality protein, and a quart daily is an important contribution to the protein requirement. A surprisingly large proportion of children do not receive an optimum of protein.

OTHER IMPORTANT FOODS

In addition to milk, the diet should include at least 1 egg, 1 serving of meat or fish, 2 vegetables, 2 fruits and at least 1 ounce of butter or fortified butter substitute. Other foods are added to satisfy the appetite and the energy requirement. Bread and cereals preferably should be of either the whole grain or the enriched variety. Children should be encouraged to eat larger amounts of vegetables and fruit than ordinarily are taken. A variety of these should be offered early in life in order to avoid formation of definite likes and dislikes.

In choosing the vegetables, tomatoes, peas, string beans, carrots, rutabagas, lettuce, spinach and other greens should be considered superior to celery, parsnips, onions, beets, eggplant and squash. All these vegetables may be used, but some from the first group should be included every day. Of the starchy vegetables and their cereal substitutes, potatoes, lima and navy beans and yellow corn provide more vitamins than white rice, macaroni and white corn. Starchy vegetables should not be substituted for the first groups mentioned, but may be fed in addition to provide needed calories.

The following recommendations are made by the national nutrition program which is promoted by official agencies.

Eat some food from each group each day:

1. Green and yellow vegetables, some raw, some cooked, frozen or canned.

2. Oranges, tomatoes, grapefruit or raw cabbage or salad greens.

3. Potatoes and other vegetables and fruits, raw, dried, cooked, frozen or canned.

4. Milk and milk products, fluid, evaporated or dried milk, cheese, ice cream, cream soups, milk puddings.

5. Meat, poultry, fish or eggs or dried beans, peas, nuts or peanut butter.

6. Bread, flour and cereals, natural whole grain or enriched or restored.

7. Butter or margarine fortified with vitamin A.

In addition to the basic 7, eat any other foods desired.

PREPARATION OF THE DIET

After the nurse has learned the food requirements of the child and how to translate these into terms of actual foods, her task has only begun. Preparing the diet, serving the tray attractively and helping the child to enjoy his food and the social experience are of equal importance.

The methods of preparation of foods for children should be the simplest possible. Meats should be cooked; potatoes, mashed or baked; vegetables, eaten either raw or boiled only until tender and seasoned with salt and butter; desserts should be simple custards, plain puddings or ice cream made with milk and eggs and egg cookies or fruits. Candies, sweets and highly starched desserts should not replace those of better nutritional value. Milk should be served plain unless great difficulty is encountered in getting the child to take a sufficient amount. In special instances, sometimes it is useful to flavor the milk with cocoa rather than omit the milk. Often children develop an interest in milk when they can pour it from a small pitcher. Lettuce and celery usually are served plain. Children usually prefer simple foods to those that are creamed or highly seasoned.

SERVING THE DIET

The nurse or the persons serving the diet should take great care to do it attractively and to have the size of the portions in keeping with the age, the size and the appetite of the child. The tray should be prepared with the individual child's capacity in mind. The hospitalized child seldom has a voracious appetite and he revolts if confronted with large amounts of food. Many children enter the hospital with definite likes and dislikes. These should be taken into account. Only the amount which the nurse believes will be eaten should be served. A child enjoys eating all his food. This statement is substantiated by the frequency with which children show their nurses their emptied plate and say, "Look. I finished it." Disliked foods often will be eaten if served in minute quantities; if they are served in large quantities, even a taste usually is refused. When large quantities are presented, the child has no opportunity to feel accomplished. When a child has learned

to accept one new food, a second one can be introduced. Gradually, in this way, the nurse can help the child become accustomed to greater variety and overcome his dislikes.

Nagging, holding up desserts and placing emphasis on uneaten food evokes antagonism and resistance instead of pleasure. It makes meal hour a miserable experience instead of one which brings enjoyment. Children enjoy helping themselves to food. If convalescent children are eating together at a table, family-style serving fosters an excellent response. They enjoy helping themselves to bread, finger foods like carrot sticks, celery or raisins and revel in using a serving spoon to take independently the amount of "seconds" that they desire.

DIETARY HABITS

When a child has had wise guidance during the early period of personality development, few difficulties will be encountered in helping him to establish good patterns of eating. However, all too frequently, parents do not recognize developmental characteristics that come with growth and fail to change their technic of guidance accordingly. Nor do they always understand the effect of the emotions on the formation of eating habits. "Feeding problems" are encountered frequently by physicians and hospital personnel.

To understand a child's problem and institute a corrective experience which will change his feelings about people and about eating, a knowledge of his background experiences within his family is essential. Children present such varied problems that no set of rules can be evolved

A DIET OF COMMON FOODS SUITABLE FOR A 12-YEAR-OLD CHILD WITH
TABULATION OF ITS CONTENT OF CERTAIN ESSENTIAL NUTRIENTS

	WEIGHT (GMS.)	CALORIES	PROTEIN (GMS.)	FAT (GMS.)	CHO (GMS.)
Milk (pasteurized), 1 qt...........976		666	34.2	38.1	48.0
Egg, 1 54		77	6.1	5.1	0.3
Meat,[1] 1 serving................. 65		130	15.9	7.3	0
Fruit,[2] 2 servings.................200		157	1.4	0.6	36.6
Nonstarchy vegetables,[3] 2 servings..185		66	4.8	0.4	10.8
Starchy vegetables or substitutes,[4] 2 servings 200		205	6.6	0.8	43.0
Enriched bread, 5 slices...........125		338	11.0	4.0	64.8
Cereal (breakfast),[5] 1 serving...... 20		76	2.1	0.5	15.9
Starchy dessert,[6] 1 serving.........120		261	4.4	9.9	38.5
Butter, 3 tblsp................... 42		300	.3	33.9	.3
Cheese 10		43	2.8	3.5	...
Peanut butter, 1 tblsp. 16		92	4.2	7.6	3.4
Sugar° 30		120	0	0	30.0
Cooking fat, 1 tblsp.............. 15		135	0	15.0	...
Cod-liver oil, 1 tsp............... 3.6		34	0	3.6	...
Total.....................		2,700	93.8		
Recommended allowance 12-year-old		2,500	70.0		

Average figures for the given food classes were determined as listed above. All figures are in grams.

Vitamin values for the foods *as served* have been used whenever available.

[1]*Meat:* Pork 75, bacon 20, ham 75, beef 75, hamburger 75, wieners 50, chicken 60, liver 25, salmon 25, fresh fish 25. Total considered as 8 servings and averaged.

[2]*Fruit:* Average of orange 100, grapefruit 100, apple (fresh) 130, apples (canned) 100, pear (fresh) 150, pears (canned) 100, peach (fresh) 100, peaches (canned) 100, plum 50, dried prunes 50, cherries (pitted) 100, strawberries (fresh) 100, pineapple (canned) 100, apricots (canned) 100, apricots (dried) 25, banana 100, watermelon 250, cantaloupe 150, grapes 100, raspberries 75, raisins 60, rhubarb 100. Total, 22 servings.

[3]*Nonstarchy vegetable:* Average of tomato 400, lettuce 50, celery 30, cabbage 150, carrots 150, beets 100, peas 200, string beans 100, spinach 50, turnips 50, squash (yellow) 50, onion 50. Total, 15 servings.

which will apply in every case. The "feeding problem" is a symptom; its cause must be found and remedied before changes in feeding behavior will be noted.

The first factor in helping the child to develop improved eating habits is to establish a constructive relationship with him and observe his behavior as a means of discovering the reasons why he has formed a pattern of resistance to eating. The child with poor feeding habits often responds well when he is placed in a group of children and when *small* portions are served and he is allowed to help himself to seconds. Placing him at the table next to a

A Diet of Common Foods Suitable for a 12-Year-Old Child with
Tabulation of Its Content of Certain Essential Nutrients *(Continued)*

Ca (Mgs.)	Fe (Mgs.)	Vitamin A (I.U.)	Thiamine (Mgs.)	Riboflavin (Mgs.)	Niacin (Mgs.)	Ascorbic Acid (Mgs.)	Vitamin D (I.U.)
1,150	0.7	1,550	0.35	1.68	1.1	12.0	35
26	1.3	550	0.05	0.14	Tr	0	25
9	2.0	880	0.385	0.245	3.3	1.2	
40	1.4	1,420	0.116	0.120	0.8	30.0	
54	1.6	5,080	0.150	0.124	1.0	34.0	
24	2.0	200	0.220	0.106	2.4	16.0	
75	2.0	0	0.24	0.15	2.2	0	
37	1.8	45	0.052	0.045	0.7	0	
56	0.7	320	0.100	0.125	0.5	0.6	
9	0.0	1,380	Tr	Tr	Tr	0	
93	0.1	170	0.010	0.060	0	0	
12	0.3	.....	0.02	0.02	2.6	0	
0	0	0	0	0	0	0	
0	0	0	0	0	0	0	
0	0	3,100	0	0	0	0	310†
1,585	13.9	14,695	1.693	2.815	14.6‡	93.8	370
1,200	12.0	4,500	1.2	1.8	12.	75.0	400

4*Starchy vegetable or substitute:* Average of potato 100, lima beans 35, corn 150, noodles 50, macaroni (cooked) 100, white rice 50, navy beans 35. Total, 15 servings.

5*Cereal, dry weight:* Average of oatmeal 20, farina 20, cornflakes 20, cream of wheat 20, Wheaties 20, shredded wheat 25, puffed rice 10. Total, 7 servings.

6*Starchy desserts:* Ice cream and 2 plain cookies, rice pudding with raisins, bread pudding, chocolate cornstarch pudding, brown betty, chocolate cake, fruit pie. Total, 7 servings, ⅔ cup each.

*Includes sugar of jam, etc.

†Value of minimum standard oil. Most oils contain a larger amount.

‡The full allowance of niacin is not necessary when sufficient milk is included in the diet, because tryptophan of milk can substitute for niacin.

child who delights in meal hours is often a great stimulus to the child who never has learned that eating can be pleasurable. If anorexia is acute, it is usually advisable for the nurse to concentrate her efforts on establishing a good relationship with him by helping him to feel safe and comfortable in his new surroundings. Factors pertaining to the meaning of food and the kind of relationships that are essential in helping children to establish good eating habits are discussed in Chapters 3 and 5.

The child who has been malnourished over long periods of time needs additional help in developing an appetite. Often these children are suffering from infections, and their anorexia has become chronic.

Their diet should be planned very carefully to include all the known stimulants to the development of appetite and it should be increased slowly.

SAMPLE DIET SCHEDULES

4 TO 7 YEARS

Breakfast

Fruit
Cereal with milk
1 egg
Milk, 8 oz. (1 glass)
Toast, cracker or zwieback with butter

Dinner

Beef, chicken, fish, liver or other meat
Mashed potato with butter
½ cup vegetable
Leaf of lettuce
1 slice of bread and butter
Simple pudding or cookie
Milk, 8 oz.

Supper

Egg or fish or liver or cottage cheese
½ cup vegetable
1 slice bread with butter
Fruit
Milk, 8 oz.

Bedtime

Glass of milk and teaspoonful cod-liver oil

8 TO 18 YEARS

Breakfast

Fruit
Cereal with milk
1 or 2 eggs
Milk, 8 oz.
Toast, crackers or zwieback with butter

Dinner

Beef, chicken, fish, liver or other meat
Mashed potato with butter
⅔ cup vegetable
Fresh vegetable or fruit
1 slice of bread with butter
Simple pudding
Milk, 8 oz.

Supper

Egg or fish or liver or cottage cheese
Baked potato or legumes
⅔ cup vegetable
1 slice of bread with butter
Fruit
Milk, 8 oz.

Bedtime

Glass of milk and teaspoonful cod-liver oil

SITUATIONS FOR
FURTHER STUDY

1. Visit a nursery school and observe the noon-meal period. How was the food served? What was the response of the children to the type of food service that was used? What did the teacher do and say during the meal period? How did her behavior affect the children's response to the meal period and to food? Do you think the kind of food service used in the nursery school would be practical for hospital use? What would be the advantages? The disadvantages? What prevents hospital personnel from instituting this type of food service?

2. To study children and the usefulness of a nursery school type of food service, place the ambulatory children at tables for meal period. Group them according to age and sit with them to serve and eat with them in order to observe the following: What contributed toward making the meal period successful or unsuccessful? Of what did pre-meal preparation consist? Did it contribute to the success of the meal period? Which children needed guidance? Why? Describe situations encountered and discuss ways of handling them. Which foods were eaten most readily? Which ones were refused consistently?

What comments were made when children were served small servings of foods that they disliked? When comments were made, what was your response? How did your servings to individual children vary? What influenced variations in serving? Did the placement of a good eater next to a poor eater bring a change in the acceptance of food by the latter? Was this meal period more successful than the ones served in the traditional service style?

3. Observe a child at the table with poor food habits. Does his physical condition influence his disinterestedness in food? What is his response when no attention is paid to his unfinished plate of food? What is his response to minute servings of all food except that which you know he particularly relishes? Does he enjoy pouring his own milk and helping himself to "seconds"? Does he eat and drink more when he is given opportunity to increase his independence? Observe the child when his parents are with him. Has their relationship influenced the development of his poor food habits? Talk to the mother to determine methods of management during the period prior to hospitalization. If his food habits improve during the period of hospitalization, what responsibility would you feel toward the child and his parents? What would be your approach to the mother? How would you counsel her?

Digestive and Nutritional Diseases

COLIC

CONSTIPATION

VOMITING

DIARRHEA

DEHYDRATION

MALNUTRITION IN INFANCY

MALNUTRITION IN CHILDHOOD

OBESITY

CELIAC DISEASE

CYSTIC FIBROSIS OF THE PANCREAS

SITUATIONS FOR FURTHER STUDY

COLIC

Infants in the first few months of life who have frequent fits of sudden crying are commonly regarded as suffering from colic. There are many theories about the nature of colic which govern the type of treatment. It is entirely possible that several factors may be responsible and that the behavior observed is merely the response of an immature infant to any of a number of types of discomfort.

Infants who suffer from colic are generally small at birth (5 to 7 lbs.). They tend to be lean with tense muscles and a nervous system which easily is triggered into a maximum response by the slightest of stimuli. During much of their day such infants are either asleep or violently protesting their discomfort. They do not remain long in the middle ground of quiet, satisfied wakefulness. The symptoms tend to be worse in the early evening and the night-time hours than they are during the day. The persistence of this type of behavior is variable. In many instances it ceases rather abruptly—often without any particular change in regimen. Such a welcome cessation may come at from 3 to 4 weeks or as late as from 3 to 4 months. The colloquial designation "3-month colic" suggests the average duration and enforces the suspicion that it is predetermined and not related to treatment.

The behavior of an infant with colic usually is suggestive of paroxysmal abdominal pain due to excessive accumulation of gas in the intestine or the stomach. Crying starts abruptly with loud screams, clenched fists and legs that are drawn up on the abdomen. During the general muscular contraction, gas may be expelled from the anus or may be belched up from the stomach. The traditional efforts to explain and treat colic center around control of the gas production within the intestinal tract.

Excessive air-swallowing often is considered as an important factor. Too rapid feeding during which the infant gulps down air is blamed sometimes. Small nipple holes or a breast that yields little milk can result in vigorous sucking and swallowing efforts which also carry an excessive amount of air into the stomach. Depending upon the individual situation, the feeding procedure may need to be altered. Frequent burping of the baby during and after feeding usually is advised. The use of carminatives such as peppermint water and fennel tea to aid in relaxation of the cardiac sphincter of the stomach is a household remedy that is not generally very effective. Enemas, suppositories and rectal tubes to relieve distention of the lower bowel are advised sometimes, but the same result usually can be achieved by turning the infant on his abdomen.

The accumulation of gas in the intestine is attributed by some to intestinal indigestion from overfeeding or from excessive use of carbohydrate, which fosters intestinal fermentation and produces gas within the lumen of the bowel. On this basis, various modifications of the amount and the type of formula are made.

Another approach is the attempt to reduce the vigor of intestinal movements by the use of drugs such as atropine and its derivatives, phenobarbital and banthine. The local application of heat by the use of a hot-water bottle also is advocated by some.

Yet another theory holds that colic is largely emotionally conditioned. The fact that many colicky infants are relieved of their distress merely by being held or permitted to suck on a pacifier is cited as evidence that the disturbance may be due to insufficient emotional satisfaction, and mothers are encouraged to give their infants additional cuddling and closeness as a temporary measure.

Whatever the importance of these various factors, at the present time it cannot be said that colic has a single etiology or appropriate treatment. The measures that are important for relief of the individual infant (and its mother) must be worked out by trial and error in each instance.

CONSTIPATION

Constipation exists when the bowels move infrequently or with difficulty or both. Usually it produces no symptoms, although there may be local pain from the passage of a large hard fecal mass. Occasionally in infancy streaks of blood are found on the outside of the stool, the blood having come from a fissure at the anus. Only rarely and only in infancy does constipation cause prolapse of the anus or the rectum. General symptoms from constipation either do not exist or are too vague to be identified.

Constipation results when the stimulus to peristalsis is insufficient or when the intestine fails to respond to a normal stimulus. Since the normal stimulus to peristalsis is food, insufficient food results in constipation. Intestinal irritability varies in different infants and children and from time to time in the same infant or child. Constipation results also when the intestinal content is of such consistency from absorption of water in the lower bowel that it is difficult for it to move onward even though peristalsis is active.

Certain anomalies of the intestinal tract lead to constipation. Constipation from such causes is uncommon as compared with those due to causes associated with food. The constipation accompanying pyloric stenosis in infancy is due to the dearth of food passing the pylorus. The constipation of megacolon is caused by mechanical interference in the lower part of the colon.

In infancy, underfeeding or persistent vomiting may cause constipation. Usually with insufficient food the stools are small and infrequent, although occasionally as a result of underfeeding the stools may be as numerous as from 8 to 10 a day. Constipation in a breast-fed baby is most frequently due to underfeeding. However, in some instances the stools are infrequent when the amount of food seems to be adequate.

When constipation is present in either a breast-fed or an artificially fed baby and the food seems to be adequate and the infant is thriving, the addition of fruits and vegetables to the diet, or an increase in the amount of these if they already are being fed, often serves to give the little increase in stimulus that is necessary. Strained orange juice usually is not laxative because the dextrose is absorbed so quickly. Prune juice is somewhat laxative.

Constipation in the artificially fed infant often may be relieved by increasing the amount of sugar in the formula. A formula high in sugar and low in milk is laxative; the reverse proportion tends to be constipating. Thus a balance between the amount of milk and the amount of added sugar is important in regulating the frequency and the consistency of the stools. The imbalance between the amounts of milk and sugar may be so great as to bring about marked and obstinate constipation. With a high-milk, low-sugar diet the lower intestinal content is alkaline in reaction, and relatively insoluble calcium and magnesium soaps form firm puttylike masses which are moved on with difficulty even though peristalsis may be active. A further disadvantage is the existence of conditions unfavorable for the absorption of calcium and fats. Because of the long stay and the slow advancement of the intestinal content, the bile pigments are changed so that the stool is a very light or even a grayish-white color. This type of constipation has been designated fat constipation, although this is not an appropriate term. If fat is eliminated from the diet, constipation ceases because the formation of soap masses is no longer possible. However, constipation is relieved with equal promptness and effectiveness by increasing the sugar or decreasing the milk protein with no change in the amount of fat. Often in this condition it is desirable to use the more laxative varieties of sugar. The liquid malt preparations, such as malt soup extract, are useful.

Constipation in the child, in addition to factors already discussed, may be produced by disregard of the impulse to go to stool or failure to bring the abdominal muscles into use during defecation, either because of inability or disinclination to make the effort. Once constipation is established, the intestinal tract may require a stimulus greater than that required normally. Children who are constipated frequently are not eating as many fruits and vegetables as they should. Sometimes an increase in the fruit and vegetable intake is all that is necessary. Regularity in habits in regard to defecation should be established. The child should be encouraged to make the effort to defecate as soon as he feels an impulse to do so.

Drugs preferably should not be used in the management of constipation. If laxatives seem to be necessary in the beginning of treatment they should be given regularly and not occasionally as apparently needed. The amount should be decreased gradually until none is being taken. For infants, magnesia magma (milk of magnesia) is effective and relatively mild. For children, phenolphthalein, magnesia magma and preparations of cascara sagrada are most useful. Castor oil should not be used for this purpose, since constipation is an after-effect of its cathartic action, and small doses definitely lead to constipation. Mineral oil by mouth is in common use but it should not be given in close relationship to meals and preferably should not be continued over long periods. It acts by keeping the intestinal content more fluid and more bulky.

A preferable way to increase the bulk and the blandness of the stool is to give any one of several available preparations that take up and retain water. One of these is dried mucillaginous material extracted from psyllium seeds; often a teaspoonful daily, mixed with water or milk, is sufficient. Another preparation with similar action is methylcellulose. Bran is widely used in the treatment of constipation and acts

by increasing the bulk of the stool; its use is held in disfavor by many physicians because it seems so often to lead to spastic colitis.

Enemas may be necessary at times to relieve difficult situations but they are too likely to lead to habitual need of increased stimulation to be useful as a regular means of relief. In addition, they may evoke rebellious feelings in the child and make him feel attacked, punished or robbed. Suppositories also may lead to habitual need and are contraindicated, both for physical and psychological reasons. Suitable massage of the abdomen often is recommended and at times may be of benefit.

VOMITING

Vomiting is much more frequent in infancy than in childhood and occurs from more trivial causes. Even though the cause is minor, the effects of vomiting are highly important to the infant. Vomiting is frequent in infancy from gastric distention and from the effects of parenteral infection; it is infrequent in childhood from these two causes. Other causes of vomiting are much the same in both infancy and childhood.

GASTRIC DISTENTION

Gastric distention from any cause results in vomiting in infancy. When the stomach is overfilled with food, it reacts by expelling the excess. Expulsion of food from this cause may be no more than a little regurgitation of a small or moderate amount of partly altered milk, which pours out of the mouth with no expulsive effort. This safety-valve action of the stomach in rejecting excessive amounts of food tends to protect the infant from the really serious consequences of overfeeding. A few infants have a small gastric capacity and are unable, without vomiting, to take all the food needed when it is offered in the usual dilutions. In such cases it is necessary to use a more concentrated food. When food is given at such short intervals that the stomach is not empty before the next feeding, vomiting often results from overfilling the stomach. When food is taken too rapidly, insufficient food leaves the stomach during the feeding, with distention and vomiting as a result.

A common cause of overdistention of the stomach is the gas that it contains in addition to food. The gas is chiefly swallowed air and may be present in large amounts. All babies swallow some air. The amount swallowed is increased when they are hungry or when the food intake is insufficient or when the milk is obtained from the nipple with difficulty. When the infant is lying on his back, the air cannot escape without first forcing out part of the fluid. Abdominal bands or clothes that are too tight have the same effect as gastric distention in producing vomiting.

IRRITATION OF THE STOMACH

Irritation of the stomach may cause vomiting at any age. It is produced sometimes in the older child by indiscretions in diet or by the ingestion of partially spoiled food. In the infant, vomiting may be caused by unusual food or by food that has "fermented" in the stomach. An excess of fat in the food of an infant prolongs the emptying time of the stomach, so that a condition favorable to bacterial decomposition is created, and vomiting may result from the irritating products formed and also from overfilling of the stomach by the cumulative bulk of one feeding and the residue of the preceding feeding. An excess of sugar is not likely to cause vomiting unless a general gastro-intestinal indigestion occurs. Intestinal indigestion is associated with decreased gastric function, both as to motility and secretion, and therefore it is frequently accompanied by vomiting. The same is true for inflammation of the intestine, such as dysentery.

OBSTRUCTION OF THE GASTRO-INTESTINAL TRACT

Obstruction of the gastro-intestinal tract of any type causes vomiting at any age. During infancy, hypertrophic stenosis of the pylorus is the most common variety of obstruction. On rare occasions obstruction in the young infant is caused by congenital atresia of the intestine, especially of the duodenum, or by other congenital malformation. Intussusception is a variety of obstruction occurring chiefly in infants. Inflammation in the abdomen, such as peritonitis, causes functional or organic obstruction at any age.

CONDITIONS OUTSIDE THE GASTRO-INTESTINAL TRACT

One of the most frequent causes of vomiting, as well as of diarrhea, in infancy is upper respiratory infection or other infection outside the intestinal tract (parenteral infection). At any age vomiting is associated with conditions affecting the central nervous system, such as tumor, hemorrhage and meningitis.

Certain allergies, especially to foods, may cause vomiting. The intoxications, such as uremia and cyclic vomiting, which are a cause of emesis, occur almost exclusively in children past infancy. Vomiting occurs at any age in association with severe coughing, especially that of whooping cough.

RUMINATION AND VOLUNTARY VOMITING

Some infants and young children are able to bring up food from the stomach at will. Others initiate vomiting by putting a hand into the mouth. When voluntary vomiting becomes a regular habit without known provocation, it is spoken of as rumination. Rumination usually occurs only in infancy. In certain instances, voluntary vomiting is a reaction of the infant or the child to unusual foods or foods that he does not like. Occasionally, vomiting develops as a result of the infant's or the child's reaction to his environment and management, such as the forcing of food. Vomiting from these latter causes is amenable to proper management, although often the environment must be changed completely to accomplish the desired result.

NURSING CARE OF INFANTS WHO VOMIT

When an infant shows a tendency to vomit, unusual care in feeding is necessary. In each case the infant's tolerance should be noted. The nursing care should be planned to eliminate unnecessary movement of the infant after feeding. Too much handling and tossing about of an infant often leads to vomiting. Treatments leading to emotional strain should neither precede nor follow feeding. The food should be kept warm and given slowly. Care in "bubbling" the baby is especially important. He should be held up after each feeding and should be patted gently on the back until the air is expelled. Holding the infant in an erect position allows the air bubble to lodge at the cardiac orifice, from which location it may escape easily without causing vomiting. Some infants have to be held up in this manner before and during feeding, as well as afterward. Placing the infant on his side and elevating the head of the bed after feeding tends to prevent vomiting and aspiration; in this position gas is expelled from the stomach more freely.

In the case of very weak babies, such as those prematurely born, vomiting is to be guarded against by every means possible. In these instances the vomitus is likely to be aspirated. The resultant pneumonia is serious and often fatal.

When vomiting occurs, skin irritation will be prevented by care of the skin of the face, behind the ears and in the folds of the neck. Charting is important. Not only is it necessary to chart the estimated amount of vomitus and the relation to feeding, but the type, the nature, the color, the consistency and the odor and the presence or the absence of nausea also may aid in diagnosis. Differentiation should be made between regurgitation, projectile vomiting and the vomiting that occurs at the time that air is expelled.

Infants who ruminate must be observed closely and provided with substitute satisfactions. Ruminator caps have been devised. These fit firmly over the chin and the throat and prevent movement of the tongue and the throat muscles which bring the food back into the mouth. At the time of feeding, the cap is loosened. Immediately after feeding the cap should be readjusted, and an effort should be made to divert the infant's attention to something that is interesting and pleasurable to him. Constant attention until the infant falls asleep or until the food has left the stomach is necessary. Such a method provides a substitute wholesome satisfaction for one that is essentially depriving.

Arm restraints often are ordered to prevent the infant from initiating vomiting with his hands. However, restraints without play materials and a close personal relationship often are not only ineffectual but also sufficiently frustrating to create additional emotional tension which tends to fix rather than eliminate the habit.

DIARRHEA

Diarrhea is a symptom having many possible causes. It is a result of increased peristalsis, the intestinal content being hurried along with diminished absorption and therefore being passed in a more or less fluid state. Increased peristalsis may result from increased irritability of the intestinal tract, from irritant action of abnormal intestinal content or from the stimulus of unusual bulk of intestinal content. Increased irritability occurs in some nervous persons under emotional stress and in those with inflammation of the intestinal tract. Irritants producing diarrhea may be indigestible or undigested foods, foods to which the intestinal tract is allergic or foods

contaminated in such a manner as to cause food poisoning. Diarrhea may be caused by impairment of absorption, such as occurs in celiac disease or pellagra, which increases the bulk of the intestinal content.

DIARRHEA IN INFANCY

Diarrhea occurs more frequently in infants than in children and often from causes that have no similar effect in the child. The effects of diarrhea tend to be more serious for the infant. In the past, diarrheal diseases caused a higher mortality rate among infants than any other disease or condition. Due to increased and more widespread knowledge of infant feeding and care, deaths of infants from diarrhea have decreased greatly. However, they are still too prevalent, especially among those in congested districts and in other unfavored social and economic groups.

Diarrhea as discussed in this section is that which occurs on a functional basis. Babies have a limited digestive capacity and a need for relatively large amounts of food. The margin between the amount of food needed and the amount that can be digested and absorbed is not large. When digestive capacity is exceeded, indigestion and diarrhea are likely to result. Digestive capacity is decreased by illness and infection; it is decreased when the hygiene of the baby is poor, as when he is overdressed in hot weather and heat is allowed to be retained excessively; it is decreased in the presence of severe malnutrition and in conditions causing impaired blood circulation, such as congenital malformation of the heart. When digestive capacity is decreased, continuance of a normal diet is likely to cause diarrhea.

Diarrhea is less frequent and less severe among breast-fed babies than among those artificially fed. The reasons for this difference are several. Human milk requires much less acidification in the stomach to prepare it for digestion and for passage beyond the stomach; secretion of acid in the stomach is decreased during illness. The bacterial content and the preparation of cow's milk may be such as to lead to digestive disturbances.

Functional or food diarrhea in infants is associated with and perhaps is caused by increased bacterial activity. Normally, the upper intestine is relatively free from bacteria, but in food diarrhea the upper intestine has been found to contain bacteria in abundance. The bacteria found are those normally present in the lower part of the tract. A possible explanation of food diarrhea is that the increased peristalsis is caused by products of excessive bacterial activity. That irritating products are present at least in the lower intestine in association with diarrhea is evidenced by the large amounts of organic acids present in diarrheal stools and the consequent excoriation of skin wherever the stool remains for a time in contact.

In extremely severe diarrhea with intoxication and dehydration, factors in addition to those discussed seem to be operating. It appears as though the body tissues generally had lost much of their ability to retain water, that they give up water which normally would be a part of their composition or normally stored and that the water thus freed leaves the body to a large extent through the intes-

tinal tract. In this condition, fluid which is administered parenterally is not retained, and after administration an increase in the stools often may be noted. In some instances this very severe type of diarrhea with failure of water retention has been found to be dependent upon certain varieties of mastoid or paranasal sinus suppuration without drainage. In these instances, as soon as adequate treatment of the infection has been established, water is retained again, and diarrhea ceases; it would seem that some toxic substance absorbed from the infection site is responsible for the diarrhea to a greater degree than is the lowered digestive function which is observed secondary to parenteral infection in general.

Prevention of Diarrhea. Diarrhea in infants is classed among the preventable diseases. A study of the enumerated causes of diarrhea makes obvious many preventive measures. Whenever possible, babies should be breast-fed, especially in unfavored socio-economic groups. In these same groups, care must be used in weaning from the breast in hot summer weather. Overdressing should be avoided, and additional fluids should be offered in hot weather. At all times the hygiene should be such as will tend to prevent infections of all kinds. Nutrition and growth progress should be supervised by a competent observer, even though the baby is well.

Symptoms. Passage of stools varies in frequency according to the severity of the disturbance. The greater the frequency, the more watery the stools. With very frequent stools the bile pigment color may be lost by dilution. Stool color changes are discussed further elsewhere. Because of speed of passage of food through the intestine, some food, particularly fat, escapes digestion or absorption. Intestinal irritation causes excessive secretion of mucus. Thus, besides water in a diarrheal stool, mucus, fatty acids and free fat may be found. A large water loss by bowel causes diminished urine output.

Weight decrease results from both food and water loss. Increased peristalsis causes discomfort and results in fretfulness, irritability and disturbed sleep. In the absence of parenteral infection, fever is only moderate and transitory, except when severe dehydration is present. Even with diarrhea secondary to upper respiratory infection, fever is often only moderate and sometimes absent.

The most serious results of severe or prolonged diarrhea are starvation and dehydration. The starvation is due to diarrheal food loss and often to associated vomiting and to subsequent therapeutic underfeeding. Some water loss always occurs in diarrhea. Frequently, the loss is great enough to cause serious or even fatal dehydration unless compensated by fluids given parenterally.

Management of Diarrhea. The management of diarrhea varies according to associated conditions and circumstances, although the general principles are the same in all instances. An occasional loose stool or a slight increase in the number of stools is not an invariable indication for a change in food, provided that the infant continues to gain and exhibits no other symptoms. In general, the indication in diarrhea is to diminish or temporarily withhold food completely. A short period without food allows the intestine to empty and permits conditions in the intestine partially or completely to return to normal. A cathartic is not indicated. Diarrhea sufficiently severe to require fasting empties the intestine adequately.

Complete deprivation of food rarely is necessary for breast-fed babies, in whom diarrhea is seldom severe. Decreasing food intake during the febrile period of infection by shortening the time at the breast, together with maintaining the fluid intake, usually suffices. When the diarrhea is more severe, boiled or acidified skimmed milk without added sugar may be substituted for part of the breast feeding. Periodic emptying of the mother's breasts is important.

In the case of artificially fed babies, moderate diarrhea does not require complete deprivation of food but only a reduction of total food, of sugar alone or of sugar and fat, depending on the severity of the diarrhea. Boiled unsweetened skimmed milk or acidified skimmed milk is a good initial food in mild diarrhea. In the more severe diarrheas, complete deprivation of food is indicated. The duration of fast depends on the severity of the diarrhea and the nutritional state of the infant. The milder disturbances may respond to the omission of one or two feedings. Rarely is a fast longer than 24 hours desirable for food diarrhea, and seldom as long as this.

Whether or not food is given, the need of the baby for water is increased. The more severe diarrheas often are associated with vomiting, making difficult or impossible the supplying of sufficient fluid by mouth. However, for most babies with food diarrhea, water may be given satisfactorily. For babies who refuse plain water, the addition of saccharin, ¼ grain to 4 ounces of water, may be satisfactory. A 5-percent solution of dextrose also is used frequently. If water or fluid is refused or vomited, it may become necessary to give suitable solutions parenterally.

The response to fast is usually favorable, although not always. Occasionally, the stools continue to be watery, even after a 24-hour fast. Although a long period of fasting may be desirable for the gastrointestinal tract, it might endanger the life of a poorly nourished infant unless food is given parenterally.

After the fast the most satisfactory food is one relatively high in milk protein, low in fat and without added sugar. Boiled skimmed milk is such a food. Often acidification is advantageous. Usually the energy intake can be increased early by the addition of dextrose. As rapidly as digestive capacity permits, whole milk may be substituted for the skimmed milk and used in quantity suitable for the age of the infant.

Protein milk has had a long-established usage in the management of diarrhea, although at present it is being used decreasingly. It consists of the curd from a quart of whole milk, plus a pint of lactic-acid skimmed milk and sufficient water to make a quart. The average composition is fat 2.5 per cent, sugar 1.5 per cent, protein 3.5 per cent; it has available 13 calories to the ounce. Protein milk is difficult to prepare but it can be purchased ready prepared in dried form. When used, it is given as the first food after fast. Sugar additions must be made early. After a sugar addition, the composition does not differ importantly from that of acidified partially skimmed fresh milk.

THE APPLE IN TREATMENT. The apple and its products have been used extensively in the past in the treatment for diarrhea, especially for older infants and young children. Originally, the treatment consisted of giving scraped raw apple, in amounts of from 1 to 4 tablespoonfuls every hour or two. Canned apple powder is available commercially and is equally effective and more convenient. It is used in a 4- to 10-per-cent solution for infants. Because pectin seems to be the effective component of the apple in the treatment of diarrhea, pectin has come into use in various forms. It is available everywhere in a 5-per-cent solution for the purpose of preparing fruit jellies. According to the age or the size of the infant, from 2 to 6 ounces of this product may be given daily. One commercial firm produces a dextrin-maltose mixture with pectin and agar for the special purpose of treating babies with diarrhea. When the diarrhea is relatively severe, the apple or pectin treatment is given after the period of fast and without other food for as long as 2 or 3 days. When the diarrhea is moderate, the pectin may be given with an appropriate milk mixture from the beginning and without fast.

DRUGS have relatively little use in the treatment of diarrhea. Cathartics are not indicated in most instances. Opium is useful at times in controlling loss of water and salts and also in relieving abdominal discomfort and permitting rest. Opium is usually given as paregoric in a dosage of 5 to 15 minims, according to the size of the baby. Phenobarbital in a dosage of from ⅛ to ¼ gr. is often useful in overcoming restlessness and irritability. Bismuth preparations often are recommended, although their usefulness is doubtful. Bismuth salts, to be effective, must be given in large amounts, since they act only mechanically by protecting the mucous membrane against irritation. Bismuth subcarbonate is greatly to be preferred to the subnitrate because of the danger of poisoning by nitrite produced from nitrate by bacteria. In the rarely encountered instances of diarrhea caused by imbalance between the sympathetic and the parasympathetic nervous control of the intestine (gastroenterospasm), atropine is a most useful remedy. The dosage is discussed under Pyloric Stenosis.

Management of Parenteral Infection. The measures that have been described for the management of babies with diarrhea concern chiefly the adjustment of the food and the care of the intestinal tract. When diarrhea is dependent on parenteral infection, much is to be accomplished by treatment of the infection. The appropriate use of antibiotics is an important part of the treatment of parenteral diarrhea.

Nursing Care. If water loss has been great, the infant usually will take fluids eagerly and in quantities that he cannot tolerate. When fluids by mouth are begun, small amounts at half-hourly intervals should be given until his tolerance has been estimated. When vomiting is present, the nursing care must be

modified according to the specific indications in each case.

Frequent changes in position are desirable in the effort to prevent intercurrent infections. Dressing the infant lightly in hot weather keeps him more comfortable and minimizes the loss of fluid by perspiration. An accurate description of each stool gives information on the infant's progress and is a guide in prescribing formulas and fluids. The nurse must be alert to the occurrence of pus or blood in the stools. When dehydration is present, a record of frequency of urination is important.

Several individualized technics are indicated. Isolation technic is desirable. After changing the diaper, the hands should be washed thoroughly before the infant's formula is handled. When diarrhea is severe, it may become advisable to take the temperature in the axilla, since the insertion of the thermometer into the rectum is irritating and causes bowel evacuation. In the endeavor to prevent redness and excoriation of the buttocks, the diapers should be changed frequently and the buttocks and the genitalia cleansed with oil on cotton. If redness or excoriation should appear, a further protection against the acid stool is afforded by a bland ointment or paste. A paste with the following composition has been found useful:

Bismuth subnitrate . . . 8 Gm. (dram 2)
Balsam of Peru. . . . . 4 cc. (dram 1)
Castor oil . . . . 4 cc. (dram 1)
Petrolatum . . . . .16 Gm. (dram 4)

Often it may be desirable to avoid contact of the skin with the stool to a greater degree and to have the affected skin exposed to warm air and light to promote healing. Keeping the infant on his abdomen gives the greatest exposure, but care must be taken to prevent irritation of the skin of the knees, the toes and the chin and, above all, suffocation. The equipment to be used for light exposure depends on what is available and to some extent on the season of the year. A bed cradle with a lamp attached in the dome serves well, or the lamp may be attached to the side of the crib with tape. The lamp should be equipped with a 25-watt bulb, protected by a shade or a wire cage and adjusted 12 inches from the infant's body. The precautions are to prevent overheating and burns. After cleansing the buttocks and the genitalia, the infant should be placed comfortably on his abdomen or on his side. With or without a bed cradle, a tent which leaves the infant's head in the open may be made. A sheet may be used to form the tent, covering the lower portion of the bed, and a folded diaper to form the front. Nursing in relation to administration of parenteral fluids is discussed under Dehydration.

Diarrhea in Childhood

Most of the diarrheas of childhood are mild and of little serious consequence. The exceptions (dysentery, typhoid fever, chronic ulcerative colitis, celiac disease) are discussed separately. Fever, heat and parenteral infections do not cause diarrhea in childhood as they do in infancy. Dietary indiscretion is the most frequent cause.

From time to time there have been observed small epidemics of what has been termed colloquially "abdominal influenza." These presumably are caused by a virus infection. Although the attacks are distressing and are associated with diarrhea, they are of short duration.

Food poisoning does not affect children as frequently as adults, because children do not eat so often at places or in circumstances likely to be associated with foods contaminated in the special ways necessary to produce this disease. The most frequent food poisoning is that produced by the growth of *Staphylococcus aureus* in foods. The foods most likely to be contaminated are those such as chicken salad, the preparation of which requires direct use of the hands, and those which, after inoculation, are kept under conditions permitting the organisms to grow. Some staphylococci have an exotoxin which under conditions of food poisoning causes severe symptoms, including diarrhea, within a few hours of ingestion. Although severe prostration results, few deaths occur.

For diarrhea of the type commonly encountered in childhood, little special treatment is called for. A laxative may be useful in cases in which dietary indiscretion is definite. Water is tolerated by mouth sufficiently well that none is necessary parenterally. A short period of rest of the alimentary tract from food often is desirable. Simple carbohydrate foods, such as cereals, crackers and toast, serve well as first foods. The apple treatment is as effective for children as for infants.

Epidemic Diarrhea of the Newborn

A highly communicable type of diarrhea in the newborn has become increasingly frequent. In some epidemics varieties of Streptococcus, Staphylococcus, Salmonella and other organisms have been found in fecal cultures. In the majority of epidemics no bacterial cause has been shown, and in several epidemics a virus has been demonstrated. Although the disease is communicable from baby to baby, it seems likely that the chief distributors are apparently healthy adult carriers. It occurs at all seasons and chiefly in the northern part of this country.

The incubation period is 5 days or less. During the invasion period the baby nurses poorly and becomes fretful and listless. After the diarrhea starts, the stools are watery and without obvious pus, blood or mucus; they often are passed explosively. The baby becomes increasingly prostrated, drowsy and restless. The cry becomes feeble. The temperature is normal, or the elevation is slight. Dehydration and acidosis develop quickly. The severity of the disease varies, but in the average case the illness is serious. The duration is from a few days to several weeks. With meticulous and expert care, most of the babies will live; however, the mortality in general is high, up to 40 per cent or more.

If the causative organism is known, appropriate sulfonamide and antibiotic treatment is indicated. While waiting for laboratory results, it is often advisable to treat with broad spectrum antibiotics on the chance that the cause may be bacterial. For the virus disease no specific treatment is yet known. In most instances it is best to withhold all oral feeding. Dehydration and acidosis are controlled by giving appropriate solutions parenterally. The fast in this condition is likely to be longer than for any other diarrheal disease; it may be a week or more before food can be given safely by mouth. In such case, appropriate supportive treatment includes parenteral administration of amino acid and glucose solutions for food, as well as electrolyte solutions for dehydration and acidosis. It is advisable to include thiamine and ascorbic acid among the nutrients supplied.

Preventive measures for this disease consist of sound nursing practice at all times and the use of aseptic technic when the disease occurs. It is largely because of epidemic diarrhea that terminal sterilization of formulas has come into use. In a hospital nursery, babies suspected of developing the condition should be removed to isolation quarters promptly and those who have been exposed should be watched closely. It is preferable also to keep babies who have been exposed isolated from those newly admitted.

DYSENTERY

Dysentery is the result of the growth of pathogenic micro-organisms in the tissues of the gastrointestinal tract. Most frequently it is caused by the dysentery bacillus, although other organisms at times are responsible. That which is caused by the typhoid bacillus and the Salmonella group is discussed in Chapter 18.

Amebic Dysentery. Amebiasis is a term applied to human infestation with *Endamoeba histolytica* whether or not diarrhea is present. This term applies to the symptomless carrier and to the carrier with mild occasional symptoms, as well as to those with acute dysentery. All these conditions are interrelated, since all these states may exist at different times in the same person. The acute disease may subside, to be followed by a carrier state and possibly by further acute attacks later.

The acute form of the disease, dysentery, is characterized by active invasion of the wall of the colon by ameba, with the formation of necrotic pockets similar to abscesses and with ultimate discharge of the necrotic material into the bowel. The acute stage is associated with nausea, vomiting, colic, abdominal pain, tenesmus, diarrhea and the passage of blood and mucus in the bile-stained fluid stool. Usually there is little or no fever. The child becomes depressed and loses strength. Spontaneous recovery may occur without special treatment.

Amebiasis is more common in adults than in children. Amebic dysentery is rare in infants in this country. Amebiasis is more common in warm than cold climates, although probably the condition is related more to primitive sanitary conditions than to climate. The form of the parasite that causes the acute phase of the disease is not communicable to reproduce the disease. The disease is transmitted by an encysted form of the ameba which occurs in carriers and in those with chronic forms of amebiasis. Only this encysted form can survive the passage through the stomach and the upper intestine. The disease is acquired through contaminated food and water, chiefly

water that has been polluted with sewage.

The diagnosis is made by finding ameba in the stools or in scrapings obtained from an ulcer site through a proctoscope. Death from this disease is uncommon in childhood. Death may occur from dehydration, hemorrhage from an ulceration, perforation of the bowel or from an overwhelming toxemia of the fulminant infection.

Until recently in the treatment of amebiasis, drugs were used which are toxic for humans but more toxic for the ameba. The drug of choice for diarrhea is emetine, given parenterally in closely controlled dosage. After the diarrhea has ceased and for those who have amebiasis without diarrhea, chiniofon is given by mouth as the usual drug of choice. Other drugs sometimes used, especially in supplementary treatment, are acetarsone and carbarsone. All these drugs are toxic and must be given with care. Recently it has been found that certain of the antibiotics are effective in both the acute and the chronic disease. Chlortetracycline is potent, but some relapses have occurred. Oxytetracycline has produced improvement in the acute disease within 72 hours and with further treatment has caused disappearance of the cystic and the vegetative forms.

Bacillary Dysentery. ETIOLOGY. Bacillary dysentery may be caused by any one of several varieties of dysentery bacilli. The Shiga type of organism in general causes the most severe illness, but it is much less common in this country than the various strains of the Flexner type. The Shiga bacillus has an exotoxin, and an effective antiserum can be prepared. This is not true of the Flexner bacilli. Bacillary dysentery is a communicable infection, with the alimentary tract the portal of entry. The source is fecal, and the organism is transmitted chiefly through food. Flies have been shown to be carriers. Numerous milk-borne and water-borne epidemics are on record. The disease is more common in summer and more common in warm than in cold climates.

The inflammation resulting from this infection is most marked in the colon and may be limited to this part of the bowel. Often the lower ileum is affected also. The extent of the inflammation varies from a simple catarrhal process in mild disease to extensive ulceration causing the passage of pus and blood.

SYMPTOMS. After an incubation period of from 2 to 3 days, the onset of the disease usually is sudden. Vomiting and diarrhea are early symptoms. The vomiting may or may not persist throughout the attack. The usual constitutional evidences of infection are present. The white blood cells are increased. Prostration and anorexia are present early. Weight loss soon becomes evident. The temperature usually is not high and may be expected to range from 99° to 102° F., except as neglected dehydration causes it to become higher. Abdominal pain and tenesmus are common. Rectal prolapse may occur. The duration of the disease is from a few days in the mildest illnesses to several weeks in the more severe, except when the course is shortened by the use of sulfonamide drugs or antibiotics.

COMPLICATIONS. The most common complications are otitis media, pyuria and pneumonia. When the dysentery infection is severe, profuse hemorrhage from the bowel or perforation of the bowel wall may occur. With severe or prolonged dysentery in those already in poor nutritional state, the effects of various deficiencies may become evident, such as nutritional edema, noma and various avitaminoses. Also, skin infections, especially about the head, may appear.

PROGNOSIS. Much of the dysentery in children in this country at present is not as severe as that observed formerly or as that which occurs in some other countries. The disease is much more serious for the infant than for the child. This is especially true of infants being cared for in a hospital because of other illness. The mortality rate among infants has ranged up to or above 30 per cent in the past. The present rate is much lower when modern therapy is used.

DIAGNOSIS in the typical disease is not difficult. It is made definitely by identifying the dysentery bacillus in cultures of pus or other material from the stools. At times dysentery has been confused with intussusception because of bloody stools. Occasionally meningitis has been the original impression because of meningismus.

TREATMENT AND NURSING CARE. Bacillary dysentery responds promptly to sulfonamides and to several of the antibiotics (chloramphenicol, chlortetracycline, oxytetracycline). With any of these preparations improvement may be noted within a few hours and relative freedom from symptoms within a day or two. With these newer remedies, the average duration of the disease has been reduced from 2 weeks to a few days.

Fasting is desirable until diarrhea decreases and vomiting ceases. When food is given, it should be of a type that will not aggravate diarrhea; this could be boiled skimmed milk with added sugar. Restoration of body fluid and electrolyte content may be necessary. Pain and tenesmus may be relieved by small doses of paregoric.

The nursing care of a child with bacillary dysentery is similar to the care of a child with diarrhea from other causes, except that more strict isolation is required. The causative organisms are abundant in the stools, and strict aseptic technic is necessary until stool cultures no longer show them. Effort should be made to discover the source of the infection. If the disease has been contracted because of negligence or ignorance in care, education of the family is desirable to prevent recurrence.

DEHYDRATION

Dehydration of the body or, as it has been termed, anhydremia results when for any reason the water intake becomes less than the water excretion. Striking examples are seen most frequently in association with severe diarrhea, especially when the diarrhea is accompanied by vomiting. It is seen in cases of pyloric stenosis in which the vomiting is so severe that practically no food or water is retained. The condition may occur also when dry breasts supply the entire fluid intake of the infant, when food and water are refused or when because of coma or for other reason the oral administration of fluid is difficult.

A relatively small proportion of the water of the body is held within the cells of body tissues; a much larger proportion is outside of and around the cells. That outside the cells is known as interstitial water. The interstitial water is labile and changes in amount with different degrees of hydration of the body. The chief reason the infant dehydrates so much more easily than the older person is that he has approximately twice as much interstitial water in proportion to the body weight. The interstitial water contains salts, chiefly sodium chloride and sodium bicarbonate in concentrations relatively constant. Neither the water nor the salts can remain in the body without the other. When water is lost, as in diarrhea, it is certain that electrolyte (salt) also has been lost. Consequently, the giving of water alone or of dextrose solution alone does not suffice to correct dehydration unless the salts are available from the food. Salt solution or Ringer's solution supplies the needed salts without dependence on the food.

The effects of dehydration are proportionate in their severity to the degree of dehydration. Especially with severe diarrhea in infants, the loss of weight (water) may be extreme and rapid. In these circumstances, the features become sharp, the eyes sunken and fixed in a stare or rolled up under half-closed lids. In infants, the fontanel is sunken. The skin is dry and has a peculiar grayish pallor. It has lost its elasticity, and folds made by picking it up flatten out slowly. Urine is scanty and highly concentrated, and small amounts of sugar and albumin may be present. The blood loses some of its plasma, and the corpuscles occupy an abnormally large proportion of the blood volume. Because of lowered blood volume the circulation is impaired, and the pulse is weak and often rapid and irregular. Fever is usually present, sometimes high, and is an effect of dehydration. With moderate dehydration, the child may be restless and excited; with greater degrees, coma occurs and frequently convulsions also.

Acidosis, often marked, is frequently present. Acidosis results in part from failure to excrete substances in the urine, chiefly acid phosphates, which normally are excreted, in part from the formation of acids, chiefly lactic, by incomplete oxidation of food materials and also in part when diarrhea is present, from the loss of base in the stools. The retention of urinary products is due to lack of water with which to excrete them. The incomplete oxidation is dependent largely on poor blood circulation. The acidosis that develops in these circumstances may be relieved by restoring the body fluid and electrolyte.

When dehydration is due to excessive vomiting unassociated with diarrhea, alkalosis rather than acidosis is likely to develop because of the loss of chloride, especially hydrochloric acid from the body. This is discussed under Pyloric Stenosis.

When dehydration is severe, and the child presents the extreme clinical phenomena described, food is contraindicated. Food cannot be digested and serves only to cause or aggravate diarrhea. When the body fluid and the blood volume have been restored, and the clinical condition is sufficiently improved, food may be given. In general, the food should be of the type described under Diarrhea.

The first treatment in dehydration is to supply water with appropriate amounts of electrolyte. Even when vomiting is not present, it is often difficult to give sufficient fluid by mouth. Parenterally, fluids may be given intravenously, subcutaneously or by way of the peritoneal cavity. The choice of routes depends largely on the preference of the physician. Each route has its advantages in special circumstances. Often larger amounts may be given intraperitoneally than subcutaneously at a single injection. As much as from 400 to 500 ml. may be given by way of the peritoneal cavity in a small baby, and the injection may be repeated as often as indicated by the degree of dehydration and the speed of absorption. Absorption becomes slower as the body need becomes satisfied.

When injecting large quantities of fluid into a vein, a safe rule is not to permit a flow greater than 5 ml. a minute. For single injections of isotonic fluid, a suitable quantity for infants and young children is 20 ml. for each kilogram of body weight (10 ml. for each pound). If the baby is extremely dehydrated, the amount can be 30 ml. or slightly more for each kilogram. If the fluid administration is to be continued over an indefinite period, the rate should not exceed 10 ml. an hour for each kilogram. Usually the amount should be less, perhaps from 6 to 8 ml., an hour for each kilogram.

The fluids used for parenteral administration are salt solution,

Ringer's solution, Darrow's buffered potassium chloride solution, Hartmann's solution,* dextrose solution and mixtures of certain of these. Salt solution and Ringer's solution supply both water and electrolyte. Dextrose is useful in supplying a small amount of food and frequently is given in addition to the salt solutions or mixed with them. Hartmann's solution is used when it is desired to correct acidosis more rapidly than would be accomplished by salt solution alone. Darrow's solution is used to replace potassium withdrawn from intracellular fluid in severe and protracted dehydration. All these solutions may be given intravenously and all, except dextrose, may be given by the other routes mentioned. Dextrose solution is slightly irritating to the tissues and preferably should not be given intraperitoneally for this reason.

The amounts of fluids mentioned in the preceding discussion as suitable are only partial guides as to the total amounts required. Eventually, sufficient fluid should be given to produce good tissue turgor and to cause a relatively normal output of urine. When the body is dehydrated, the urine is concentrated. One of the indications of hydration is the passage of thin urine. An excess of water in the

---

*The Hartmann's solution referred to here consists of a solution of neutral sodium lactate to which have been added the chlorides of sodium, potassium and calcium. It differs from Ringer's solution chiefly in that it contains chloride in no greater concentration than occurs in the blood and it contains sodium lactate as potential alkali.

body may be as harmful as a deficiency. If the amount administered continues to be in excess of that excreted, the tissues become edematous, and the circulation is overburdened. Serious effects are evident in dilation of the heart and edema of the lungs, and death may result from such damage.

When dextrose solutions are used in appreciable quantity the need for the B vitamins, especially thiamine, is increased, usually beyond the supply unless special attention is given to the intake.

In many children with dehydration, a need for transfusion exists because of underlying and associated conditions. In such instances, the transfusion should not be given until the child is hydrated.

The technics of obtaining blood for chemical examination and for administering fluids are discussed in Chapter 6.

MALNUTRITION IN INFANCY

Extreme malnutrition in infancy has been known by the terms marasmus, infantile atrophy, decomposition and athrepsia. Of these terms, athrepsia, meaning lack of food, best fits the condition, which is essentially a starvation. Extreme malnutrition may be the result of prolonged underfeeding. It also may be the result of emotional deprivation which interferes with food intake. In other instances, malnutrition results from loss of food through vomiting or diarrhea, and perhaps through associated therapeutic underfeeding. In still other instances it is found in association with chronic infections. Infections decrease available food by decreas-

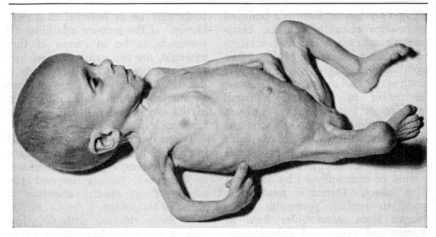

FIG. 91. An infant with severe malnutrition.

ing appetite and lowering powers of digestion and by increasing the combustion of food within the body, thus causing a disproportion between the food available and that required.

In all the conditions stated, the amount of food absorbed from the intestinal tract is inadequate to meet the needs of the infant. Since the infant must continue to burn food, such foods as are available in the body are used. Thus the fat deposits disappear, and emaciation becomes apparent. Probably every organ in the body suffers by loss of material for combustion. The volume of the blood is diminished because part of its protein has been burned. Because of depletion and poor circulation the digestive glands have decreased capacity. As a consequence, less food can be ingested without the production of a gastrointestinal disturbance. With continued disproportion between absorption and combustion, there comes a time when the infant is able to digest and absorb successfully only a portion of the amount of food actually required. When food is given within the limits of digestive ability, the stools are normal in character. Diarrhea is induced easily, either by increase in food in an attempt to cause gain in weight or by intercurrent infections.

An athreptic infant has decreased resistance to infections and is subject to infections of all kinds, notably pyelitis, bronchitis, upper respiratory infections and furunculosis. Infection thus becomes a part of a cycle in the production of increasing degrees of malnutrition. Continued combustion of essential body tissues must be fatal eventually.

The appearance of an extremely malnourished infant is striking. Emaciation is the prominent feature. The eyes are sunken, but alert; the cheek bones prominent; the facial appearance is that of an aged person (Fig. 91). The fat at the center of each cheek disappears late because its composition differs from that of other fat deposits. These "sucking pads" are present in all but the most severely malnourished. The bony skeleton becomes more prominent over the entire body. The hands and the feet become clawlike; the skin is often of paper thinness, hanging in folds. The skin at first is pale and later a characteristic grayish white. The head appears too big for the body, because the brain continues to grow even though certain other parts of the body waste.

Other characteristics also may be prominent. Hunger may be great in the beginning and difficult to satisfy. As emaciation continues, hunger may disappear. In extreme cases the cry is feeble, the heart rate is slow, the heart sounds are weak and the body temperature becomes subnormal. As emaciation increases, activity of the baby decreases, and the basal metabolic rate becomes lower. Growth in body length (skeletal growth) continues at a retarded rate long after growth in weight has ceased, but even growth in length eventually ceases and after it has stopped it does not start again until growth in weight has continued for weeks.

The most obvious features of marasmus are those caused by deficiency in calories. However, other deficiencies may become evident. Nutritional anemia is relatively common. Nutritional edema occurs occasionally as a result of protein deficiency. Rigidity of the muscles, especially those of the legs and the neck, which is observed occasionally, has been attributed to niacin deficiency. Xerophthalmia from vitamin A deficiency has been observed.

Rickets rarely occurs because of the slowness of bone growth.

As activity of the baby decreases, the possibility of development of bedsores increases. These are most likely to appear on the head, but may occur at any pressure point. Thrush is relatively common. Severely athreptic infants sometimes are subject to periods of collapse or syncope, in which they may die. The syncope is accompanied by large and sudden weight (water) loss, lowered body temperature, low heart rate and increased impairment of circulation. Such syncopal attacks frequently are associated with unsuspected hidden infections such as mastoiditis.

Prevention

The measures for prevention of malnutrition in infancy are much the same as those stated for the prevention of diarrhea. Breast feeding should be encouraged, especially in unfavored groups. The baby should be under competent supervision as to growth progress, diet, emotional and physical hygiene. Infections should have prompt and appropriate treatment.

Treatment

Food. If an athreptic infant is to recover, it is essential that the amount of food ingested be increased to a point at which the infant will gain. At the same time it is necessary to keep the food within the limits of digestive capacity. Satisfaction of both these therapeutic indications is sometimes most difficult. The food requirement is high. As much as from 200 to 250 calories for each kilogram of body weight (100 to 120 calories to the pound) daily may be necessary. The digestive capacity is low, and food in excess of the capacity is a potent cause of diarrhea and consequent further weight loss. In meeting this therapeutic problem, considerable care must be taken in the choice of food, and such measures should be employed as tend to increase the ability of the infant to utilize the food successfully.

SELECTING FOOD. In the selection of food a type should be chosen that is easily digestible, one that offers a medium relatively unfavorable to bacterial growth. It is desirable also to use a concentrated food, since vomiting is very likely to occur if the large amount of food needed is offered in customary dilution. Two types of food meet these requirements fairly well. When human milk is available, it may be fortified by the addition of dried milk and further modified to advantage by partial acidification. When only cow's milk is available, a good preparation is undiluted acidified whole milk with added carbohydrate. When a tendency to diarrhea exists, somewhat less sugar and fat than customary should be given, or the added sugar may be changed to a type quickly absorbable, such as dextrose. At times it is desirable to increase the food value of the cow's milk formula by the addition of dried skimmed milk. Too much attention should not be given to moderately increased frequency of the stools if the baby is making good gains in weight and the condition is satisfactory otherwise.

Moderate dehydration is common in athrepsia even in the absence of diarrhea. Loss of interstitial fluid is characteristically a part of the loss of body weight in malnutrition. Replacement of this fluid and its maintenance in interstitial tissues are two of the first essentials in recovery. Parenteral administration of fluid from time to time as indicated is helpful in hastening recovery.

Transfusion. The ability of the infant to utilize food may be increased by restoring the blood volume by means of transfusions. Transfusions hasten recovery and often permit recovery in an otherwise hopeless case. A suitable amount of blood to give at one time is 20 ml. for each kilogram of body weight. In extreme malnutrition, several transfusions at intervals of several days to a week are indicated.

NURSING CARE

The body temperature of athreptic infants must be guarded very much, as in the case of prematurely born infants, although seldom is an incubator necessary. If additional clothing fails to supply the necessary warmth, a lamp-heated bed (see under Diarrhea) is useful. Preventing infections, careful feeding and close observation for signs of collapse comprise the specific physical care.

The baby with marasmus must have abundant emotional warmth given with each feeding. He needs extra cuddling, sucking, interest and care which helps him to feel that those in the world are giving and responsive to his needs. Every effort should be made to supply him with continuity of maternal care.

MALNUTRITION IN CHILDHOOD

The fundamental causes of malnutrition in the child are the same as those discussed in the case of the infant. However, relatively few older children become malnourished because of vomiting and diarrhea. Therapeutic underfeeding is not common. The child has more control than the infant over the kind and the quantity of food eaten. Parenteral infections do not have as severe an adverse effect in the child as in the infant.

In order that a child be well nourished, it is necessary that enough available food be ingested, digested and absorbed to meet all metabolic needs. When the amount of food ingested or the amount absorbed is deficient, growth or increase in weight likewise is deficient. An intake that is adequate under normal conditions may become inadequate with excessive activity or insufficient sleep. Low food intake is likely to be encountered under the following conditions: prematurely satisfied appetite, emotional disturbance, the presence of certain physical defects and improper food and eating habits.

APPETITE

Certain children, particularly nervous and sickly children, evidence an appeased appetite after the ingestion of only small quantities of food. Others of this class at times seem to have no appetite. Poor hygiene, such as insufficient stimulation and personal interest, excessive clothing or lack of fresh air and sunshine, may lead to poor appetite. Excessive fatigue also may be a factor. Such physical defect as a carious tooth may make eating uncomfortable, so that hunger scarcely will be satisfied. Chronic infection usually diminishes appetite and fre-

quently causes increased combustion of food in the body.

IMPROPER FOOD

An example of decreased intake due to improper food is the drinking of coffee instead of milk. Sweets before or at the beginning of a meal diminish the appetite. An excessive consumption of milk may abolish the appetite for other foods. If the diet is deficient in various nutritional essentials, decreased appetite is likely to result. Thiamine particularly is related to appetite. Nutritional anemia also is a cause of poor appetite.

ENVIRONMENT AND TRAINING

The causative factors that have been enumerated are important in varying degree in individual cases. However, all of them are relatively unimportant in the majority of instances as compared with the influence of environment and training. The most conspicuously and persistently poor appetites are found in children who are living under excellent hygienic conditions and have had their physical defects attended to, but their mealtime is characterized by nagging and overattention in regard to food. This parental attitude reacts harmfully in several ways. Frequently, it arouses antagonism on the part of the child to the extent that the emotional disturbance produced by the mere mention of food causes the child to forget what little hunger he may have had. In other instances, the child has found that refusal of food is the easiest and surest way of getting the increased attention which he so much desires and needs. That anorexia is wholly functional in the majority of instances has been demonstrated abundantly.

SYMPTOMS

Malnutrition often is associated with other symptoms beside the disproportion between body weight and height. Often malnourished children are irritable; they demand to be entertained rather than find something they themselves can do. They seem to be consumed with anxiety which depletes their supply of energy and brings fatigue. Often their sleep is restless. They tend to be timid. Because of easy and frequent fatigue, undernourished children tend to assume a fatigue posture, which usually is one of lordosis and round shoulders. A disinclination toward mental exertion is encountered, which may simulate mental retardation, even though the mental capacity is inherently excellent. The undernourished child has increased susceptibility to infections.

TREATMENT

In order to correct malnutrition, the underlying physical and psychological causes must be found and corrected. Foci of chronic infection should be eradicated. Relief from anxiety must be provided. Sufficient sleep must be obtained. A rest hour in the middle of the day is beneficial. When all these things have been done, the child is ready to gain. The remaining problem is to bring about the ingestion of sufficient and proper food. This is not always easy. Proper training in food habits is by far the most important factor. Such training is discussed elsewhere, but it may be emphasized here that the easiest and most

uniformly successful method of correcting poor food habits is to begin by making a radical change in the environment of the child. The mother will need help to gain insight into the needs of her child and to bring changes in her feelings toward him and the guidance that he requires.

It has been found that undernourished children make better weight and growth gains when the diet is relatively low in fat and high in carbohydrate. If the diet is complete in all essentials, the more rapid growth with the high sugar diet is associated with increase of good normal tissue, and not with high water retention as might be presupposed. In the examples of diets given in illustration, fat is kept low, and much of the energy value is derived from dextrose. Butter is permitted on bread to make it palatable. Ice cream may be given from time to time. The amount of dextrose to be given in 24 hours varies from 1/3 cup (1 1/3 ounces avoirdupois) in the first diet to ½ cup (2 ounces by weight) in the second diet. It is given in the fruit juices or any other appropriate vehicle in the diet. An even larger quantity of dextrose may be given if it is well taken in addition to the specified diet.

Drug Tonics

It may be stated as a general rule that drug tonics have little or no effect on the appetite. Although anorexia is a result when thiamine deficiency exists, the effect of thiamine administration is not noticeable when the anorexia is the result of an emotional disturbance.

DIET FOR MALNUTRITION ACCOMPANIED BY ANOREXIA

FIRST DIET	LATER DIET
Small portions	High calorie diet for age

Breakfast	*Breakfast*
Fresh fruit	Fresh fruit
Buttered toast	Buttered toast with jam
Skimmed milk, 6 oz.	Skimmed milk, 8 oz.
	Cereal with undiluted evaporated milk
	Egg and strip crisp bacon

9 A.M.	*9 A.M.*
Tomato juice, 4 to 6 oz.	Tomato juice, 4 to 6 oz.
Dextrose	Dextrose

Noon	*Noon*
Small amount of meat or chicken	Meat, average serving
Leafy vegetable	Potato with butter
Buttered toast with jelly	Leaf of lettuce
Fresh fruit and plain cookie	Buttered bread and jelly
Skimmed milk, 6 oz.	Pudding or fruit with dextrose
	Skimmed milk, 8 oz.

2 P.M.	*2 P.M.*
Orange juice, 6 oz.	Orange juice or milk
Dextrose	Dextrose

Supper	*Supper*
Egg or egg and crisp bacon	Egg or cottage cheese or liver
Vegetable	Rice cooked in milk
Buttered toast	Vegetable, fresh or cooked
Fresh fruit	Buttered bread
Skimmed milk, 6 oz.	Fruit and 2 cookies
	Skimmed milk, 8 oz.

8 P.M.	*8 P.M.*
Vitamin concentrate	Vitamin concentrate
Glass of fruit juice with dextrose	Glass of skimmed milk or fruit juice with dextrose

OBESITY

Obesity is the result of the ingestion and the absorption of food in excess of the body's energy needs. The need may be relatively small and the amount of food average, or the need may be average and the food excessive. In either case the result is the same. This generalization applies in all instances of obesity.

The amount of food energy needed by the body is determined by the amount of energy necessary for basal metabolism, growth and activity. The one component of this group subject to great variation in childhood is activity. An amount of food satisfactory for an active child would cause obesity in an inactive child of the same age. Striking illustrations are found in children confined to bed for long periods by conditions which do not impair appetite. A child who becomes obese from any cause frequently exercises decreasingly as the obesity progresses, thus increasing the disproportion between the amount of food required and that ingested.

A familial or individually inherent tendency to obesity has been assumed to exist; obesity occurs with the ingestion of average amounts of food. In such persons, the obesity is said to be from endogenous causes; that is, causes within the body such as superior utilization of food in contrast with the exogenous cause of excessive intake. Evidence for the existence of endogenous obesity is meager, and it seems likely that inactivity is the chief cause of obesity when the food intake is not excessive. The occurrence of obesity in families and in several generations may be due more to familial dietary habits of generous food intake than to inheritance of endogenous factors.

Endocrine Dysfunction

Despite a widespread belief to the contrary, obesity is caused by endocrine dysfunction in few, if any, instances. The thyroid and the pituitary glands are the ones commonly held responsible for endocrine obesity. In hypofunction of either of these glands, retarded growth is a characteristic feature, whereas accelerated growth almost constantly is associated with obesity in childhood. Obese children are taller than the the average for their age, and their skeletal development (bone age) is in advance of that normally expected.

Froehlich's syndrome is frequently stated as the diagnosis in cases of obesity in childhood, especially in boys. True Froehlich's syndrome is a result of pituitary disease and includes retarded growth with small stature, girdle distribution of fat and retardation in sexual development. The basal metabolic rate usually is normal, although it is thought to be low for reasons discussed subsequently. The obesity is caused by inactivity or increased food intake or both. Froehlich's syndrome is rare. The sexual infantilism of ordinary obesity is only apparent, not real. The genitalia are buried in fat; they are seen to be of normal size for the age when the fat is pushed aside. The apparent infantilism disappears at puberty.

Basal Metabolic Rate

Estimations of basal metabolic rate made in the customary manner give values for the obese child less than the average which has been accepted as normal, whereas the true rate for obese children usually is greater than average. The weight of the child enters into the customary calculation. In the obese child a large proportion of the weight is from fat. Actually, the basal rate is in proportion to the amount of active or heat-producing tissue and is wholly unrelated to the fat of the body. The heat-producing tissues are increased above the average in the obese child, but the relative increase is not so great as that of the fat. The obese child may have from 30 to 40 per cent less heat-producing tissue than the average child in proportion to the body weight. Such a child might have a true basal rate of plus 20 per cent or more, yet have a minus value by customary calculations. Customary methods of estimation serve satisfactorily only when the body is of average proportion.

From the preceding discussion it is evident that obese children show evidence of abundant nutrition by accelerated growth; they have an increased metabolic rate; they mature earlier than average. Such findings are not compatible with concepts of endocrine causation of obesity.

SYMPTOMS

The symptoms associated with obesity are few. The tendency to decreased activity has been mentioned. Sometimes the posture becomes faulty in the endeavor to carry with greater ease the extra load of fat (Fig. 92). In occasional instances, ingestion of water is increased abnormally. Medical advice is most commonly sought because of the social and psychological problems that result from the child's being markedly different from his associates.

DIAGNOSIS

When an obese child comes under care, the possibility of endocrine dysfunction is excluded. If the stature and the bone age are in excess of the average, endocrine diseases commonly held responsible for obesity are not present. The basal metabolic rate may be determined but must be interpreted with caution. In any case, the food energy intake is in excess of the need. Sometimes this excess is not obvious and is denied by the parent and the child. However, it usually is revealed by detailed observation of the child's diet. A diet may be relatively low in bulk and yet high in energy value, particularly if fruits and vegetables are present in minimum quantity. Some children obtain an excess of food between meals.

TREATMENT

In the usual case of obesity, the indications are to decrease the food intake and to increase the energy output. Energy output is increased by exercise. The type and the intensity of the exercise must be fitted to the child. For the markedly obese, attempts at violent exercise may be actually harmful, although activity may be made increasingly strenuous as the child becomes thoroughly accustomed to it. Decrease in the amount of food is much more rapidly effective in reducing weight than is increased exercise.

For the child who is young and only moderately obese, it may be satisfactory to reduce the diet only enough to maintain the weight at a fairly constant level over a prolonged period. During this period the child is growing and eventually will be of suitable weight for the height and the age. For the markedly obese, this procedure is not satisfactory because many of these children weigh more than they should were they fully grown. In such circumstances it is desirable to remove at least some of the excess fat. This objective is accomplished only by supplying food in such reduced quantity that the body fat must be burned to supply the necessary energy. When the regimen is managed carefully, a loss of from 2 to 3 pounds of body fat a week may be brought about with safety and at the same time permit increasing activity.

Low-Calorie Diets for Obesity

Child of 6 or 7 years 1,000 calories	Child of 10 or 12 years 1,200 calories
Breakfast	*Breakfast*
½ orange 1 egg 8 ounces skimmed milk	Whole orange 1 egg· 8 ounces skimmed milk ½ slice bread or small potato
Noon	*Noon*
2 ounces lean beef ½ cup vegetable Leaf of lettuce Ripe peach 8 ounces skimmed milk	3 ounces lean meat 2/3 cup vegetable Lettuce Ripe peach 8 ounces skimmed milk ½ slice toast
Supper	*Supper*
Egg or meat ½ cup vegetable ½ slice bread Fresh fruit 8 ounces skimmed milk	Egg or meat Celery 2/3 cup vegetable Fresh fruit ½ slice bread 8 ounces skimmed milk
Evening	*Evening*
8 ounces skimmed milk Vitamin concentrate	8 ounces skimmed milk Vitamin concentrate

Even though the diet is greatly reduced in energy value, it must be "complete" at all times. Reliance is placed on the stores of body fat for some of the energy, but all other nutritional essentials must be supplied. The full requirement of protein, minerals and vitamins must be furnished, and sufficient carbohydrate must be present in order that fat may not be called on for fuel in excess of the ability of the body to burn it completely. In the beginning of a reduction regimen, it is advisable to start with a diet which is only slightly below the calculated average requirement in energy, and then to make the decrease gradually until the desired rate of loss in weight is reached. Weight loss that is too rapid is undesirable and presumably harmful.

These sample diets have been used for children of the ages stated. Such diets always must be adjusted to the individual child and increased or decreased according to rate of weight loss. The older child could have a glass of skimmed milk at bedtime, if hungry.

Psychic Aspects

Certain psychic aspects of obesity often are important for successful management. In many instances, the excessive eating that has produced the obesity is part of an emotional and compensatory mechanism in a child poorly adjusted to his environment. In such instances, relief of the maladjustment is necessary in order to obtain permanent results from treatment.

CELIAC DISEASE (CHRONIC INTESTINAL INDIGESTION)

Celiac disease is a term applied to a chronic functional disorder prevalent from the second to the fifth year, in which the chief fault lies in inability to absorb fat and digest starch. When a customary diet is ingested, bulky, frothy, foul, semiliquid stools result. The stools are composed chiefly of unabsorbed food. Continued failure to absorb sufficient food leads to failure of growth and to malnutrition, often extreme (Fig. 93). The food deficiency is not only of calories but also of any or all nutritional essentials. Thus, deficiency diseases in addition to malnutrition may become evident.

Anatomic examination of the intestinal tract reveals nothing striking other than a greatly dilated colon, which is chiefly responsible for the characteristic protuberant abdomen. When fat is fed in customary amounts, a large proportion appears in the stools, even though most or all of it has been split by digestive enzymes. These children are able to absorb and use monosaccharides, but starch is acted on by bacteria with aggravation of the indigestion. Marked and rapid fluctuations in weight due to instability of body water are commonly observed when the disease is not under dietary control.

A few children have symptoms essentially identical with those of celiac disease, in whom the fault is chiefly inability to digest starch; fats may be tolerated when starch is omitted from the diet. Such children require the same type of management as those with typical celiac disease.

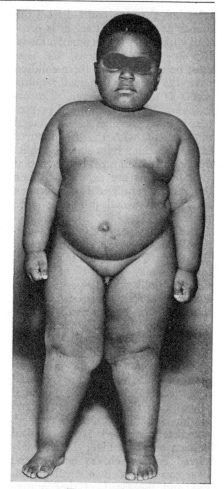

Fig. 92. Obesity.

Celiac disease is to be distinguished from cystic fibrosis of the pancreas. This condition is discussed subsequently.

TREATMENT

Although no agreement exists as to cause, celiac disease responds satisfactorily to nutritional management. Since fats and starch are not tolerated, they are omitted from the diet to as great an extent as is practical with a diet from common foods. Despite these omissions, the diet must be complete, for these children have the same nutritional requirements as healthy children. The caloric requirement is supplied by protein and simple sugars; the mineral requirement, with the exception of iron, is obtained from skimmed milk. Special attention must be given that vitamin needs are supplied. When the various requirements have been met, normal growth progress will be made.

Initial diets depend on the severity of the symptoms and the age of the child. For an infant, an initial formula may consist of boiled skimmed milk with 10-per-cent dextrose or banana powder addition, these sugars being used because monosaccharides and invert sugars are absorbed more promptly without fermentation. Protein milk, so frequently recommended for early treatment of celiac disease, has too great a fat content to be well tolerated when the disturbance is severe. Within a day or two, finely mashed, completely ripened raw or baked banana can be added. Later, finely sieved cottage cheese and ground liver can be added in small quantities and increased. Either orange juice in customary amounts or ascorbic acid, 25 to 50 mg., should be given to satisfy the need for vitamin C. The equivalent of a teaspoonful of cod-liver oil in a water-dispersible concentrate of vitamins will satisfy the daily need for these two nutrients. Increased amounts of vitamin B complex are indicated. Sometimes intramuscular injections of vitamin B complex and crude

liver extract are given. It has been reported that more rapid recovery has been made by the use of additional sources of vitamin B, and it has been suggested that celiac disease may be caused by deficiency of one or more components of these preparations. Folic acid has been found especially useful in sprue, a condition in adults similar to celiac disease in young children.

Puréed fruits and vegetables may be added early, provided that those containing significant amounts of starch are withheld. Ground chicken and meat also may be added early. As recovery occurs, foods containing fat are added first, and those containing starch are added last. Eggs and whole milk would be included in the group of fat-containing foods. Potato and cereal foods would be the final additions in the return to a normal diet.

When celiac disease occurs in a child of preschool age, the initial formula will comprise the same foods in larger amounts, supplementary foods being increased more rapidly in variety and quantity as their tolerance is noted. The extra dextrose that is given to bring the energy intake up to the requirement can be offered as a 10-per-cent solution flavored with orange or other tart fruit juice. When distributed appropriately between meals, dextrose is well utilized and does not aggravate the diarrhea. Dextrose also can be added to the milk, as described for the infant. The ability to utilize fat returns before that for starch. When the disturbance has been severe, even one white cracker or a spoonful of potato may cause diarrhea of several days' duration in a child who recently

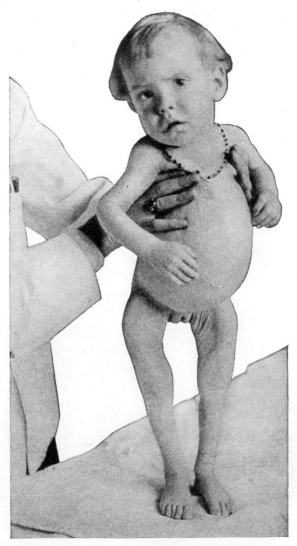

FIG. 93. Severe malnutrition from celiac disease.

has been brought under good control.

With this type of diet, evidence of improvement is indicated promptly by a change in the type of stools. Nervous manifestations, such as irritability and fretfulness, become less apparent, and the child begins to show a gain in weight (Fig. 94). Increase in height, which previously had been stopped or re-

tarded greatly, begins after a period proportionate to the severity of malnutrition.

NURSING CARE

The child with celiac disease needs protection, understanding of his feelings pertaining to food deprivation and care which alleviate his symptoms of distress. He is malnourished and anemic and requires

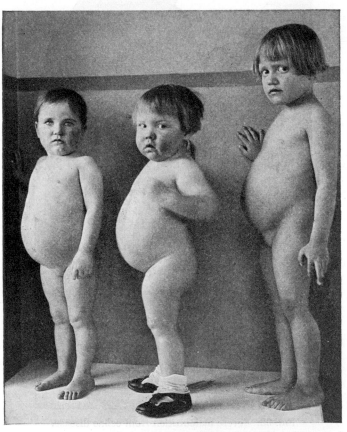

FIG. 94. Three children with celiac disease who are making good growth progress under treatment. The child in the center is the same as in Fig. 93.

good hygiene to prevent infections. He perspires freely, tends to lie in one position and is prone to develop respiratory infections that increase his indigestion. His temperature is often subnormal, his extremities are cold, and dressing him warmly is required for his protection.

When the child first comes under care, his appetite may be capricious, and he needs warm, thoughtful feeding experiences. Foods should be given to him slowly in small amounts and with no attempt to force him beyond his interest for it. As the dietary regimen is instituted, marked change in digestion and desire for food will be noted. The kinds and the amounts of food eaten and the child's behavior during feeding are observations that should be made and recorded. After the initial period when new foods are added to the diet, the stools, the degree of abdominal distention and the child's disposition should be noted to determine the tolerance to each one. Stools must be described accurately, for they are a guide in prescribing the diet. Should symptoms of indigestion be increased, the new food should be eliminated temporarily from the diet. Although appetite may be great, new foods should be introduced slowly, for unless digestion has improved, hastily introduced foods increase bulk and do little to improve the child's nutritional state.

When the child is hungry and is deprived of food, he will react to his frustration with anger or rage. Food has great meaning to a child. To be deprived of the satisfaction that comes from an adequate intake evokes feelings which may be expressed in many different ways. The child may express his feelings tempestuously or he may feel punished and withdraw. Some children completely deny their cravings, hate the impulse that strives for satisfaction and develop anorexia and vomiting. The child with celiac disease needs freedom to complain and to relieve his feelings concerning the deprivation that he is experiencing. The infant will scream with fury when he is hungry; the older child will voice his feelings with words if he is permitted to do so. Pent-up feelings and anxiety are minimized when the child is able to express his feelings with crying or words and he feels his nurse's sympathetic understanding. Providing sympathetic understanding is one of the most important factors in the nursing care of the child with celiac disease.

For diagnostic purposes the proportion of ingested fat excreted in the stools is determined while the child is receiving a diet with an amount of fat customary for a normal child. Such a study may be made for a period of 24 hours or longer. During the period chosen, the amounts and the kinds of foods must be recorded accurately. The beginning of the stool collection period is marked by passage in the stool of carmine given previously by mouth. The dye is tasteless and can be given in a portion of the milk; the time of ingestion of the carmine must be recorded. Beginning with the first appearance of the dye, all stools are saved until the carmine appears again after ingestion of a second capsule given exactly 24 hours, or other longer time period chosen, after ingestion of the first. The stools should be placed in a covered container in a laboratory refrigerator. The normal child excretes approximately 10 per cent of the ingested fat in the stool, while the child with celiac disease may excrete as much as from 50 to 70 per cent or even more.

In celiac disease, nervous instability accompanies symptoms of indigestion. The child usually is inhibited and rarely expresses his aggression overtly. His play is passive and meager. He fatigues easily and is peevish, withdrawn, depressed and precocious. Infantile habits, such as thumb-sucking and dependence on certain objects or toys, frequently are noted. The child needs study to find methods of approach that will bring him comfort. The nurse who understands his irritability, mood changes and regressive behavior and is patient gives him security and comfort. Until his physical condition improves, no attempt to divert his attention from his infantile habits should be made. When he is suffering from indigestion, he needs all the emotional satisfactions that he can get. Gradually, as he begins to gain in weight and improve generally, interest in his surroundings and a need for increased stimulation will become evident. His dependence on infantile satisfactions will decrease as he finds satisfaction in play and in his relationship with others.

The period of hospitalization and subsequent supervision is a long one, for often it is several years before a completely normal diet can be ingested safely. Before the child leaves the hospital, the mother needs to understand the child's dietary regimen, his need for general hygienic measures to prevent infection and for follow-up medical examinations. These points must be emphasized, for many of these children die because of lack of adequate supervision. On the other hand, a mental hygiene approach must be maintained. If a mother is frightened rather than helped to become more aware of her child's needs, she may protect her child so completely that changes in environment result which prevent the child from participating in normal play experiences with other children. With good supervision and care these children recover completely.

The mother of a child with celiac disease often needs help to relinquish her overprotective methods of guidance. A history of difficult feeding experiences from birth often is elicited from the mother. Frequently, the mother has responded to her crying, hungry baby with feelings of self-reproach. A crying, hungry baby disturbs the most experienced, well-adjusted mother. It is a reproach or a symbol of her failure to provide the motherliness that her infant requires. Overprotectiveness is the most natural response to such feelings. The mother of a child who has had a digestive disturbance early in life needs empathy. She needs relief from feelings of guilt and also help to find means of instituting the dietary regimen in such a way that both she and her child obtain the satisfactions that they require. A preschool child will have feelings of resentment when he is deprived of foods that he sees his parents and siblings eating. A mother who can accept his feelings of resentment and provide delicacies which are made especially for him not only will meet her child's need but also will obtain gratification herself. Cookies can be made of dried fruit or egg whites and artificial sweetening, and ice cream and cakes can be made of gelatin. Diabetic candies are received enthusiastically by children, and their use minimizes the negative feelings that arise when such children discover that they cannot have what other children are given.

CYSTIC FIBROSIS OF THE PANCREAS (MUCOVISCIDOSIS)

The term cystic fibrosis of the pancreas is used to include not only characteristic changes in the pancreas but also other abnormalities, chiefly in the lungs. The condition is congenital and is inherited as a recessive trait; it frequently occurs in several children of the same family.

In this condition the secretion of the mucous glands of the body is thick and viscid. For this reason the name mucoviscidosis often is used. The thick secretion occludes the ducts of the pancreas, producing absence of pancreatic enzymes in the intestine and causing subsequent atrophy and fibrosis of the pancreas. It is the absence of pancreatic secretion in the intestine that produces the characteristic indigestion of this condition. In the bronchi the thick mucus impairs movement of the cilia so that it cannot be moved upward in a normal manner. Frequently and recurrently, it obstructs smaller bronchi, causing atelectasis or emphysema, depending on whether the obstruction is complete or partial. The abnormal condition of the lungs leads to repeated attacks of pneumonia and eventually to fibrosis or bronchiectasis.

Nutrition and general health suffer. Fat and starch cannot be digested, and considerable impairment of protein digestion occurs; thus, ordinary food is utilized poorly. Absorption and utilization are further affected adversely by the repeated infections that occur. Malnutrition and retarded growth result.

SYMPTOMS

Symptoms are present at birth or soon thereafter. In a few instances, as a result of lack of digestive enzymes the meconium remains so thick that it cannot be passed, and intestinal obstruction results; this condition is known as meconium ileus. In most instances the disease is more insidious in its onset. Both the bronchial and the pancreatic abnormalities may be apparent at birth; either condition may become obvious before the other. The first bronchial symptom is cough, which is frequent and persistent. Roentgenograms of the chest at this early stage may show little or nothing abnormal; they may reveal emphysema or atelectasis. Later changes in the lungs depend on recurring infections; these are repeated attacks of pneumonia and subsequently increasing bronchiectasis. Usually the first evidence of digestive difficulty is failure to gain weight. Moderate diarrhea may be present early. Eventually, the stools become bulky and foul. The fat of the diet appears in the stools, and if starch is fed, the stools are frothy. Thus the stools resemble those of celiac disease.

DIAGNOSIS

Diagnosis is made by finding absence of tryptic activity in the stools or in secretions removed by catheter from the duodenum and also by finding extremely viscid duodenal secretions. Corroborative evidence may be obtained by demonstrating low blood levels of viamin A after a test dose in oily solution by mouth and low levels of amino acid in the blood after a test meal of protein.

PROGNOSIS

Prognosis is poor in most cases, regardless of the kind of care given. Some die in the first few months, others live for several years, but few live beyond the period of childhood. Even though nutrition often may be managed with fair success, the increasing lung changes eventually lead to death.

TREATMENT

Treatment consists chiefly of management of nutrition and of the recurring lung infections. The diet should be low in fat and starch and should consist chiefly of protein and simple sugars. If unmodified protein is used, pancreatin given with it aids in its digestion. Sometimes protein hydrolysates are used, since they require no further digestion. Dextrose is well absorbed and is an aid in meeting the energy requirement. The fat-soluble vitamins preferably are given in water-miscible form. In the treatment of lung infections as they occur, reliance is placed chiefly on the antibiotics. At times the sulfonamides are useful. The antibiotics may be given by inhalation spray in addition to other routes. Because of the serious consequences of infection, often such children are kept upon a continuous dose of prophylactic sulfadiazine or broad-spectrum antibiotic.

Duodenal Catheterization

The following equipment is necessary: radiopaque catheter No. 10 to 12 French, medicine glass of water, 20 ml. syringe, an indicator, test tubes, adhesive tape and elbow restraints. After the restraints have been applied to prevent removal of the tube, the catheter is lubricated with water and passed through the nose and the stomach and into the duodenum. Fluid is aspirated through the tube, and its reaction is tested: gastric secretion is acid, and duodenal content is alkaline. If the fluid is definitely alkaline (pH above 7), the infant is examined fluoroscopically to verify the position of the catheter. If the fluid has a pH of less than 7 by indicator, the head of the bed is elevated, the infant is restrained on his right side, the catheter is inserted an inch or two further, and the upper end is made secure to the infant's face with adhesive tape. Fluid is withdrawn, and its reaction is tested at intervals until an alkaline reaction indicates that the end of the catheter has passed into the duodenum. After fluoroscopic verification of the position, fluid is withdrawn. The material obtained from the duodenum in cases of cystic fibrosis is very viscid and sticks to glass. The finding of such material is pathognomonic of cystic fibrosis. The fluid is tested for tryptic activity. Successive dilutions are made, usually up to 1:100. These are tested with gelatin. A simple procedure is to apply a large drop of the fluid of the various dilutions to the gelatin surface of a photographic film and incubate for 1 hour. In the presence of tryptic activity, the treated portion of the gelatin digests and leaves a clear spot on the film. The test for tryptic activity in the stool is carried out in the same manner as with duodenal secretion. Early in cystic fibrosis, tryptic activity may still be present and disappear later.

SITUATIONS FOR FURTHER STUDY

1. A normal infant 6 months old is being cared for in an underprivileged home. On visiting this home during the early summer months, what parent counseling would aid in the prevention of diarrhea?

2. In caring for an infant with diarrhea, what symptoms would indicate acidosis?

3. A child 2 years old is being discharged from the hospital after a dysentery infection. If you visit this home prior to his discharge, what observations would you make, and what would you help the parents to learn about his care at home?

4. If in visiting a home you found an 8-year-old child severely malnourished and highly nervous and unhappy, how would you approach the problem of giving aid to this child and his family? How would you study the problem? What information would you secure that would be helpful to the physician in treating this child? What community resources are available to provide the care that this type of child requires?

5. Study a preschool child with celiac disease. What personality characteristics did he show when he first came into the hospital? In conversation with the parents discover the symptoms that led them to seek medical assistance. Determine how these symptoms altered their guidance of the child. Compare his behavior now with the behavior observed when he first came into the ward. How has your guidance of him changed during this period? In what way have you attempted to help the mother to accept his changing needs?

BIBLIOGRAPHY

Aldrich, C. A., Sung, C., and Knop, C.: The crying of newly born infants, J. Pediat. **27**:428, 1945.

Anderson, D. H.: Cystic fibrosis of the pancreas, *in* The Practice of Pediatrics, ed. by Joseph Brenneman, Hagerstown, Md., Prior, 1948.

Babbitz, Matilda: Bobby has celiac disease, Am. J. Nursing **53**:322, 1953.

Barber, W. W.: Celiac disease, Am. J. Nursing **36**:660, 1936.

Black, E. W., and Poncher, H. G.: Inhalation therapy in pediatrics, Am. J. Dis. Child. **76**:169, 1948.

Bruch, H.: Obesity in childhood, physiologic and psychologic aspects of the food intake of obese children, Am. J. Dis. Child. **59**: 739, 1940.

Farber, Sidney: Pancreatic function and disease in early life. V. Pathologic change associated with pancreatic insufficiency in early life, Arch. Path. **37**:238, 1944.

Fraiberg, Selma: Counseling for the parents of the very young child, Social Casework **35**:47, 1954.

Gibbs, G. E., and Smith, Kathryn: Cystic fibrosis of the pancreas, Am. J. Nursing **49**:783, 1949.

Mayo, Merle: Nursing care in bacillary dysentery, Am. J. Nursing **50**: 304, 1950.

Prugh, D. G.: A preliminary report on the role of emotional factors in idiopathic celiac disease, Psychosom. Med. **13**:220, 1951.

Ribble, Margaret: The Rights of Infants, New York, Columbia, 1943.

Deficiency Diseases

GENERAL DISCUSSION

Deficiency of any, several or all of the nutritional essentials may exist through lack of ingestion or failure of utilization. Deficiency of each of these materials produces its own peculiar symptoms and signs by which it may be recognized when sufficiently severe. Many of the deficiency diseases are discussed in this chapter; others are discussed elsewhere. Deficiency of food energy is discussed under Malnutrition; hemorrhagic disease dependent on deficiency of vitamin K is discussed under Diseases of the Newborn; cheilitis, keratitis and visual disturbances dependent on deficiency of riboflavin and the results of vitamin A deficiency are included in the general discussion of vitamins. The effects of calcium deficiency are mentioned in the discussion of the minerals.

The therapy for the deficiency diseases included in this chapter is discussed under each disease. A good general rule for the vitamin deficiencies is to give therapeutically approximately 10 times the normal allowance until the symptoms of deficiency have disappeared. Subsequently, only the normal allowance is required, and this amount, except in the case of vitamin D, should be obtained from the foods of a good diet rather than from special vitamin preparations. The promiscuous taking of vitamins is greatly overdone and much of it represents waste.

BERIBERI

Beriberi results from deficiency of thiamine (vitamin B_1) The disease is common in parts of the world where polished rice constitutes a large part of the diet. It is not common in this country. In most parts of the country it occurs among children less often from low intake of thiamine than from failure of absorption, as in chronic diarrhea.

SYMPTOMS

Beriberi usually is insidious in its onset, being the result of a long-continued partial deficiency of thiamine. Only after a period of vague and indefinite symptoms does the disease become fully manifest. During the prodromal period, the complaints made are referable to many systems, but most prominently to the nervous system. The mental symptoms are such as to lead to a diagnosis of neurosis. Undue anxiety is shown, along with lassitude, general weakness, easy fatigue and lack of interest in normal activities and personal care. Irritability and inattentiveness may be present.

After beriberi is fully developed, the symptoms are referable chiefly to the peripheral nerves, the heart and the alimentary tract. The gastrointestinal tract shows altered motility, with constipation more often than diarrhea. Anorexia is constant, and nausea and vomiting may be present. The signs of peripheral neuritis appear, preceded and accompanied by burning, tingling and numbness of the hands and the feet. Tenderness is present over the nerve trunks and the calves. Muscle weakness may be marked. The muscle of the heart also becomes weakened, the symptoms being the same as those of myocarditis from other causes and may include rapid heart rate, dyspnea, pain over the heart and thready pulse.

Sometimes generalized edema is present. Then the disease is known as wet beriberi in contradistinction to the dry beriberi unassociated with edema. No doubt the myocardial changes contribute to the production of edema, but it is not clear that these are the sole cause. Wet beriberi is likely to be a more acute disease than dry beriberi, with rapid onset of the acute symptoms and sometimes with sudden death.

TREATMENT

Beriberi responds dramatically to thiamine. For those severely ill, parenteral administration may be desirable; otherwise, the oral route is satisfactory. For infants, 10 mg. daily in divided dose is ample, and for older children, twice this amount. Half the amounts stated are adequate when the disease is mild. After the symptoms have disappeared, the normal daily allowance is all that is required, except when the disease is dependent on chronic diarrhea which persists. It is seldom that deficiency of any component of the vitamin B complex exists alone; consequently, the treatment with thiamine should be supplemented by administration of the complex or food materials containing it, such as yeast. Complete rest in bed is necessary, at least until full recovery from the myocardial disease.

PELLAGRA

Pellagra is caused by dietary deficiency of niacin (nicotinic acid), a member of the vitamin B complex. It is endemic in southeastern United States, southern Europe, and a few other regions. Where it is endemic, it exists at least in a latent form throughout the year. It becomes manifest notably in the spring, the symptoms increase in frequency and severity until early summer and then recede to the winter low level. Deficiency of niacin usually is partial rather than absolute. The effects of partial deficiency appear to be cumulative. With each successive year of deficiency the recurring manifestations are more apparent and more severe. In the first two years of life, gross lesions are uncommon. They increase in frequency with the age in pellagrous families. The severe disease of many adults had its beginning in childhood.

The occurrence of pellagra is dependent on dietary habits. A typical diet of a pellagrous family in southeastern United States is greatly restricted in variety and includes chiefly salt fat pork, corn bread and syrup. It is lacking in vegetables, fruit, lean meat, milk and eggs. It is deficient in almost all nutritional essentials. Whole corn meal contains a moderate amount of thiamine and other members of the vitamin B complex but contains little niacin. Also corn protein is deficient in tryptophan, an amino acid that decreases to some extent the need for niacin. Babies of pellagrous mothers usually must be weaned early because of lack of milk. The subsequent diet usually is unsatisfactory. The children take over the dietary habits of the family. Once these habits are established, they are difficult to change, regardless of availability of better foods.

In this country the death rate, and presumably the incidence, of pellagra reached a peak about 1928. The decline since that time has been attributed largely to extensive use of dried yeast.

SYMPTOMS

The symptoms of niacin deficiency in its earliest stages are vague and ill-defined, but with continued deficiency the manifestations characteristic of pellagra make their appearance.

Alimentary Tract. Lesions of the mucous membranes of the alimentary tract are usually the first to appear. The changes are those of inflammation, and the most characteristic visible changes occur in the tongue. A subjective sensation of burning precedes and accompanies an intense glossitis. The tongue becomes very red, swollen and smooth. Inflammation of the mouth and the gums usually is present also. The gums become red and ulcerated, much of the ulceration being caused by Vincent's organisms (see Vincent's Angina). Similar inflammatory lesions may be present in the pharynx and the stomach, and more or less throughout the alimentary tract. Anorexia and abdominal pain develop early. Enteritis and proctitis cause diarrhea with foul watery stools. Abdominal pain becomes severe, and distention is marked. Intensity of inflammation necessary to produce diarrhea is not as common in children as in adults. Many children have only soreness of the tongue and the lips and abdominal pain. Often they are constipated, with only occasional attacks of diarrhea during the spring and the summer. There have been instances of babies in whom only diarrhea was present. Exacerbations of the alimentary symptoms of pellagra and the appearance of the characteristic dermatitis occur concurrently.

Genito-urinary Tract. The mucous membranes of the genito-urinary tract' also may become affected, and the lesions may become manifest as urethritis or vaginitis. In association with these lesions, as in the case of those in the mouth, Vincent's organisms grow profusely.

Skin Lesions. The skin lesions of pellagra are due to an inflammation similar to that produced by sunburn. They are initiated by exposure to the sun and they tend to heal gradually if sunshine is excluded. Because exposure to sunshine usually is symmetrical, the dermatitis also is symmetrical. It occurs in its characteristic form on exposed parts, especially the back of the hands and the neck. On the arms it extends up to the line of the sleeve. Coincident with the appearance of lesions on parts exposed to the sun, or subsequently, a somewhat different type of dermatitis may appear on unexposed parts subject to irritation. The parts commonly affected are the elbows, the knees and the ankles, where the affected skin remains dry, and the axillae and the perineum, where a moist type of dermatitis appears. The characteristic lesions on exposed parts pass through the same stages as do those of sunburn, though the course is slower and more chronic. The initial redness deepens, and pigment is deposited gradually. The older the lesion the greater the brownish pigmentation. The skin becomes thickened, rough and scaly. In some instances, seldom in childhood, the initial inflammation is sufficiently severe to produce large blisters. In practically all instances, the edges of the area of inflammation are sharply demarcated. A sensation of burning is present in the early stages.

Nervous and Mental Symptoms. The nervous and mental symptoms of pellagra increase in number and severity with continuation through years of niacin deficiency and recurring attacks of manifest pellagra. The more severe varieties of mental disturbances, such as mental confusion, delirium, mania and dementia, observed in adults, are not commonly present in the child. The milder nervous symptoms shown by the child may be due as much to chronic illness as to more specific effect on the nervous system, if not more. The children become tired and apathetic and lacking in normal childhood interest. Because of their physical status and consequent inability to concentrate, they do poorly in school. They become irritable, fretful and apprehensive and sleep restlessly.

NUTRITIONAL STATUS

The general nutritional status of pellagrous children is poor. Because of inadequate diet and poor health with anorexia, the children are undernourished in both stature and weight.

DIAGNOSIS

The diagnosis of manifest pellagra is made by finding the characteristic glossitis or dermatitis, or both. The diagnosis of niacin deficiency is more difficult in children who may have minimum skin lesions or none. Such children may have gastro-intestinal symptoms, weight loss, weakness, depression and a multiplicity of vague subjective symptoms, none of which is diagnostic. With these symptoms, psychoneurosis may be diagnosed erroneously. Deficiency should be suspected if such symptoms occur in a child of a pellagrous family, even in the absence of diagnostic signs. A therapeutic test may cause prompt improvement.

PROGNOSIS

The prognosis in children with treatment is excellent, much better than in adults. Response to treatmen is prompt, often dramatic. With or without treatment, and with continued dietary deficiency, the recurrences become increasingly severe and eventually lead to death.

TREATMENT

The treatment consists primarily of giving niacin or preparations containing it. Either niacin or its amide is given in a dosage of from 50 to 300 mg. daily, depending on the size of the child and the severity of symptoms. It is given best in divided doses, 10 mg. at a time for the small child and 20 mg. for the older child, in order to obtain better absorption and to avoid unpleasant subjective sensations which may occur with larger doses.

Dried brewers' yeast also is effective. An appropriate amount for a child up to 6 or 7 years is 45 Gm. daily, for an older child 60 Gm. The yeast may be mixed with milk. It is given in divided doses.

Niacin deficiency seldom exists alone. Consequently, attention must be paid to the entire diet. Deficiency manifestations most commonly associated with pellagra are those caused by lack of other members of the vitamin B complex, particularly thiamine. Symptomatic treatment, such as parenterally administered fluids for dehydration and transfusion for anemia and severe malnutrition, is to be given as indicated.

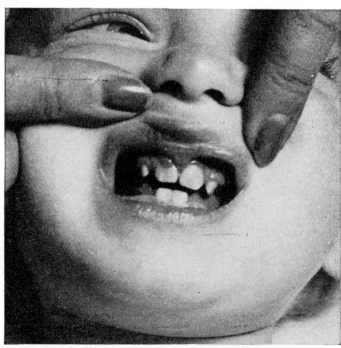

FIG. 95. The characteristic gum changes of scurvy.

SCURVY (SCORBUTUS)

Scurvy is caused by deficiency of ascorbic acid (vitamin C) in the diet. Scurvy occurs only in those whose diet is abnormally restricted. For this reason, scurvy is rare in children and adults. In infancy, the diet is much more limited and it is chiefly at this period that scurvy occurs. At present, scurvy is uncommon even in infancy as compared with former years. Most mothers now know that the artificially fed baby should have orange juice or some equivalent source of ascorbic acid. Even without a special source of ascorbic acid, the diet usually is not completely devoid of this material. This partial deficiency causes scurvy to appear somewhat later than if the deficiency were absolute. Scurvy is rare in the first 6 months and has its highest incidence in the second 6 months. It disappears as soon as foods containing vitamin C are included in the diet.

Symptoms

In its early stages, preceding the clinical signs by which it may be recognized, scurvy is characterized by indisposition, fretfulness, pallor, diminished appetite and failing nutrition. Pulse and respiration rates are increased. These symptoms continue through the manifest phases of the disease. The important manifestations are a tendency to hemorrhage and changes in the bones.

The hemorrhages of scurvy occur through the capillaries because of loss of cement substance between the cells of the capillary walls and because of arrested growth of connective tissue and its collagen-supporting structure. They are not caused by any change in the blood. Hemorrhage may occur in many places. Blood may appear in the urine or the stool. Small hemorrhages may appear within the skin, the appearance often resembling the effect of a bruise. Hemorrhage occurs in the gums and is usually limited to the site of erupted teeth. The gums become dark and swollen and bleed easily. Their appearance is strikingly suggestive, almost diagnostic, of scurvy (Fig. 95).

The bone changes are dependent in part on hemorrhage, but the important diagnostic changes as shown by roentgenograms are produced by impaired growth of osteoblasts and capillaries, especially at the points of growth of the bones. No difficulty exists in the deposit of mineral in the newly formed bone, but the newly calcified bone is not converted to trabeculated bone in a normal manner. As a result, there is present an abnormally heavy line of calcification immediately beyond a zone of rarefaction caused by impaired osteoblastic activity. For the same reasons, the trabeculae of the bones become thinner and less well defined in roentgenograms. Bone-marrow cells may largely disappear, a factor in addition to hemorrhage in producing anemia. In advanced scurvy, epiphyseal separation may occur from slight trauma.

The characteristic hemorrhages in bones are subperiosteal and in the long bones. They start at the growing end of the bone and strip off the periosteum, producing subperiosteal hematomas.

One of the characteristics of scurvy is pain and tenderness of the extremities, especially of the legs. The baby resents handling, the legs are not moved voluntarily, and pa-

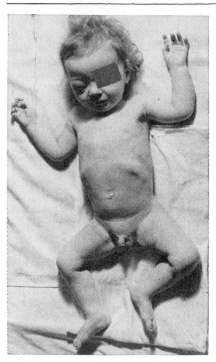

Fig. 96. Illustrating the characteristic posture of an infant with scurvy and periorbital hemorrhage.

ralysis is simulated, and the thighs and the legs are held flexed with outward rotation at the hips (Fig. 96).

Moderate anemia is constantly present in scurvy, and severe anemia may develop. Slight fever is often present, and the temperature may be as high as from 102° to 103° F. when the disease is acute.

DIAGNOSIS

The diagnosis of frank scurvy is seldom difficult. Scurvy with pseudoparalysis is easily differentiated from diseases causing true paralysis by careful observation. Most hemorrhagic diseases other than scurvy which occur in infancy have characteristic blood changes. Roentgenograms show definitely diagnostic changes in the bones.

TREATMENT

Scurvy responds quickly to ascorbic acid, whether given in crystalline form or as foods naturally containing this material. The pain and acute symptoms are relieved within a few days. A longer period is required to recover from anemia and nutritional and bone changes. For the first few days of treatment, from 100 to 200 mg. of ascorbic acid may be given daily in divided doses. Subsequently, the normal allowance is sufficient.

NURSING CARE

All procedures are associated with pain when the infant first comes under care. Nearing his bed often produces reactions of fear. Gentleness in handling is important. If taking up the infant for feeding is accompanied by excessive pain and poor acceptance of food, it is reasonable to feed him in bed with his head elevated. As soon as the acute symptoms subside, holding the infant for feeding should be resumed. Because of pain on motion, the infant tends to lie in one position, a symptom which must be kept in mind in attempts to prevent intercurrent infection. As much of the needed care as possible should be given at one time; avoidable handling should be eliminated. When upper bedclothing is used, the weight should be reduced by the use of a bed cradle.

RICKETS (RACHITIS)

ABNORMAL METABOLISM OF CALCIUM AND PHOSPHORUS

Rickets in all instances is a result of abnormal metabolism of calcium and phosphorus. In most instances, the abnormality is caused by vitamin D deficiency. Other causes are discussed under Late Rickets.

Rickets can occur only when growth is active. The counterpart of rickets in those fully grown is osteomalacia. The more rapid the growth the more likely is rickets to develop. The most rapid growth occurs in infancy, and it is almost exclusively among infants that rickets occurs as a deficiency disease. By histologic examination of necropsy material, Park has found evidence of rickets in 46 per cent of children between 1 month and puberty. If rickets occurs to such an extent among children past infancy, it is not recognizable during life by present criteria. However, when criteria other than the development of rickets are used, evidence is abundant that vitamin D deficiency occurs in childhood with great frequency.

Rickets is more common in artificially fed than in breast-fed babies. It occurs chiefly in the temperate zones, where babies may have long periods without sunshine. It is more common in dark-skinned races because some of the ultraviolet rays are filtered out by the pigment. Rickets is not common in the tropics, even in dark-skinned races with the poorest of diets. Rickets is seasonal. It begins to be active when babies are more closely housed for the winter. Its activity is at its height in the northern hemisphere in March and subsides as babies are allowed sunshine again in the spring.

The disturbance of calcium and phosphorus metabolism is evidenced by poor retention of these materials by the body, by abnormal blood levels of calcium, phosphorus and phosphatase, and by faulty mineralization of bones. Normally, the blood of an infant contains from 10 to 12 mg. of calcium and from 5 to 7 mg. of phosphorus for each 100 cc. of serum. When rickets is present and active, the blood calcium may be expected to be from 9 to 10 mg. and the phosphorus less than 4 mg. for each 100 cc. When the product of the calcium and the phosphorus values is less than 30, rickets is present and active. The occasional finding of very low calcium and normal or high phosphorus is explained subsequently under Tetany. Phosphatase is an enzyme which increases in the blood in proportion to the severity of the rickets.

BONES

The growth in length of the long bones takes place in the shaft at its junction with the epiphysis. This area of growth change is the metaphysis. The normal process of increase is by growth of cartilage cells (osteoid tissue) and mineralization of these cells at such a rate that only a thin layer of osteoid tissue is present. In rickets, the deposit of calcium and phosphate in the newly grown cartilage is deficient. The roentgenogram shows a raggedly calcified bone end. The osteoid tissue continues to grow, producing enlargement of the end of the bone by overgrowth or a mushrooming effect of pressure on soft tissue. Enlarge-

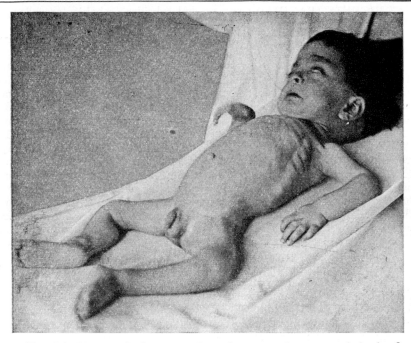

Fig. 97. Very marked active rickets, showing enlargement of the head from "bossing," a marked "rosary," enlarged epiphyses and inability to stand or sit.

ment of the bone end becomes apparent on inspection and palpation. This same process produces small knobs at the junction of the ribs with the cartilage near the sternum. Because of their distribution, these enlargements have been designated collectively a rachitic rosary (Fig. 97).

The shafts of the long bones eventually become soft from lack of mineral and they may bend according to the direction in which stress is put on them (Fig. 98). The pull of the diaphragm on the softened ribs, particularly when combined with nasal obstruction, causes deformities of the chest, the most common of which is

depression of the ribs at the line of attachment of the diaphragm (Harrison's groove). Softening of the spine may result in scoliosis or kyphosis. The bones of the skull sometimes become sufficiently soft to permit indentation by the finger as though made of stiff parchment. This condition is known as craniotabes and occurs chiefly in the occipital bones. Sometimes overgrowth occurs on the parietal and frontal bones of the skull, producing bosses and giving to the skull a somewhat square shape. Rickets causes delay in eruption of teeth and in closing of the fontanel. Whatever the bone changes may be as a result of rickets,

they tend to occur similarly and
equally on the two sides of the body.

MUSCLES

Muscles as well as bones suffer in
rickets. As rickets advances, the
muscles show a general weakness
and loss of tone. Because of these
changes, sitting, standing and walking are delayed, or the baby may
retrogress in these acts if they were
already established. The abdominal
wall is relaxed, and the abdomen
protrudes when the child is erect.
Constipation may result from loss
of muscle strength. Ligaments about
joints may become lax and permit
unusual mobility. Sometimes the
spleen is enlarged by simple hyperplasia, and the liver may be increased in size.

OTHER SYMPTOMS

The more marked of the bony
changes which have been described
are to be noted only when rickets
is well advanced. In many instances,
the resultant changes are milder
when vitamin D deficiency is not
great or has been of short duration.
The onset of rickets is insidious, and
the earliest stages present no characteristic or diagnostic symptoms except for moderate changes in the
calcium, the phosphorus and the
phosphatase in the blood. At no
time is pain or discomfort a part of
rickets. Rachitic infants often show
lowered resistance to infections, particularly respiratory infections.

DIAGNOSIS

The diagnosis of active rickets is
made by finding the characteristic
changes in roentgenograms of bones
or abnormal blood levels of calcium
and phosphorus, or both. Also,

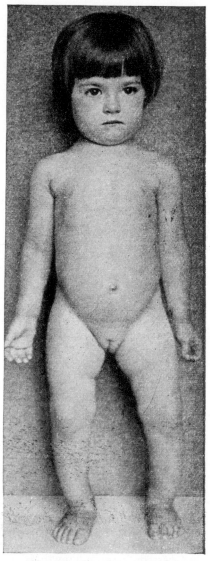

FIG. 98. Showing some of the
deformities of rickets. This child
shows anterior bowing of the
legs, enlargement of the epiphyses
at the wrists and moderate "bead-
ing" of the ribs.

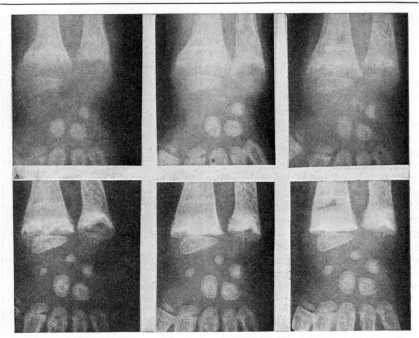

Fig. 99. Showing various stages in the healing of active rickets. The increase of calcification as observed from time to time is evident.

blood phosphatase is increased above the normal. Rachitic changes are found roentgenographically at the wrist when they are evident in any other bones.

PROGNOSIS

Rickets is not a direct cause of death, though it may be a contributing factor by predisposing to other diseases. With rare exceptions, rickets subsides, even without treatment, by the time the period of infancy has passed, because growth is not so rapid, and the child can get more sunshine under his own power. The deformities of rickets may persist. There is considerable tendency for moderate deformities to disappear in the period from 2 to 5 years of age. Severe deformities remain unless corrected by operative or mechanical means. Some deformities, such as those of the chest, are not easily amenable to corrective procedures.

TREATMENT

The treatment of rickets consists primarily of the administration of Vitamin D. The larger the dosage the more quickly the healing process begins. Since the baby is not ill and no emergency exists, moderate rather than massive dosage is preferable. Vitamin D in the amount of from 1,500 to 3,000 units daily may be expected to produce evidence of recovery in the blood in about a week, and in the bones in approximately 2 weeks (Fig. 99). Some of the high-potency cod-liver oils contain 900 units to the teaspoonful. Of these, from 2 to 3 teaspoonfuls daily suffice. Concentrated preparations may be preferred to low-potency oils because of the bulk of oil required for the larger doses. In any case, a large dosage serves a useful purpose only until the healing process has well begun; thereafter a maintenance dose of from 300 to 400 units daily is adequate. Except for correction of existing dietary faults, no other treatment is necessary in most instances.

In a few instances, corrective appliances may be desirable during the healing stage of rickets and subsequently. These appliances would be for the correction of deformity such as bowlegs or knock-knees. Operative correction of deformity, if necessary, is deferred until the rickets has healed completely.

The mercury arc quartz lamp is not used as much as formerly in the treatment of rickets, though it is effective if used. A suitable procedure is to expose the baby at first 3 minutes at a distance of 120 cm. from the lamp. The time is gradually increased to 20 minutes, and the distance from the lamp decreased to 75 cm. The increment of increase in time may be 2 minutes. Exposure may be made daily in the beginning, 3 times a week subsequently. Bone healing may begin within 2 weeks of starting treatment.

Nursing Care

Infants with rickets need frequent change in position to prevent upper respiratory infection and head deformities. Prevention of infection is an important part of the care of a rachitic infant. Exposure to drafts should be avoided, and the head should be kept dry when head sweating is present.

When rickets is severe, weight bearing on the lower extremities is undesirable until healing has occurred. Body restraints may be necessary for the older infant. They must be applied sufficiently tightly to accomplish the purpose, yet loosely enough to permit such activity as cannot be harmful. To prevent deformity, a firm mattress should be provided, as well as a back support, if the child is allowed to sit.

Occasionally, enemas may be necessary. Their need may be lessened by giving additional fluid between feedings and by massaging the weakened abdominal muscles.

When giving vitamin D concentrates, it is preferable to drop the preparation directly on the infant's tongue. In this way the nurse can be certain that he has received the required amount. Until the infant has become accustomed to its taste and consistency, cod-liver oil should be given in small amounts from a glass, a medicine dropper or a spoon. Infants learn quickly to enjoy the oil, especially if it is offered without an attitude of repugnance on the part of the adult. Mixing the oil with fruit juice is unnecessary and inexpedient. It is more desirable to help the infant to accept each new food in its natural and undisguised form.

Sun baths may be given to hasten recovery if rickets should be active in warm weather. Complete exposure is possible after a period of acclimating the infant to the outdoors.

and to direct sunshine. Exposure should be gradual; great care should be taken to prevent burning the tender skin of the infant. Protection of the eyes from direct sunlight can be accomplished by the placement of the crib and by bed awnings of dark heavy material. A sheltered part of the roof or the porch should be selected to avoid strong currents of air on the exposed infant.

Rickets in Childhood (Late Rickets)

Older children sometimes show bone changes similar to those observed in infantile rickets. The similarity exists in the nature of the bone deformities, in the roentgenographic evidence of rickets and in the amounts of calcium, phosphorus and phosphatase in the blood. By all these criteria the condition is rickets. However, in few instances in this country is clinically recognizable rickets caused by dietary deficiency.

Severe dietary deficiency presumably was the cause of rickets reported in children of central Europe after World War I. For normal bone mineralization not only must vitamin D be present, but there must also be appropriate amounts of calcium and phosphorus. Rickets has been reported in India among high-caste girls who were kept closely housed under the system of purdah during late childhood and adolescence.

Late rickets is uncommon in this country. When it does occur, it is nearly always due to some metabolic disturbance which is unrelated to the intake of minerals and vitamin D and makes normal retention of calcium and phosphorus impossible. Several varieties of such disturbances have been recognized. Infantile rickets usually does not last long enough to produce permanent stunting of growth, whereas late rickets dependent on a metabolic disorder is a chronic disease, and stunted growth is a common occurrence.

In some instances of late rickets, the difficulty seems to lie in a defect in the mechanism by which vitamin D promotes the utilization of calcium and phosphorus. In these cases, response is observed when the intake of vitamin D is greatly increased. The necessary increase may be so great that only a small margin exists between the therapeutic and the toxic dose. Children under treatment must be observed frequently and carefully.

Chronic acidosis from any cause is likely to produce rickets. In this condition, calcium is used to help neutralize the excessive amounts of acid. In most of these instances, improvement or recovery occurs with the continued administration of alkali.

Renal rickets is a term applied to rickets observed in association with chronic nephritis. Usually some acidosis is present, causing increased excretion of calcium, but an equally important factor is the failure to excrete phosphates. The increased concentration of phosphate in the body affects adversely the deposition of calcium in bone.

Other metabolic causes exist. Some of them are obscure and the underlying cause is difficult to find. A high-milk, high-vitamin diet is of benefit in most instances.

TETANY (SPASMOPHILIA)

Tetany is a condition of general hyperirritability caused by a lowered calcium level in the blood or by lack of availability of the calcium that is present.

ALKALOSIS

Alkalosis may cause tetany by affecting adversely the availability of the calcium of the blood. Severe vomiting unaccompanied by diarrhea, as with pyloric stenosis, causes alkalosis, sometimes of sufficient degree to produce tetany.

CHRONIC NEPHRITIS

Chronic nephritis is often associated with retention of phosphate. The greater the increase of phosphate in the blood the less the availability of blood calcium. Also, chronic nephritis is accompanied commonly by acidosis. Acidosis causes increased excretion of calcium but also increases the anti-tetany effect of that which is present. In most instances, the favorable effect of acidosis on calcium availability compensates for the unfavorable effect of phosphate retention. This compensation disappears if the acidosis should be wholly corrected by alkali administration: then tetany would appear. In a few instances, tetany of the newborn has been shown to be caused by kidney dysfunction or by dehydration in the first days of life, giving rise to retention of materials normally excreted by the kidneys. The resultant phosphate retention causes some decrease in the calcium content of the blood and makes less available the remainder.

PARATHYROID GLANDS

The parathyroid glands are concerned with the maintenance of a normal blood-calcium level. When these glands are removed or destroyed, or when their secretion is deficient, the calcium of the blood is decreased, and tetany appears. In childhood, tetany from this cause occurs chiefly in the neonatal period. The reason for its occurrence at this time is overactivity of the mother's parathyroids during pregnancy, with consequent inhibition of the activity of the parathyroids of the fetus, the result being that for a short time after birth the infant suffers from lack of this hormone from his own glands.

RACHITIC TETANY

While the preceding conditions can and do cause tetany, vitamin D deficiency is much the most common cause in childhood. This type of tetany occurs only in infants and young children and only in the presence of rickets, though at times the external evidence of rickets is meager. Tetany has the same seasonal and age incidence as rickets, since the underlying causes are identical. One of the first effects of vitamin D in rickets is an increase in the phosphorus content of the blood and a decrease in the calcium. If the amount of vitamin D is adequate, and if the dosage is continued, the lowering of calcium is small and transitory. However, if vitamin D administration is brief and in small dosage, the blood calcium continues low. Thus the taking of a rachitic baby into the sunshine on a pleasant spring day may cause tetany if the procedure is not repeated consistently.

SYMPTOMS

As a result of the general nervous irritability in tetany, three clinical manifestations are common: general convulsions, local spasm of the larynx and contracture of the hands and the feet. Usually all three symptoms are not present in the same infant. One may have convulsions; another, laryngospasm; and still another, carpopedal spasm. The convulsions do not differ from those of a cerebral type from any other cause. In laryngospasm, the larynx is drawn together by the adductor muscles. The force of expiration is sufficient to overcome this pull so that no expiratory obstruction exists. The difficulty in inspiration varies from an inspiratory crow due to a partially closed larynx to complete cessation of breathing because of complete closure of the larynx. Laryngospasm occurs in short attacks, and, though very alarming, rarely causes ⋆death from asphyxia. Between attacks the infant seems to be in his usual state of health. In carpopedal spasm, the hands and the feet assume a characteristic position. Without associated pain or discomfort, the fingers are held stiffly, slightly flexed at the knuckles, thumb stiff and held straight inside the palm, and the wrists slightly flexed. The feet are held in as similar a position as their anatomy allows. Carpopedal spasm may be transitory or it may persist for days at a time.

A child with tetany may have the appearance of excellent health. The slightest causes, or even no apparent cause, may serve to initiate an attack of laryngospasm or a convulsion.

DIAGNOSIS

Neither a convulsion nor an attack of laryngospasm is diagnostic, since both conditions may occur from other causes. Typical carpopedal spasm occurs in no other condition. The diagnosis of tetany is made definitely by finding a low level of calcium in the blood. When the blood calcium is from 7 to 8 mg. for each 100 cc., tetany is latent, and clinical symptoms do not appear unless some extra stimulus, such as a febrile illness, is given. With a calcium value of 6 mg. or less, symptoms occur with no extra stimulus.

In making a clinical diagnosis, certain signs of nervous irritability are useful:

Chvostek's sign is tested by tapping over the branches of the facial nerve in front of the ear. A positive response is a quick contraction of the muscles supplied by the branch of the nerve tapped.

Trousseau's sign is elicited by constricting tightly the middle of the upper arm by hand or by a tourniquet for 30 seconds or more. If the test is positive, the hand assumes the position of carpal spasm already described (Fig. 100).

Erb's sign is elicited by determining the amount of electric current necessary to produce a muscular contraction when an electrode is applied over a nerve. The test is usually applied to an arm or a leg. The test is positive when the amount of electricity required to produce a contraction is less than that required normally.

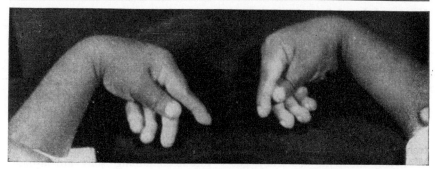

Fig. 100. Showing the characteristic position of the hands in the carpal spasm of tetany.

PROGNOSIS

The chances of death from tetany are not great, but it may occur as a result of suffocation from laryngospasm or from cardiac failure in either a convulsion or an attack of laryngospasm. While low blood calcium results in increased irritability of nerves, the effect on heart muscle is that of a depressant. Death may be averted in all instances by the application of appropriate emergency measures as soon as the diagnosis is made.

TREATMENT

The measures described for the treatment of rickets will also cure tetany, but a week or more of such treatment may be necessary before improvement is noted. The manifestations of tetany cannot be allowed to continue for such a length of time. The oral administration of acid-producing salts, such as calcium or ammonium chloride, in doses of from 10 to 15 grains 4 or 5 times a day, will produce the desired effect usually in about 12 hours. Presumably, the acid-producing salts act by increasing the ioniz-ation and the availability of such calcium as already is present in the blood. The medication must be continued until the vitamin D has caused increase in the blood-calcium level.

Usually an immediate effect is desired. This may be accomplished by a parenteral injection of either a calcium or a magnesium salt. Calcium salts preferably are given only intravenously. Either the chloride or the gluconate may be used; the chloride is very irritating when given either subcutaneously or intramuscularly. Often intramuscular injection is to be preferred. For this purpose magnesium sulfate, 10 to 15 grains, in solution serves well. Magnesium has the same effect on tetany as calcium. The effect of a single injection usually lasts until the oral medication becomes effective. If it does not, a second injection may be necessary. Excessive amounts of magnesium cause serious depression of respiration. Calcium is an antidote for this effect of magnesium.

SIMPLE GOITER

Simple goiter is the result of enlargement of the thyroid gland and is caused by deficiency of iodine. Iodine is an essential part of the thyroid secretion, part of which is a colloid material. In the attempt to compensate for deficiency, the colloid material is produced in excess within the gland acini, with the result that the acini are dilated, and the entire gland becomes enlarged.

When iodine deficiency is extreme, goiter may occur at any age. With only moderate deficiency, goiter is likely to develop only at times of metabolic stress. Puberty in girls and pregnancy are among the most potent causes of stress leading to goiter production. Goiter may occur with chronic or protracted acute disease, such as tuberculosis and typhoid fever. Goiter is much more frequent in girls than in boys. Simple goiter is always preventable by an adequate intake of iodine. If the thyroid gland already is increased in size, iodine administration stops the enlargement and frequently causes a decrease to normal size.

The amount of iodine required for normal function of the thyroid gland is minute. One mg. of sodium or potassium iodide a week is sufficient to maintain normal thyroid secretion in an adult. Because this amount may be too small in case of metabolic strain, an intake of at least 5 mg. weekly is desirable. The maximum storage capacity of the adult thyroid is approximately 125 mg. (2 grains), and the average content from 10 to 15 mg. (40 to 60 mg. for each 100 Gm.). Only when the iodine content of the thyroid decreases below 10 mg. for each 100 Gm. does the gland begin to enlarge. The need of the child is proportionate to that of the adult on the basis of weight.

Food is the logical and natural source of iodine. However, food cannot contain iodine when produced in regions where the soil is deficient in this material. Sea foods are rich in iodine. Nuts and butter fat contain a relative abundance. Among the food plants, green leaves have the highest content and cereals the lowest. The majority of foods rich in iodine when produced on iodine-containing soils are usually not imported into regions where goiter is prevalent.

For regions where goiter occurs, some effective means of iodine supply is desirable. Iodine is effective when administered in any form or manner. It need not be given daily. A year's supply may be given at intervals of from 4 to 6 months if the total dosage for the period be distributed over a period of from 10 days to 2 weeks. In the past, a few cities have practiced periodic iodization of the water supply. Such a method, however is not applicable to rural communities. Iodine administered as medication has been much used in school prophylaxis. This procedure has much to commend it, but it reaches only a portion of the population. Mixing iodine with table salt which is distributed commercially is a simple method of supplying those who elect to use this variety of salt. The iodine is ingested as part of the food, the intake is small but well distributed throughout the year, the whole family is affected, and the method is applicable in all communities. Commercial iodized salt contains 1 part of sodium or potassium iodide to each 10,000 parts of salt.

Objection has been raised in some quarters to the promiscuous, unsupervised ingestion of iodine even in the minute quantities necessary to supply the known requirement for this nutritional essential, though no objection has been made to people's living in regions where larger amounts of iodine are constantly ingested. The reason given for the objection is the possibility of overproduction of the thyroid hormone in some cases. It is generally granted that this supposed danger does not exist if the full requirement for iodine has been supplied since early childhood, and that its existence is rare in any circumstances in the period of childhood. It is certain that persons for whom iodine may be considered dangerous are relatively few. There exists a divergence of opinion in regard to the dangers of the suggested iodine dosage for these few. The fact remains that iodine is a nutritional essential.

NUTRITIONAL ANEMIA

Anemia which results from a long-continued ingestion of a diet low in iron sometimes is designated *nutritional anemia*. The most severe of the nutritional anemias occur almost exclusively in infancy. Some infants receive for many months a diet of little else than milk, which is a poor source of iron. The resultant anemia appears insidiously and may become extreme before measures are taken for its correction. The occurrence of infections hastens the development of anemia or aggravates it if present. The anemia present is of a hypochromic microcytic type and is a part of a larger group classified under this term. It responds to therapy with iron. Transfusions are useful in promoting more rapid recovery when the anemia is severe. Only

small amounts of iron, either in food or as medication, are required for prevention.

NUTRITIONAL EDEMA

The body is compelled to burn its own tissues when the energy intake is less than the requirement. Eventually, the body reservoirs of fat disappear, and some of the body protein is broken down for energy production. If the amount of protein in the diet is low at the same time, some of the protein tissues of the body must be broken down to provide the necessary amino acids for renewal of more essential protein tissues. In severe or long-continued depletion, the body protein destroyed includes that of the blood plasma. When the blood protein, particularly the albumin fraction, becomes low, edema results. When edema occurs as a result of protein depletion, it is designated *nutritional edema*. During World War I it was known also as *war edema,* having been the result of the famine of war conditions.

Nutritional edema is insidious in its onset, usually being the result of many months of deficiency. The edema may be local or general, depending on the degree of deficiency. Edema from low blood protein may result also from wasting diseases of various types in which the intake and the absorption of energy and protein do not equal the need; it is the type of edema that occurs in nephrosis. This type of edema is to be distinguished from that resulting from cardiovascular disease, as in glomerular nephritis and in heart disease with decompensation.

The only treatment required for starvation edema is the giving of a good diet. In other instances, the underlying disease, such as chronic diarrhea or celiac disease, requires appropriate management.

DENTAL CARIES

It is considered appropriate to include tooth decay among the deficiency diseases. The cause of this condition is controversial, but observers agree that the content of the diet is the chief determining factor in the production or the prevention of dental caries. Divergence of opinion exists as to whether the dietary factors operate only externally on the teeth by their effect on the oral environment or operate internally through the nutrition of the tooth.

Sugar has been held to be an important contributing factor to tooth decay by supplying a nutrient medium for the growth of caries-producing bacteria in the mouth. However, evidence exists that dental caries may be expected to stop despite large intakes of sugar when the diet is complete. Evidence exists also that the better the quality of the diet the less the desire of children for sweets. The voluntary ingestion of excessive sweets is circumstantial evidence that the diet is not complete.

It seems to be an acceptable belief on the basis of existing evidence that when the diet contains all the known essentials in adequate amounts, sound teeth will not become carious, and decay already present will cease. No doubt bacteria and their growth products play a role in causing dental caries, but this factor apparently is of little importance when the dietary regimen is good. The teeth are protected by a good diet even though the

dental hygiene is poor. However, good oral hygiene is desirable for other obvious reasons.

No one dietary factor alone is responsible for tooth decay or its prevention. Dental caries has been reduced in observation groups by the addition of calcium and phosphorus (milk) to the diet; it has been reduced by the addition of vitamin D. A close correlation has been shown between the amount of sunshine and tooth decay. Vitamin C also is important. Fluorine in minute amounts also acts preventively. These same factors plus vitamin A are important for the formation of sound teeth during the time of their development.

The diet advised in the preceding pages as one suited to the needs of the child has been shown repeatedly to be effective in the prevention and the arrest of dental caries. This type of diet is one which every child should have, not because it will arrest caries but because it is complete. A special diet for the benefit of the teeth is quite unnecessary. Even more unnecessary are the various mineral preparations which have been advocated for this purpose.

The exposed soft dentin of the tooth cavities of active caries becomes hard, and the caries is arrested in approximately 2 months after the institution of a good diet. Sometimes one is confronted with the paradox of a child with carious teeth and a mother who states sincerely that the child is receiving all the articles of a suggested diet list. Usually a record of foods actually eaten proves to the mother that she has been mistaken. Also, close dietary supervision of such a child in a hospital serves the same purpose.

Occasionally one encounters children who have defective absorption, particularly of the fat-soluble vitamins, and have dental caries despite a good diet. Such children require special management.

Poor teeth are not inherited. The familial predisposition to dental caries frequently observed is only apparent and is due to faulty food habits in the family. Nutritional disturbances and improper feeding habits in infancy may and frequently do lead to defects in the structure of unerupted permanent teeth. These defects may be such as to cause the teeth to be more susceptible than usual to those factors that cause decay. Nevertheless, even the most defective of these teeth will not become carious after eruption if the diet is good at all times. Active decay in teeth is dependent on causes operating in the present and the recent past. These causes, when present, have a greater effect on defective teeth than on those well formed, but the activating cause is unrelated to tooth development. Of all the teeth, the first permanent molars are most frequently affected by caries. A possible explanation is that the structure of these teeth often tends to be poorer than that of other teeth, for the reason that these are the only teeth of which the exposed parts (crowns) are formed entirely in that period (from birth to 2½ years) when nutritional disturbances are most common.

The great prevalence of dental caries among children of all classes and economic levels is an indication of the frequency with which the diet is defective. When 80 per cent or more of our population have a disorder dependent on a faulty diet, no doubt can remain that the usual concept of a good diet needs modification.

SITUATIONS FOR FURTHER STUDY

1. In teaching a mother methods of giving vitamin concentrates and orange juice to a young infant, what points would you include?

2. What instructions would you give a mother when she inquired about a method of giving sun baths to her 2-month-old infant?

3. By what process does tetany develop in healing rickets?

4. By what methods can nutritional anemia be prevented?

BIBLIOGRAPHY

Committee on Dental Health, Dental Caries; a survey of the literature, National Research Council Publication No. 225, Washington, D. C., 1952.

Eliott, M. M., and Park, E. A.: Rickets, in Brenneman's Practice of Pediatrics, Hagerstown, Md., Prior, 1948, vol. I, Chap. 36.

McIntosh, R., Infantile Scurvy, in Brenneman's Practice of Pediatrics, Hagerstown, Md., Prior, 1948. Vol. I, Chap. 35.

Index

Abdomen, distention, from megacolon, 256
   from paralytic ileus, in pneumonia, bacterial, primary, in infants, 305
  in pellagra, 722
  in typhoid fever, 565
  eruption (rose spots), in typhoid fever, 565
  protuberant, in celiac disease, 711
Abruptio placentae, producing anoxia in fetus, 212
Abscess(es), brain, diagnosis, differential, from tumor of brain, 405
  from otitis media, acute, 286
  "cold," 575
  lung, from foreign bodies in bronchus, 293
  multiple, in pneumonia, staphylococcus, 308
  peritonsillar, with tonsillitis, acute, 283
  retropharyngeal, 283-285
   diagnosis, 284
    differential, 284
   nursing care, 284-285
   symptoms, 283-284
   treatment, 284
  tuberculous, 575
Acarus scabiei as etiologic agent, scabies, 432
Accidents, cerebral, permanent damage, 21-22
  prematurity from, 222
  prevention, 27
Acetone bodies, in urine, in vomiting, recurrent, 607-608
Achromycin therapy, 194
  meningitis, influenza bacillus, 413
Acid(s), aceto-acetic, 609
  acetone, 609
  amino, in digestion in small intestine, 635
   in proteins, 619-620

Acid(s) *(Continued)*
  carbonic, 347, 609
  citric, addition to formula in artificial feeding of infant, 657, 672
  folic, requirement in diet, 630
  folinic (citrovorum factor), requirement in diet, 630-631
  hydrochloric, role in gastric digestion, 634
  hydroxybutyric, 609
  lactic, 609
   addition to formula in artificial feeding of infant, 669-672
  nicotinic. *See* Niacin
  organic, as waste products of body, 347
  pantothenic, requirement in diet, 631
  sources, 508-509
Acid-base balance, physiologic considerations, 172-173
Acidosis, 608-613
  buffer substances of blood, 609
  chronic, rickets from, 732
  definition, 608-610
  in dehydration, 700
  in diabetes mellitus, 469-470, 476-478
   death from, 470, 476, 482
   mechanism of development, 476
   symptoms 476
   treatment, 476-478
  diagnosis, 611
  loss of base by bowel, 610-611
  in nephritis, chronic, 357
  prognosis, 611
  role of kidneys, 609
  from salicylate therapy, 329
  sources of acid, 608-609
  symptoms, 611
  therapeutic, 611
  treatment, 612-613
  types, acetone-body, 610
  in uremia, 349
Acne vulgaris, 448-449
Acrodynia, 601-604
  etiology, 601

Folic acid (*Continued*)
  therapy, anemia, 489
    nutritional, 492
    hypoplastic anemia from, 493
Folinic acid (citrovorum factor), anemia from disturbance of normal metabolism, 492
Fontanels, 49
Food(s), allergy, 599
  poisoning, diarrhea from, 695
    from Salmonella infection, 567
Forceps marks on newborn, temporary, 206
Forehead, acne vulgaris, 448
Foreign body(ies), in alimentary tract, 264
  bronchi, 293
  esophagus, 264
  eye, conjunctival sac, inflammation from, 456-457
  or materials, ingestion or inhalation, death from, 27
  pharynx, 264, 293
  respiratory tract, 293-295
  stomach, 264
Fracture(s), in birth, 216
  clavicle, in birth, 216
  humerus, in birth, 216
  skull, 423
    linear, in birth, 216
Fredet-Rammstedt operation for pyloric stenosis, 252
Friedreich's ataxia, 421
Friendships, with peers, school-age period (6 to 10 years), 97, 98
Froehlich's syndrome, as etiologic factor in obesity, 708
Fruit, addition to milk in artificial feeding of infant, 665, 666, 674
Frustration, in earliest months of life, as injurious, 59
  in family interpersonal relationships, socialization period (3 to 6 years), 90-91
  personality growth through, school-age period (6 to 10 years), 97-98
Furmethide therapy, stimulation of bladder contraction in poliomyelitis, 535
Furunculosis, 221, 429-430, 525

Galactose, conversion from complex sugar in digestion in small intestine, 635
Gamma globulin, as prophylaxis, measles, 26

Gantrisin, 190
Gargoylism, 419
Gastritis, in pellagra, 722
Gastro-enteritis, differential diagnosis from appendicitis, 268
Gastro-intestinal tract, obstruction, vomiting from, 688
  period required for passage of food, 635
  See also Alimentary tract
Gastrostomy, atresia of esophagus, 247-248
Gaucher's disease, 419
Gavage feedings, acrodynia, 604
  poliomyelitis, bulbar, 537
  in prematurity, 231-233
  in tetanus, 555
Gengou and Bordet, identification of etiologic agent of pertussis, 555
Genitalia, burns, 439
  diseases, scabies, 432
  female, external, inflammation, in mumps, 531
  of newborn, hormonal effects, 211
  male, malformations, 372-374
    cryptorchidism, 372-373
    epispadias, 373
    hydrocele, 373
    hypospadias, 373-374
    phimosis, 374
    preputial adhesions, 374
    undescended testicle, 372-373
  of newborn, 210-211
    circumcision, 210-211
    hydroceles, 210
  nursing care, in nephrosis, 355
Genito-urinary system, bladder. *See* Bladder
  diseases, 348-375
  kidneys. *See* Kidney(s)
Genito-urinary tract, infections, 362-372
  penis, 371-372
  pyuria. *See* Pyuria
  urethra, male, 372
  vulvovaginitis. *See* Vulvovaginitis
  lesions, in pellagra, 722
  lower, malformations. *See* Congenital anomalies, genito-urinary tract, lower
Gentian violet therapy, burns, 437, 438
  impetigo contagiosa, 429
  pinworm infestation, 269
  smallpox pustules, 526
  stomatitis, aphthous, 245
  thrush, 246
German measles. *See* Rubella